BASIC ORTHOPAEDIC BIOMECHANICS
Second Edition

BASIC ORTHOPAEDIC BIOMECHANICS
Second Edition

Editors

Van C. Mow, Ph.D.
Professor of Mechanical Engineering and Orthopaedic Bioengineering
Departments of Mechanical Engineering and Orthopaedic Surgery
Director, Center for Biomedical Engineering
Columbia University
New York, New York

Wilson C. Hayes, Ph.D.
Maurice E. Mueller Professor of Biomechanics
Harvard Medical School
Director, Orthopedic Biomechanics Laboratory
Department of Orthopedic Surgery
Beth Israel Deaconess Medical Center
Boston, Massachusetts

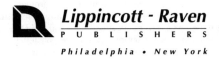

Lippincott - Raven
PUBLISHERS
Philadelphia • New York

Acquisitions Editor: Danette Knopp
Developmental Editor: Juleann Dob
Manufacturing Manager: Dennis Teston
Production Manager: Maxine Langweil
Associate Managing Editor: Kathleen Bubbeo
Production Service: Colophon
Cover Designer: Patricia Gast
Indexer: Indexing Research
Compositor: Lippincott–Raven Electronic Production
Printer: Maple Press

Printed in the United States of America

9   8   7   6   5   4   3   2   1

Library of Congress Cataloging-in-Publication Data
Basic orthopaedic biomechanics / [edited by] Van C. Mow, Wilson C.
   Hayes. — 2nd ed.   p. cm.
      Includes bibliographical references and index.
      ISBN 0-397-51684-3
      1. Orthopedics.   2. Human mechanics.   I. Mow, Van C.   II. Hayes,
   Wilson C.
      [DNLM: 1. Biomechanics.   2. Orthopaedics.   WE 103 B312 1997]
RD732.B35   1997
616.7–dc21
DNLM/DLC   97-1336
for Library of Congress   CIP

Care has been taken to confirm the accuracy of the information presented and to describe generally accepted practices. However, the authors, editors, and publisher are not responsible for errors or omissions or for any consequences from application of the information in this book and make no warranty, express or implied, with respect to the contents of the publication.

The authors, editors, and publisher have exerted every effort to ensure that drug selection and dosage set forth in this text are in accordance with current recommendations and practice at the time of publication. However, in view of ongoing research, changes in government regulations, and the constant flow of information relating to drug therapy and drug reactions, the reader is urged to check the package insert for each drug for any change in indications and dosage and for added warnings and precautions. This is particularly important when the recommended agent is a new or infrequently employed drug.

Some drugs and medical devices presented in this publication have Food and Drug Administration (FDA) clearance for limited use in restricted research settings. It is the responsibility of the health care provider to ascertain the FDA status of each drug or device planned for use in their clinical practice.

Contents

Contributing Authors

Kai-Nan An, Ph.D.   *Professor of Bioengineering, Mayo Medical School, Mayo Clinic, Biomechanics Laboratory, Division of Orthopaedic Research, Mayo Foundation, Rochester, Minnesota 55905*

Thomas P. Andriacchi, Ph.D.   *Department of Orthopedic Surgery, Rush-Presbyterian-St. Luke's Medical Center, Chicago, Illinois 60612*

Hannu T. Aro, M.D., Ph.D.   *Department of Orthopaedic Surgery, University of Turku, Turku, Finland*

James A. Ashton-Miller, Ph.D.   *Biomechanics Research Laboratory, Department of Mechanical Engineering and Applied Mechanics, University of Michigan, Ann Arbor, Michigan 48109-2125*

Gerard A. Ateshian, Ph.D.   *Associate Professor, Departments of Mechanical Engineering and Orthopaedic Surgery, Columbia University, New York, New York 10032*

Gordon W. Blunn, Ph.D.   *Department of Biomedical Engineering, University College London, Royal National Orthopaedic Hospital Trust, Stanmore, Middlesex HA7 4LP, United Kingdom*

Mary L. Bouxsein, Ph.D.   *Instructor in Orthopaedic Surgery, Harvard Medical School, Orthopaedic Biomechanics Laboratory, Beth Israel Deaconess Medical Center, Boston, Massachusetts 02215*

Edmund Y. S. Chao, Ph.D.   *Orthopaedic Biomechanics Laboratory, Johns Hopkins University, Baltimore, Maryland 21205-2196*

Farshid Guilak, Ph.D.   *Assistant Professor, Department of Surgery, Division of Orthopaedic Surgery, Duke University Medical Center, Durham, North Carolina 27710*

Wilson C. Hayes, Ph.D.   *Maurice E. Mueller Professor of Biomechanics, Harvard Medical School, Director, Orthopedic Biomechanics Laboratory, Department of Orthopedic Surgery, Beth Israel Deaconess Medical Center, Boston, Massachusetts 02215*

Rik Huiskes, Ph.D.   *Professor of Musculoskeletal Biomechanics, Vice Chairman for Research, Institute of Orthopaedics, University of Nijmegen, 6500 Nijmegen, The Netherlands*

Debra E. Hurwitz, Ph.D.   *Department of Orthopedic Surgery, Rush-Presbyterian-St. Luke's Medical Center, Chicago, Illinois 60612*

Kenton R. Kaufman, Ph.D.   *Co-Director, Biomechanics Laboratory, Mayo Clinic, Rochester, Minnesota 55905*

Glen A. Livesay, M.S. *Research Engineer, Musculoskeletal Research Center, Department of Orthopaedic Surgery, University of Pittsburgh, Pittsburgh, Pennsylvania 15213*

Van C. Mow, Ph.D. *Professor of Mechanical Engineering and Orthopaedic Bioengineering, Departments of Mechanical Engineering and Orthopaedic Surgery, Director, Center for Biomedical Engineering, Columbia University, New York, New York 10032*

Raghu N. Natarajan, Ph.D. *Department of Orthopedic Surgery, Rush-Presbyterian-St. Luke's Medical Center, Chicago, Illinois 60612*

Anthony Ratcliffe, Ph.D. *Associate Professor of Orthopaedics Biochemistry, Columbia University, Head, Biochemistry Section, New York Orthopaedic Hospital Research Laboratory, and Department of Orthopaedic Surgery, Columbia University, New York, New York 10032*

Thomas J. Runco, B.S. *Research Engineer, Musculoskeletal Research Center, Department of Orthopaedic Surgery, University of Pittsburgh, Pittsburgh, Pennsylvania 15213*

Robert Sah, Ph.D. *Assistant Professor, Department of Bioengineering, University of California, San Diego, La Jolla, California 92093*

Albert B. Schultz, Ph.D. *Biomechanics Research Laboratory, Department of Mechanical Engineering and Applied Mechanics, University of Michigan, Ann Arbor, Michigan 48109-2125*

Lori A. Setton, Ph.D. *Assistant Professor, Department of Biomechanical Engineering, Duke University, Durham, North Carolina 27708*

Louis J. Soslowsky, Ph.D. *Assistant Professor of Surgery and Mechanical Engineering and Applied Mechanics, Orthopaedic Research Laboratories, University of Michigan, Ann Arbor, Michigan 48109-0486*

Nico Verdonschot, Ph.D. *Assistant Professor of Musculoskeletal Biomechanics, Director, Joint Replacement Biomechanics, Institute of Orthopaedics, University of Nijmegen, 6500 HB Nijmegen, The Netherlands*

Peter S. Walker, Ph.D. *Professor, Department of Biomedical Engineering, Institute of Orthopaedics, University College London, Royal National Orthopaedic Hospital Trust, Stanmore, Middlesex HA7 4LP, United Kingdom*

Savio L-Y. Woo, Ph.D. *Ferguson Professor and Director, Musculoskeletal Research Center, Department of Orthopaedic Surgery, University of Pittsburgh, Pittsburgh, Pennsylvania 15213*

Edmund P. Young, M.D. *Research Fellow, Musculoskeletal Research Center, Department of Orthopaedic Surgery, University of Pittsburgh, Pittsburgh, Pennsylvania 15213*

Preface to the First Edition

Great strides have been made in the advancement of orthopaedic surgery during the 30 years since Sir John Charnley's successful development of the total hip replacement. Today, total joint replacements for joints such as the knee, shoulder, and elbow are part of the daily routine of the orthopaedic surgeon. This clinical basis has developed a strong need for basic science knowledge on such topics as forces acting in the extremities and axial skeleton; the stress–strain behaviors of bone, tendons, ligament, cartilage, and knee meniscus; lubrication of joints; mechanics of fracture fixation, mechanics of bone–prosthesis interactions; and prosthesis design.

Indeed, an explosion of knowledge has taken place in orthopaedic research that closely parallels the clinical needs in orthopaedic surgery. As a result, scientific research in these areas has been exciting and has led to an ever-increasing number of well-trained professionals in the engineering and biomedical sciences. The difficult and challenging problems necessitate an interdisciplinary approach and demand knowledge of both biology and mechanics, and these basic studies have melded into a single discipline known as orthopaedic biomechanics. Unfortunately, the sheer amount of new information may be daunting to the beginning student. This is true for the engineering student interested in orthopaedic biomechanics and for the orthopaedic resident in training who aspires to pursue orthopaedic research. This book distills the progress made in orthopaedic biomechanics over the past 20 years into a single volume presented in a format suitable for teaching both orthopaedic residents and engineering students. The book is aimed at senior level engineering students wishing to pursue biomechanics research and at orthopaedic residents, with a basic engineering background, pursuing biomechanics research. In some chapters, problems have been provided to emphasize important topics.

Van C. Mow, Ph.D.
Wilson C. Hayes, Ph.D.

Preface

The first edition of *Basic Orthopaedic Biomechanics* was published in 1991—only six years ago. It was written by leading authors in the field of orthopaedic biomechanics, with the goal of providing a baseline of information for biomechanics students, orthopaedic residents, and others wishing to have some in-depth knowledge of the basic sciences that underlie the field of orthopaedic surgery. We are pleased that this book has received wide acceptance, and, indeed, it can be found on the desks of serious orthopaedic biomechanists worldwide. However, many new developments have occurred since 1990, when the original contributed chapters were completed. It seemed appropriate to organize and write a revised second edition that would include two new areas, which have since received intense scrutiny, and to include an important subject that was inexplicably omitted from the first edition.

The two new areas included in this second edition are "Physical Regulation of Cartilage Metabolism," by Farshid Guilak, Robert Sah, and Lori A. Setton, and "Quantitative Anatomy of Diarthrodial Joint Articular Layers," by Gerard A. Ateshian and Louis J. Soslowsky. Both areas have come into their own, each with a sizable number of researchers. A new chapter, "Biomechanical Principles of Total Knee Replacement Design," by Peter S. Walker and Gordon W. Blunn, has also been added. Many chapters have been greatly expanded to keep abreast of the new developments in their respective areas, including significant new results in articular cartilage biomechanics; friction, lubrication, and wear of diarthrodial joints; and biomechanics of artificial joints—the hip. Thus, we hope that this second edition of *Basic Orthopaedic Biomechanics* will continue to provide the required basic science information for students of orthopaedic biomechanics.

Van C. Mow, Ph.D.
Wilson C. Hayes, Ph.D.

Acknowledgments

We thank the authors for their outstanding contributions to this volume. We also thank our editor at Lippincott–Raven Publishers, Danette Knopp, for her patience and constant encouragement during the preparation of this second edition. Also, we wish to acknowledge again Mary Martin Rogers, now President of Lippincott–Raven Publishers, for inviting us to publish our first edition with Raven Press in 1991.

Finally, we gratefully acknowledge the editorial assistance of Robert J. Foster and our orthopaedic resident fellows and bioengineering students for their critique, without which this book could not have been finished.

Basic Orthopaedic Biomechanics, 2nd ed.,
edited by Van C. Mow and Wilson C. Hayes.
Lippincott–Raven Publishers, Philadelphia © 1997.

Chapter 1

Analysis of Muscle and Joint Loads

Kai-Nan An, *Edmund Y.S. Chao, and †Kenton R. Kaufman

*Department of Bioengineering, Mayo Medical School, Mayo Clinic,
Biomechanics Laboratory Division of Orthopaedic Research, Mayo Foundation, Rochester,
Minnesota 55905;*Orthopaedic Biomechanics Laboratory, Johns Hopkins University, Baltimore,
Maryland 21205-2196; and †Biomechanics Laboratory, Mayo Clinic, Rochester, Minnesota 55905*

Human joints are subjected to a wide range of forces during the activities of daily living. Even for relatively sedentary individuals, joint forces can be several times body weight during activities such as slowly climbing stairs, standing on one leg, or rising from a chair. With athletic activity such as running, jumping, or lifting weights, however, these joint forces can increase to as high as 10 to 20 times body weight. Because of the magnitude of these forces, it is all the more remarkable that most human joints can undergo many millions of loading cycles without significant degradation and that we can usually continue well into old age without clinical symptoms of joint damage. And yet, in some individuals, the control mechanisms that normally protect our joints from excessive loads break down, thereby initiating a cycle of joint degeneration known as osteoarthritis. Although the protective mechanisms responsible for maintaining joint integrity are not well characterized, and the initiating factors associated with joint degeneration are poorly understood, it is generally agreed that abnormal joint forces play a central role in the process. Thus, if for no other reason than to understand the etiology of degenerative joint disease, it is crucial to understand those factors leading to such large forces across human joints.

An improved understanding of joint forces is important in many other areas of orthopaedics as well. In total-joint-replacement arthroplasty, the wear and deformation of the articulating surface, the stress distribution in the implant, the mechanical behavior of the bone–implant interfaces, and the load-carrying characteristics of the remaining bone are intimately related to the joint loads. Postoperative rehabilitation after total joint arthroplasty or internal fixation of fractures can also be strongly influenced by the joint forces applied during the course of therapy. As an example, until it was appreciated that straight-leg-raising exercises can subject the hip to forces of several times body weight, such exercises were commonly used to maintain joint mobility and muscle tone soon after total hip replacement. The loads encountered by the human body are also of obvious importance in determining the possible mechanism and prevention of injury during occupational or sports activities.

In this chapter, we review and summarize methods for determining muscle and joint loads. To provide background, we first present some basic definitions and mathematical operations associated with the analysis of vectors, because forces are vector quantities. We then develop the concepts of static equilibrium and summarize methods used to analyze joint forces in light of the fact that there is generally cocontraction of synergistic muscles acting across the joint. After reviewing the available experimental methods for validating the theoretical predictions of joint forces, we summarize currently accepted magnitudes of joint forces for various joints and activities.

DEFINITIONS AND BASIC CONCEPTS

There are a number of fundamental concepts and definitions that are required as a foundation for an understanding of joint forces. Scalars are those fundamental physical quantities that require only a single number to specify. Examples include volume, mass, density (kg/m^3), electric charge (coulombs), and speed (m/sec). By contrast, vectors require specification of both magnitude and direction. Examples include force, velocity, acceleration, and displacement.

Degrees of freedom is a term in mechanics that describes the ability of an object to move in space. The number of degrees of freedom (DOF) of a system is the number of independent coordinates that must be specified to define the location and orientation of the object. A rigid body in space without any constraint has six degrees of freedom. This means that three coordinates of reference points on the body are needed to specify its location and three angles of a set of reference axes on the body are needed to specify its orientation. However, if the motion of the rigid body is somehow limited, the number of degrees of freedom is reduced.

An axle free to rotate within a bearing has a single degree of freedom because only a single angle of rotation is required to specify its position completely. A coin resting on a table has three degrees of freedom: it can translate in two directions and it can rotate about an axis perpendicular to the table. Three quantities (x and y coordinates and an angle θ) are therefore required. Frequently, joint movements are also described in terms of degrees of freedom. The hip, able to rotate around three axes in a stationary person, has three degrees of freedom; the elbow and forearm system, able to rotate about both flexion–extension and pronation–supination axes, has two; and the interphalangeal joints of the thumb and finger have one.

Forces

Force represents the action between two bodies. A force can be exerted by actual contact or indirectly at a distance, as in the case of gravitational force. In mechanics, the resultant force acting on a body is related to the mass of the body and the way in which the velocity of the body changes with time. In the standardized Système International (SI), a newton (N or nt) is defined as the force that causes linear acceleration of a mass of 1 kg at 1 m/sec².

Weight is the force with which a given mass is attracted toward the center of the earth. The earth's gravity accelerates any mass at 9.8 m/sec². Thus, a 1-kg mass weighs approximately 9.8 N on earth. Inertia is an inherent characteristic of matter that resists any change in the state of motion. Inertia varies directly with the mass: the greater the mass, the greater the inertia; thus, the leg has greater inertia than the forearm.

Moments

Moment (M) represents the tuning, twisting, or rotational effect of a force. Any off-axis force, applied at a distance from an actual or potential axis of rotation of an object, tends to cause angular acceleration, velocity, and displacement. Human motions are the result of the moments applied by muscles that cross the joints on which they act. A moment is defined as the product of a force and the perpendicular distance between the line of action of the force and the axis of rotation (Fig. 1A). Moment in SI units is therefore expressed in units of newton-meters (Nm). A moment is a vector quantity with (a) a magnitude given by the product of the force times the lever-arm distance from the force to the center of pivot and (b) direction defined by the "right-hand rule" (Fig. 1B). To apply the right-hand rule, one curls the fingers of the right hand in the direction that the force would rotate the object, and then the thumb points in the direction of positive moment. Note that the direction of a moment is along the axis of rotation (or potential rotation) and thus perpendicular to the plane in which the twisting force is applied. Moment arm, or the distance used in calculating the moment, is the perpendicular distance from the action line to the actual or potential pivot point of the system, regardless of the state of motion.

The moment arm (*d*) must not be confused with the action arm of the force. The action arm (*a*) is the direct distance along the structure from the point of force application to the pivot point. It may be the same, but more often it is a greater distance than the actual moment arm (*d*). In Fig. 2, note that the action arm (*a*) and moment arm (*d*) are different when the force is not applied perpendicular to the structure.

Newton's Laws and Static Equilibrium

Three fundamental laws of mechanics were formulated by Newton, and these provide a convenient basis for our discussion of force equilibrium. Conceptually, the first law states

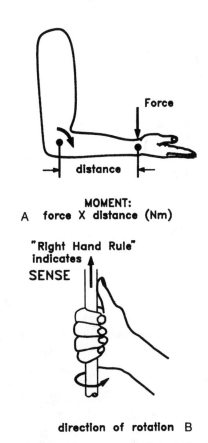

FIG. 1. (A) Moment represents the rotation effect of a force applied at a distance from an axis of rotation. **(B)** The direction of a moment is given by the right-hand rule.

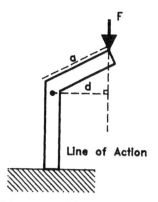

FIG. 2. Moment arm (*d*) versus action arm (*a*). The action arm is the direct distance along the structure, whereas the moment arm is the perpendicular distance from the line of action of the force to the axis of rotation.

that if the resultant force acting on a body is zero, then the body will either remain at rest or move with a constant velocity. The second law states that if the resultant force acting on the body is not zero, then the body will have an acceleration proportional to the magnitude and the direction of the resultant force. The third law states that the forces of action and reaction between bodies in contact have the identical magnitude and same line of action but opposite sense.

Equilibrium is a condition that exists when there are no unbalanced resultant forces or moments acting on an object that would tend to cause linear accelerations (in the case of unbalanced forces) or rotational accelerations (in the case of unbalanced moments). This situation can, in fact, be viewed as a special case of Newton's second law, because when the unbalanced forces and moments are zero, the object is not accelerating or, for our purposes, is at rest. A rigid body is thus said to be in equilibrium when the external forces acting on the rigid body form a system in which the total or resultant force is equivalent to zero. (In a more general sense, this statement is also true for dynamic conditions when inertial forces are acting, but this is beyond the scope of our discussion.)

In performing a force analysis of a rigid-body system, it is essential to consider all the forces acting on the body and to exclude any forces or moments that are not directly applied on the body. In a free-body diagram, the body (or part of a body) is isolated from the environment, and the environment is replaced by forces acting on the system.

Three-point correction and immobilization of a long bone fracture is a simple clinical example that can be used to introduce the concept of static equilibrium (Fig. 3). The forces A and B act downward and must be resisted or the body will move downward. A third force, the reaction force, acting upward, is supplied by the structure at the fulcrum supported by the ground. Thus, the forces are in static equilibrium. Each force may or may not produce a moment, an entity that must be considered separately. The force A acting over distance *c* also produces a moment (A*c*) acting to cause

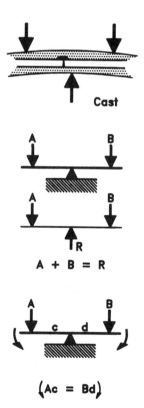

FIG. 3. Three-point immobilization in a cast. The forces, A and B, are resisted by the reaction, R. The net counterclockwise moment, *Ac,* equals the net clockwise moment, *Bd.*

counterclockwise rotation. To achieve rotational (moment) equilibrium, A*c* must equal the moment that acts in the clockwise direction B*d*. Reaction (R) does not produce a moment because it is considered the pivot point. One can vary the forces and distances, but as long as the product of force and distance remains the same, equilibrium will be maintained. Calculations of this kind can be used to determine whether or not equilibrium exists, or, if we know already that a system is in equilibrium, we can work backward to determine unknown forces.

Inverse Dynamic Problem

When a limb segment is functioning either statically or dynamically, two types of loads occur. Externally, the segment experiences loads directly applied through contact and also inertial loads that result from the movement of the limb and the joint. Internally, the muscular, capsuloligamentous, and bony articulating systems provide loads to counterbalance the externally applied loads. Usually, for dynamic problems (Fig. 4A), a solution of the rigid-body motion is sought because all loading conditions are defined. Although the initial value problem is complex, and sometimes mathematical solutions are difficult to obtain, accurate results can be achieved numerically using a digital computer.

In biomechanics, however, the motion of the musculoskeletal system under controlled body activities can be easily and accurately measured. For example, gait analysis can be used to describe the motion of the body. Because the unknown muscle and joint forces cannot easily be measured, they must be determined mathematically (Fig. 4B). This type of problem is known as the "inverse dynamic problem" in which the motion is known and the forces and moments required to produce the motion are calculated. The inverse method is used extensively for the dynamic analysis of the human musculoskeletal system (17).

COMPOSITION AND RESOLUTION OF FORCES

In solving internal force problems in biomechanics, we must take into account all the forces that are acting on the body of interest. Such analyses of forces may be approached in two ways. When we have two or more forces acting in the same plane and at the same point, we often wish to show their combined effect as a single force, the force resultant. This approach is often referred to as the composition of forces. Occasionally we must also replace a single force by two or more equivalent force components. This process is called the resolution of forces. Both approaches may be solved by graphic or algebraic methods.

The graphic method of combining forces utilizes a vector diagram in which the forces are represented by arrows, with the length of the arrow representing the magnitude of the

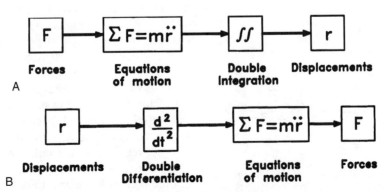

FIG. 4. (A) Direct dynamic problem. **(B)** Inverse dynamic problem.

force and the arrowhead representing the direction. Using the graphic method requires that the magnitude be drawn exactly to scale and that the direction be indicated precisely.

The algebraic method makes use of algebraic equations and utilizes trigonometric concepts. As with the graphic method, it is desirable to have a free-body diagram that shows all the forces that are acting. However, some of the forces are unknown in magnitude and may also be unknown in direction. The first step is to draw a free-body diagram and place all the known forces on it in their proper locations. Then, we determine where an unknown force might be acting. To aid us, we use Newton's third law, which says that for every action there must be an equal and opposite reaction. If an object is held in the hand, and we remove the object, we must replace it by a force at the point of contact (Fig. 5).

Because the magnitudes of the forces that exist among several bodies in contact are unknown, and in some cases we do not even know whether they exert a pull or a push on the body under consideration, it is necessary to introduce a vector to represent the force (with the arrowhead representing the assumed direction). If the assumed direction is incorrect, the sign in the algebraic solution of the problem will be negative, which indicates that the force is acting in the opposite direction.

Combination of Force Vectors

Simple mechanics experiments show that any set of coplanar concurrent forces may be replaced by a single force having the same effect as that of the given forces. This single force, obtained by combining the given forces, is called the resultant force. Vectors may be combined by addition and subtraction. Vectors are added by joining the head of one vector to the tail of the next vector while retaining the magnitude and direction of each vector. The resultant vector is represented by the distance between the last head and the first tail. Thus, specification of the components of a vector is equivalent to specification of the vector itself.

Resolution of Force Vectors

As we have seen, the addition (or subtraction) of two or more vectors results in a new vector. Conversely, any vector may be broken down or resolved into several components, the combined action of which is equal to the original vector. Because there is no unique way in which a vector may be resolved, a vector can have an infinite number of components. Most frequently, vectors are resolved into components at right angles to each other. Each component represents the projection of the vector onto the x, y, z coordinate axes. Thus, specification of the three components of a vector is equivalent to specification of the vector itself. In general, because vectors are three-dimensional quantities, three components are required. In the following, however, we restrict our discussions to the simpler case of force vectors in a plane. In the planar case, a force vector is resolved into two perpendicular components.

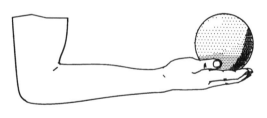
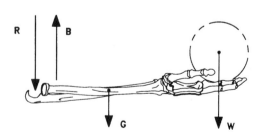

FIG. 5. Free-body diagram. **W**, weight in the hand; **G**, gravitational pull on the forearm; **B**, upward force of biceps muscle; **R**, reaction force of the humerus against the ulna.

There are many applications for vector resolution of forces in static problems related to orthopaedics. In regard to joint function, resolution of the applied muscle force can show what component of the muscle force produces a specified motion and what component produces joint compression or stabilization. For example, consider the force exerted by the ground on the heel at heel-strike. Resolving the force vector relative to a ground reference frame would determine what portion causes a vertical reaction force on the floor and what portion is resisted by friction.

Finally, because right triangles are easy to solve for unknowns using trigonometry, rectangular components of vectors often are determined as a first step in mathematical solutions to many problems involving forces. For example, in planar equilibrium problems involving multiple forces at various angles, it is frequently necessary to resolve each force into x (horizontal) and y (vertical) components. These components usually are written as F_x and F_y, respectively.

Graphic Resolution and Combination of Vectors

Force vectors may be represented and manipulated graphically. Consider the deltoid muscle pulling on the abducted arm with a force of 100 N. The line of action of the force makes an angle of 20° with the humerus (Fig. 6). We wish to find the vertical and horizontal

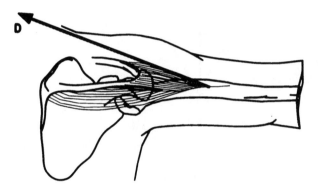

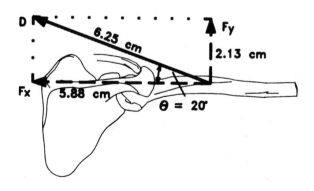

Given: D = 100N
Let: 0.25cm = 4N
Then: D = 6.25cm
So: Fx = 5.88cm = 94N
           and Fy = 2.13cm = 34N

FIG. 6. Graphic method of vector resolution. The force of the deltoid can be represented by a vector. The resultant vector can be resolved or broken down into two components acting at right angles to each other. The horizontal and vertical components are determined by drawing the vector components to scale.

components of the force. By selecting a linear unit of measurement to represent a unit of force, such as 0.25 cm to represent 4 N of force, and by constructing a line of the appropriate length at an angle of 20° to the humerus, one can determine the horizontal and vertical components of the force D. This is done by constructing a right triangle in which the hypotenuse is the vector representing the force in the deltoid, the vertical side is the rotatory component, and the horizontal side is the stabilizing component. The horizontal and vertical force components are determined by carefully

measuring the lengths of the respective sides of the triangle and converting those amounts to force values. This is done by using the conversion factor (0.25 cm equals 4 N force). The values obtained are 94 N horizontal force component and 34 N vertical force component. This illustration shows how a vector quantity can be resolved into its components using graphic methods.

The combination of vectors to form a resultant vector may also be accomplished graphically using a parallelogram. The sides of the parallelogram are linear representations

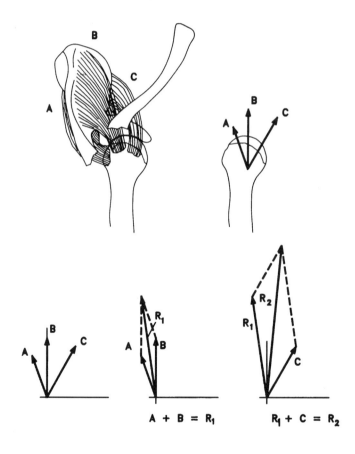

A + B = R₁   R₁ + C = R₂

A = M. infraspinatus
B = M. supraspinatus
C = M. subscapularis

FIG. 7. Parallelogram method used for determining the resultant of three or more forces applied to the same point. R_1 is the resultant of the combined forces **A** and **B**. R_2 is the resultant of the combined forces R_1 and **C**: **A** + **B** + **C** = R_2.

of the two vectors. From a convenient point, two lines are drawn to scale, with the correct angle between them—that is, the same angle that actually exists between the two vectors. By using these two lines as two sides of a parallelogram, the other two parallel sides are constructed by simple geometry (Fig. 7). The diagonal is then drawn from a point of application to the opposite corner. This diagonal represents both the magnitude and the direction of the resultant vector.

When one wishes to determine the result of three or more vectors acting at one point, a similar procedure is followed (Fig. 7). The resultant of two of the vectors is found. A second parallelogram is then constructed using the third vector as one side and the resultant of the first two vectors as the second side. The resultant vector of this second parallelogram is the resultant of all three vectors (Fig. 7).

Trigonometric Resolution and Combination of Vectors

Although the graphic method can sometimes be useful, its accuracy is difficult to control, and it only applies to concurrent force systems. Nonconcurrent force systems produce a resultant moment. A more accurate and efficient approach makes use of trigonometric relationships to combine and resolve vectors. Any vector may be resolved into horizontal and vertical or rectangular components if trigonometric relationships for the right triangle are employed. In the previous example of the deltoid muscle (Fig. 8), we can find the horizontal force (F_x) and the vertical force (F_y) by constructing a right triangle. With the magnitude of the force (D) as the hypotenuse of the triangle, the vertical and horizontal components of the force become the vertical and horizontal

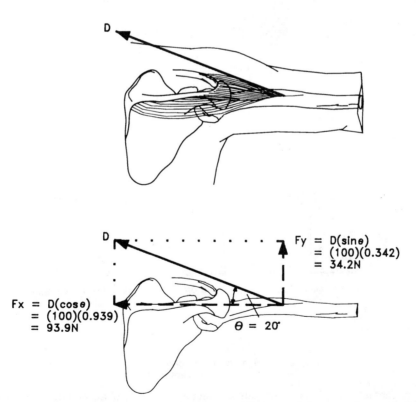

FIG. 8. Resolution of deltoid force, **D**, into a rotatory component, F_y, and stabilizing component, F_x. Angle of force application, Θ, is 20°.

sides of the triangle. To obtain the values of F_x and F_y the sine and cosine functions are used:

$$F_x = D \cos 20° = 100 \times 0.939 = 93.9 \text{ N}$$

$$F_y = D \sin 20° = 100 \times 0.342 = 34.2 \text{ N}$$

To reverse the procedure, we could find D by recalling that the square of the hypotenuse of a right triangle is equal to the sum of the squares of the other two sides, or

$$D^2 = F_x^2 + F_y^2$$

$$D = \sqrt{F_x^2 + F_y^2} = \sqrt{93.9^2 + 34.2^2} = 100 \text{ N}$$

This also provides a means to check if the components F_x and F_y are correctly calculated.

If more than two vectors are involved, or if they are not at right angles to each other, the resultant may be obtained by first determining the x and y components, R_x and R_y, for each individual vector and then summing these individual components to obtain the x and y components of the resultant force. Once these x and y components are known, the magnitude and direction of the resultant may be obtained by the relationship $R^2 = R_x^2 + R_y^2$ and $\theta = \tan^{-1} (R_y/R_x)$.

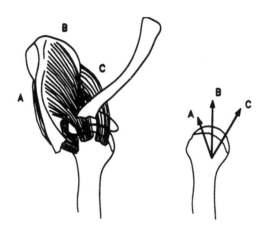

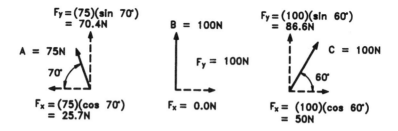

A = M. infraspinatus
B = M. supraspinatus
C = M. subscapularis

FIG. 9. Trigonometric combination of summed vectors. The sum of all x components becomes the horizontal vector component, and the sum of all y components becomes the vertical vector component.

Example 1. Consider the rotator cuff, where three muscles, the infraspinatus, supraspinatus, and subscapularis, pull on the humerus. We are interested in determining the resultant force of these muscles and its resultant direction (Fig. 9). To solve this problem trigonometrically, the horizontal and vertical components of each muscle must be determined first. The infraspinatus acts with a magnitude of 75 N at an angle of 70° from the horizontal. The vertical component for the infraspinatus is

$$F_y = A \sin \theta = 75(0.9397) = 70.5 \text{ N}$$

and the horizontal component is

$$F_x = -A \cos \theta = -(75)(0.3420) = 25.7 \text{ N}$$

The negative sign indicates that the horizontal component acts in the minus x direction. The supraspinatus acts with a magnitude of 100 N in the vertical direction only. Thus, $F_x = 100$ N, and $F_y = 0$ N. The subscapularis has a magnitude of 100 N and a direction of 60° from the horizontal. So, the vertical component for the subscapularis is

$$F_y = C \sin \theta = 100(0.866) = 86.6 \text{ N}$$

and the horizontal component of the subscapularis is

$$F_x = C \cos \theta = 100(0.5) = 50 \text{ N}$$

The y component of the resultant effect of the three muscles is obtained by summing the effects of each muscle in the y direction. The Greek letter sigma (Σ) is usually used to indicate summation. In this notation, the resultant y component (R_y) is

$$R_y = \Sigma F_y = 70.5 + 100 + 86.6 = 257.1 \text{ N}$$

Similarly, the resultant component (R_x) is the sum of the x values for the three muscles:

$$R_x = \Sigma F_x = -25.7 + 0 + 50 = 24.3 \text{ N}$$

As we have seen, a knowledge of the horizontal and vertical components makes it possible to determine the resultant vector. A triangle is formed, and the Pythagorean theorem is used to find the hypotenuse:

$$R = \sqrt{R_x^2 + R_y^2} = \sqrt{24.3^2 + 257} = 258.1 \text{ N}$$

The line of action, θ, of the resultant is

$$\theta = \tan^{-1}(R_y/R_x) = \tan^{-1}(257/24.3) = 84.6°$$

from the positive x direction. Thus, the composite muscle pull is 258 N pulling at an angle of 84.6° from the horizontal. This example demonstrates that the combined effect of several forces acting on a single bone can be determined by finding the force resultant.

STATIC EQUILIBRIUM

An object is said to be in equilibrium when no unbalanced forces or moments are acting on it and it is not accelerating with respect to a reference system. Strictly speaking, an object that is moving at constant velocity is also not accelerating, but for our purposes, an object in equilibrium can be assumed to be at rest, i.e., neither translating nor rotating. Knowing that a body is in static equilibrium allows us to determine unknown muscle and joint forces.

To demonstrate this, we will consider only forces acting in a plane but should again keep in mind that forces actually occur in three dimensions. However, in many instances the main features of a joint force problem can be captured with a two-dimensional analysis. For an object to be in equilibrium, there are two sets of conditions that must be satisfied: translational equilibrium and rotational equilibrium.

Translational Equilibrium

An object in translational equilibrium has no unbalanced forces acting that would tend to cause the object to accelerate in the x, y, or z direction. For the two-dimensional case in the xy plane, this means that there must be no unbalanced forces acting in either the x or the y direction. Note that this is equivalent to requiring that both the x and y components of the resultant force acting on the object are zero. Thus, translational equilibrium requires that the vector sum of forces (i.e., the force resultant) must be equal to zero. It is possible, however, for there still to be unbalanced moments. Hence, even though there may be translational equilibrium, this does not automatically ensure rotational equilibrium. This is discussed in the next section.

The condition for translational equilibrium can be written $\Sigma F = 0$. This is a vector equation standing for two equations:

$$\Sigma F_x = 0$$

$$\Sigma F_y = 0$$

In this notation, a component is positive if it points along the positive axis and negative if it points in the other direction.

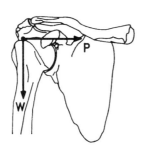

A.

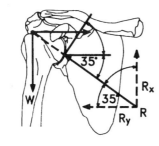

B.

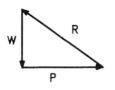

C.

FIG. 10. Static forces on the glenohumeral joint during standing.

Example 2. As an example, let us see what force is needed to maintain the position of the upper limb in Fig.10A. Suppose the slope of the glenoid fossa at the point of joint contact is 35° from the horizontal, and the weight of the upper limb is 50 N.

Questions: What is the force in the supraspinatus and joint capsule that is necessary to prevent subluxation of the humeral head? What is the joint reaction force?

Solution: A free-body diagram is drawn (Fig. 10B), with the x axis parallel to the direction of the force of gravity. By using vector analysis, we can determine the magnitude of the muscle force and the direction and magnitude of the glenohumeral joint reaction force. We must know the magnitude, the direction, and line of action of the pull of gravity, W, and the direction and line of action of the supraspinatus muscle and the joint capsule. The direction of the joint reaction force, R, is assumed to be perpendicular to the joint surface because healthy articular cartilage surfaces transmit nearly no frictional forces parallel to the joint surface.

The reaction force, R, can then be resolved into two components. The horizontal component is $R_y = R \cos 35°$. The vertical component is $R_x = R \sin 35°$. Then the equilibrium equations are:

$$\Sigma F_y = P - R_y = P - R \cos 35° = 0$$

and

$$\Sigma F_x = R_x - W = R \sin 35° - W = 0$$

which give

$$R = W/\sin 35° = 50/0.574 = 87.1 \text{ N}$$

and

$$P = R_y = R \cos 35° = (87.1)(0.819) = 71.3 \text{ N}$$

The graphic solution is illustrated in Fig. 10C.

Rotational Equilibrium

For an object to be in rotational equilibrium, there must be no unbalanced moments acting that would tend to cause rotation. Consider two forces that are parallel to one another (Fig. 3). To be in translational equilibrium, the sum of the combined forces, A + B, must be opposed by the upward force, R (Fig. 3). In this situation, however, a second condition of equilibrium must be introduced to ensure that rotation does not occur. As we have seen, a force acting on a rigid body at a distance from a fixed point tends to cause the body to rotate. In Fig. 3, we can see that the force A produces a counterclockwise moment around the fixed point, whereas the force B produces a clockwise moment. We have already defined the perpendicular distance from the line of application of a force to the axis of rotation as the moment arm of the force. From your experience on a teeter-totter, you probably found that to balance, the heavier person had to sit closer to the center than the lighter one. This illustrates the combined importance of both the distance from the axis at which the force is acting and the magnitude of the force itself. An increase in either its magnitude or its distance from the pivot point increases the tendency of the force to cause rotation about the pivot.

For the body to be in rotational equilibrium, the sum of moments about a point must be equal to zero ($\Sigma M = 0$). That is, the sum of the clockwise moments (ΣM_{cw}) plus the sum of the counterclockwise moments (ΣM_{ccw}) must equal zero. Thus, the body is in rotational equilibrium if the algebraic sum of all the moments is zero:

$$\Sigma M = 0$$

or

$$\Sigma M_{cw} = \Sigma M_{ccw}$$

Example 3. Consider the flexed forearm that is holding a ball, as shown in Fig. 11. Gravity pulls downward on the forearm and the ball, while the biceps muscles pull upward. Because the lever arms of G and W are greater than that of B, the force B must be larger to counterbalance the moment exerted by the forces G and W. With the biceps muscles supporting the forearm at 90° of elbow

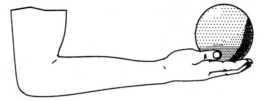

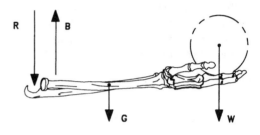

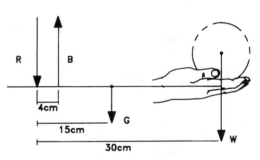

FIG. 11. A parallel force system acting on the forearm.

flexion, the lever arm is the perpendicular distance from the tendon to the axis of the elbow joint. In this instance, the lever arm is anatomically fixed, but the magnitude of the muscle force can be varied to alter the moment. The biceps muscle provides a counterclockwise force opposed by the clockwise forces of gravity and the weight, both acting about an axis of rotation at the elbow joint.

Suppose the forearm weighs 15 N, its center of mass is 15 cm from the elbow joint, the weight weighs 20 N and is placed in the hand at 30 cm from the elbow center, and the biceps muscle has a lever arm of 3 cm. The elbow joint is the axis of rotation (or potential rotation). Note that the reaction force produces no moment about the elbow because its distance from the axis is zero ($R \times 0 = 0$). To solve for the unknown force B, the moments produced by each force are added algebraically. From rotational equilibrium, we may write:

$$(G \times 15 \text{ cm}) - (W \times 30 \text{ cm}) - (B \times 3 \text{ cm}) = 0.$$

In this example, we take the clockwise moments of G and W as positive and the counterclockwise moment of B as negative. From rotational equilibrium, we write

$$(15 \text{ N}) (15 \text{ cm}) - (20 \text{ N}) (30 \text{ cm})$$
$$- (B \text{ N}) (3 \text{ cm}) = 0$$

$$825 \text{ N-cm} - 3 B \text{ N-cm} = 0$$

$$B = 275 \text{ N}$$

Note that in this example one could instead assume the potential axis of rotation to be at the point of application of the force B. In that case, one could instead solve for the elbow joint reaction force R. This illustrates that in using the rotational equilibrium condition, it makes no difference which axis is used for the purpose of summing moments. We will also see in the next section that the combined use of both translational and rotational equilibrium allows solution for both R and B.

General Planar Force Systems

In many situations, the forces acting on a body are neither parallel nor concurrent. This is described as a general force system. Both translational and rotational equilibrium need to be maintained in a general force system. Thus, the equations are

$$\Sigma F_x = 0$$

$$\Sigma F_y = 0$$

$$\Sigma M = 0$$

These equations, referred to as the planar equilibrium conditions, simply say that for an object to be in equilibrium in a plane, the sum of the forces acting in the x and y directions must be zero and the sum of the moments acting about any axis must be zero. If there are no forces in a particular direction, then obviously there are no unbalanced forces in that direction, and the equilibrium condition for that direction is satisfied. In the example of Fig. 11, we can apply the planar equilibrium conditions. Because there are no forces acting in the x direction, we have

$$\Sigma F_x = 0$$

or

$$0 = 0$$

Summing forces in the y direction:

$$\Sigma F_y = 0$$

$$-R + B - G - W = 0$$

Here, R, G, and W are taken as negative because they all act in the negative y direction. Because B is known from the above discussions of rotational equilibrium to be 275 N, we can determine the remaining unknown R from

$$R = B - G - W$$

$$= 275 - 15 - 20 \text{ N}$$

$$= 240 \text{ N}$$

The positive sign indicates that we have correctly assumed that R acts in the negative y direction.

The above example involves a particular case of planar force systems in which all forces are parallel. The situation becomes slightly more complex when nonparallel forces occur.

Example 4. Consider the example of the biceps muscle acting on the forearm when the elbow is not at a 90° angle but when the forearm is 30° below the horizontal and the biceps inserts at an angle of 45° with the forearm (Fig. 12). The muscle insertion is 3 cm from the elbow joint, the 15-N forearm weight is centered 15 cm from the elbow, and a 20-N weight is held in the hand 30 cm from the joint center. With the forearm position other than horizontal, the gravitational forces do not

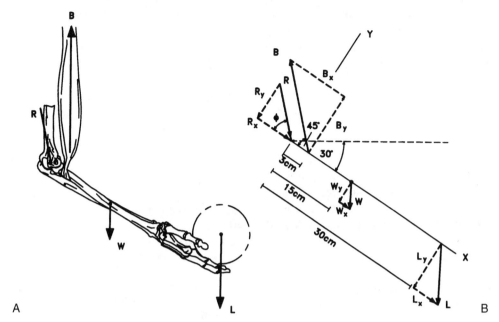

FIG. 12. Static forces about the elbow joint when the forearm is 30° below the horizontal.

act at 90° to the limb but instead at an angle defined by the orientation of the limb with respect to the vertical. However, these gravitational forces can be resolved into components both perpendicular to and parallel to the limb. Similarly, with the change in position, the biceps muscle does not act at 90° to the forearm. However, again, the biceps force may be resolved into components perpendicular to and parallel to the forearm. The key to solving for the unknown magnitude of the biceps force (note that we know the direction) and the unknown magnitude and direction of the elbow reaction force is to resolve all forces into x and y components that are taken as parallel to and perpendicular to the forearm. In the new x and y axis system, the planar equilibrium conditions can then be used as above to solve for the unknown forces and directions.

Question: What is the muscle force needed to maintain the forearm position 30° below the horizontal? What are the elbow joint reactions?

Solution: Again, we draw a free-body diagram as shown in Fig. 12B. Because the pull

of gravity and the muscle insertion are not perpendicular to the forearm, we must find their x and y components in the directions shown in Fig. 12B. The weight components perpendicular to the forearm, W_y and L_y, form 30° angles with the force of gravity, W, and the load, L. Thus, $W_y = W \cos 30°$. The muscle force is at an angle of 45° to the forearm, so $B_y = B \sin 45°$. Assuming the x axis to lie along the forearm, we use the elbow joint as the axis of rotation and solve for the sum of moments around this point (taking counterclockwise moments as positive).

$$\Sigma M = 0$$

$$(B_y \times 3 \text{ cm}) - (W_y \times 15 \text{ cm})$$
$$- (L_y \times 30 \text{ cm}) = 0$$

$$(B_y \times 3 \text{ cm}) - (W \cos 30° \times 15 \text{ cm})$$
$$- (L \cos 30° \times 30 \text{ cm}) = 0$$

$$(B_y \times 3 \text{ cm}) - (15 \text{ N} \times 0.866 \times 15 \text{ cm})$$
$$- (20 \text{ N} \times 0.866 \times 30 \text{ cm}) = 0$$

$$(B_y \times 3) - (195) - (520) = 0$$

$$B_y = 714/3 = 238 \text{ N}$$

The rotatory component of the muscle has a magnitude of 238 N, producing a counter-clockwise moment. The magnitude of B can then be found from the trigonometric relationship

$$B_y = B \sin 45°$$

$$238 = B\,0.707$$

$$B = 337 \text{ N}$$

For the joint reaction force, we use the sum of the force components acting both along and perpendicular to the forearm, i.e., $\Sigma F_x = 0$ and $\Sigma F_y = 0$. First, summing forces in the x direction, we have

$$\Sigma F_x = B_x - W_x - L_x - R_x = 0$$

However, we know the values of B, W, and L from simple trigonometry:

$$B_x = B \cos 45° = 337 \times 0.707 = 238 \text{ N}$$

$$W_x = W \sin 30° = 15 \text{ N} \times 0.5 = 7.5 \text{ N}$$

$$L_x = L \sin 30° = 20 \text{ N} \times 0.5 = 10 \text{ N}$$

We then substitute these values in order to solve for R_x

$$(-238) + (7.5) + (10) + R_x = 0$$

$$(-220.5) + R_x = 0$$

$$R_x = 220.5$$

Using a similar approach, we sum forces in the y direction.

$$\Sigma F_y = B_y - W_y - L_y - R_y = 0$$

$$(238) + (-13) + (-17) + R_y = 0$$

$$208 - R_y = 0$$

$$R_y = -208$$

The magnitude of the joint force, R, is found using the Pythagorean theorem:

$$R = \sqrt{R_x^2 + R_y^2}$$

$$= \sqrt{(220.5)^2 + (-208)^2} = 303 \text{ N}$$

We determine the direction by using one of the trigonometric functions:

$$\tan \theta = R_y/R_x$$

$$\theta = \tan^{-1}(-208/220.5)$$

$$\theta = \tan^{-1}(-0.943) = -43°$$

The direction is to the right and downward at a 43° angle with the x axis.

To summarize, when an object is known to be at rest, the equations of equilibrium may be applied. However, care must be taken in constructing a free-body diagram in order to show all forces acting. These forces must be represented as vectors (showing their direction), with letters being assigned to them to represent their magnitudes. If we are to arrive at the correct solution, all forces pertinent to the problem must be included. Steps in the solution of the equilibrium problem are:

1. Select the free body appropriate to the solution of the problem.
2. Draw the free-body diagram.
3. Choose coordinate axes and the axis to be used for summing moments.
4. Substitute the forces from the free-body diagram into the pertinent equations of equilibrium ($\Sigma F = 0$; $\Sigma M = 0$).
5. Solve the equations of equilibrium to obtain the unknown values.

Intersegmental Load

Braune and Fischer (16) proposed that body segments such as the trunk, shank, and forearm could be modeled as a limited system of rigid bodies. Although limb segments are never absolutely rigid and deform under the loads to which they are subjected, these deformations are usually small and do not appreciably affect the conditions of equilibrium or motion under consideration. These body segments can also be assumed to be interconnected at the joints. In such a model, the laws of three-dimensional rigid-body mechanics can be used to calculate the resultant forces and moments between the segments. If the displacement histories and mass properties of the segments are known, then the intersegmental force and moment acting on the limb can be solved by applying the equations of motion for the system. These equations are more general representations of the simple force and moment equations we have used above. However, in this case, we use dynamic equations based on consideration of linear and angular moment. In the Newtonian approach, a free-body diagram must first be obtained. The equations of motion for the isolated free-body segment have the following general form:

$$\Sigma \vec{F}_c = m(d\vec{r}_c/dt)$$

$$\Sigma \vec{M}_A = \dot{\vec{H}}_A + m(\vec{r}_A \times \vec{r}_c)$$

where $\Sigma \vec{F}_c$ is the force vector acting on the body, $\Sigma \vec{M}_A$ the resultant moment vector about point A, $\dot{\vec{H}}_A$ the rate of change of angular momentum about point A, $\vec{r}_A$ the absolute velocity of point A, $\vec{r}_c$ the absolute velocity vector of the center of gravity, C, and m the mass of the free-body segment.

It is usually desirable to write an equation involving the moments about the joint center, A, because this equation will not contain the unknown reaction force at A. An intersegmental resultant force and moment can be described at the proximal and distal ends of each body segment. These forces and moments are the net kinetic effect that the adjoining body segments have on each other. It is important to note that these intersegmental resultants are conceptual kinetic quantities that do not necessarily represent any single anatomic structure. Rather, the intersegmental resultant represents the vector sum of all the forces in the anatomic structures and the vector sum of all the moments produced by those forces. It is important to remember that the intersegmental resultant can be determined uniquely from the known kinematics, inertia, and external loads. The anatomic structures consist of the muscle, ligament, and articular surface contact. The problem of calculating the force within the anatomic structures can be thought of as a "distribution problem."

DISTRIBUTION PROBLEM

Consider a planar model of the elbow (Fig. 13). This model consists of three muscles—

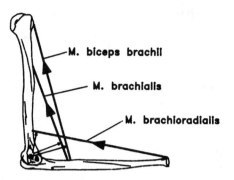

FIG. 13. A planar-functioning joint with three possibly active flexor muscles; the angles of inclination between biceps brachii, brachialis, and brachioradialis are 80.3°, 68.7°, and 23.0°, respectively, from the x axis.

the biceps (BIC), brachialis (BRA), and brachioradialis (BRD)—resisting the applied force, F. With the forearm in the position shown, the lever arms of the biceps, brachialis, and brachioradialis are 4.6 cm, 3.4 cm, and 7.5 cm, respectively. The 15-N forearm weight is centered 15 cm from the elbow, and a 20-N weight is held in the hand 30 cm from the joint center as shown in Fig. 11. The unknown elbow joint reaction force components are J_x and J_y. Because the pull of gravity and the weight are perpendicular to the forearm, their lever arms are 15 cm and 30 cm, respectively. Again, taking clockwise moments as positive, we use the following equations to solve for the muscle forces.

$$\Sigma M = 0$$

$$-4.6F_{BIC} - 3.4F_{BRA} - 7.5F_{BRD} + (15 \times 15) + (20 \times 30) = 0$$

$$4.6F_{BIC} + 3.4F_{BRA} + 7.5F_{BRD} = 825$$

$$\Sigma F_x = 0$$

$$-F_{BIC} \cos 80.3° - F_{BRA} \cos 68.7° - F_{BRD} \cos 23.0° + J_x = 0$$

$$J_x = 0.17F_{BIC} + 0.36F_{BRA} + 0.92F_{BRD}$$

$$\Sigma F_y = 0$$

$$F_{BIC} \sin 80.3° + F_{BRA} \sin 68.7° + F_{BRD} \sin 23.0° - J_y = 0$$

$$J_y = 0.99F_{BIC} + 0.93F_{BRA} + 0.39F_{BRD}$$

Note that there are only three equations, but there are five unknowns. Three of the unknowns are muscle forces, and two are joint reaction forces. In this case, there are an infinite number of solutions that could satisfy the equations, and the problem is to know which solution is the correct one. In reality, muscles act synergistically to control joint position, and thus, the usual situation is that several muscle forces act across a joint simultaneously. Finding how the total force is distributed among these muscles is sometimes referred to as the distribution problem. Such problems are also called indeterminate because the number of independent equations available for their solution is less than the number of unknowns. In this case, additional assumptions must be made in order to achieve a solution for the unknown distribution of forces. In order to distribute the forces in the muscles and joint to obtain a unique solution, two methods are commonly employed: (a) the reduction method and (b) the optimization method.

Reduction Method

The goal of the reduction method is to reduce the degree of redundancy until the number of unknown forces is equal to the number of equations. This can be achieved by reducing the number of unknown forces (ignoring muscles and/or grouping muscles with similar function) or by increasing the number of equations (for example, by assuming a known force distribution between muscles) based on anatomic consideration and physiological observation through electromyography, for instance.

Several uses of the reduction method to solve the distribution problem have appeared in the literature. The first of these works (59) describes predictions of muscle forces about the hip during locomotion and are made to estimate the articular surface contact force at the hip. In this study, the general distribution problem at the hip was made determinate through several simplifying assumptions. The muscles crossing the hip were combined into several

functional groups: (a) long flexors, (b) short flexors, (c) long extensors, (d) short extensors, (e) abductors, and (f) adductors. The force magnitude transmitted by these six muscle groups combined with the three components of articular surface contact force comprise nine unknown scalar quantities. Previous reports of the electromyographic activity were cited to demonstrate that there is little antagonist muscle action, and thus only muscle agonists were considered. Despite these simplifications, the possibility of activity in both long and short flexors and extensors still made the problem indeterminate. A solution could be obtained, however, by assuming activity in only one flexor (either the long or short, but not both) and one extensor. A determinate solution was obtained in each instance, and the expectation was that the true solution would lie between these two solutions.

With methods adapted from these techniques, a more comprehensive study of the human knee joint was conducted by Morrison (54). One of the most significant conclusions of Morrison's work was that the maximum joint force at the knee during walking was in the range of two to four times body weight, the average value being 3.0 times body weight. The forces acting in the mediolateral direction were generally much smaller, with a mean value of 0.26 times body weight. Solutions to the indeterminate problem were found by anatomic or functional simplification.

The reduction method is useful because of its simplicity and its ability to provide some valuable quantitative insight into the mechanics of posture and movement. However, the anatomic simplifications that are inherent in this method may necessitate considerable effort, and the mechanical action of the individual muscles is obscured. For a detailed analysis and calculation of individual muscle forces, a more powerful approach called the optimization method is often used.

Optimization Method

An alternative method for solving the indeterminate problem is to seek an optimum solution (i.e., a solution that maximizes or minimizes some process or action). In this method, a solution to the redundant equation system is obtained by formulating an objective function and utilizing a mathematical optimization technique. The objective function provides the basis for comparison of candidate solutions.

The "best" solution is sought by the optimization algorithm. The optimization approach is based on the assumption that load sharing between the muscles is unique during learned motor activities and that the neurologic control of muscle action is governed by certain physiological criteria that guarantee "efficient" muscle actions. The objective function should correspond to these physiological criteria. Intuitively, it seems reasonable that the controlled process of human locomotion involves a process of optimization. This general notion was first mentioned by the Weber brothers (73), who stated that humans walk in the way that costs us the lightest energy expenditure for the longest time and gives the best results. For a particular physical activity to be performed with a large number of potential force-carrying structures at a joint, an individual may exercise considerable discretion in generating force in the actively controlled muscles. The criteria that the individual chooses, either consciously or unconsciously, to determine the control of muscle action may vary considerably with the nature of the physical activity to be performed and the physical capabilities of the individual. Muscle control in sprint running may serve to maximize velocity, whereas in walking, the control process may serve to maximize endurance. In a painful pathologic situation, such as degenerative joint disease, muscular control may serve to minimize pain. If this pain occurs as a result of joint surface pressure, the appropriate optimization criterion may be to minimize the articular surface contact force. Muscular control may also serve to minimize the forces transmitted by passive joint structures such as ligaments. The possible optimization criteria are many, and the choice of a criterion to solve a particular distribution problem may not be obvious.

To solve an optimization problem, its format has to be specified. This is done by (a) defining the cost function (the function to be optimized), (b) identifying the constraint functions, (c) specifying the design variables, and (d) setting the appropriate bounds for the design variables. The formulation of this method can be summarized as follows:

minimize $J = f(x_1, x_2, \ldots, x_n)$
subject to $g_j(x_1, x_2, \ldots, x_n)$ for $j = 1, 2, \ldots, m$
and $0 \leq x_i \leq U_i$ for $i = 1, 2, \ldots, n$

where J is the optimal criterion (cost function) and can be linear or nonlinear. The function g represents the equations of motion and certain equality constraint relationships. The x_i stands for the independent variables, which are the unknown joint and muscle forces. These variables may also be subject to inequality constraints. With either linear or nonlinear functions, the optimization problem can be solved by a number of numerical schemes that may be implemented on digital computers.

It is important to understand both the mathematical behavior and the physiological significance of this general method of solving the indeterminate distribution problem. The way in which an optimal solution is found and the general characteristics of that solution are best introduced by a simple example.

Example 5. Consider the problem:

minimize $J = 2x + y$
subject to $2x - y = 4$
$x + 3y \leq 9$
$x \geq 0$
$y \geq 0$

A graphic representation of this problem and its solution are shown in Fig. 14. The penalty function, described by the line $2x - y$ = constant as it decreases, moves into the constraint area defined by the lines $2x - y = 4$, $x + 3y = 9$, $x \geq 0$, and $y \geq 0$. It continues to move until it intersects the inequality constraint line, $y \geq 0$. Any further movement of this line would violate the $y \geq 0$ constraint; therefore, the minimum value of the penalty function has been found at $x = 2$ and $y = 0$.

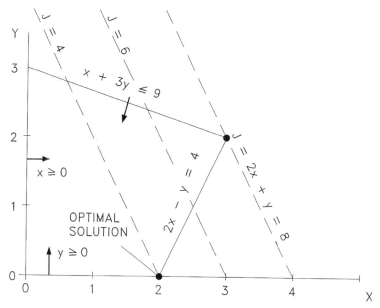

FIG. 14. Graphic solution of the indeterminate distribution problem (see text).

Optimal Criteria

Optimal solutions in joint force problems can be found as functions of muscle forces, ligament forces, and articular surface contact forces. However, the selection and justification of optimal criteria has been a major problem. Optimization criteria are grouped according to whether linear or nonlinear optimization methods are used. Further, these criteria may include single or multiple objective functions.

Linear Criteria

Mathematical formulations of physiological criteria for load sharing began appearing about 25 years ago. MacConaill (51) defined a principle of minimal total muscular force, which postulated that no more muscular force than is both necessary and sufficient to maintain a posture or perform a motion would be used. Accordingly, this would minimize the sum of the muscle forces, namely, ΣF_i.

This sum of muscle forces as the objective function in computations has been used ex-

tensively (60,68). Unfortunately, because of the specific characteristics of linear programming, the results of a linear criterion are not always physiologically consistent, and this has been noted by most investigators. When a planar model for a single joint is used, minimization of a linear objective function will result in the prediction that only one muscle (the muscle with the largest lever arm) is active. However, in most activities, several muscles crossing the joint are active simultaneously.

One way to improve the predictions of muscle forces with linear criteria is to formulate additional constraints. An inequality constraint that limits the stress in each muscle was used by Crowninshield (21), Crowninshield and Brand (22), Pedotti et al. (60), and Patriarco et al. (57). Usually, it is assumed that the maximum physiological stress is the same for each muscle. The use of this constraint results in the prediction that a muscle starts to be active when another muscle reaches its maximum stress. Initially, only the muscle with the largest arithmetic product of moment arm and physiological cross-sectional area is active until it reaches its limit, at which moment the muscle with the second largest product is selected, and so forth (26). Crowninshield (21) defined a maximum stress and was able to model synergistic muscle action. Patriarco et al. (57) formulated an additional equality constraint to enforce synergism between two muscles by assuming equal stresses in these muscles. It should be noted that when a sufficient number of the constraints are formulated, the problem becomes deterministic.

Recently, several new approaches that involve minimizing muscle intensity have been suggested. Schultz et al. (67) developed lumbar trunk models that minimized the compression on the spine while, at the same time, minimizing maximum muscle contraction intensity. They obtained solutions to the problem by solving a sequence of linear programs, each with a different upper bound of muscle intensity selected by a stepwise procedure. They began with low muscle intensities that led to infeasible models and gradually increased the muscle intensity until the first feasible solution was found. The difficulties of this approach were its substantial computational requirements and instability of solutions as intensity values were changed. In spite of these shortcomings, this model provided results that were in better agreement with experimental measurements than those provided by less sophisticated models.

An et al. (5) suggested an improved technique based on minimizing the upper bound of muscle stress. In this approach, additional inequality conditions were introduced, namely,

$$F_i/PCSA_i \leq \sigma$$

The left-hand side represents the "stress" on the ith muscle, where F_i is the force and $PCSA_i$ is the physiological cross-sectional area of the ith muscle. The single variable, σ, on the right-hand side represented the upper bound for all of the muscle stresses. The unique solution for distributing muscle forces was then obtained by minimizing σ.

These approaches make use of the linear optimization method and therefore guarantee that the solution will converge on a global minimum. The popularity of linear objective functions is partially a result of the fact that linear optimization problems can be readily solved with the simplex method (24), resulting in a unique solution. The simplex algorithm is easy to use and is available in commercial software packages. Nonlinear formulations are not so easily addressed. There are no algorithms available that can guarantee a unique solution to the general nonlinear programming problem.

Nonlinear Criteria

Nonlinear objective functions can predict synergistic muscle activity, even without the formulation of additional constraints. Gracovetsky et al. (33) defined an objective function as the sum of squared shear stresses in the vertebral column and predicted forces during weight lifting. For the analysis of walking, Pedotti et al. (60) used the sum of squared muscle forces, ΣF_i^2.

Several investigators have sought to characterize the relationship between muscle force and endurance experimentally. They have concluded, in general, that the endurance time is approximately inversely proportional to the quantitative value of muscle force raised to some power. However, there exists a large spread in the reported values of this exponent. Combining these approaches with the work of Fick (30), who showed that an approximately proportional relationship exists between a muscle's maximum exertional capability and its physiological cross section, Crowninshield and Brand (22) proposed that maximum endurance can be expressed as a function of the muscle stress. The cost function for maximum endurance was written as the sum of muscle stresses raised to the third power.

Multiple Performance Criteria

Recently, Bean et al. (9) presented a novel scheme for the use of linear programming to calculate muscle contraction forces in models describing musculoskeletal system biomechanics. They suggested a two-objective problem with two sequential linear programs as follows. First, as in An et al. (5), minimize the upper bound of muscle stress. Let the optimal muscle intensity value from this solution be I^*. Second, solve a linear program to minimize the sum of the muscle forces using I^* as the muscle intensity limit. Thus, the first linear program determines the lowest muscle intensity value that allows feasible solutions. The second linear program chooses among these solutions to minimize muscle force. Hence, this scheme addressed both the stated objectives.

Constraints

In order to model the musculoskeletal system adequately, equality and inequality constraints are needed. The equality constraints arise from the need to satisfy force and moment equilibrium. The inequality constraints arise from the fact that individual muscles only produce tensile forces, and these forces are further limited by the muscle physiology.

Dynamic Equilibrium Constraints

Determination of the dynamic equilibrium constraints of the musculoskeletal model requires calculation of the time-dependent external forces (intersegmental loading), which are then balanced by the time-dependent internal (muscle, ligament, and joint) forces. The force and couple are estimated from kinematic and kinetic information by first finding the position and orientation of the body segments (assumed again to be rigid) as a function of time. The linear and angular velocities and accelerations are calculated by successive differentiation. The kinematic data are then integrated with the forces and moments acting on the limb to derive the equations of motion, and these are then solved for the proximal intersegmental force, F_p, and moment, M_p. The intersegmental loading describes the external force system acting on the limb.

Under quasistatic conditions, where inertial forces and moments are negligible, the external force system is balanced by the internal force system acting on the limb. The muscle forces required to generate the joint torques are found from the orientations of the ligament during movement. The origins and insertions of the muscles are scaled to the limb dimensions of the individual whose motion patterns are under investigation. The external force system is balanced against the internal force system, resulting in the dynamic equilibrium constraints:

$$\sum_{i=1}^{m} \left| \vec{F}_i^M \right| \vec{\tau}_{ik} + \vec{F}_k^J + \vec{F}_k^L = \vec{F}^P; \; k = 1,3$$

$$\sum_{i=1}^{m} \left| F_i^M \right| (\vec{r}_i \times \vec{\tau}_i)_k + \vec{M}_k^J + \vec{M}_k^L = \vec{M}^P; \; k = 1,3$$

where
$\vec{F}^P, \vec{M}^P$ = intersegmental force and moment
$\vec{F}_i^M$ = muscle force of ith muscle
$\vec{F}_k^J, \vec{M}_k^J$ = joint contact force and moment
$\vec{F}_k^L, \vec{M}_k^L$ = ligament force and moment
$\vec{\tau}_{ik}$ = unit force vector of ith muscle
$\vec{r}_i$ = location of ith muscle insertion with respect to the joint center.

Muscle Force Constraints

Because muscles exert force only in tension and not in compression, a proper muscle force solution requires imposition of this muscle force constraint (45). This constraint requires that any individual muscle must have a force greater than or equal to zero and less than some upper limit (45–48). Thus:

$$0 \le F_i^M \le (F_i^a + F_i^p)(PCSA_i \cdot \sigma)_i = 1, m \; \ldots \ldots$$

The upper bound for the ith muscle, F_i^M, is determined by the muscle stress limit, σ, the physiological cross-sectional area ($PCSA_i$), the normalized muscle active force correction, F_i^a, for the length–tension and force–velocity relationships, and the normalized muscle passive force characteristics, F_i^p. This constraint is considered a means of incorporating physiological information into the musculoskeletal model.

Example 6. Consider a simple two-dimensional analysis of weight lifting at the wrist with the upper arm vertical and the elbow flexed to 90°. Based on the free-body analysis of the forearm isolated at the elbow joint, the moment equilibrium equation in flexion–extension motion is $M = \Sigma r_i F_i$, in which M represents the intersegmental moment caused by the externally applied load in the plane of flexion–extension about the elbow joint center. The moment arms of the ith muscle for the nine muscles considered are listed in Table 1. Obviously, the problem formulated is an indeterminate one in which only one equation is available for the nine unknown variables of the muscle forces, F_i.

The optimization method was used for resolving this indeterminate problem. The most commonly used objective or cost functions to be minimized in the optimization methods are (a) the summation of muscle force; (b) the summation of muscle stress; (c) the summation of the square of muscle force; and (d) the summation of the square of the muscle force, F_i, by the corresponding muscle physiological cross-sectional area ($PCSA_i$), as shown in Table 1. Among these four objective functions, the first two consist of the linear combination of the unknown variables, F_i; thus, the problem could be simply solved by using the linear programming method. On the other hand, the last two objective functions consist of the nonlinear combination of the unknown variables, and

TABLE 2. *Comparison of optimization method for muscle and joint force determination (in the unit of applied force at the distal ulna)*

Muscle	Min F_i	Min S_i	Min F_i^2	Min S_i^2	Min σ: $S_i \leq \sigma$
BIC			1.4	2.5	1.8
BRA		9.5	1.0	4.6	2.9
BRD	4.3		2.3	0.4	0.6
FCR			1.5	0.1	0.8
ECRL			0.9	0.4	0.9
ECRB			0.8	0.2	0.7
ECU			0.4	0.1	0.6
TRI					
Joint	4.0	8.6	6.8	6.9	6.5

Abbreviations: min, minimizing criterion; F_i, muscle force; S_i, muscle stress; σ, upper bound of muscle stress.

more complicated nonlinear optimization methods have to be adopted.

As shown in Table 2, by using the summation of muscle force and summation of muscle stress as the minimizing criteria, only one muscle is predicted to carry forces in each of the solutions. This is characteristic of the use of linear programming with no inequality constraints; i.e., the number of nonzero variables equals the number of equality constraint equations. However, if additional inequality constraints are considered, this particular limitation can be eliminated.

To minimize the summation of muscle forces, the muscle that has the largest moment arm, namely the brachioradialis muscle, was selected in the solution. On the other hand, in order to minimize the summation of muscle stress, the muscle that has the largest product of moment arm and *PCSA*, namely the brachialis muscle, was selected in the solution. Again, when nonlinear combinations of the unknown variables are used as minimizing criteria, more than one muscle can be calculated to carry force in the solution. As shown in Table 2, the number of muscles that carry nonzero force is predicted when nonlinear optimization is used. The results of muscle force, as well as the resultant joint reaction forces, compared favorably with those obtained by use of the summation of the square of muscle stress as the minimizing criterion.

TABLE 1. *Physiological cross-sectional area (PCSA) and the associated flexion–extension moment arms (r) of the elbow muscles at 90° of flexion*

Muscle	PCSA (cm²)	r (cm)
Biceps (BIC)	4.6	4.6
Brachialis (BRA)	7.0	3.4
Brachioradialis (BRD)	1.5	7.5
Triceps (TRI)	18.8	−2.0
Flexor carpi radialis (FCR)	2.0	0.5
Extensor carpi ulnaris (ECU)	3.4	1.3
Extensor carpi radialis longus (ECRL)	2.4	2.9
Extensor carpi radialis brevis (ECRB)	1.5	−0.1

MECHANICAL PARAMETERS OF THE MUSCLE TENDON STRUCTURE

In the above force equilibrium equations, the coefficients of the muscle force represent the components of the unit vector of the muscles in the respective coordinate axes. In the moment equilibrium equations, the coefficients of the muscle forces represent the three components of the moment arm of the muscle force vector about the joint center with respect to the three axes. To establish a realistic model, these parameters must be determined from anatomic specimens. The experimental techniques to determine orientations and moment arms of muscle line of action can be divided into three broad categories (6): (a) geometric measurement, (b) tendon and joint displacement, and (c) direct load measurements.

In the geometric measurement method, one locates the paths of the tendon and muscle at the joint in terms of the joint coordinate system and then calculates the orientations and moment arms of the lines of action of the muscles or tendon (3,14). This can be done by direct digitization, biplanar radiography, and serial cross-sectioning. From the data of geometric measurement, the orientation of the muscle line of action can then be calculated from the positional vectors of the origin and insertion across the joint, $\vec{r}_o$ and $\vec{r}_i$, respectively:

$$e_i = \frac{\vec{r}_i - \vec{r}_o}{|\vec{r}_i - \vec{r}_o|}$$

The associated moment arms can be calculated as:

$$R = \vec{r}_i \times \vec{e}_i$$

The tendon and joint displacement method is mainly for determining moment arms using the relationship between the tendon excursion and the angular joint displacement:

$$\partial E / \partial \Theta = R$$

where E is the tendon excursion caused by rotation of the joint, Θ is the amount of joint rotation, and R is the moment arm of the tendon. To implement this approach, an electrogoniometer is used to monitor the angular displacement and an electropotentiometer to measure the tendon excursion simultaneously during joint rotation. From the curve of the tendon and joint displacement obtained, the slopes at various joint angles throughout the range of joint motion can be derived, and these represent the moment arms about the center of rotation of that particular muscle in the plane of motion.

The rationale for direct load measurement is very simple. Muscles create forces that are transmitted through the joint to the distal segment. If the forces and moments created on the distal segment can be monitored when these muscles are active, then the coefficients in the force and moment equilibrium equations can be obtained.

Each of the experimental techniques has its own merit as well as disadvantage. Geometric measurement provides not only the moment arm but also the orientation of the line of muscle action. This method is best suited for the situation in which a tendon crosses a joint with well-defined pulley constraints and a known joint center of rotation. Otherwise, it is difficult to select the optimal location along the tendon path to represent the line of action. The tendon–joint displacement method is probably the least involved in terms of experimental procedures. Furthermore, the experiment requires rotation of the joint throughout its whole range of motion to obtain data at multiple joint configurations. However, this method provides data on the moment arms only in the plane of rotation. The major advantage of this method is that the moment arm can be accurately measured without *a priori* knowledge of the axis or center of rotation. Direct load measurement, theoretically, should provide the most reliable information on these mechanical parameters. However, experimentally, this method is more demanding. It requires not only a sensitive load transducer but also rigid fixation of the skeletal system during the experiment.

PHYSIOLOGICAL MUSCLE PARAMETERS

The ability of the body to generate externally effective forces depends on the interrelationship of the geometric arrangement of the bony levers and the dynamics of muscular contraction. As actuators of the musculoskeletal system, muscles are critical elements, and their physiological properties must be included.

Physiological Cross-Sectional Area

The moment arm of a muscle merely indicates the efficiency of the muscle for rotation of the bony segment about that particular joint axis. The force that can actively be generated by each muscle is proportional to the physiological cross-sectional area (2,15). The physiological cross-sectional area (PCSA) is obtained by dividing the muscle volume by its true fiber length. The rationale for this assumption is simply that the cross-sectional area of muscle is proportional to the number of its fibers, and the individual muscle fiber is the basic element that generates the active tension. The relationship between the force a muscle can generate and its cross-sectional area is expressed as a proportional constant related to the upper bound of the muscle stress. A wide range of values for this constant has been reported, perhaps as a result of wide differences in the cross-sectional area measurements reported.

Muscle Stress

The relationship between the force a muscle can generate and its cross-sectional area can be expressed as a constant, σ, the muscle stress limit. Many authors have expressed the stress developed by a muscle in terms of the ratio of maximum isometric force to physiological cross-sectional area. It is clear, however, that absolute muscle stress does not have much meaning unless the conditions under which it is measured are carefully specified. First, the force developed depends on muscle length. Second, the PCSA must account for obliquity of the muscle fibers. It is reasonable to assume the existence of such constraints because the tensile strength of muscle fibers is limited. This constraint expresses condi-

tions that prevent tendon rupture and avulsion of the tendon–bone junction. It is usually assumed that the maximum stress is the same for each muscle.

The tensile strength of human skeletal muscle has long been a subject of interest. In 1910, Fick (30) reported that human skeletal muscle exerts an absolute stress of 1 MPa (= 10^6 N/m^2 = 145 psi). Estimates of maximum muscle effort have ranged from 0.1 to 1.0 MPa (43). The wide range makes it imperative that any model developed to calculate joint and muscle forces have the flexibility to account for improved estimates of these fundamental physiological parameters. In addition, the available evidence indicates that there is no marked difference in the intrinsic strength of the contractile material of fast and slow muscle fibers (18,43).

Index of Architecture

Steno (72) described the geometry of muscles, using diagrams to give a clear picture of the way a series of muscle fibers join a tendon and the way in which the tendon becomes progressively thicker as it accepts more and more fibers. Brand et al. (13) and An et al. (2) confirmed these general principles. They found that the length of fibers is surprisingly constant throughout each individual muscle. The generally fusiform shape of many muscles gives a false impression of unequal fiber lengths. When a muscle is looked at *in situ*, a few fibers might appear to extend from one end of muscle to the other, and some appear to reach only part way along its length. However, when the muscle is displayed with the fibers aligned, most of the fibers are about equal in length and uniform in thickness. Further, they all reach from the bone or tendon of origin to the tendon of insertion.

A schematic representation (Fig. 15) shows that a muscle consists of a number of fibers arranged in parallel between two tendon plates. The fibers lie at an angle to the direction of induced motion. Two measurements can be taken at muscle optimum length. The length of a single fiber is defined as the mean

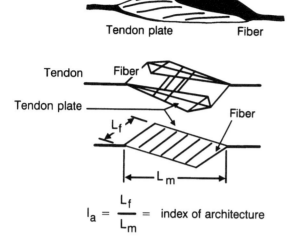

$$i_a = \frac{L_f}{L_m} = \text{index of architecture}$$

FIG. 15. Muscle architecture. Three-dimensional arrangement of muscle fibers and tendon plates *(top)*. Schematic representation of muscle architecture *(center)*. Important architectural parameters of muscle fiber length, L_f, and muscle belly length, L_m, define the index of architecture, i_a *(bottom)*.

fiber length. The distance from the proximal to distal tendon is defined as the muscle belly length. Woittiez et al. (75) defined the ratio of the mean fiber length to the muscle belly length at muscle optimum length as the index of architecture, i_a. Because muscles are obviously three-dimensional structures, the above classification represents a simplification. Despite this, the index of architecture is an important parameter to describe the relative fiber length of muscles.

Length–Tension Relationship

When skeletal muscle is stimulated, it is rapidly activated, changing from passive tissue into dynamic tissue capable of developing force. During stimulation, the length of the muscle may decrease, increase, or remain the same, depending on the external opposing forces acting on the muscle. The dynamic characteristics of stimulated skeletal muscle are best determined from isotonic and isometric experiments. The isometric force developed by a stimulated muscle restrained from movement is a function of muscle length. When skeletal muscle is tetanized and allowed to shorten against an isotonic load from a fixed initial length, its velocity of shortening is a function of the external isotonic force and the length of the muscle.

Blix (12), using isolated frog muscles, first demonstrated the relationship between the resting length of a muscle and the tension it could generate when contracting. These data form the Blix curve, which demonstrates the relationship of total muscle force, passive stretch force, and muscle contractile force to the length of the muscle.

A fundamental relationship exists between the tension that a muscle is capable of developing during contraction and the existing length of the muscle. Because of the elastic nature of the connective tissues, a muscle isolated from the body will assume a certain length to which it will return if passively stretched and released. This length, defined as the rest length, is the length at which the tension in the inactive whole muscle is zero (18). The optimum length is defined as the length at which maximum isometric tetanic tension may be developed and is between 100% and 120% of the rest length.

It has been demonstrated that in an isolated muscle fiber (32) or intact skeletal muscle (8), the active tension developed in a tetanic contraction is maximum at the optimum length and decreases at greater and lesser lengths. The active length–tension curve of whole muscle has a longer descending than ascending limb (55). Woittiez et al. (75) pointed out that asymmetry in the active force–length relationship is expected because of rotation of the muscle fibers and also for muscles with variation in the length of their fibers.

While developing the length–tension relationship for whole muscle, Woittiez et al. (75) attempted to account for differing muscle architecture. The muscles with considerable pennation had greater fiber angles, greater physiological cross section, and a narrower active and steep passive length–force relationship. Overall, the force output was a function of the inclination of the muscle fibers. The relative fiber length of muscles, an important aspect of their architecture, was characterized by the index of architecture, i_a. However, the mathematical function utilized by Woittiez was parabolic. The real shape of the length–tension relationship is more complex (32,63). Huijing and Woittiez (40) noted that deviation from a parabola may occur and that incorporation of more complex length–tension relationships into muscle models is indicated.

From the data in the literature, a mathematical model for the muscle active tension–length relationship has been developed (44). This model considered the muscle architecture and is defined as

$$F_\ell(\varepsilon, i_a) = \exp\left\{-\left[\frac{(\varepsilon + 1)^{0.9643(1-1/i_a)} - 1.0}{0.35327(1 - i_a)}\right]^2\right\}$$

$$for\ i_a < 1$$

$$F_\ell(\varepsilon, i_a) = \exp\{-[2.727177 \times \ln(\varepsilon + 1)]^2\}$$

$$for\ i_a = 1$$

where F_ℓ is the normalized active muscle tension, i_a, is the muscle architecture index, and ε is the muscle strain. This muscle model can be used to predict the normalized active muscle force, F, as a function of the muscle strain, ε, and the index of architecture, i_a (Fig. 16).

Force–Velocity Relationship

There have been many attempts to relate the velocity of shortening of an isotonically contracting skeletal muscle to the force it develops (isotonic force–velocity curve). As the speed of shortening increases, the muscle force de-

creases. Perhaps the best-known relationship between force and velocity of muscular contraction is Hill's equation (37). Hill's equation was originally used to describe frog muscles at 0°, but it applies to human muscles at body temperature as well (74). Hill's equation indicates a hyperbolic relationship between muscle tensile force and velocity. The higher the load, the slower is the contraction velocity. The higher the velocity, the lower is the tension. This is in direct contrast to the viscoelastic behavior of a passive material, for which higher velocity of deformation calls for higher forces. Therefore, the active contraction of a muscle has no resemblance to the viscoelasticity of a passive material. The force–velocity relationship is determined by the rate of breaking and reforming the cross bridges, with higher rates producing less effective bonds (31).

If a load greater than the maximum isometric force is applied to a muscle, the muscle lengthens at a velocity related to the load, P. The surprise is that the steady speed of lengthening is much smaller than would be expected from an extrapolation of Hill's equation to the negative velocity region. In fact, Katz (42) found that $-dP/dv$, the negative slope of the force–velocity curve, is about six times greater for slow lengthening than for slow shortening.

Hatze (36) described a continuous force–velocity relationship:

$$F_v(\dot{\eta}) = 0.1433\{0.1074 + \exp[-1.409 \sinh(3.2\dot{\eta} + 1.6)]\}^{-1}$$

in which F_v = normalized active muscle tension from the force–velocity relationship, $\dot{\eta}$ = normalized contractile element velocity. This relationship is shown in Fig. 17. The muscle velocity, $\dot{\eta}>$, may be calculated based on the coordinates of muscle origin and insertion and the relationship of joint movements.

In addition, Woittiez et al. (75) studied muscles of differing architecture but equal optimum length. They found that normalizing the force–velocity relations of muscles with respect to maximal active force and maximal velocity of shortening deletes all effects of architecture. Therefore, the equation does not

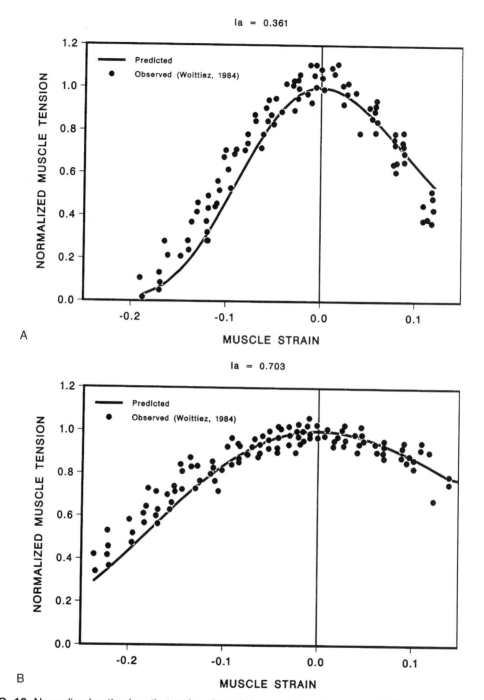

FIG. 16. Normalized active length–tension data of the medial gastrocnemius **(A)** and semimembra-
nosus **(B)** based on the data of Woittiez (75), compared to the length–tension relationship predicted
by the muscle model given in the text.

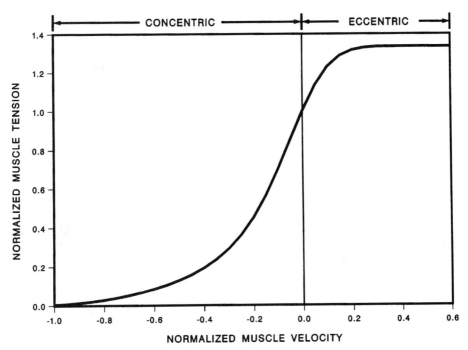

FIG. 17. Normalized muscle force–velocity relationship for concentric and eccentric contractions. (From Hatze, ref. 36, with permission.)

need to be modified for differing muscle architecture.

EXPERIMENTAL VALIDATION

There have been many attempts to verify the theoretical calculations of muscle and joint forces. These methods include indirect determinations of muscle force based on electromyography and direct tendon force measurement using tendon force transducers. For joint force measurements, instrumented implants as well as strain gauge devices have been used. Direct measurement of musculoskeletal force has been attempted for more than two decades. Strain gauge measurement, used primarily on bone, has been limited to animal studies. Tendon and ligament tension has been monitored with special force transducers for humans during intraoperative procedures. Instrumented prosthetic devices have also been used in human patients.

Tension in ligaments and tendons has been studied both *in vitro* and *in vivo*. A majority of the *in vivo* experiments were conducted in animals with the measurement data transmitted through the skin and transcutaneous tissue. Force transducers have also been designed for tendon tension measurement in humans during carpal tunnel surgery under local anesthesia. The transducer was clamped over the tendon, and the tendon tension was measured directly. The thumb and finger flexors were found to have forces ranging between 100 and 200 N, or one to three times the pinch force in simulations of the normal condition. Such measurements not only are useful to validate predicted theoretical results but also could provide useful assessment intraoperatively during tendon transfer procedures.

Instrumented prostheses have also been used to measure joint forces directly. Rydell (66) first instrumented a noncemented Moore hip endoprosthesis to record the *in vivo* joint contact force in hip-replacement patients. Maximum hip joint force was found to be 2.3 to 3.3 times the body weight during weight bearing. A similar study was performed using an instrumented hip nail with a telemetry system to transmit the bending load at the upper end of the femur, based on which the hip joint force was calculated. Even for non-weight-bearing activities during the early postoperative period, hip joint forces were found to be well above the body weight of the patient. Kilvington and Goodman (49) instrumented an "English" total hip femoral component with a telemetric data-transmitting system. Single-axis hip joint loading data at 4, 12, and 42 days postoperatively were collected for single-leg stance and walking activities. These *in vivo* measurements were substantially lower than those predicted using theoretical methods.

Recently, *in vivo* measurements of the hip joint load and acetabular pressure were performed with instrumented devices utilizing the most advanced technology for data acquisition and transmission. Hip joint force varied from 0.86 to 2.19 times the body weight for activities of rising from a seated position to standing, unsupported single-leg stance, and crutch walking. Acetabular pressures were recorded from 2.7 to 4.4 MPa for minor activities around bed. These data appear to be closer to those of theoretical predictions (10,11,25,38).

Measurement of intramuscular pressure is an alternative method to estimate muscle forces and validate joint force predictions. The method is based on the assumption that intramuscular pressure reflects the total muscle force, i.e., the sum of both the active contraction and passive stretch. Intramuscular pressure measurement during gait has been performed to correlate the timing and intensity of muscle contraction (48). Two types of systems are available for recording intramuscular pressure. One system is fluid-filled, and the other system uses a fiber-optic transducer. Fluid-filled systems are sensitive to hydrostatic artifacts and may be used only with limited types of movement that do not involve limb position changes relative to the horizontal plane. In contrast, a fiber-optic transducer system is not sensitive to hydrostatic artifact and has been shown to be ef-

fective for measuring intramuscular pressure during exercise.

ELECTROMYOGRAPHY

The application of electromyography (EMG) for verification of theoretical results has been widely adopted. The relationship between electric activity and muscle activity was first reported by Galvani in the late 18th century. He recognized that frog muscle could be stimulated to contract by applying an electric current. In the mid-1800s, the function of human muscles was systematically determined by individually stimulating them with galvanic currents. The converse of electric stimulation is that contracting muscles also evoke an electric signal. Based on work with the biceps muscle in synoplastic amputees, Inman et al. (41) concluded that the integrated EMG (IEMG) parallels the tension in human muscle contracting isometrically. These reports raised hopes that EMG signals, appropriately analyzed, could lead to direct estimates of muscle and joint forces. However, the relationships between EMG signal and muscle force in situations other than controlled isometric contractions have proven to be extremely complex. The EMG, nevertheless, can play a role in the understanding of muscle forces in two different ways: processed EMG signals can be used (a) to directly estimate muscle force or (b) to validate mathematical estimates of muscle activity.

Estimating Muscle Forces from EMG Signals

The use of EMG signals to directly estimate individual muscle activity during function is based on the assumption that the quantitative relationship between EMG signal (appropriately processed or analyzed) and muscle forces are known or can be determined. The relationship between muscle force and surface EMG during voluntary contractions in the absence of fatigue has been the subject of considerable controversy. Experimentally, a linear relationship was observed by Lippold (50) during voluntary isometric contractions of the triceps surface group. Many investigators have confirmed this observation for both isometric and constant-velocity isotonic contractions of various muscles. In addition, a nonlinear relationship has also been found. It is not clear whether the discrepancies between these results arise because of anatomic and physiological differences in the particular muscles employed or because of distortions introduced by the recording techniques and differences in various experimental procedures used. Many factors can affect the relationship between muscle tension and the EMG signal. Discrepancies may result from difference in technique and signal processing or differences in fiber composition and recruitment patterns of the muscle. In addition, the type of muscle contraction, either isometric or isotonic, and the condition of fatigue may also affect the relationship.

When the EMG is used experimentally for indirect force estimation, two significant biomechanical considerations are required for the derivation of force–EMG relationships (4). First, a mathematical model that provides the decomposition of the measured external force on the limb into individual components of force is required. The development of this model can be achieved by considering the force and moment equilibrium at the joint. Second, and most important, all of the muscles that cross the joint must be included in the analytic model because these muscles may create moments during joint movement. Otherwise, the regression analysis to derive the relationship between EMG and muscle tension may result in erroneous conclusions. Conceptually, this approach of using EMG to determine muscle force is appealing. However, at the present time, it is of limited utility because of the inherently complex (and as yet unknown) relationships between EMG signal and muscle force during complex activities.

The EMG Signal as a Validation

The second use of EMG is as a validation tool. Muscle activity (force) is estimated mathematically and then simply compared to the presence or absence of EMG signal at a particular time in an activity under study. The mathematical solution may be considered to be temporally validated (but not quantitatively validated) if there is qualitative agreement. Good agreement also tends to suggest that the physiological rationale on which the mathematical solution is based is reasonable. This method of temporal validation has been used by several researchers (21,60,67,69) with more or less reasonable agreement of mathematical predictions and EMG signals. Such validation is subject to limitations. First, a threshold of activity must be established to avoid the problem of minor signals that reflect physiologically insignificant contractions. Any threshold level is somewhat arbitrary and may inappropriately include certain muscle activity in the solution or exclude muscle activity from it. Second, the solution may be mathematically feasible and follow the EMG constraint but still be physiologically unreasonable. Third, the kinematic and kinetic data that are the basis for the muscle force predictions and the EMG signal should be obtained simultaneously because EMG signals can vary considerably from trial to trial, even for a given activity in a given person.

JOINT FORCES DURING DAILY ACTIVITIES

The musculoskeletal system provides structural support for the human body. With the aid of muscular actions, the human body can perform complicated limb movements through the numerous articulating joints. In performing such movements, the joints can be subjected to very large forces. In past years, both of the analytic and experimental methods discussed in this chapter have been used by numerous investigators to calculate and to measure the loads encountered by the joints in various activities of daily living and professional tasks. A sample of the available literature concerning forces transmitted through the joints in the body is presented in Tables 3 and 4. The magnitude of these forces depends on the joint and the type of loading and activity being performed. Within each table, the activity that produces that level of force is described.

Joint forces of the upper extremities are not trivial (Table 3). During powerful pinch and grasp functions, 20 to 30 kg of compressive forces are expected in the finger and thumb joints. The forces through the elbow and shoulder joints could be as high as a few times body weight. The hip joint forces have been calculated and measured with instrumented devices (Table 4). During normal gait, these forces can reach a peak of two to three times body weight.

SUMMARY

Estimation of the forces on muscle, tendon, ligament, cartilage, and bone are necessary for understanding the etiology of musculoskeletal disorders and for developing improved joint replacements. Numerous analytic and experimental methods are available to predict these muscle and joint forces. The analytic approach is formulated as an inverse dynamics problem in which the kinematic parameters are measured in order to calculate the intersegmental joint forces and moments. Distribution of the intersegmental forces and moments within the anatomic structures, including muscle and ligaments, is an indeterminate problem. Both optimization methods and the reduction method have been utilized to resolve this problem. Experimentally, instrumented implants and transducers have also been used to measure joint and tendon forces directly. Electromyographic and intramuscular pressure measurements are available for predicting the muscle forces indirectly.

TABLE 3. *Joint forces of upper extremities*

Source	Joint	Function	Force (N) Axial	Force (N) Shear
An et al. (5)	Finger			
	DIP	Pinch	70–280	5–30
		Grasp	120–325	20–65
	PIP	Pinch	120–475	25–65
		Grasp	30–190	5–40
	MCP	Pinch	95–380	45–200
		Grasp	80–260	60–220
Cooney and Chao (19)	Thumb			
	IP	Pinch	70–280	4–20
		Grasp	130–240	35–45
	MCP	Pinch	120–475	30–145
		Grasp	470–700	19–61
	CMC	Pinch	240–950	30–145
		Grasp	850–1640	15–200
Mayo (unpublished data)	Wrist			
	Radial/carpal	Grasp		504–1386
		Push-up		830–1450
	Ulnar/carpal	Grasp		140–385
Amis et al. (1)	Elbow			
	Ulnar/humeral	Lift		750–3000
		Push		1500–2500
	Radial/humeral	Lift		1500–3500
		Push		900–1250
Poppen and Walker (62)	Shoulder			
	Glenohumeral	Lift arm strenuously	630	300
		Abduction	2800	2500

Abbreviations: CMC, carpometacarpal; DIP, distal interphalangeal; IP, interphalangeal; MCP, metacarpophalangeal; PIP, proximal interphalangeal.

TABLE 4. *Hip joint force*

Source	Activity	Force (× BW)[a]
McLeish and Charnley (52)	One-legged stance	1.8–2.7
Rohrle et al. (65)	Gait, 0.8 m/sec	4.1
	Gait, 1.2 m/sec	5.5
	Gait, 1.6 m/sec	6.9
Crowninshield et al. (20)	Gait	4.3
Pierrynowski (61)	Gait	4.7
Brand et al. (15)	Gait, male	5.2
	Gait, female	5.0
Seireg and Arvikar (69)	Gait	5.4
Hardt (34)	Gait	5.7
Paul (58)	Gait	5.8
Davy et al. (25)	Gait, single-limb stance	2.6–2.8
	Gait, double-limb stance	1.0
	Stair climbing	2.6
Bergmann et al. (11)	Slow walking	2.6–3.0
	Abduction/ adduction in bed	0.3–0.5
	Lifting leg in bed	1.5

[a]BW, body weight.

In general, the muscle and joint forces in the human musculoskeletal system are much larger than the externally applied loads. This is mainly because the effective moment arms of the muscles around joints are relatively smaller than those of the applied external loads. In reviewing and interpreting the results in the literature, attention must be paid to the assumptions used in the analytic models and limitations involved in the experimental measurements.

REFERENCES

1. Amis, A. A., Dowson, D., and Wright, V. (1980): Elbow joint force predictions for some strenuous isometric actions. *J. Biomech.,* 13:765–775.
2. An, K. N., Hui, F. C., Morrey, B. F., Linscheid, R. L. and Chao, E. Y. (1981): Muscles across the elbow joint: a biomechanical analysis. *J. Biomech.,* 14(10):659–669.
3. An, K. N., Chao, E. Y., Cooney, W. P. III, and Linscheid, R. L. (1979): Normative model of human hand for biomechanical analysis. *J. Biomech.,* 12:775–788.
4. An, K. N., Cooney, W. P., Chao, E. Y., Askew, L. J., and Daube, J. R. (1983): Determination of forces in extensor pollicis longus and flexor pollicis longus of the thumb. *J. Appl. Physiol. Respir. Environ. Exercise Physiol.,* 54:714–719.
5. An, K. N., Kwak, B. M., Chao, E. Y., and Morrey, B. F. (1984): Determination of muscle and joint forces: A new technique to solve the indeterminate problem. *Trans. ASME,* 106:364–367.
6. An, K. N., Takahashi, K., Harrigan, T. P., and Chao, E. Y. (1984): Determination of muscle orientation and moment arms. *Trans. ASME,* 106:280–282.
7. An, K. N., Kaufman, E. Y., and Chao, E. Y. (1989): Physiological considerations of muscle force through the elbow joint. *J. Biomech.,* 22:1249–1256.
8. Banus, M. G., and Zetlin, A. M. (1938): The relation of isometric tension to length in skeletal muscle. *J. Cell. Comp. Physiol.,* 12:403–420.
9. Bean, J. C., Chaffin, D. B., and Schultz, A. B. (1988): Biomechanical model calculations of muscle contraction forces: a double linear programming method. *J. Biomech.,* 21(1):59–66.
10. Bergmann, G., Graichen, F., and Rohlmann, A. (1993): Hip joint loading during walking and running, measured in two patients. *J. Biomech.,* 26(8):969–990.
11. Bergmann, G., Rohlmann, A., and Graichen, F. (1990): Hip joint force during physical therapy after joint replacement. *Trans. Orthop. Res. Soc., New Orleans,* 15:2.
12. Blix, M. (1894): Die lange and die spannung des muskels. *Skand. Arch. F. Phys.,* 5:149–206.
13. Brand, P. W., Beach, R. B., and Thompson, D. E. (1981): Relative tension and potential excursion of muscles in the forearm and hand. *J. Hand Surg.,* 6(3):209–219.
14. Brand, R. A., Crowninshield, R. D., Wittstock, C. E., Pedersen, D. R., and Clark, C. R. (1982): A model of lower extremity muscular anatomy. *J. Biomech. Eng.,* 104:304–310.
15. Brand, R. A., Pedersen, D. R., and Friederich, J. A. (1986): The sensitivity of muscle force predictions to changes in physiological cross-sectional area. *J. Biomech.,* 19(8):589–596.
16. Braune, W., and Fischer, O. (1872): Concerning the center of gravity of the human body with reference to the equipment of the German infantryman. *Abh. Koenigl. Saechs. Ges. Wissenschaft,* 15.
17. Chao, E. Y., and Rim, K. (1973): Application of optimization principles in determining the applied moments in human leg joints during gait. *J. Biomech.,* 6:497–510.
18. Close, R. I. (1972): Dynamic properties of mammalian skeletal muscles. *Physiol. Rev.,* 52(1):129–197.
19. Cooney, W. P., and Chao, E. Y. (1977): Biomechanical analysis of static forces in the thumb during hand function. *J. Bone Joint Surg.,* 59A:27–36.
20. Crowninshield, R. D., Johnston, R. C., Andrews, J. G., and Brand, R. A. (1978): A biomechanical investigation of the human hip. *J. Biomech.,* 11:75–85.
21. Crowninshield, R. D., (1978): Use of optimization techniques to predict muscle forces. *J. Biomech. Eng.,* 100:88–92.
22. Crowninshield, R. D., and Brand, R. A. (1981): A physiologically based criterion of muscle force prediction in locomotion. *J. Biomech.,* 14:793–801.
23. Dahlkvist, N. J., Mayo, P., and Seedham, B. B. (1982): Forces during squatting and rising from a deep squat. *Eng. Med.,* 11(2):69–76.
24. Dantzig, G. B. (1963): *Linear Programming and Extensions.* Princeton University Press, Princeton.
25. Davy, D. T., Kotzar, G. M., Brown, R. W., Heiple, K. G., Goldberg, V. M., Heiple, K. G., Jr., Berilla, J., and Burstein, A. H. (1988): Telemetric force measurements

across the hip after total arthroplasty. *J. Bone Joint Surg.,* 70A:45–50.

26. Dul, J., Johnson, G. E., Shiava, R., and Townsend, M. A. (1984): Muscular synergism-II. A minimum-fatigue criterion for load sharing between synergistic muscles. *J. Biomech.,* 17(9):675–684.

27. Ellis, M. I., Seedham, B. B., and Wright, V. (1979): Forces in the knee joint whilst rising from normal and motorized chairs. *Eng. Med.,* 8:33–40.

28. Ellis, M. I., Seedham, B. B., and Wright, V. (1984): Forces in the knee whilst rising from a seated position. *J. Biomed. Eng.,* 6:113–120.

29. Ericson, M. O., and Nisell, R. (1986): Tibiofemoral joint forces during ergometer cycling. *Am. J. Sports Med.,* 14(4):285–290.

30. Fick, R. (1910): *Handbuch der Anatomie des Menschen,* Vol. 2. Veriag von Gustav Fischer, Jena.

31. Freivalds, A. (1985): *Incorporation of Active Elements into the Articulated Total Body Model.* Publication No. AAMRL-TR-85-061, U.S. Air Force/AFSC, Aeronautical Systems Division, Wright-Patterson AFB, OH.

32. Gordon, A. M., Huxley, A. F., and Julian, F. J. (1966): The variation in isometric tension with sarcomere length in vertebrate muscle fibres. *J. Physiol. (Lond.),* 184:170–192.

33. Gracovetsky, S., Farfan, H. F., and Lamy, C. (1977): A mathematical model of the lumbar spine using an optimization system to control muscles and ligaments. *Orthop. Clin. North Am.,* 8:135–153.

34. Hardt, D. E. (1978): Determining muscle forces in the leg during normal human gait—an application and evaluation of optimization methods. *J. Biomech. Eng.,* 100:72–78.

35. Harrington, I. J. (1976): A bioengineering analysis of force actions at the knee in normal and pathological gait. *Biomed. Eng.,* 11:167–172.

36. Hatze, H. (1981): *Myocybernetic Control Models of Skeletal Muscle.* University of South Africa, Pretoria.

37. Hill, A. V. (1938): The heat of shortening and the dynamic constants of muscle. *Proc. R. Soc. Lond.,* 126B:136–195.

38. Hodge, W. A., Fijan, R. S., and Carlson, K. L. (1986): Human *in-vivo* acetabular pressure measurement: a one-year update. *Trans. Orthop. Res. Soc. New Orleans,* 11:436.

39. Huberti, H. H., and Hayes, W. C. (1984): Patellofemoral contact pressure. *J. Bone Joint Surg. [Am.],* 66A(5):715–724.

40. Huijing, P. A., and Woittiez, R. D. (1985): Notes on planimetric and three-dimensional muscle models. *Neth. J. Zool.,* 35(3):521–525.

41. Inman, V. T., Ralston, H. J., de Saunder, J. B., Feinstein, B., and Wright, E. W. (1952): Relation of human electromyogram to muscle tension. *EEG Clin. Neurophysiol.,* 4:187–194.

42. Katz, B. (1939): The relation between force and speed in muscular contraction. *J. Physiol.,* 96:45–64.

43. Kaufman, K. R. (1988): *A Mathematical Model of Muscle and Joint Forces in the Knee During Isokinetic Exercise.* Ph.D. Dissertation, North Dakota State University, Fargo, ND.

44. Kaufman, K. R., An, K. N., and Chao, E. Y. S. (1989): Incorporation of muscle architecture into the muscle length–tension relationship. *J. Biomech.,* 22:943–948.

45. Kaufman, K. R., An, K. N., Litchy, W. J., and Chao, E.

Y. S. (1991): Physiological prediction on muscle force I: Theoretical formulation. *Neuroscience,* 40(3):781–792.

46. Kaufman, K. R., An, K. N., Litchy, W. J., and Chao, E. Y. S. (1991): Physiological prediction on muscle force II: Application to isokinetic exercise. *Neuroscience,* 40(3):793–804.

47. Kaufman, K. R., An, K. N., Litchy, W. J., Morrey, B. F., and Chao, E. Y. S. (1991): Dynamic joint forces during knee isokinetic exercise. *Am. J. Sports Med.,* 19(3):305–316.

48. Kaufman, K. R., and Sutherland, D. H. (1995): Dynamic intramuscular pressure measurement during gait. *Oper. Tech. Sports Med.* 3(4):250–255.

49. Kilvington, M., and Goodman, R. M. F. (1981): *In vivo* hip joint forces recorded on a strain-gauged "English" prosthesis using an implanted transmitter. *Eng. Med.,* 10:175–187.

50. Lippold, O. C. J. (1952): The relation between integrated action potentials in a human muscle and its isometric tension. *J. Physiol. (Lond.),* 117:492–499.

51. MacConaill, M. A. (1967): The ergonomic aspects of articular mechanics. In: *Studies on the Anatomy and Function of Bones and Joints,* edited by F. G. Evans, pp. 69–80. Springer, Berlin.

52. McLeish, R. D., and Charnley, J. (1970): Abduction force in the one-legged stance. *J. Biomech.,* 3:191–209.

53. Morrison, J. B. (1969): Function of the knee joint in various activities. *Biomed. Eng.,* 4:573–580.

54. Morrison, J. B. (1970): The mechanics of the knee joint in relation to normal walking. *J. Biomech.,* 3:51–61.

55. Muhl, Z. F. (1982): Active length–tension relation and the effect of muscle pinnation on fiber lengthening. *J. Morphol.,* 173:285–292.

56. Nisell, R., Ericson, M. O., Nemeth, G., et al. (1989): Tibiofemoral joints forces during isokinetic knee extension. *Am. J. Sports Med.,* 17:49–54.

57. Patriarco, A. G., Mann, R. W., Simon, S. R., and Mansour, J. M. (1981): An evaluation of the approaches of optimization models in the prediction of muscle forces during human gait. *J. Biomech.,* 14(8):513–525.

58. Paul, J. P. (1965): Bio-engineering studies of the forces transmitted by joints. In: *Engineering Analysis in Biomechanics and Related Topics (II),* edited by R. M. Kenedi. Pergamon Press, Oxford, p. 369.

59. Paul, J. P. (1967): Forces transmitted by joints in the human body. *Proc. Inst. Mech. Engrs.,* 181(3J):8–15.

60. Pedotti, A., Krishnan, V. V., and Stark, L. (1978): Optimization of muscle-force sequencing in human locomotion. *Math. Biosci.,* 38:57–76.

61. Pierrynowski, M. R. (1982): *A Physiological Model for the Solution of Individual Muscle Forces During Normal Human Walking.* Ph.D. Dissertation, Simon Fraser University, Vancouver, British Columbia.

62. Poppen, N. K., and Walker, P. S. (1978): Forces at the glenohumeral joint in abduction. *Clin. Orthop. Rel. Res.,* 135:165–170.

63. Ramsey, R. W., and Street, S. F. (1940): The isometric length–tension diagram of isolated skeletal muscle fibers of the dog. *J. Cell Comp. Physiol.,* 15:11–34.

64. Reilly, D. T., and Martens, M. (1972): Experimental analysis of the quadriceps muscle force and patellofemoral joint reaction force for various activities. *Acta Orthop. Scand.,* 43:126–137.

65. Rohrle, H., Scholten, R., Sigolotto, C., and Sollbach, W.

(1984): Joint forces in the human pelvis–leg skeleton during walking. *J. Biomech.,* 17(6):409–424.

66. Rydell, N. W. (1966): Forces acting on the femoral head prosthesis. *Acta. Orthop. Scand. [Suppl.],* 88.

67. Schultz, A., Haderspeck, K., Warwick, D., and Portillo, D. (1983): Use of lumbar trunk muscles in isometric performance of mechanically complex standing tasks. *J. Orthop. Res.,* 1(1):77–91.

68. Seireg, A., and Arvikar, R. J. (1973): A mathematical model for evaluation of forces in lower extremities of the musculoskeletal system. *J. Biomech.,* 6:313–326.

69. Seireg, A., and Arvikar, R. J. (1975): The prediction of muscular load bearing and joint forces in the lower extremities during walking. *J. Biomech.,* 8:89–102.

70. Smidt, G. L. (1973): Biomechanical analysis of knee flexion and extension. *J. Biomech.,* 6:79–92.

71. Smith, A. J. (1972): *A Study of Forces on the Body in Athletic Events with Particular Reference to Jumping.* Ph.D. Thesis, Leeds, England.

72. Steno, N. (1667): Elementorum myologiae specimen s. musculi descriptio geometrica. In: *Opera Philosophico,* Vol. 2, edited by V. Maar, p. 108. Copenhagen, 1910. Quoted in Bastholm, E. (1950): *The History of Muscle Physiology.* Copenhagen: Ejnar Munksgaard.

73. Weber, W., and Weber, E. (1836): *Mechanik der Menschlichen Gehwerkzeuge.* W. Fisher-Verlag, Gottingen.

74. Wilkie, D. R. (1950): The relation between force and velocity in human muscle. *J. Physiol. (Lond.),* 110:249–280.

75. Woittiez, R. D., Huijing, P. A., Boom, H. B. K., and Rozendal, R. H. (1984): A three-dimensional muscle model: a quantified relation between form and function of skeletal muscles. *J. Morphol.,* 182:95–113.

76. Zernicke, R. F., Garhammer, J., and Jobe, F. W. (1977): Human patellar-tendon rupture. A kinetic analysis. *J. Bone Joint Surg. [Am.],* 59A:179–183.

Basic Orthopaedic Biomechanics, 2nd ed.,
edited by Van C. Mow and Wilson C. Hayes.
Lippincott–Raven Publishers, Philadelphia © 1997.

2

Musculoskeletal Dynamics, Locomotion, and Clinical Applications

Thomas P. Andriacchi, Raghu N. Natarajan, and Debra E. Hurwitz

Department of Orthopedic Surgery, Rush-Presbyterian-St. Luke's Medical Center, Chicago, Illinois 60612

KINEMATICS OF MOTION: BASIC DEFINITIONS

Kinematics is the study of motion (10). Kinematics is used to describe displacement, velocity, and acceleration with respect to time without reference to the cause of the motion. In the analysis of human locomotion, kinematic techniques have been used to study body movements. The segments of the body are usually considered as rigid links. Although there are many types of kinematic measurements that can be used to quantify locomotion, relative segmental angular motions have been the most frequently used. For example, the temporal patterns of the angle between the thigh and the shank (knee flexion motion) during the gait cycle provide a good indicator of human locomotion function. Kinematic measurements of the angles between adjacent limb segments, the relative segmental angles, have been applied extensively (18,19,34,40) in studies of walking and other activities of daily living. However, in many instances, the anatomic definitions of angular joint movements are potentially ambiguous and not kinematically rigorous. This section provides some basic kinematic definitions and indicates general applications to locomotion studies.

Types of Motion of a Rigid Link

General three-dimensional motion of a rigid body is defined by six independent quantities: three translational motions and three rotational motions. Subclassification of motion can be defined as the following:

1. Translational motion is motion of a body in which a straight line drawn between two

points on the body maintains the same direction during the motion. During translational motion, all the particles forming the rigid link move along parallel lines. If these paths are straight lines, the motion of the rigid link is said to be a rectilinear motion; if the paths are curved lines, the motion is a curvilinear translation.

2. Rotation about a fixed axis is motion of a rigid link in which all points on the link move in parallel planes along circles centered on the same fixed axis.

3. General plane motion of a rigid link is motion in which all points on the link move in parallel planes. Plane motion that is neither a rotation nor a translation is referred to as a general plane motion.

4. Motion about a fixed point is a three-dimensional motion of a rigid link attached to a fixed point.

5. General motion is rigid body motion that does not fall in any of the above categories. This motion requires six independent measures.

Because of the wide range of possible types of motion, care must be taken in describing or interpreting the biomechanics of human movement. The type (linear or angular) of movement, the reference frame, as well as the dimensions of the movement (degrees of freedom) must be defined. The general movement of an object is defined by a vector quantity that is a combination of both linear and angular displacement. A linear displacement is any change in motion that occurs along a straight line. An angular displacement is any change in motion of the body that results in rotation of the body. The movement of a joint can be described in terms of relative linear and angular displacements of one bone segment with respect to the adjacent segment. For example, the total movement of the femur with respect to the tibia can be described as a combination of three linear displacements and three rotations.

Velocity is the time rate of change of displacement. Linear velocity is expressed in units of length per time (m/sec). Angular velocity is expressed in units of angular measure per time (e.g., radians/sec). Because velocities are vector quantities, both magnitude and direction must be specified.

Acceleration is the time rate of the change of velocity. Linear acceleration is expressed in units of length per time squared (e.g., m/sec^2). Angular acceleration is the time rate of change in angular velocity (e.g., radians/sec^2). Accelerations are also vector quantities, and again, both magnitude and direction must be specified.

In describing the motion of a rigid body, one must specify a frame of reference because the motion will be different when viewed from other frames of reference. For example, consider the planar (sagittal plane) measurement of knee flexion angle (Fig. 1). Typically, during functional measurement, both the tibia and the femur are moving with respect to a coordinate system fixed in the laboratory. Thus, depending on the reference frame used, the angle of the tibia and the femur could be defined in a number of ways. As shown in Fig. 1, the angle α defines the position of the tibia with respect to a frame of reference fixed in the laboratory; similarly, angle β defines the angle of the femur with respect to the fixed reference frame, and the angle γ is the position of the femur measured with respect to a reference frame fixed in the tibia. It should be noted that although both the tibia and the femur are moving, the analysis of the relative movement of the femur with respect to the tibia essentially treats the tibia as a fixed reference frame and describes the movement of the femur with respect to that reference frame.

For example, goniometric measurements give relative segmental angles because one end of the goniometer is fixed in the distal segment with the other end attached to the proximal segment. Thus, the angular movement between the two segments is provided. Optical measurements usually provide segmental motion with respect to a fixed reference frame. The angle γ, the angular movement of femur with respect to tibia, can be calculated by merely taking the difference between the movements of the two segments

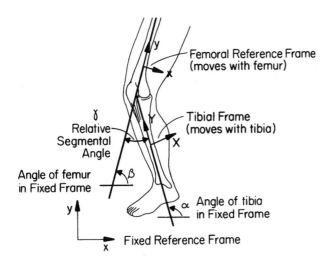

FIG. 1. Relative angular position with respect to a fixed reference frame.

with respect to the fixed reference frame. Therefore, in the example above, γ would equal $\alpha - \beta$. The above example provides a planar analysis of angular motion. Complete three-dimensional analysis is significantly more complicated and will be discussed subsequently.

Example: Relative Segmental Angles During Gait

The complexity of kinematic analysis increases substantially from a planar analysis to a complete three-dimensional analysis. Typically, limb segments are treated kinematically as rigid bodies for most biomechanical applications. The motion of a rigid body in three-dimensional space is described by six independent degrees of freedom, three translational and three rotational. The complexity of the analysis arises from the three-dimensional description of rigid body position. Among the technical difficulties is the fact that large rigid-body rotations cannot be treated as vectors. Large rigid-body rotations do not obey the mathematical principles of transformation, independence, and interchangeability of operations that vectors obey. Typically, to address the problem of angular displacements and position measurements in rigid bodies, a Euler angle

system is used (24). The sequence of the Euler angle definition is important in uniquely defining the position of a rigid body and must be taken into consideration. A detailed discussion of the problems involved in describing three-dimensional motion is beyond the scope of this text. The purpose here is to make the reader aware of the potential difficulties. The relevance to biomechanical application has been described and summarized in several articles (18,26).

Figure 2 illustrates a case in which three-dimensional axes have been defined in terms of anatomic definitions (18). A critical aspect of these definitions is the appropriate choice of fixed and floating axes. Again, for further detail on the theory and application of these methods, the reader is referred elsewhere (18, 24,26,31). The relative segmental angular measurements conventionally used to describe limb movement during gait are reported for the hip, knee, and ankle. These measurements are obtained using both electrogoniometric and optical methods (22,41). The temporal characteristics of these segmental angles are quite reproducible during normal gait. To illustrate, the common features of the sagittal plane motion of the hip, knee, and ankle during the stance and swing phases of gait can be divided into eight segments. During the stance phase, the events are described as initial contact, loading

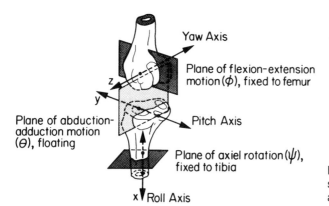

FIG. 2. Illustration of three-dimensional axes defined in terms of anatomic definitions (8).

response, midstance, terminal stance, and pre-swing. The swing phase is described in terms of initial swing, midswing, and terminal swing. At initial contact during the stance phase, the hip is flexed approximately 20°, the knee is near full extension, and the ankle is slightly plantarflexed (Fig. 3). As the limb moves into a loading response phase, the hip joint extends, the knee joint flexes, and the ankle dorsiflexes. At midstance, the hip joint continues to extend from its initially flexed position, the knee joint reaches a relative maximum, and the ankle re-

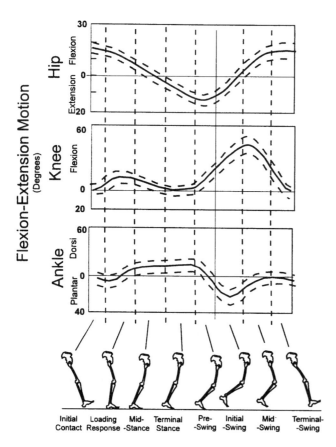

FIG. 3. The position of the hip, knee, and ankle during gait. The stance phase is divided into five segments, and the swing phase is divided into three segments. The curves represent the normal patterns of motion for the hip, knee, and ankle. The position of the limb below the curves illustrates the position of the pelvis, thigh, and shank segments as they would be observed during each of these phases of the gait cycle. The normal sequence of events is quite regular and reproducible, as indicated by the relatively narrow bandline segments around the solid bars, which represent the average of the normal motion patterns.

mains in a dorsiflexed position. As the limb goes into terminal stance, the hip reaches an extended position, the knee flexes in preparation for the swing phase, and the ankle plantarflexes. During the initial swing phase, the hip and knee flex while the ankle moves toward dorsiflexion from an initially plantarflexed position. In the final portion of the swing phase, the hip reaches maximum flexion, the knee extends in preparation for heel strike, and the ankle plantarflexes.

It is important to note that the narrow band around each of the motion curves (Fig. 3) at the hip, knee, and ankle suggest that the characteristics of these patterns do not vary substantially during normal gait (34). However, care must be taken in measuring certain peak amplitudes because it has been shown that these values are related to walking speed.

The sagittal plane angles described above can be reproducibly measured using reflective markers placed on the skin. However, other planar motions such as motion in coronal and transverse planes have been studied using target markers fixed to intracortical traction pins attached to the limb segments (33). High-speed cameras can be used to measure three-dimensional coordinates of the target markers. From these measurements it is possible to define motions of the lower limb segments in three dimensions. The average pattern of abduction–adduction of the tibiofemoral joint is (Fig. 4a) uniphasic (33). During the major portion of stance phase, the knee joint remains abducted by a small amount (1°). During the swing phase, the knee joint abducts to a mean peak value of 6° and returns to a value of 1° of abduction just before heel strike. The knee rotates to an average maximum less than 5° of internal or external rotation during the stance phase (Fig. 4b). During swing phase, the knee reaches a maximum of about 9° of external rotation.

The translational motion of the tibia with respect to the femur is important and has a close relationship with the sagittal plane motion of the knee joint (33). These linear mo-

tions are measured relative to their positions at heel strike. During the stance phase, an initial medial shift occurs, followed by a lateral shift (Fig. 4c). During the swing phase, the tibia continues the medial shift. The tibial shift in the medial–lateral direction occurring during the stance and swing phases produces tibial excursions of about 5.6 mm. When the knee joint flexes, the tibia slides medially, and when it extends, the tibia moves laterally, closely matching the flexion–extension of the joint. The linear posterior drawer motion amounts to 3.6 mm during stance phase (Fig. 4d), whereas during the swing phase, a much larger posterior drawer motion of 14.3 mm is observed. Once again, the pattern of drawer motion of the tibia exhibits a striking similarity with the flexion–extension behavior of the knee joint. The distraction–compression of the knee joint shows a pattern similar to both shift and drawer (Fig. 4e). The maximum distraction occurs twice, once during the stance phase and once again during the swing phase. Both of these maxima occur when the flexion of the knee joint attains a maximum value.

More complete analysis of total joint movement (six degrees of freedom) can be obtained when fixtures or markers are applied directly to the bone. This minimizes errors in displacement measurements related to deformation. Techniques such as this have been employed (32) using a six-degree-of-freedom linkage system. Recently, photometric techniques (51) have been applied to kinematic studies of cadaver knee joints (14) using metallic markers embedded in bone.

It is important to consider the overall application in evaluating the technical aspects of kinematic techniques. The biomechanical application should dictate the degree of kinematic complexity needed in the analysis. As previously noted, most analyses assume a limb segment to be a rigid body. Further, for *in vivo* evaluation such as gait analysis, goniometer or marker systems are usually placed externally on the skin rather than attached directly to the bone. Thus, precise measurement of complete six-degree-of-free-

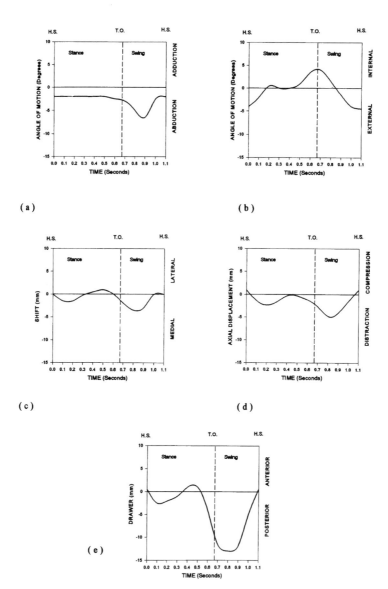

FIG. 4. Pattern of tibiofemoral joint angular and linear displacements during level walking (33). It is plotted starting from heel-strike and ends with heel-strike of the ipsilateral limb. The line represents the average of individual patterns. The tibiofemoral relative linear displacements were obtained based on the motions of the most proximal point of the medial intercondylar eminence on the tibia with respect to the motion of deepest point of the intercondylar fossa of the femur: **(a)** abduction–adduction; **(b)** internal–external rotation; **(c)** shift in medial–lateral direction; **(d)** draw in the anterior–posterior direction; **(e)** distraction–compression in the axial direction.

dom segment movement is often not possible or feasible during large-scale motions like those that occur during gait. However, there are many applications where approximate techniques for measuring relative segmental movements are appropriate and have been employed using both goniometers (18,19,34) and optical methods (40) for studies of both normal and clinical populations.

The study of joint kinematics provides one with the motion of the limb segments but not the forces and moments that are transmitted across joints. The study of kinetics attempts to provide such information.

KINETICS: EXTERNAL FORCES ON LIMB SEGMENTS, MASS, AND INERTIA

An understanding of the kinetics of human movement is fundamental to the understanding of the musculoskeletal system. The motion of the musculoskeletal system is the result of a balance between those forces and moments that act external to the body and the forces and moments that act internally.

Before one can begin to analyze the forces acting at different joints in the human body during human movement, some basic definitions and assumptions must be made. In most studies of locomotion, as noted before, the limb segments are assumed to be rigid. This simplifies the analysis because the structure is assumed not to deform under load. Forces acting on the rigid body may be classified as either external forces or internal forces. External forces represent the action of other bodies on the rigid body under consideration. In gait analysis, ground reaction forces, gravitational forces, and inertial forces are taken as external forces. Internal forces are responsible for holding together the component parts that make up the rigid body. For example, the forces that hold together the shank and thigh are called internal forces. Force will be expressed in units of Newtons (N). The moment of a force about an axis measures the tendency of the force to impart to the body a rotational motion about a fixed axis. A moment of a force will be expressed in units of Newton-meters (Nm).

Inertia is a body's resistance to acceleration. Inertial resistance to linear acceleration depends on mass, whereas resistance to angular acceleration depends on geometry and mass distribution (and is generally referred to as mass moment of inertia). The mass moment of inertia must be referenced to a coordinate system. A more detailed discussion of mass moment of inertia can be found in many basic texts on mechanics (10).

The analysis of forces and associated motion is a branch of mathematics called dynamics. Newton's second law of motion links the kinematics of a body to its kinetics. This law may be stated as follows: "If the resultant force acting on a body is not zero, the body will have an acceleration proportional to the magnitude of the resultant and in the direction of this resultant force."

Calculation of Intersegmental Forces and Moments

General Approach

Newton's second law makes it possible to solve for intersegmental forces and moments. The foot–ground reaction forces are usually measured using a force plate. The weight and inertial forces are often approximated by modeling the leg as a collection of rigid segments representing the thigh, shank, and foot. Limb motion is measured using various types of optoelectronic methods. To illustrate the computational procedure, assume each segment is symmetric about its principal axes and that the angular velocity and acceleration about the longitudinal axis of the segment are negligible.

The following is a description of how Newton's second law of motion is used in calculating external intersegmental forces and moments at different joints during human locomotion. The first step in this process involves the establishment of a model. The model we are describing here is a link model (Fig. 5a) in which inertial properties for each rigid segment are lumped at its mass center (a lumped mass approximation). The second step in the process involves the measurement of the external ground reaction forces, some method for approximating limb segment inertial properties, and a method of locating the three-dimensional position of the joint centers in space and time.

Once these data are obtained, the analysis begins with a free-body diagram for each of the segments (Fig. 5b). The free-body dia-

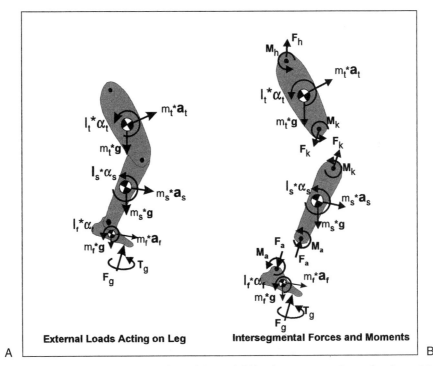

External Loads Acting on Leg

A

Intersegmental Forces and Moments

B

FIG. 5. (A) Link model. The model consists of three rigid body segments: foot, shank, and thigh. The known forces and moments are the ground reaction force and moment, inertial forces and moments, as well as gravitational forces on the three rigid bodies. **(B)** Free-body diagram. Free-body diagrams for the three rigid links are shown here. The calculations proceed from the distal to proximal end and start at the foot. With the help of rigid-body equilibrium equations, the force and moment at the ankle are calculated. The force and moment at the distal end of the shank are equal and opposite to the force and moment at the ankle. With the distal force and moment of the shank known, the proximal end force and moment are then calculated.

gram includes the intersegmental forces and moments at the joint centers and the inertial forces and moments and gravitational forces acting at the center of mass of the segment. The calculations start at the foot because the only unknown intersegmental force is at the ankle and then proceeds from distal to proximal. Segmental equilibrium equations are written at the mass center using Newton's second law of motion. Unknown intersegmental forces and moments at the proximal end of the segment are obtained from the solution of these equilibrium equations. Once the intersegmental forces and moments are calculated at the ankle, they are applied to the next segment as an equal and opposite force and moment at the distal end of the segment (shank). The process continues with solving for the

unknown intersegmental forces and moments at the proximal end of the segment.

Details of the Calculation

The free-body diagram for each of the rigid segments is shown in Fig. 5b. The governing equations for the ankle can be expressed as two vector equations representing six scalar equations. The first vector equation represents the equilibrium of the rigid body under external forces. The second vector equation represents the moment equilibrium equation. Bold letters indicate vectors quantities. Each of these vector equations has three components, one along each of the global axes: x, y, and z.

The two vector equations of equilibrium for the foot (subscript f) are given as

$$\sum \mathbf{F} = \mathbf{m}_f a_f \qquad (1)$$

(force equilibrium equations) and

$$\sum \mathbf{M} = \mathbf{I}_f \alpha_f \qquad (2)$$

(moment equilibrium equations, in which moments are taken about the center of mass of the rigid body), where m_f is the mass of the foot, $\mathbf{I}_f$ the moment of inertia, $\mathbf{a}_f$ the linear acceleration of the mass center, and α_f the angular acceleration.

The forces and moments at the distal end ($\mathbf{F}_g$ and $\mathbf{T}_g$) of the foot are the ground reaction forces and moment measured by the force plate. The intersegmental forces and moments at the ankle ($\mathbf{F}_a$ and $\mathbf{M}_a$) are unknowns. The mass center is located at a distance of $r_{cm,p}$ and $r_{cm,d}$, respectively, from the proximal and distal ends of the rigid body.

To solve for the intersegmental force ($\mathbf{F}_a$) at the ankle, apply the force equilibrium equation for a rigid body as follows:

$$\mathbf{F}_a + \mathbf{F}_g + m_f \mathbf{g} = m_f a_f \qquad (3)$$

where $\mathbf{g}$ is the acceleration by gravity. Thus, the intersegmental force at the ankle is given by

$$\mathbf{F}_a = m_f a_f - \mathbf{F}_g - m_f \mathbf{g} \qquad (4)$$

To solve for the intersegmental moment at the ankle, the moment equilibrium equation for the rigid body is written as

$$\mathbf{M}_a + \mathbf{T}_g + (\mathbf{r}_{cm,p} \times \mathbf{F}_a) + (\mathbf{r}_{cm,d} \times \mathbf{F}_g) = \mathbf{I}_f \alpha_f \quad (5)$$

Thus, the intersegmental moment at the ankle is given by

$$\mathbf{M}_a = -\mathbf{T}_g - (\mathbf{r}_{cm,p} \times \mathbf{F}_a) - (\mathbf{r}_{cm,d} \times \mathbf{F}_g) \\ + \mathbf{I}_f \alpha_f \quad (6)$$

The above method of calculating the intersegmental forces and moments at the ankle joint can be extended to calculate intersegmental forces and moments at the knee joint. The equations remain the same except the subscript a (ankle) in the equations is replaced by k (knee). Further, because we now know the intersegmental forces and moments at the ankle joint, subscripts g (ground) and a (ankle) are to be replaced by a (ankle) and k (knee), respectively.

The rigid body (currently the shank is assumed as the rigid body) on which the forces and moments at the distal end ($\mathbf{F}_a$ and $\mathbf{M}_a$) are known from the previous calculations (equations 4,6). The forces and moments at the proximal end ($\mathbf{F}_k$ and $\mathbf{M}_k$) are assumed to be unknown. The shank has a mass of m_s, the mass center is located at a distance of $r_{cm,p}$ and $r_{cm,d}$, respectively, from the proximal and distal ends of the rigid body. The shank is assumed to move with an acceleration of $\mathbf{a}_s$. The subscript s in the following equations (7–10) indicates that the segment under consideration is the shank.

The force equilibrium equation for the rigid body is

$$\mathbf{F}_k + \mathbf{F}_a + m_s \mathbf{g} = m_s \mathbf{a}_s \qquad (7)$$

Thus, the intersegmental force at the knee is given by

$$\mathbf{F}_k = m_s \mathbf{a}_s - \mathbf{F}_a - m_s \mathbf{g} \qquad (8)$$

where $\mathbf{F}_a$ is given in equation 4.

The moment equilibrium equation for the rigid body is written as:

$$\mathbf{M}_k + \mathbf{M}_a + (\mathbf{r}_{cm,p} \times \mathbf{F}_k) + (\mathbf{r}_{cm,d} \times \mathbf{F}_a) = \mathbf{I}_s \alpha_s (9)$$

Thus, the intersegmental moment at the knee is given by:

$$\mathbf{M}_k = -\mathbf{M}_a - (\mathbf{r}_{cm,p} \times \mathbf{F}_k) \\ - (\mathbf{r}_{cm,d} \times \mathbf{F}_a) + \mathbf{I}_s \alpha_s \quad (10)$$

The above method of calculation of forces and moments at the knee joint can also be extended to calculate intersegmental forces and moments at the hip. The equations remain the same except that the subscript s in the equations is replaced by t (thigh). Further, because we now know the forces and moments at the knee joint, subscripts a and k are to be replaced by k and h, respectively. Thus, the force at the hip is given by:

$$\mathbf{F}_h = m_t \mathbf{a}_t - \mathbf{F}_k - m_t \mathbf{g} \qquad (11)$$

Similarly, the moment at the hip joint is given by:

$$\mathbf{M}_h = -\mathbf{M}_k - (\mathbf{r}_{cm,p} \times \mathbf{F}_h) \\ - (\mathbf{r}_{cm,d} \times \mathbf{F}_k) + \mathbf{I}_t \alpha_t \quad (12)$$

The preceding three-dimensional example is an application of the rigid-body equations to solve for the intersegmental forces and moments at any joint. The analysis is done from distal to proximal. The unknown intersegmental loads are solved sequentially at the ankle, knee, and hip. The intersegmental load at the distal segment is applied with equal magnitude and opposite direction to the distal joint of the next segment up the limb. This leaves one unknown force, the proximal intersegmental load. In the next section, we will see how the intersegmental forces and moments at the joints can be used to calculate the internal forces, i.e., muscle and internal joint reaction forces.

Example 1: Application of kinetics to gait analysis. This example illustrates the basic steps used to calculate the intersegmental forces and moments at the ankle and knee joints from measurements of limb segment displacements, body mass, and ground reaction forces during gait (Fig. 6). For this example, the forces and moments acting on the segments in the sagittal plane alone will be considered. The foot is assumed to be of negligible mass compared to the mass of the shank. The ground reaction forces, ground reaction moment, inertial forces of the shank

TABLE 1. *Numerical values for Example 1: application of kinetics in gait analysis*

Description	Symbol	Value
Knowns		
Ground reaction force		
Vertical	F_g^v	700 N
Horizontal	F_g^h	150 N
Lever arms		
Floor to ankle		
Horizontal	h_1	0.13 m
Vertical	v_1	0.10 m
Ankle to center of mass of the shank		
Horizontal	h_2'	0.06 m
Vertical	v_2'	0.16 m
Knee center to center of mass of the shank		
Horizontal	h_2''	0.09 m
Vertical	v_2''	0.12 m
Shank weight	mg	28 N
Inertial forces		
Shank mass (m) × horizontal acceleration (a_h)	ma_h	0.7 N
Shank mass (m) × vertical acceleration (a_v)	ma_v	3.3 N
Shank inertia (I) × angular acceleration (α)	$I\alpha$	0.06 Nm
Unknowns		
Force at ankle		
Horizontal	F_a^h	150 N
Vertical	F_a^v	700 N
Moment at ankle	M_a	106 Nm
Force and moment at shank		
Distal end		
Horizontal force	F_d^h	150 N
Vertical force	F_d^v	700 N
Moment	M_d	106 Nm
Proximal end		
Horizontal force	F_p^h	149.3 N
Vertical force	F_p^v	696.7 N
Moment	M_p	43.16 Nm

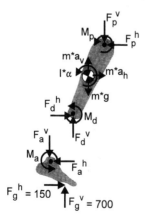

FIG. 6. Sagittal plane intersegmental forces and moments at ankle and knee joints. Intersegmental forces at the ankle and knee joints as well as the ground reaction force are resolved in the horizontal and vertical directions. Note that the inertia forces and moments of the foot are neglected.

(both linear and angular), distance of ankle from floor, and length of shank are known. Because the current example deals with forces in only one plane (the sagittal plane), the forces are expressed in horizontal and vertical components. The vertical component of force is denoted by a superscript of *v*, and the horizontal component is denoted by a superscript of *h*. The numerical values for this example are given in Table 1.

Thus, the force equilibrium equation for the foot segment can be rewritten as

$$F_a^h + F_g^h = 0$$

$$F_a^v + F_g^v = 0$$

Substituting the known values of $F_g{}^h$ and $F_g{}^v$ into the above equations, the external forces at the ankle along horizontal and vertical directions can be obtained. The numerical solution is given in Table 1.

The moment equilibrium equation for the foot is reduced to

$$M_a + F_g{}^h \cdot v_1 + F_g{}^v \cdot h_1 = 0$$

where h_1 and v_1 are the horizontal and vertical distances of the ankle joint from the position of the ground reaction force. Table 1 contains the numerical value of this moment.

In regard to the analysis of the forces and moments in the shank, at the distal end the forces will be equal and opposite in nature to those acting at the ankle. Thus, $F_d{}^h = F_a{}^h$, and $F_d{}^v = F_a{}^v$. Now, if we write the force equilibrium equations for the shank along horizontal and vertical directions, respectively,

$$F_d{}^h - F_p{}^h = ma_h$$

from which the unknown force $F_p{}^h$ is calculated, and

$$F_d{}^v - F_p{}^v = ma_v$$

from which the unknown force $F_p{}^v$ is calculated.

The moment equilibrium equation is written about the center of mass of the shank and given as

$$F_d{}^h \cdot v_2' - F_d{}^v \cdot h_2' + F_p{}^h \cdot v_2'' - F_p{}^v \cdot h_2'' + M_d + M_p = I\alpha$$

where h_2' and v_2' are the horizontal and vertical distances, respectively, of the center of mass of the shank from the ankle joint. The corresponding horizontal and vertical distances, respectively, of the center of mass of the shank from the knee joint are h_2'' and v_2''. In the above equation, all quantities are known except M_p. The results are shown in Table 1.

Equilibrium Between External and Internal Forces

Equilibrium requires a balance between intersegmental forces and internal forces such that there is no change in the state of rest or motion of the body. For locomotion studies, the state of equilibrium at the joint is of relevance. The intersegmental forces and moments calculated by the methods described in Example 1 must be balanced by a set of forces and moments acting internally to maintain equilibrium. These internal forces are generated primarily by muscle contraction, passive soft tissue stretch, and articular reaction forces. Equations of equilibrium can be resolved into a total of six equations (three forces and three moments). Thus, in three dimensions, it is only possible to solve for six unknowns. In general, there are more internal forces (unknowns) than equations, thereby rendering the problem statically indeterminate. Thus, a unique solution for individual muscle forces is not possible without further assumptions. However, it is possible to reduce the problem, with appropriate assumptions, to a case in which there are an equal number of unknowns and equations. The problem thus becomes statically determinate and can be solved. Important insight into the forces sustained by internal structures has been gained using this approach (30,38,39,48).

Example 2. Statically determinate analysis. To illustrate how a statically determinate analysis can be used to calculate internal forces, let us consider a two-dimensional statically determinate example. The external as well as internal forces are treated as scalar quantities as opposed to being considered vectors. The free-body diagram in Fig. 7 contains the external forces (known) and the internal forces (unknown) acting on the knee joint. The external vertical and horizontal components of the forces, $F_p{}^v$ and $F_p{}^h$, have been explicitly calculated in the previous example. The external moment, M_p, acting at the knee has also been calculated explicitly and is tending to flex the knee. The internal forces acting at the knee include the vertical component of the tibial–femoral contact force, $F_c{}^v$, and the vertical and horizontal components of the quadriceps muscle force, $F_q{}^v$ and $F_q{}^h$, which are all unknown.

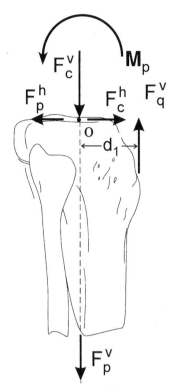

FIG. 7. Free-body diagram of external and internal forces acting at the center of the knee on the tibial plateau. This problem is statistically determinate because there are three unknowns, which can be determined from the three equilibrium equations of the rigid body.

For the purpose of this example, we will not consider the horizontal component of the quadriceps force.

One approach to simplifying the problem would be to assume that the hamstring muscles are inactive because the external moment tends to flex the joint and would be balanced by the quadriceps muscles. The problem then becomes statically determinate because there are three unknowns, horizontal and vertical forces contact and the vertical quadriceps force, and three independent equations of equilibrium. The contact point between the tibia and femur is assumed to be at the center of the tibial plateau.

Summing forces in a vertical direction gives:

$$-F_c^v + F_q^v + F_p^v = 0$$

Summing forces in a horizontal direction gives:

$$F_c^h - F_p^h = 0$$

Summing moments at the center of contact on the tibial plateau to eliminate the unknown contact force, we obtain:

$$F_q^v \cdot d_1 - M_p = 0$$

where d_1 is the distance from the vertical component of the contact force F_c^v to the vertical component of the quadriceps force F_q^v.

The equations of equilibrium contain three unknown forces, which are the vertical components of the quadriceps, F_q^v, the contact force F_c^v, and the horizontal component of the contact force F_c^h. Mathematically, the system consists of three linearly independent equations with three unknowns and is therefore statically determinate. Numerical values are provided in Table 2.

The external moment that tends to flex the knee is balanced by the vertical component of the quadriceps force, F_q^v, acting at a distance d_1 from the tibial–femoral contact point, 0. In general, this situation, in which the external moment acting at the joint is balanced by internal moments generated by muscle forces, occurs with most joints. Muscles are in mechanically efficient positions to balance external moments at the joints and usually provide the largest portion of the internal joint moment. As a result, large joint reaction forces are generated primarily from muscle contraction.

For the case in which antagonistic muscle activity is present, the problem again becomes

TABLE 2. *Numerical values for Example 2: statically determinate analysis*

Description	Symbol	Value
Knowns		
External reaction force and moment		
Vertical force	F_p^v	697 N
Horizontal force	F_p^h	149 N
Moment	M_p	43.2 Nm
Unknowns		
Quadriceps force (vertical)	F_q^v	1080 N
Tibiofemoral contact force		
Vertical force	F_c^v	382 N
Horizontal force	F_c^h	149 N

statically indeterminate (the equations of equilibrium cannot be solved explicitly) because the number of unknowns exceeds the number of equations. Sophisticated mathematical models incorporating additional information have been used to solve these problems.

Techniques for Solving the Indeterminate Problem

The techniques illustrated in Examples 1 and 2 have been used to predict muscular forces at the joints. In a three-dimensional statically determinate analysis of the knee joint, Morrison (38) developed a method for determining tibial–femoral contact force and forces developed in various muscle groups during level walking. The muscles acting at the knee joint were grouped into the hamstrings, gastrocnemius, and quadriceps muscles, and the ligaments into the cruciate and collateral ligaments. The maximum joint contact force occurring during gait was calculated to be four times body weight with a mean maximum value of 3.3 times body weight. This approach simplified the problem of determining muscle forces by grouping various muscles and by assuming no antagonistic muscle action.

The indeterminate nature of the problem was first addressed by Seireg and Arvikar (49), who developed a mathematical model of the lower extremities to predict muscle forces using linear optimization techniques. In this method, a system of linear equations in which the number of unknowns exceeds the number of equations is combined with an optimization criterion, which seeks to either maximize or minimize an objective function. In this study, various objective functions were considered to evaluate muscular forces during static leaning and stooping postures. As an extension of their previous work, Seireg and Arvikar (50) applied their model to examine muscle forces during quasistatic walking. Maximum knee joint forces for quasistatic walking were reported to be 7.1 times body weight. This was approximately twice the knee joint force reported by Morrison (39).

Crowninshield (20) discussed certain limitations of optimization methods including anatomic simplifications and problems associated with estimating antagonistic muscle activity. He concluded that present optimization methods to predict muscle activity are, at best, a first attempt to model a highly complex optimization process.

In an attempt to study the muscular-force optimization problem, Pedotti (43) formulated four biological optimization criteria for the solution of muscle forces during level walking. The most feasible criterion selected was the sum of squares of (actual force)/(maximum force) for all muscles at each instant of time. The maximum force was based on a relationship between force and velocity of muscular contraction known as Hill's equation (2,27). The results presented for normal level walking show good agreement between muscle force and EMG for the 11 muscles considered in the analysis. The knee joint was modeled as a hinge joint; hence, the moving contact between the tibia and femur was not considered.

Another class of optimization problems exists for nonlinear systems. The techniques for solving this class of problem varies, and no general method exists that can guarantee a global optimum in a finite number of steps, as does linear programming. Using a nonlinear optimization scheme, Crowninshield and Brand (21) developed a muscle model that utilized as a criterion the maximum endurance of musculoskeletal function. Results obtained from level walking, using this criterion, agreed qualitatively with EMG measurements.

In a study conducted by Patriarco (42), the significance of the various factors that contribute to the formation of a muscle force were considered, and an optimization solution was evaluated. Two relevant factors included the precision of the kinematic data acquisition systems and the intermediate processing needed to calculate the muscle moment arms and external moments. It was also determined that the ultimate source of deficiencies in many gait models is incomplete information about the physiological function and the role of the individual muscles during the gait cycle.

The problem of determining muscle forces during gait is very complex. The methods for solving the statically indeterminate problem with more than six unknowns for a three-dimensional model described above are further complicated when inherent features such as mechanical and physiological aspects are incorporated. For example, at the knee joint, both the mechanical tibial–femoral articulation and the physiological features of the muscles must be taken into consideration. From a mechanical aspect, the motion of the knee joint constantly changes the contact point between the articulating surface formed by the distal portion of the femur and the proximal portion of the tibia. This moving contact point changes the effective length of the lever arm of the forces generated by the muscles. This is an important intrinsic mechanical characteristic of the knee. It has been shown (35) that the relative movement of the articular surfaces to the knee joint provides a mechanical advantage that reduces the quadriceps force necessary to extend the knee joint.

Another important characteristic that influences the force generated by muscle is that the maximum force depends on the velocity of contraction and the muscle length. At low velocities, muscles can exert high forces. At high velocities, the potential of a muscle to exert force diminishes. This relationship between force and velocity is given by Hill's equation and is fundamental to muscle mechanics.

The kinetics of normal walking indicates certain optimal conditions from a viewpoint of muscular demand. The largest demands on muscles occur at the point of the gait cycle where the muscle has its greatest length (origin to insertion) and is contracting at zero velocity. According to Hill's equation, a muscle working at zero velocity can generate its maximum force. Variations from the kinematics of normal gait would likely change this delicate relationship among muscle force, length, and velocity of contraction and, thus, produce a less energy-efficient gait.

The above discussion illustrates the complexity of determining muscle forces using statically indeterminate models combined with optimization criteria that may vary depending on activity, level of fatigue, or pathologic conditions. Thus, these techniques must be applied with care. Yet, an approximate knowledge of muscle and joint forces can be derived from external measurements of joint reaction moments.

Example 3: Frontal plane moments (adduction) and the distribution of load across the knee joint. This example illustrates the relationship between the intersegmental forces and moments acting at the knee joint and the distribution of loads across the medial and lateral plateaus of the knee. In particular, there is a moment tending to adduct the knee throughout the major portion of stance phase (Fig. 8). This moment is countered internally by muscle forces (F_m) and lateral soft tissue forces (passive and active) balancing the reaction forces at the knee joint. The following describes the application of a model (48) that can be used to approximate the loads on the medial and lateral plateaus of the tibia (Fig. 8).

Model description. The model (48) is similar to Morrison's (38). Input to the model consists of knee flexion angle, external flexion–extension moments, abduction–adduction moments, and axial and anterior–posterior loads. The model differs from that of Morrison's in that

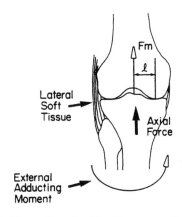

FIG. 8. The external adducting moment was resisted by the minimum sagittal plane muscle force (F_m) and axial load acting over (l). Pretension in the lateral soft tissues would maintain equilibrium if the muscle force were insufficient (48).

the point of contact changes with knee flexion, the cruciate ligaments resist only anterior–posterior shear forces, and collateral ligaments resist only abducting–adducting moments. The movement of the tibial–femoral contact and the resulting changes in muscle moment arms are modeled by a third-order polynomial relating the angle of knee flexion to the tibial–femoral contact point (23). The medial–lateral location of the tibial–femoral contact remains fixed at 25% of the tibial width from the knee joint center on each plateau, while the anterior–posterior contact changes with flexion (23,30). The average width of the tibia is taken as 80 mm. A linear relationship is assumed to exist between the knee flexion angle and the inclination of the patellar ligament with the long axis of the tibia (37). In common with Morrison's model, the three muscle groups in this model consist of the quadriceps, hamstrings, and gastrocnemius. The quadriceps resists the net external flexion moment, and the hamstring and gastrocnemius resist the net external extension moment. The activity of the flexor–extensor muscle is assumed to be dependent on the direction of the external moment. The force in the iliotibial band resulting from contraction of the tensor fascia latae and gluteus maximus, along with the tensile forces in the lateral collateral ligament and capsular forces, are grouped together and referred to as lateral soft tissue pretension.

It can be shown from the moment equilibrium equation that if the externally applied moment increases, and the assumption is made that the ratio of antagonist to agonist muscle force remains constant, the forces in the quadriceps and hamstring muscles must increase proportionately. The contribution of antagonistic muscle activity increases the load at the joint because the force in the agonist muscles must increase to counteract the contribution to the internal moment of the antagonistic muscle activity. Thus, if no antagonistic muscle activity is present, the moment magnitude and direction reflect the lower bound of muscle force and joint force. The presence of any antagonistic activity increases both the muscle and joint forces. Thus, in the

current example, the minimum force in a muscle group to balance the net external flexion or extension moment can be calculated. The joint reaction force is the vector sum of the active muscle force plus the ground reaction force resolved along the axis of the tibia.

The external adducting moment is balanced by muscle group forces plus the axial load (Fig. 8) acting about the medial contact. If the adducting moment is not resisted by the summed muscle force and axial load, then lateral soft tissue tension (active or passive) is used to maintain equilibrium.

Prediction of joint and muscle forces. From the model, the total joint reaction for a normal subject during normal level walking consists of three peaks (Fig. 9). The first peak, just following heel strike with a magnitude of approximately three times body weight, is the result of the hamstrings, the second the quadriceps, and the third the gastrocnemius. The resulting joint reaction force, as predicted without antagonistic muscle activity, therefore represents a lower bound. It should be noted that the minimum muscle force is not sufficient to balance the adducting moment (Fig. 8), and thus, either antagonistic muscle activity or lateral soft tissue pretension is needed to prevent lateral joint opening. Thus, both passive and active lateral forces are

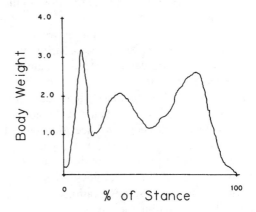

FIG. 9. The total joint reaction for a normal subject during walking consisted of three peaks. The first peak is a result of the hamstrings, the second the quadriceps, and the third the gastrocnemius (48).

TABLE 3. *External measurements and internal predictions*

		Normal group
Adduction moment	(input)	3.30 ± 0.67% (bw × ht)
Flexion moment	(input)	1.81 ± 0.65% (bw × ht)
Extension moment	(input)	2.86 ± 0.82% (bw × ht)
Axial load	(input)	1.01 ± 0.08 bw
Extensor muscle force	(output)	0.75 ± 0.26 bw
Flexor muscle force	(output)	1.65 ± 0.46 bw
Medial joint reaction	(output)	2.25 ± 0.39 bw
Lateral joint reaction	(output)	0.91 ± 0.24 bw
Lateral pretension	(output)	0.50 ± 0.18 bw

needed to balance the adducting moment during walking to maintain the knee with dynamic lateral stability.

The average extensor and flexor muscle force, medial and lateral joint reactions, and lateral soft tissue pretension were calculated with the help of the model for a group of normal subjects (Table 3). The normal subjects had a biphasic flexion–extension moment pattern that demanded muscle activity to oscillate between the flexors and the extensors (23). The knee moment pattern used for this example favored the flexors. As a result, the average peak flexor motor force was nearly twice that of extensor muscle force. Medial joint reaction force was also found to be more than two times larger than the reaction on the lateral joint at the knee.

Thus, a critical interaction between dynamic muscle forces and pretension forces in the lateral soft tissues is needed to stabilize the knee joint during walking. A minimum muscle force (no antagonist) to maintain equilibrium is insufficient to balance the adduction moment and keep the knee joint closed laterally. Cocontraction of antagonistic muscle action and/or pretension in the passive soft tissue is needed for dynamic joint stability during walking. These observations suggest a possible explanation for the presence of antagonistic muscle action during normal walking. A high adduction moment in a patient with lateral laxity could lead to a condition in which the joint opens laterally and transfers

the entire joint reaction through the medial compartment.

JOINT MOMENTS IN LOCOMOTION

An analysis of the temporal characteristics of the moments acting at the joints of the lower extermity during walking and other activities of daily living demonstrates characteristic patterns. These patterns include predictable phasic changes in the magnitude and direction of the joint moment during the walking cycle (Figs. 10 and 11). To differentiate variations detected in gait among individuals from variations in individual body sizes, the moment magnitudes shown are reported as a percentage of body weight times height [%(bw × ht)]. This normalization assumes that the moments, typically measured in Newton-meters (Nm), are proportional to the height and weight of an individual. Thus, differences detected among individuals would be associated with differences in gait rather than body size.

Flexion–Extension Moment Patterns During Walking: Normal Variability

The appropriate application of the joint moment to the study of normal and abnormal function requires an understanding of the variability that can be expected in a normal population. Shown in Fig. 10 are the flexion–extension moment patterns at the hip, knee, and ankle throughout the stance and swing phases of gait. Also included in Fig. 10 in tabular form are the variations in pattern of the joint moment during level walking obtained from the analysis of 316 stride cycles taken from 29 normal subjects over a range of slow, normal, and fast walking speeds.

The hip has the most reproducible characteristics of flexion–extension moments of the three major joints. At heel strike, the external moment tends to flex the hip joint, reaching a maximum value just before midstance. The pattern reverses direction after midstance to a moment tending to extend the joint. This sinusoidal pattern was found at all

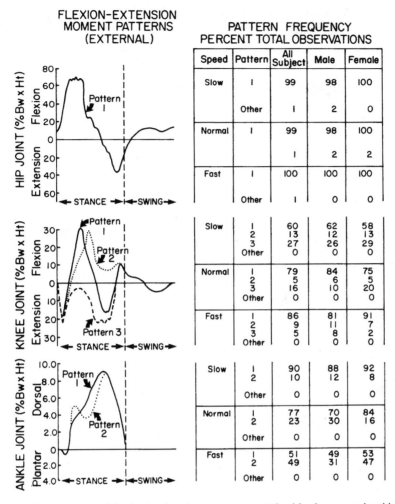

FIG. 10. The patterns of flexion–extension moments at the hip, knee, and ankle (9).

walking speeds and among both male and female subjects. The maximum magnitude of moments at the hip was greatest in the direction tending to flex the joint, although the overall pattern was fairly symmetric.

The most frequently occurring pattern for the knee (Pattern 1) is present in approximately 80% of all stride cycles at a normal walking speed. This pattern is biphasic, tending to produce extension at heel strike, flexion through midstance, extension in late stance, and flexion just prior to toe-off. The deviations from the most frequently occurring pattern take place during middle stance phase. Pattern 2, occurring in 5% of the nor-

mal observations for the normal walking speed, tends to flex the knee during the entire portion of the middle stance. Pattern 3, which occurs in approximately 15% of the observations, tends to extend the knee during the entire portion of middle stance phase. The predominance of Pattern 1 seems to be dependent on walking speed. At a slower walking speed, there was an increase in the frequencies of Pattern 2 and Pattern 3. At faster walking speeds, there was less variability in the flexion–extension pattern, with the majority of the observations tending toward Pattern 1. The change to Pattern 1 at higher speeds was especially true among the

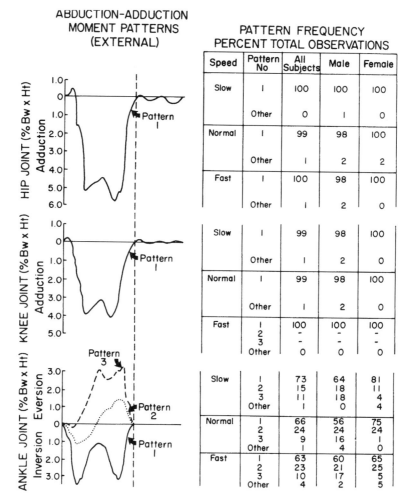

ABDUCTION–ADDUCTION
MOMENT PATTERNS
(EXTERNAL)

PATTERN FREQUENCY
PERCENT TOTAL OBSERVATIONS

Speed	Pattern No	All Subjects	Male	Female
Slow	I	100	100	100
	Other	0	I	0
Normal	I	99	98	100
	Other	I	2	2
Fast	I	100	98	100
	Other	I	2	0
Slow	I	99	98	100
	Other	I	2	0
Normal	I	99	98	100
	Other	I	2	0
Fast	I	100	100	100
	2	-	-	-
	3	-	-	-
	Other	0	0	0
Slow	I	73	64	81
	2	15	18	11
	3	11	18	4
	Other	I	0	4
Normal	I	66	56	75
	2	24	24	24
	3	9	16	I
	Other	I	4	0
Fast	I	63	60	65
	2	23	21	25
	3	10	17	5
	Other	4	2	5

FIG. 11. The patterns of abduction–adduction moment at the hip, knee, and ankle during level walking (9).

female subjects, where the predominance of Pattern 1 increased from 58% at a slow speed to 91% of the total observations at a fast speed.

The two patterns of the flexion–extension moment at the ankle were similar. Both patterns tended to dorsiflex the ankle throughout the entire portion of stance phase. The only difference between the two patterns was the change in slope in Pattern 2 just before mid-stance phase. There was a greater tendency toward the Pattern 2 characteristics as walking speed increased in both male and female subjects.

Adduction–Abduction Moment Patterns During Walking

The patterns of abduction–adduction moments at the hip, knee, and ankle are quite reproducible, with only one pattern present for all subjects at all walking speeds (Fig. 11). There is an abduction moment at the hip at heel strike, which reverses immediately to adduction throughout the entire period of stance phase. A similar pattern is observed at the knee. The ankle demonstrates the most variablility, with the most frequently occurring pattern appearing in 66% of the observations.

This pattern is associated with the moment that would tend to invert the ankle throughout stance phase.

Amplitudes of Moment Patterns as a Function of Walking Speed

As previously illustrated, the magnitude of the moment pattern can be related to the magnitudes of the net muscle force and internal joint reaction forces. Using this relationship, the relative magnitudes of the moments during various activities can be used as an indicator of forces acting on the joint. For example, the magnitude of the flexion–extension moments has been shown to be dependent upon walking speed. Because the internal forces are related to the joint moments, the internal forces acting on the joints can also be expected to vary with walking speed.

This speed dependency is present at the hip, knee, and ankle joint (Fig. 12). The flexion moment has the greatest dependency on speed, exhibiting a nearly threefold increase as the walking speed approximately doubles. The only moment component that does not substantially change with walking speed in the sagittal plane is the moment tending to plantarflex the ankle. The other components of the moments, for abduction–adduction and internal–external rotation, do not substantially change with walking speed.

To provide estimates of the actual moments that occur during walking, the normalized values of moment (Fig. 10) can be converted to actual values. For example, the average bw × ht formula for the male portion of the population represented in Figs. 10 through 12 is 1370 Nm, whereas the average bw × ht for the female population is 990 Nm. Thus, if one were to take the magnitude of the hip flexion moment at a normal walking speed as 9%(bw × ht), this represents an average flexion moment magnitude at the hip of 123 Nm for a man of average size and 89.1 Nm for a woman of average size.

It should be noted that the normalized data shown in Fig. 10 show no statistical difference between the moment magnitudes for the male and female population for the flexion–extension components. The only differences that appear in the moment magnitudes after normalization between the men and women are in the moments tending to adduct the hip and knee joints. The moment is approximately 8% greater at the knee and 4% greater at the hip for the female subjects. These differences are present during all walking speeds and seem to

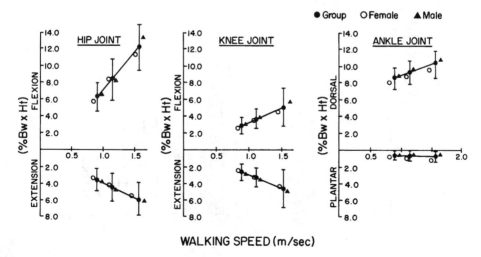

FIG. 12. An illustration of the walking speed dependence of the flexion–extension moments at the hip, knee, and ankle (9).

reflect differences in pelvic structure between men and women. The women with relatively larger pelvises probably have a relatively higher moment tending to adduct the hip and the knee. Clearly, normalization that accounts only for height differences does not account for other types of structural differences.

Moment Magnitudes During Level Walking

The largest moments in the joints of the lower extremities occur in directions tending to flex the hip and dorsiflex the ankle. These flexion moments at the hip and ankle are more than twice the magnitude of the flexion moment that occurs at the knee for a walking speed of 1.2 m/sec (Fig. 13). Assuming equal muscle lever arms at the hip, knee, and ankle, these differences suggest that the extensor musculature at the hip and the muscles involved in plantarflexion at the ankle sustain greater forces than the knee extensor musculature for normal walking. Again, it should be noted that the patterns described during level walking are measured external to the joint and use the fundamental principles of mechanical equilibrium to determine a lower boundary for the muscle forces.

The dorsiflexion moment at the ankle joint is sustained through nearly the entire portion of stance phase (Fig. 10). Thus, in addition to having the largest magnitude, it is sustained for the greatest duration. Hence, the endurance of the calf muscles is important because they sustain a large force for a relatively long time during the gait cycle. From Fig. 10, it is apparent that the flexion–extension oscillations about the zero axis are generally associated with low maximum moments as well as moments sustained for only short periods during normal gait. It appears that this normal pattern of loading, associated with midstance knee flexion to approximately 20°, minimizes knee joint load-

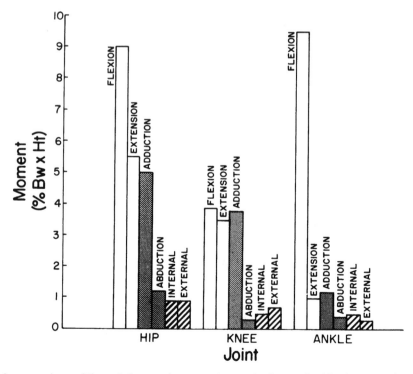

FIG. 13. A comparison of the relative peak moment magnitudes at the hip, knee, and ankle during level walking.

ing. It will be shown in the following section that this efficient biphasic pattern at the knee changes when an abnormal gait is present.

The relative magnitudes of the flexion–extension, abduction–adduction, and internal–external rotation moments are also illustrated in Fig. 13. As can be seen, with the exception of the ankle, the moment tending to adduct each joint is of comparable magnitude to the flexion or extension moments. At the knee, the magnitude of this moment is slightly larger than either of the flexion–extension moments and probably represents one of the major factors influencing the loads at the knee joint. The adduction moment in Fig. 13 results primarily from the medial offset of the body's center of mass and the medial and lateral acceleration and deceleration of the center of mass during walking. An adduction moment on the limb tends to force the ankle medially and, without internal resistance, would thrust the knee into increasing varus. Thus, it is this moment component that causes the medial compartment of the knee to bear a higher load than the lateral compartment (46). Approxi-

mately 60% to 80% of the total compressive load transmitted across the knee is on the medial compartment.

Moments During Activities of Daily Living

The largest moments during most activities of daily living are in directions tending to flex the joints. This type of limb motion places demands on the extensor antigravity muscles of the joint's extremity. A comparison of the maximum flexion moments during walking, ascending stairs, descending stairs, rising from a seated position, and jogging indicates a substantial variation in the peak values at each of the joints (Fig. 14). At the hip and knee, walking produces the lowest flexion moment, whereas the lowest flexion moment at the ankle occurs when rising from a seated position. Using the magnitude of the moment during walking as a basis, comparison of the relative muscular efforts can be made. For example, the flexion moment at the hip during walking is

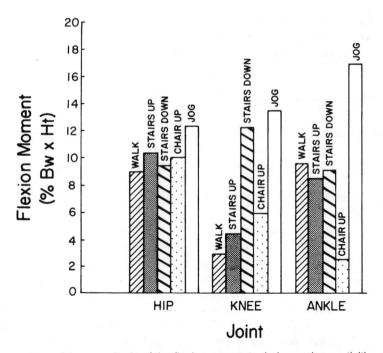

FIG. 14. A comparison of the magnitude of the flexion moments during various activities of daily living.

approximately 9%(bw × ht). This magnitude increases slightly to 10%(bw × ht) during stair climbing and to approximately 12%(bw × ht) during jogging. Thus, the range of joint loadings is relatively uniform during a variety of activities of daily living, with an approximately 30% increase in joint loads experienced during jogging over the base level for straight walking. The knee joint, with a relatively small flexion moment during level walking, sustains substantial increases during several activities including descending stairs and jogging. The large increases in the flexion moment at the knee joint for descending stairs and jogging are likely associated with the high incidence of patellofemoral problems in individuals involved in middle- and long-distance running as well as the difficulty in descending stairs for those with patellofemoral problems. It is likely that the relative increase (by approximately a factor of five) in flexion moment during jogging over the nominal level of walking values is more important on a comparative basis than the absolute magnitude. For example, the ankle dorsiflexion moment during jogging is higher than the flexion moment at the knee. However, the relative increase in the dorsiflexion moment sustained during jogging as compared to level walking is only by a factor of two as compared to the fivefold increase seen in the knee flexion moment.

CLINICAL APPLICATIONS

The quantitative analysis of human locomotion can be a useful method for improving our understanding of various musculoskeletal diseases and injuries. In many cases, the functional changes associated with an injury or disease result from an adaptation to the condition rather than as a direct result of the mechanical change associated with the pathologic or anatomic change. For example, in patients with knee ligament injuries, such as an anterior cruciate ligament rupture, walking may not produce an abnormal anterior drawer on the tibia because the subject can stabilize the knee using muscular substitution. Thus, the gait adaptation would be associated with a compensatory mechanism that provides muscular stabilization. These types of dynamic adaptations appear during locomotion and, in most cases, represent the manifestation of the pathologic condition and thus require an interpretation of the adaption. Pathologic stimuli such as pain, instability, or muscle weakness can cause dynamic adaptations. Often, a biomechanical analysis of the adaptation reflects the nature of the underlying pathology. Another example is the case of the Trendelenburg gait. The adaptation in this situation is the avoidance of stress in the abductor muscles of the hip by shifting the body weight over the center of the hip joint, thereby eliminating the need for the abductors to balance the moment because of the offset of bodyweight.

An understanding of the cause and effect of functional adaptations is extremely important for the development of methods for training, rehabilitation, and treatment of functionally impaired individuals. The purpose of this section is to illustrate some aspects of our current knowledge of biomechanical functional adaptations and to discuss the clinical implications of these adaptations.

Total knee replacements. An analysis of level walking in patients following total knee replacement provides an excellent example of the use of several types of parameters for the evaluation and analysis of function. There are a large number of parameters that can be measured during walking. These gait measures range from fundamental measures of time and distance to motion (kinematics) and forces (kinetics). The choice of which gait measurements to use depends on the intended application. These three general classes of gait measurements (time–distance, kinematics, and kinetics) can be applied to an evaluation of patients with total knee replacement. Time–distance measurements include measures of stride length, walking speed, and cadence. These are important measures of normal and abnormal walking (44). Stride length (distance between consecutive unilateral heel strikes) is one of the simplest and most sensitive indicators of walking abnormalities. It is important to note that stride length is dependent on walking speed (25); thus, in comparing measurements among normals and individuals with walking disabilities, it is important to account for differences in walking speed. For example, the relationship between stride length and walking speed for normal individuals is relatively linear and reproducible. It has also been shown that recovery of function from surgical reconstructions, such as total knee replacement, can be evaluated by comparing the overall stride length–walking speed relationship over a range of walking speeds. An improvement in walking ability is indicated by the stride length–walking speed relationship approaching normal between the 3- and 6-month postoperative gait evaluations (Fig. 15). The range of speeds selected by the patients are substantially less than normal, and without examining the relationship of stride length to speed, it would be extremely difficult to make comparisons between patients and normals or between the patients' observation at 3 and 6 months.

Time–distance parameters, although extremely efficient in evaluating quantitative changes in the overall characteristics of walking, do not provide specific information that can be related to the cause of the walking ab-

normality. For example, it has been shown (5) that the stride length–walking speed relationship does not fully return to normal following total knee replacement (Fig. 15). Patients continue to walk with a shorter than normal stride length when differences in walking speed are taken into account. This observation suggests that patients with total knee replacement, in spite of a successful clinical result, do not completely recover normal function during level walking. The cause of these functional differences cannot, however, be obtained from simple stride length measurements.

Measurement of joint kinematics can be used to quantify specific joint involvements in walking disabilities (47). In particular, relative segmental angles are joint specific and have been used to quantify changes in patterns of motion related to specific joints. Consider again the example of the gait of patients with total knee replacement. In addition to the shorter than normal stride lengths, these patients have reduced knee flexion (7,47) during the midportion of stance phase (Fig. 16). The normal midstance knee flexion is approximately 20° at an average speed, whereas patients, in spite of a pain-free clinical result, tend to walk with less than 10° of midstance

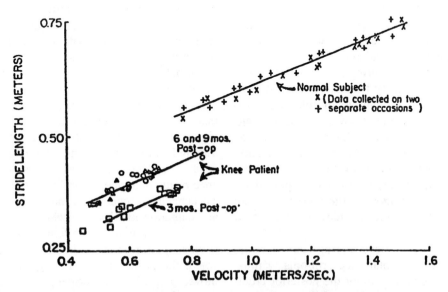

FIG. 15. An illustration of the normal stride length–walking speed relationship in comparison to the measurements taken from a postoperative patient with total knee replacement (5).

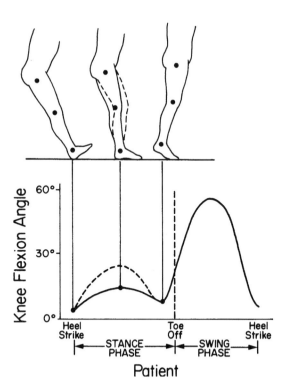

Patient

FIG. 16. An illustration of the change in midstance knee flexion angle following total knee replacement.

knee flexion. Thus, it appears that the adaptation to knee reconstruction is associated with a subtle inhibition in knee flexion. This type of kinematic analysis permits the localization of the adaptation to the knee joint and to the specific phase of the gait cycle, but at present it does not provide an explanation for the mechanism of this adaptation.

Joint moments during locomotion can also be used to identify the nature and cause of functional abnormalities in total knee replacement. As indicated previously, the magnitude and direction of the flexion–extension moment can be related to muscular function and to joint loading. In patients with total knee replacement, it has been reported (7, 52) that the moment at the knee joint is an important measure to identify functional changes.

A study of patients during stair climbing (4,6) following total knee arthroplasty illustrates the contribution of the posterior cruciate ligament to normal knee function. Patients have been tested with designs that range from

the early Geomedic and Polycentric to the newer Miller/Galante and posterior stabilized total condylar designs. These design groupings include posterior cruciate-retaining, -sacrificing, and -substituting designs.

Examination of the stair-climbing differences between the cruciate-substituting and -retaining designs indicates that the functional abnormality in patients with the cruciate-sacrificing designs is associated with a forward lean of the body (Fig. 17) in such a way that the moment tending to flex the knee during stair climbing is substantially reduced. This reduction in the moment tending to flex the knee reflects either a weakness or avoidance of the quadriceps during stair climbing. This change in function has been described as an adaptation to a knee in which the normal posterior movement of the femur on the tibia (rollback) with flexion is inhibited in designs where the posterior cruciate ligament is removed (Fig. 17). This normal posterior movement of the tibiofemoral contact provides a larger lever arm for the quadriceps mecha-

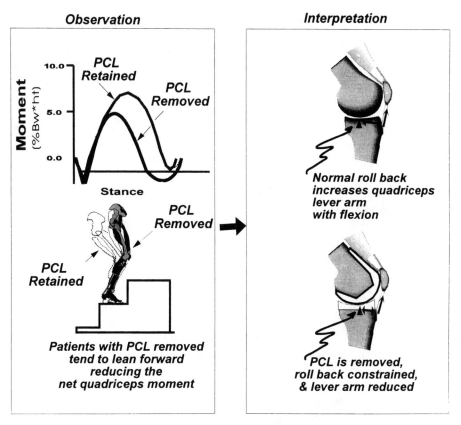

FIG. 17. Examination of the stair-climbing differences between the cruciate-substituting and -retaining designs.

nism as the knee flexes. If this mechanism is lost through either constraint of the articulating surface or removal of the posterior cruciate ligament, the normal rollback is inhibited. The normal interaction between tibiofemoral contact motion has also been demonstrated in cadaver studies (6,23). The passive kinematics of the knee influence the efficiency of active muscle function by changing the moment arm of various muscles as the knee is flexed.

Functional evaluation in high tibial osteotomy. Gait analysis has been used to evaluate patients with varus gonarthrosis prior to and following treatment with high tibial osteotomy. The fundamental premise of this procedure (36) has been that the varus deformity places an increased stress on the medial compartment of the knee and that this stress is, in part, responsible for the symptoms of the degenerative process as well as for accelerating the degeneration. The rationale for the treatment of medial compartment arthritis with high tibial osteotomy is, therefore, to reduce the stress on the medial compartment of the knee. The procedure is particularly suitable for the younger patient because it is more conservative than other treatment modalities such as total joint arthroplasty. The results, however, have been somewhat variable and unpredictable (28). It has been assumed that the amount of stress on the medial compartment is proportional to the degree of varus deformity measured by standing x-rays (36). However, the dynamic loads that occur during walking may play a more important role than do the static loads resulting from varus malalignment (46).

This observation is based on a study of patients tested in the gait laboratory before a high tibial osteotomy and at yearly intervals following treatment (46,54). The investigation focused on the dynamic peak adduction moment at the knee, with the analysis based on the relationship described earlier relating the adduction moment to the stress on the medial side of the knee. One might predict that patients with a large varus deformity would have a higher than normal adduction moment. However, a preoperative gait analysis indicated that only about one-half of the patients had a higher than normal adduction moment ("high adduction moment" group) in spite of the varus deformity at the knee joint.

The clinical outcome of the treatment of patients with varus gonarthrosis with high tibial osteotomy has been related to the magnitude of the adduction moment measured in the gait laboratory before surgery (46,54). Patients were grouped on the basis of the magnitude of their preoperative adduction moment; they were considered to have "high" adduction moments if the adduction moment exceeded 4%(bw × ht). Thus, it was possible for approximately one-half of the patients to adapt their gait dynamically to reduce the normal loading across the knee joint. All other patients were classified as having a "low" adduction moment. Approximately one-half of the patients in the original study group had an adduction lower than 4%(bw × ht). Thus, it was possible for approximately one-half of the patients to adapt their gait dynamically to reduce the normal loading across the knee joint.

Following surgery, the adduction moment was reduced in both groups. However, the average postoperative adduction moment in the "low" adduction moment group was still significantly lower than the average adduction moment in the "high" adduction moment group (Fig. 18). The two groups were indistinguishable based on preoperative knee score, initial varus deformity, immediate postoperative correction, age, and weight. In a follow-up of between 3 and 8.9 years after surgery, the patients in the "low" adduction moment group had significantly better clinical outcome (Fig. 18). The passage of time caused a decline in the clinical results in both the "high" and "low" adduction moment groups. However, the patients who had a low preoperative adduction moment maintained a better clinical result than did patients in the "high" adduction moment group at an average of 6 years. Further, 79% of the knees in the "low" adduction moment group

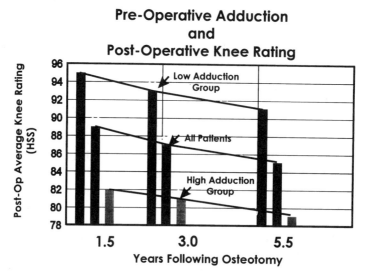

FIG. 18. Postoperative knee adduction moments and postoperative knee rating.

had maintained valgus correction, whereas only 20% of the knees in the "high" adduction moment group remained in valgus alignment.

The adaptive mechanism used by some patients to reduce the adduction moment has been related to a shorter stride length and an increased external rotation (toe-out) of the foot during stance phase. The adaptation using the toe-out mechanism altered the adduction moment during gait. The mechanics of this technique simply involved moving the ground reaction vector closer to the center of the knee joint and, thus, reducing the lever arm of the external ground reaction force.

It is possible for patients to reduce the dynamic loading on the medial compartment of the knee. Preoperative gait analysis provides a means of detecting which patients develop these adaptive mechanisms. Gait analysis can be used as an additional means of selecting patients who have a higher probability of a good result with a high tibial osteotomy. It also provides a basis for training patients to lower the loads at the knee joint and slow the progression of degenerative changes or increase the probability of a better result with a high tibial osteotomy.

Function following anterior cruciate ligament disruption. Another example of an adaptive mechanism involves the analysis of patients with complete rupture of the anterior cruciate ligament (ACL) of the knee. Patients with an ACL-deficient knee typically have difficulties with movements involving lateral thrust or rotatory loads at the knee joint. However, some patients are able to perform these activities in spite of an ACL-deficient knee. Patients with ruptured ACLs have been tested during level walking, jogging, ascending stairs, and more stressful activities such as running and pivoting (11,53). When the results of patient tests are compared with those from normal subjects, several common characteristics of functional changes in patients with ACL-deficient knees from normal were observed.

Interestingly, the greatest change from normal was during level walking. The char-

acteristics of the gait abnormality were common to most patients with ACL-deficient knees and reflected a change in the flexion–extension moment at the knee joint. The patients with the ACL-deficient knee had a significantly lower than normal net quadriceps moment during the middle portion of the stance phase of walking. This type of gait has been interpreted as a tendency to avoid or reduce the demand on the quadriceps muscle and has been called a "quadriceps avoidance" gait (3,11–13). This "quadriceps avoidance" in ACL-deficient patients may seem surprising because the demand on the quadriceps muscles is relatively low during walking. However, despite the relatively low loads on the knee that occur during level walking, 75% of the patients in a recent report had the "quadriceps avoidance" gait, and 25% had a normal biphasic flexion–extension moment (Fig. 19). It is important to note that the magnitude of the net quadriceps moment reduction during walking was more than 100% relative to normal. This net reduction in the quadriceps moment could also be interpreted as an increase in the hamstring activity relative to quadriceps activity. As the angle of knee flexion increases, the hamstring can provide a dynamic substitute for the quadriceps.

Further analysis during the jogging and stair-climbing activities suggests that quadriceps weakness was not an explanation for the "quadriceps avoidance" pattern seen during level walking. The net quadriceps moment was approximately 4.5 times greater than normals during jogging when compared to level walking (Fig. 14). Patients had approximately a 25% reduction in the net quadriceps moment during jogging, and there was more than a 100% reduction from normal during level walking (Fig. 20). During stair climbing, when the net quadriceps moment was still substantially larger than in level walking, the patients and normal subjects had essentially the same pattern and magnitude of quadriceps moment. Thus, it is not likely that this result was an indication of quadriceps weakness.

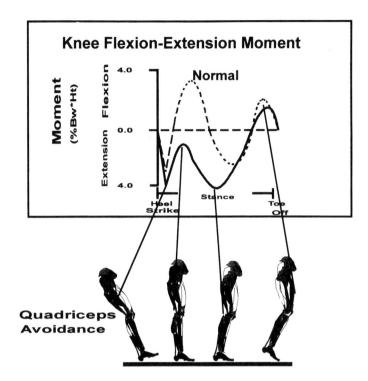

FIG. 19. Knee flexion–extension moment pattern for the "quadriceps avoidance" patient group.

An explanation for the functional changes associated with the loss of the ACL can be related to the anterior pull of the patellar ligament when the knee is near full extenstion. The "quadriceps avoidance gait" seen in patients with ACL deficiencies was greatest during level walking when the knee was near full extension. Quadriceps contraction produces an anteriorly directed force on the tibia when the knee is near full extension. The anterior pull of the patellar mechanism is reduced as the knee approaches 45° of flexion and reverses beyond 45° of flexion. It appears that patients adapt to the absence of the ACL by minimizing the demand for quadriceps activation when the knee is near full extension. This observation would explain the functional differences in normal subjects and patients with ACL-deficient knees. In activities in which the knee flexes beyond 45°, the pull of the extensor mechanism is actually a secondary restraint to the anterior drawer of the tibia. Thus, patients with ACL-deficient knees tend to use normal or more than normal quadriceps activities in stair climbing where the maximum demand on the quadriceps occurs at about 60° of knee flexion.

Running injuries and joint moment magnitudes. An analysis of the joint loading during jogging can be used to evaluate some of the mechanisms of the overuse injury occurring in middle- and long-distance runners (8). Overuse injury results from cyclic loading of the joint with sufficient magnitude to produce injuries when applied over a large number of cycles. This overuse pattern differs from a traumatic injury in which the load is substantially higher and is of sufficient magnitude to cause injury during a single occurrence.

The knee—in particular, the patellofemoral joint—is a frequent site of overuse injury patterns in middle- and long-distance runners (29). Other frequent sites of overuse injury in runners are the iliotibial band, Achilles tendon, and metatarsal heads (8). Shown in Fig. 21 are three portions of the running cycle in-

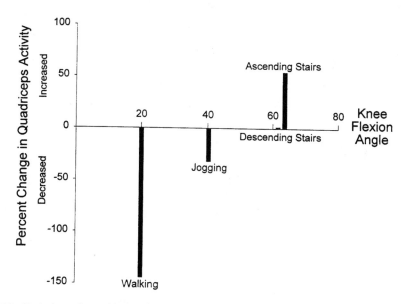

FIG. 20. Variation of quadriceps function in different activities as a percentage of normal.

cluding the foot-strike, midsupport, and preswing configurations of the limbs and torso. At foot-strike, the hip and knee are slightly flexed, and the foot contacts the ground dorsiflexed. During running, the body has a more vertical posture at heel-strike with slightly more hip and knee flexion than during level walking. Landing in this flexed position provides a potential for absorbing the higher impact that occurs during running. An analysis of the intrinsic loading at the knee at foot-strike indicates compressive and posteriorly directed force components and a moment that tends to flex the joint. As the body moves forward to the midsupport phase, the axial force reaches a maximum of two times body weight, the posterior shear reaches body weight, and the moment tending to flex the knee approaches 15%(bw × ht). Again, it should be noted that this maximum knee flexion moment is greater than five times the moment that normally occurs during level walking. As the limb moves to the preswing position, the hip and knee joints extend and the ankle plantarflexes.

Also shown in Fig. 21 is the configuration of the limb in the frontal plane during the three phases of the support phase of running. At foot-strike, there is a medially directed shear of 8% body weight as well as a moment tending to abduct the knee and internally rotate the joint. At midsupport, the shear reverses direction to a maximum of 8% body weight directed laterally, the internal rotation reaches a maximum of 2%(bw × ht), and the moment tending to adduct the knee reaches a maximum of 6.5%(bw × ht). As the body moves toward preswing, internal rotation, abduction–adduction and the medially directed force continue in the same direction but reduce in magnitude before the foot leaves the ground.

A comparison of the maximum loads at the knee that occur during running (3 m/sec) and walking (1.2 m/sec) indicates that the moment tending to flex the knee increases the most. This increase in flexion moment can be related to an increase in quadriceps force, patellofemoral contact force, and joint compressive force. Therefore, there appears to be a correspondence between the frequency of running injuries to the knee joint and the increase in magnitude of the flexion moment over that which occurs during level walking. Similarly, the large adduction moment at the hip increases the iliotibial band stress, and the dorsiflexion moment at the

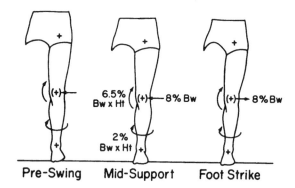

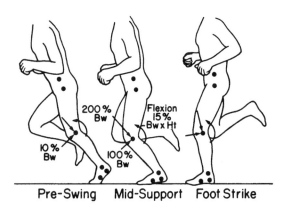

FIG. 21. An illustration of the limb configuration during running.

ankle stresses the Achilles tendon. Clearly, structures that are more highly stressed during running are operating in a range where any perturbation (such as change in distance, speed, or shoe style) may be sufficient to alter the delicate balance between healing and repair mechanisms associated with the overuse injury. Thus, it is important to first describe, and then evaluate, any adaptations to these perturbations, because they may cause increased loading to already high loads.

It is hoped that the examples above provide a broad although by no means inclusive overview of the types of clinical orthopaedic problems where the application of biomechanical principles, as briefly described in this chapter, may aid in the understanding of the body's response to such abnormal or disease states.

PROBLEMS

1. A person at the gym is going to strengthen his or her quadriceps muscles by doing a series of leg extension exercises.

Case 1: Assume that the femur is at a right angle to the tibia and that the weight exerts an external force, F, which acts perpendicular to the tibia through the ankle joint at a distance, d_1, to the center of the tibial plateau. Calculate the external moment generated at the knee in response to the force, F, at the ankle and the mass of the shank, m. The distance from the ankle to the center of the knee joint is $d_1 = 0.4$ m, the weight lifted is F = 400 N, and the mass of the shank is m = 2.89 kg.

Case 2: Assume that the leg is fully extended. Use the same values given for Case 1. The distance from the mass center to the tibial plateau is $d_2 = 0.1$ m.

2. Using the result for the external reaction moment at the knee obtained from Problem 1, calculate the internal force in the quadriceps muscle necessary to balance the external reaction moment when the knee joint is flexed at 90° and when it is at full extension. Assume that the quadriceps is the only muscle acting and that the distance from the quadriceps muscle force to the tibial–femoral contact point is $d = 0.02$ m. Calculate the force in the quadriceps muscle if the distance from the quadriceps force, $F_q{}^v$, to the tibial–femoral contact point, 0, is $d = 0.04$ m. Refer to Fig. 7 in the text.

3. A person steps across a force platform in a gait analysis laboratory. At heel-strike, the floor exerts a vertical reaction force on the foot measured by the force platform to be $F_g{}^v$ = 700N with a horizontal component, $F_g{}^h$ = 100N. Neglecting the inertial forces, determine the external reaction forces at the hip joint. The configuration of the lower limb at heel-strike is shown in the figure. All distances are measured from either the vertical or horizontal components of the ground reaction force and are labeled. The weight of the thigh ($F_{wt}{}^v$ = 70N) and shank ($F_{ws}{}^v$ = 29N) are located at the mass center of the thigh and shank, respectively.

REFERENCES

1. Advisory Committee on Artificial Limbs, National Research Council (1953): *The Pattern of Muscular Activity in the Lower Extremity During Walking.* Prosthetic Devices Research Project, Institute of Engineering Research, University of California, Berkeley, Series II, Issue 25.
2. Abbot, B. C., and Wilkie, D. R. (1953): The relation between velocity of shortening and the tension length curve of skeletal muscle. *J. Physiol.,* 120:214–223.
3. Andriacchi, T. P. (1990): Dynamics of pathological motion: Applied to the anterior cruciate deficient knee. *J. Biomech.,* 23(Suppl.):99–105.
4. Andriacchi, T. P., and Galante, J. O. (1988): Retention of the posterior cruciate ligament in total knee arthroplasty. *J. Arthroplasty,* 3:S13–S19.
5. Andriacchi, T. P., Ogle, J. A., and Galante, J. O. (1977): Walking speed as a basis for normal and abnormal gait measurements. *J. Biomech.,* 10:261–268.
6. Andriacchi, T. P., Galante, J. O., and Draganich, L. F. (1985): Relationship between knee extensor mechanics and function following total knee replacement. In: *Pro-*

ceedings lst Annual Meeting of the Knee Society, edited by L. Dorr, pp. 83–94. University Park Press, Baltimore.
7. Andriacchi, T. P., Galante, J. O., and Fermier, R. W. (1982): The influence of total knee replacement design on walking and stairclimbing. *J. Bone Joint Surg.,* 64A: 1328–1335.
8. Andriacchi, T. P., Kramer, G. M., and Landon, G. C. (1985): The biomechanics of running and knee injuries. In: *American Academy of Orthopaedic Surgeons, Symposium on Sport Medicine, The Knee,* edited by G. Finerman, pp. 23–32. C. V. Mosby, St. Louis.
9. Andriacchi, T. P., and Strickland, A. B. (1985): Lower limb kinetics applied to the study of normal and abnormal walking. In: *Biomechanics of Normal and Pathological Human Articulating Joints, NATO ASI Series, Series E: No. 93,* edited by N. Berme, A. E. Engin, and K. M. Correia Da Silva, pp. 83–102. Martinus Nijhoff, Dordrecht.
10. Beer, F. P., and Johnston, E. R. (1972): *Vector Mechanics for Engineers: Dynamics,* second edition. McGraw-Hill, New York.
11. Berchuck, M., Andriacchi, T. P., Bach, B. R., Jr., and Reider, B. R. (1990): Gait adaptations by patients who have a deficient ACL. *J. Bone Joint Surg.,* 72A:871–877.
12. Birac, D., Andriacchi, T. P., and Bach, B. R., Jr. (1991): Time related changed following ACL rupture. In: *Transactions of the 37th Annual Meeting of the Orthopaedic Research Society, Section 1,* p. 231.
13. Branch, T. P., Hunter, R., and Donath, M. (1989): Dynamic EMG analysis of anterior cruciate deficient legs with and without bracing during cutting. *Am. J. Sports Med.,* 17:35–41.
14. Blankervoort, L., Huiskes, R., and de Lange, A. (1986): The helical axes along the envelope of passive knee joint motion. In: *Transactions of the 32nd Annual Meeting of the Orthopaedic Research Society,* 12:410.
15. Bresler, B., and Frankel, J. P. (1953): The forces and moments in the leg during level walking. *Trans. Am. Soc. Mech. Eng.,* 48A:62.
16. Cappozzo, A., Figura, F., and Marchetti, M. (1976): The interplay of muscular and external forces in human angulation. *J. Biomech.,* 9:35–43.
17. Cavanaugh, P. R., Pollock, M. L., and Landa, J. (1977): A biomechanical comparison of elite and good distance runners. *Ann. N. Y. Acad. Sci.,* 301:328–345.
18. Chao, E. Y. S. (1980): Justification of triaxial goniometer for the measurement of joint rotation. *J. Biomech.,* 13:989–1006.
19. Chao, E. Y., Laughman, R. K., and Stauffer, R. N. (1980): Biomechanical gait evaluation of pre- and postoperative total knee replacement patients. *Arch. Orthop. Traumat. Surg.,* 97:309–317.
20. Crowninshield, R. D. (1978): Use of optimization techniques to predict muscle forces. *ASME J. Biomech. Eng.,* 100:88–92.
21. Crowninshield, R. D., and Brand, R. A. (1981): A physiologically based criteria of muscle force prediction in locomotion. *J. Biomech.,* 14:793–801.
22. Dillman, C. J. (1975): Kinematic analyses of running. In: *Exercise and Sport Sciences Review,* Vol. 3, edited by J. H. Wilmore, pp. 193–218. Academic Press, New York.
23. Dragnich, L. F., Andriacchi, T. P., and Anderssoln, G. B. J. (1987): Interaction between intrinsic knee mechanics and the knee extensor mechanism. *J. Orthop. Res.,* 5: 539–547.
24. Goldstein, H. (1950): *Classical Mechanics,* first edition. Addison–Wesley, Reading, MA.

25. Grieve, D. W. (1968): Gait patterns and the speed of walking. *Biomed. Eng.,* 3:119–122.
26. Grood, E. S., Sontay, W. J. (1983): A joint coordinate system for the clinical description of three-dimensional motions: application to the knee. *ASME J. Biomech. Engng.* 105:136–144.
27. Hill, A. V. (1953): The mechanics of active muscle. *Proc. R. Soc. Lond.,* 38:57–76.
28. Insall, J. N., Joseph, D. M., and Msika, C. (1984): High tibial osteotomy for varusgonarthrosis. *J. Bone Joint Surg.,* 66A(7):1040–1048.
29. James, S. L., Bates, B. T., and Osternig, L. R. (1978): Injuries to runners. *Am. J. Sports Med.,* 6(2):40–50.
30. Johnson, F., Scarrow, P., and Waugh, W. (1991): Assessment of loads in the knee joint. *Med. Biol. Eng. Comput.,* 19:237–243.
31. Kettelkamp, D. B., Johnson, R. J., Smidt, G. L., Chao, E. Y. S., and Walker, M. (1970): An electrogoniometric study of knee motion in normal gait. *J. Bone Joint Surg.,* 52A(4):775–790.
32. Kinzel, G. L., Hall, A. S., and Hillberry, B. M. (1972): Measurement of the total motion between two body segments I: Analytical development. *J. Biomech.,* 5:93–105.
33. Lafortune, M. A., Cavanagh, P. R., Sommer, H. J., and Kalenak, A. (1992): Three-dimensional kinematics of the human knee during walking. *J. Biomech.,* 25: 347–357.
34. Lamoreux, L. (1971): Kinematic measurements in the study of human walking. *Bull. Prosth. Res.,* 10–15:3–84.
35. Lindahl, O., and Movin, A. (1967): The mechanics of extension of the knee joint. *Acta Orthop. Scand.,* 38: 226–234.
36. Maquet, P. (1980): The biomechanics of the knee and surgical possibilities of healing osteoarthritic knee joints. *Clin. Orthop. Rel. Res.,* 146:102–110.
37. Mathews, L. S., Sonstegard, D. A., and Henke, J. A. (1977): Load bearing characteristics of the patellofemoral joint. *Acta Orthop. Scand.,* 48:511–516.
38. Morrison, J. B. (1968): Bioengineering analysis of force actions transmitted by the knee joint. *Biomed. Eng.,* 3: 164–170.
39. Morrison, J. B. (1970): The mechanics of the knee joint in relation to normal walking. *J. Biomech.,* 3:51–61.
40. Murray, M. P., Drought, A. B., and Kory, R. C. (1964): Walking patterns of normal men. *J. Bone Joint Surg.,* 46A:335–360.
41. Murray, M. P., Brewer, B. J., and Zuege, R. C. (1972): Kinesiologic measurements of functional performance

before and after McKee–Farrar total hip replacement. *J. Bone Joint Surg.,* 54A(2):237–256.
42. Patriarco, A. G., Mann, R. W., Simon, S. R., and Mansour, J. M. (1981): An evaluation of the approaches of optimization models in the prediction of muscle forces during human gait. *J. Biomech.,* 14:513–525.
43. Pedotti, A., Krishner, V. V., and Stark, L. (1978): Optimization of muscle-force sequencing in human locomotion. *Math. Biosci.,* 38:57–76.
44. Perry, J. (1974): Clinical gait analyzer. *Bull. Prosthet. Res.,* 10–22:188–192.
45. Perry, J., Hoffer, M. M., Giovan, P., Antonelli, D., and Greenberg, R. (1974): Gait analysis of the triceps surae in cerebral palsy: a preoperative and postoperative clinical and electromyographic study. *J. Bone Joint Surg.,* 56A(3):511–520.
46. Prodromos, C. C., Andriacchi, T. P., and Galante, J. O. (1985): A relationship between gait and clinical changes following high tibial osteotomy. *J. Bone Joint Surg.,* 67A(8):1188–1194.
47. Rittman, N., Kettelkamp, D. B., Pryor, P., Schwartzkopf, G. L., and Hillbery, B. (1981): Analysis of patterns of knee motion walking for four types of total knee implants. *Clin. Orthop. Rel. Res.,* 155:111–117.
48. Schipplein, O. D., and Andriacchi, T. P. (1991): Interaction between active and passive knee stabilizers during level walking. *J. Orthop. Res.,* 9:113–119.
49. Seireg, A., and Arvikar, R. J. (1973): A mathematical model for evaluating forces in lower extremities of the musculo-skeletal system. *J. Biomech.,* 6:313–326.
50. Seireg, A., and Arvikar, R. J. (1975): The prediction of muscular load sharing and joint forces in the lower extremities during walking. *J. Biomech.,* 3:51–61.
51. Selvik, G. (1974): A roentgen stereophotogrammetic method for the study of the kinematics of the skeletal system. Dissertation, University of Lund, Sweden.
52. Simon, S. R., Trieshmann, H. W., Burdett, R. G., Ewald, F. C., and Sledge, C. B. (1983): Quantitative gait analysis after total knee arthroplasty for monarticular degenerative arthritis. *J. Bone Joint Surg.,* 65A(5):605–613.
53. Tibone, J. E., Antich, T. J., Fanton, G. S., Moynes, D. R., and Perry J. (1986): Functional analysis of anterior cruciate ligament instability. *Am. J. Sports Med.,* 14: 276–284.
54. Wang, J. W., Kuo, K. N., Andriacchi, T. P., and Galante, J. O. (1990): The influence of walking mechanics and time on the results of proximal tibial osteotomy. *J. Bone Joint Surg.,* 72-A:905–909.

Basic Orthopaedic Biomechanics, 2nd ed.,
edited by Van C. Mow and Wilson C. Hayes.
Lippincott–Raven Publishers, Philadelphia © 1997.

3

Biomechanics of Cortical and Trabecular Bone: Implications for Assessment of Fracture Risk

Wilson C. Hayes and Mary L. Bouxsein

Department of Orthopedic Surgery, Harvard Medical School, and Orthopedic Biomechanics Laboratory, Beth Israel Deaconess Medical Center, Boston, Massachusetts 02215

Bone is the primary structural element of the human body. It serves to protect vital internal organs and provides a framework that allows the skeletal motions that are necessary for survival. Bone is also unique among structural materials in that it is self-repairing and can alter its properties and geometry in response to changes in mechanical demand (70, 145,152,153). Although the hypertrophy that occurs in skeletal muscle in response to heavy exercise or disuse is obvious, it is less apparent that bone is also remarkably responsive to the mechanical demands imposed. Bone density reductions are known to occur with aging, disuse, and certain metabolic conditions. Increased bone density occurs with heavy exercise and after treatment with certain therapeutic agents. Moreover, changes in bone geometry are observed during fracture heal-

ing, with aging, with exercise, and after certain operative procedures. Understanding these phenomena, which appear to be adaptive, stress-related events, has been a central focus of bone physiology and biomechanics for over a century.

Many of these adaptive phenomena appear to be directed toward restoring and maintaining the structural integrity of the skeleton despite changes in the mechanical environment—a kind of biomechanical homeostasis. Fracture healing and increased bone density with chronic exercise are obvious examples. Less obvious is the possibility that the cross-sectional geometry of long bones might change with aging in order to compensate for age-related reductions in bone density and mechanical properties. In fact, epidemiologic evidence indicates that the reductions in bone density and strength that are known to occur with age in cortical bone are not accompanied by dramatic increases in the incidence of shaft fractures among the elderly, suggesting that compensatory mechanisms are, in fact, at work. However, such homeostatic, compensatory mechanisms do not appear to be sufficient to protect the aging skeleton against fractures at other skeletal sites such as the hip, spine, and distal radius. The incidence of such fractures has increased dramatically in recent years.

Because of their associated mortality and morbidity, hip fractures are a cause for particular concern. In the United States alone, more than 250,000 hip fractures and 500,000 vertebral fractures occur each year among persons over 45 (120). Nearly 33% of women and more than 17% of men will experience a hip fracture if they live to age 90. Death rates in patients with a hip fracture are 12% to 20% higher than those in persons of similar age, race, and sex (68,69,73,78,96,149). The estimated annual cost of medical and nursing services related to hip fractures is over $10 billion (64,115,116a). Moreover, continued growth in the elderly population can be expected to cause the number of hip and vertebral fractures to increase dramatically, because fracture incidence rates increase exponentially with age. In fact, some have suggested that, if current demographic and incidence trends continue, the number of hip fractures may well double or triple by the middle of the next century (35,72). Comparable trends can be expected for vertebral fractures. By any measure, these age-related fractures are a public health problem of crisis proportions. Without successful national initiatives aimed at reducing their incidence, the implications for allocations of health resources in this and the next century are staggering.

The design and implementation of intervention efforts aimed at reducing the number of age-related fractures depends on an adequate understanding of those etiologic factors that cause the incidence rates of hip and vertebral fracture to increase among the elderly. Surprisingly, given the importance of the problem, there are fundamental questions about these etiologic factors, which remain unresolved. The predominant view is that age-related bone loss, or osteoporosis, is the most important determinant of fracture risk, and indeed, many studies have shown dramatic decreases with age in the density and strength of bone. Despite this, others have suggested that factors associated with the increased incidence of falling among the elderly make a more important contribution to fracture risk. Two lines of indirect evidence tend to support this view. First, most densitometric indicators of osteoporosis of the proximal femur have failed to discriminate between hip fracture patients and age- and gender-matched controls, a finding that suggests that other confounding factors must be at work. Second, intervention efforts designed to increase bone density through the use of estrogen replacement therapy, calcium supplementation, or exercise have at best yielded only modest reductions in hip fracture incidence.

In the face of this conflicting evidence, Melton and Riggs (94) suggested that *both* reduced skeletal strength and an increased propensity for fall-related trauma among the elderly are together important determinants of age-related fracture risk. However, the relative importance of age-related bone strength reductions and increased traumatic loading is unclear (54). If the relative risk associated with age-related reductions in bone strength were shown to be dominant, then intervention efforts aimed at maintaining bone density would appear to be appropriate. If, however, trauma associated with falling were shown to dominate hip fracture risk, then the focus should be on intervention efforts designed to reduce the high incidence of falls or the severity of those falls that do occur.

To a significant extent, data are available that allow us to address this question of relative risk. The mechanical properties of both cortical and trabecular bone and how they change with age and reductions in density are relatively well understood. Information is also available on the geometric changes in long bones that occur with age. There is also a growing body of data on the strength of whole bones and of certain subregions such as the proximal femur and vertebrae. Evidence is also becoming available regarding the forces to which skeletal regions such as the hip and spine are subjected, both during the activities of daily living and as a result of a traumatic event such as a fall. Viewed in the appropriate context, these data allow some preliminary inferences regarding the relative risk associated with bone loss and trauma in the etiology of hip and vertebral fracture among the elderly.

To provide this context, this chapter begins with an introduction to the structure and composition of bone and then summarizes, from the engineering discipline known as strength of materials, the concepts that can be used to describe the mechanical behavior and failure characteristics of bone as a tissue and of whole bones as structures. With this material as background, some of the most important data on the tissue-level mechanical properties of cortical and trabecular bone are reviewed, emphasizing what is known about age-related changes in these properties. Data from the use of noninvasive imaging techniques such as quantitative computed tomography (QCT) to determine mechanical properties of trabecular and cortical bone are also reviewed. This is followed by a summary of the available data on the structural behavior of whole bones, focusing in particular on fracture of the proximal femur and vertebrae and on the use of dual-energy x-ray absorptiometry (DXA) to estimate fracture risk of these regions. Then, based on these data, we return to the question of age-related fractures and demonstrate what inferences can be drawn regarding mechanisms that appear to protect the elderly against shaft fractures but allow dramatic increases in incidence rates for fractures of the hip and spine (3).

STRUCTURE AND COMPOSITION OF BONE

Bone is one of a number of the connective tissues described elsewhere in this volume. As with the other connective tissues, bone tissue consists of cells embedded in a fibrous organic matrix (in this case, osteoid), which is primarily collagen (90%) and 10% amorphous ground substance (primarily glycosaminoglycans and glycoproteins). Osteoid comprises approximately 50% of bone by volume and 25% by weight. The characteristic rigidity and strength of bone derive from the presence of mineral salts that permeate the organic matrix. The mineral phase comprises approximately 50% of bone by volume and 75% by weight. The principal constituents of bone mineral are calcium phosphate and calcium carbonate, with lesser quantities of sodium, magnesium, and fluoride. The mineral components consist mainly of hydroxyapatite $[Ca_{10}(PO_4)_6(OH)_2]$ crystals and amorphous calcium phosphate. Bone apatite crystals are approximately 50 to 100 angstroms (Å) long and are arranged in an orderly pattern within the collagen network.

Bone collagen is the same type I collagen found in dermis, tendon, and fascia. Because of the presence of stable intermolecular cross-links, bone collagen is extremely insoluble in the solvents commonly used to extract collagen from connective tissues. The cells of bone include osteoblasts (bone-forming cells), osteoclasts (bone-resorbing cells), and osteocytes (bone-maintaining cells). Osteocytes represent osteoblasts trapped by secretion of the extracellular matrix. During bone formation, uncalcified osteoid is secreted by osteoblasts. Hydroxyapatite crystals then precipitate in an orderly fashion around collagen fibers present in the osteoid. Although the osteoid rapidly becomes about 70% calcified within a few days, maximal calcification occurs only after several months.

Whole bones are composed of two types of bony tissue (Fig. 1). Cortical bone comprises the diaphysis of long bones and the thin shell that surrounds the metaphyses. Trabecular bone in the metaphyses and epiphyses is continuous with the inner surface of the metaphyseal shell and exists as a three-dimensional, interconnected network of trabecular rods and plates. The trabeculae divide the interior into intercommunicating pores of varying dimensions, thereby resulting in a struc-

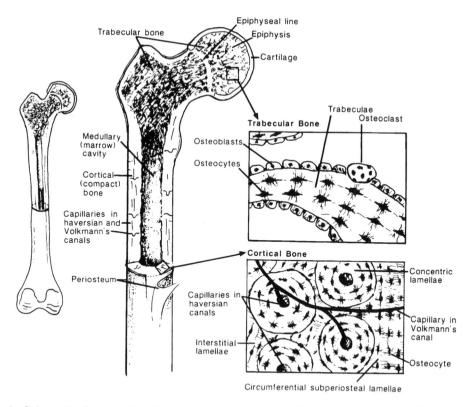

FIG. 1. Schematic diagram of cortical and trabecular bone. (From Hayes, ref. 59, with permission.)

ture of variable porosity and density. A network of rods produces low-density, open cells, while a network of plates can result in higher density, nearly closed cells (50). The classification of bone tissue as cortical or trabecular is based on relative density, i.e., the ratio of specimen density to that of fully dense cortical bone (usually assumed to have a density of 1.8 g/cc). The relative density of trabecular bone varies from 0.05 to about 0.7, corresponding to porosities that range from about 30% to more than 90%. The relative density of cortical bone ranges from about 0.7 to about 0.95. Obviously, the distinction between low-density cortical bone and high-density trabecular bone is somewhat arbitrary.

During growth and throughout life, there is a continuous and highly regulated process of bone resorption by osteoclasts followed by osteoblastic deposition of new bone. All bone formed by this process is called secondary bone to distinguish it from the first bone (primary bone) formed in a region through endochondral ossification or direct subperiosteal deposition. Three types of primary bone are found in humans: (a) circumferential lamellar bone; (b) woven-fibered bone; and (c) primary osteons. At birth, cortical bone consists largely of woven-fibered bone with randomly arranged collagen bundles and large, irregularly shaped vascular spaces lined with osteoblasts. The osteoblasts deposit successive layers (lamellae) of new bone and thus progressively reduce the volume of the vascular spaces. The resulting convoluted areas occupying what were previously vascular channels are called primary osteons. These primary osteons are generally (but not always) parallel to the long bone axis and may contain one to several vascular canals. On the periosteal surface, the diameter of long bone is increased during growth by the deposition of new primary lamellar bone consisting of an orderly arrangement of collagen fibers.

In the adult, remodeling continually changes the internal architecture of bone. The process is initiated by osteoclastic resorption to create longitudinally oriented tubular channels. Osteoblasts on the surfaces of these channels then deposit successive layers of lamellar bone until the diameter of the cavity is reduced to a small, singular vascular canal. The newly formed layered lamellar cylinders surrounding a longitudinally oriented vascular canal are called secondary osteons or Haversian systems. Unlike primary osteons, secondary osteons are always bounded by cement lines formed where osteoclastic activity ceases and osteoblastic bone formation begins. Such cement lines are strongly basophilic, contain little or no collagen, and exhibit a high content of inorganic matrix. The irregular areas of bone between secondary osteons are referred to as interstitial bone and consist of the remnants of woven-fibered bone, circumferential lamellar bone, or primary and secondary osteons that previously occupied the area.

Normal cortical bone in the adult human consists of regions of secondary osteons bounded on the endosteal and periosteal surface by circumferential lamellar bone. Woven-fibered bone is found only during rapid bone formation such as with fracture healing, hyperparathyroidism, and Paget's disease. Lamellar bone consists of alternating sheets (each with a characteristic collagen fiber orientation) of about 7 μm thickness separated by thin interlamellar cement layers of about 0.1 μm thickness. Thus, at both the microstructural level (where osteons and circumferential lamellae are formed from layers of fibers with alternating orientations) and at the whole bone level (where the diaphysis is formed by longitudinally oriented secondary osteons), cortical bone exhibits a number of the features of fiber-reinforced engineering composites.

The microstructural features of trabecular bone have received considerably less attention than those of cortical bone. Individual trabecular plates and rods are composed primarily from interstitial bone of varying composition, although on occasion lamellar trabecular plates and osteonal trabecular rods are found. The architectural features of trabecular bone are remarkably similar to porous engineering foams, and indeed, many of the features of its mechanical behavior can be described using techniques first developed for characterizing the mechanical behavior of porous foams (49,50). It has also long been suspected that the morphology and density of trabecular bone are related to the stresses imposed during the activities of daily living (39,145,152). Although the laws by which form follows function have not been comprehensively described, the general assumption is that the direction of trabecular orientation is related to the directions in which the imposed stresses reach maximum and minimum values (principal directions). If the loads are about equal in all directions, trabecular bone tends to form approximately equiaxed cells. If one load is much larger then the others, the trabecular cell walls tend to align and thicken in the directions that will best support the load (50). It is also generally accepted that the density of trabecular bone depends on the magnitude of the imposed load. In regions where trabecular loading is low, trabeculae tend to form a rodlike network of open cells. As the loads increase, the cell walls thicken and spread so that they resemble perforated plates (50). However, there is considerable uncertainty as to which of the many time-varying loads the bone experiences most influences trabecular architecture. It has also been suggested that mechanisms exist for integrating loading information so that trabecular architecture and density are influenced by both the number and magnitude of loading cycles (6,7,20).

BASIC BIOMECHANICAL CONCEPTS

The relationships between the mechanical behavior of bone tissue as a material and the structural behavior of whole bones suggests that the biomechanics of bone should be approached at two levels (60,61,71). At the tissue level, standardized mechanical tests on uniform specimens of bone can be performed to determine the material properties of the tissue. The structural behavior of whole bones or bone subregions (which represent organized constructs of bone tissues in complex geometric arrangements) can also be studied. In this context, bone fracture represents failure of both bone tissue at the material level and the whole bone at the structural level. To understand the complex relationships between failure of bone tissue and fracture of the whole bone requires a critical analytic step involving calculation of the internal stresses (force intensities) in the whole bone. This step in turn involves knowledge of the material properties of the involved tissues and of the geometric features of the whole bone and of the loads being applied. Once the internal stresses are known, they can be compared to the strength properties of bone tissue to provide an assessment of fracture risk. Thus, the process of failure (or fracture) prediction involves: (a) characterization of tissue-level material properties; (b) information on bone geometry; (c) knowledge of the loads being applied; (d) an analysis (which incorporates geometric and loading information) of the internal stresses; and (e) a comparison of the predicted stresses against the known strength properties at the tissue level. If the predicted stresses exceed the known strengths, the bone is at high risk of fracture under the assumed loading conditions.

In the next sections we define some of the biomechanical concepts required to predict bone fracture (and thus assess fracture risk) under a variety of simplified loading conditions. We first use the simple case of axial loading in tension to define stress, strain, modulus, and strength and to contrast the material behavior of bone as a tissue with the structural behavior of whole bones. We then examine bending and torsional loading as ways to introduce important geometric concepts that can be used to characterize the geometry of long bones.

Axial Loading: Material Versus Structural Behavior

When forces are applied to any solid object, the object is deformed from its original dimensions. At the same time, internal forces are produced within the object. The relative deformations created at any point are referred to as the *strains* at that point. The internal force intensities (force/area) are referred to as the *stresses* at that point. When a bone is subjected to forces, these stresses and strains are introduced throughout the structure and can vary in a complex manner. To avoid some of these complexities and demonstrate some important mechanical concepts, it is useful to focus on a regular structure loaded under well-defined conditions (Fig. 2a). Similar specimens of regular geometry are used to determine the material properties of bone tissue.

In Fig. 2a, a cylindrical bar of length L and a constant cross-sectional area (A) is shown subjected to pure tensile force (F). As load is applied, the cylinder begins to stretch. This situation can be described by analogy to the simple equation that describes stretching of a spring:

$$F = kx \tag{1}$$

where F is the applied force, x is the change in length or elongation of the spring, and k is the spring constant or stiffness of the spring. Inverting this simple relationship ($x = F/k$) demonstrates that with a very stiff spring (high k), the elongation x is small for a given applied force. The analogous relation for stretching of the cylinder is:

$$\Delta L = FL/AE \tag{2}$$

where (ΔL) is the elongation of the cylinder, L is the original unstretched length, A is the cross-sectional area, F is the force, and E is a factor (which we will subsequently define as the modulus) that describes whether the material is rigid (such as with steel) or flexible (as with rubber). According to the simple relationship shown in equation 2, the elongation (ΔL) is directly proportional to the applied force and to the original length and inversely

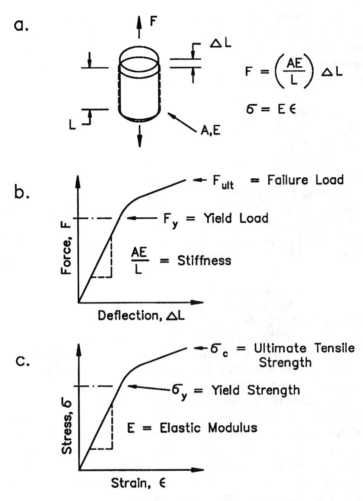

a.

$$F = \left(\frac{AE}{L}\right) \Delta L$$

$$\sigma = E \epsilon$$

b.

F_{ult} = Failure Load

F_y = Yield Load

$\frac{AE}{L}$ = Stiffness

Force, F

Deflection, ΔL

c.

σ_c = Ultimate Tensile Strength

σ_y = Yield Strength

E = Elastic Modulus

Stress, σ

Strain, ϵ

FIG. 2. Material versus structural behavior: **(a)** compressive loading of a cylinder of trabecular bone (with length L and cross-sectional area A) results in a deflection ΔL; **(b)** plot of force versus deflection defines structural behavior because specimen geometry influences the stiffness AE/L and the ultimate load F_{ult}; **(c)** plot of stress versus strain defines material (or tissue-level) behavior because the effects of geometry have been eliminated. (From Hayes et al., ref. 63, with permission.)

proportional to the cross-sectional area and to factor E. Note also from Fig. 2 and equation 2 that the total elongation (ΔL) depends both on the original length and on the cross-sectional area of the bar.

We can plot a force–deflection curve to represent the structural behavior of the cylindrical bar (Fig. 2b). A cylinder of bone tested in tension would yield a linear region (also known as the elastic region) followed by a nonlinear region where "yielding" occurs and there is an internal rearrangement of the structure, often involving damage accumulation. After yielding, nonelastic deformation occurs until finally fracture results in the loss of load-bearing capacity of the bar. The load at which yielding occurs is referred to as the yield load, F_y. The load at which failure occurs is called the ultimate or failure load, F_{ult}. It is particularly important to note that a force–deflection curve describes the behavior of the structure because the curve would differ for a cylindrical bar of different cross-sectional area or different length (eq. 2).

To provide a standardized representation of the mechanical behavior of the material (as opposed to the behavior of the structure), we plot a normalized curve known as a stress–strain curve (Fig. 2c). This normalizes the force–deformation relationship (i.e., eliminates the influence of the geometry of the cylinder) by dividing the applied force (F) by the cross-sectional area (A) and the deformation (ΔL) by the original length (L). We define this internal force intensity as stress (σ). The units of stress are Newtons per square meter (N/m^2) or Pascals (Pa). [1 N = 0.225 lb force; 1 Pa = 145.04×10^6 lb per square inch (psi).] We often express stress in terms of megapascals (MPa) (1 MPa = 1×10^{-6} Pa) or gigapascals (GPa) (1 GPa = 1×10^9 Pa).

The ratio of the elongation to the original length is defined as the strain (ε). Note that strain is a nondimensional quantity. In a stress–strain curve (Fig. 2c), the slope of the linear elastic region is referred to as the modulus (E). Because the modulus is defined as the slope of the stress–strain curve in the elastic region, and because the units of stress are megapascals and strain is nondimensional, the units of modulus are the same as those of stress (MPa or GPa). In the stress–strain curve, the material yields at a stress level known as the yield strength (again with units of megapascals). Ultimately, the material fractures at a stress level known as the fracture strength or ultimate tensile strength (units of megapascals). Note that the stress–strain representation allows us to compare different materials in terms of both the slope of the stress–strain curve and these strength parameters. From such stress–strain curves, the modulus of steel is shown to be approximately 10 times that of cortical bone. The ultimate tensile strength of steel is approximately five times that of cortical bone.

Example 1. Axial stiffness. The results of a nondestructive (i.e., fully elastic) tensile test of a small circular cylinder of bone removed from the femoral diaphysis of an adult man yields the force–deformation curve shown in Fig. 2b. Assume that the cylinder is of cross-sectional area A, length L, and modulus E.

What happens to the force–deformation curve when we cut the specimen in half (so that L becomes $L/2$) and repeat the test? Derive an expression for the ratio of the new to the old slopes of the two force–deformation curves.

Solution. Rewriting equation 1 in the form ($y = mx$) where m is the slope, we have

$$F = (AE/L)\Delta L$$

The slope (AE/L) of the force–deformation curve is known as the *axial stiffness*. Written this way, it is immediately apparent that the slope increases directly with increasing A and E and decreases with increasing L. Thus, the ratio of the new to the old axial stiffness is

$$m'/m = [AE/(L/2)]/(AE/L) = 2$$

The axial stiffness of the shorter cylinder is therefore twice that of the original. It is therefore immediately apparent that different force–deformation curves result from cylinders of different geometries even though the material (as reflected by the modulus E) remains the same. Thus, a force–deformation curve describes structural behavior since it reflects not only the material but also the geometry of the specimen. By contrast, a stress–strain curve describes only the material behavior because the geometric influences have been eliminated by the normalization process.

Beam Bending: Areal Moment of Inertia

Bones of the appendicular skeleton are long, slender, slightly curved elements that are loaded primarily by compressive forces applied at the joints. Because of this gentle curvature, bones are subjected to a combination of axial compressive forces and bending forces. It is therefore instructive to focus first on these two loading cases separately and then to examine how these load cases can combine to produce the general loading patterns of whole bones. We have already discussed the axial loading case for tension (Fig. 2). Compressive loading is analogous except that the deformation ΔL is now a shortening of the rod. The magnitude of this shortening is still given by $\Delta L = FL/AE$, with the associated compressive stress being given by F/A. By convention, compressive stresses are assumed to be negative, and tensile stresses are positive.

In engineering, long slender structures that are designed to resist transverse or bending loads are referred to as *beams*. Examples are the I-beams commonly used in civil engineering structures such as bridges or highway overpasses. Such beams are long in comparison to their cross-sectional dimensions and, for this reason, are similar to the long bones of the appendicular skeleton. A beam can be subjected to bending loads in a number of ways, including the application of two sets of forces near the beam ends (Fig. 3). This loading configuration, known as four-point bending, subjects the central section of the beam to a constant bending moment (of M = Fa) and is often used in the laboratory for studying the biomechanics of fracture healing. To make this loading situation clearer, imagine grasping a meterstick near its ends in such a way that the thumb and fingers apply the forces and the meterstick is flexed into a bowed shape. The deflection of the midpoint of the beam can be found from elementary strength of materials and is tabulated in engineering handbooks. The midspan deflection is given by the relationship shown in Fig. 3 involving the geometric characteristics of the beam and the location of the applied forces (as expressed by L and a), the magnitude of applied forces, the modulus E of the beam material, and a new quantity I known as the *areal moment of inertia*. This geometric parameter expresses the characteristics of the distribution of the cross-sectional area in relation to a transverse axis. It reflects, for instance, the large differences in bending resistance of the meterstick bent when it is held flat versus when it is held on edge. We return below to a further discussion of this geometric parameter.

Note, however, that there are similarities between the expressions used to characterize axial and flexural loadings (eq. 2 and Fig. 3). In both cases, the deformations are directly proportional to the applied forces and to certain geometric features of the structure. In both cases, the deformations are inversely proportional to a combination of parameters reflecting material stiffness E and a geometric feature of the cross section. In axial loading, we called this combination AE the *axial rigidity*. In bending (or flexure) we call this combination EI, the *flexural rigidity*.

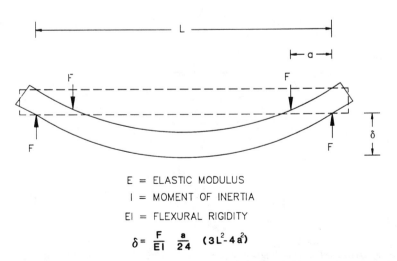

E = ELASTIC MODULUS
I = MOMENT OF INERTIA
EI = FLEXURAL RIGIDITY

$$\delta = \frac{F}{EI} \frac{a}{24} (3L^2 - 4a^2)$$

FIG. 3. Flexural (bending) loading of a beam. The midspan deflection is inversely proportional to the flexural rigidity, *EI*. (From Hayes and Gerhart, ref. 61, with permission.)

To visualize the internal forces or stresses that occur in a beam, imagine holding the ends of the meterstick and bending it so as to produce a convex surface on one side and a concave surface on the other side. It can be shown that the material on the convex side of the beam is subjected to tensile (or stretching) strains. The material on the concave side is subjected to compressive strains. This suggests that at some point between the two surfaces, the strains are zero (i.e., the original length of the beam is unchanged). This location is referred to as the neutral axis. For a beam of one material, the *neutral axis* is at the geometric centroid of the beam. The strains produced at any cross section of the beam also result in stresses at that cross section. The concave side of the beam is subjected to compressive stresses while the convex side experiences tensile stresses (Fig. 4). It can be shown from elementary strength of materials that the linear variation in stress across the cross section is given by

$$\sigma = \pm My/I \tag{3}$$

where M is the bending moment at the cross section, y is the distance from the neutral axis, and I is the areal moment of inertia. The $\pm$ sign is used to indicate that one surface of the beam is subjected to tensile stress (+) and one to compression (−). Notice that the maximum stresses are experienced by the material on the surface of the beam. If the bending forces are increased until the beam begins to fracture, the fracture will be initiated at the surface of the beam where the stresses are highest. For a beam in four-point bending (Fig. 3), the bending moment $M = aF$, and thus the maximum bending stress, is given by

$$\sigma = \pm Fac/I \tag{4}$$

where F is the applied force, a is the distance between the forces applied at each end, c is the distance from the neutral axis to the beam surface, and I is the areal moment of inertia. The $\pm$ sign is again used to indicate that one

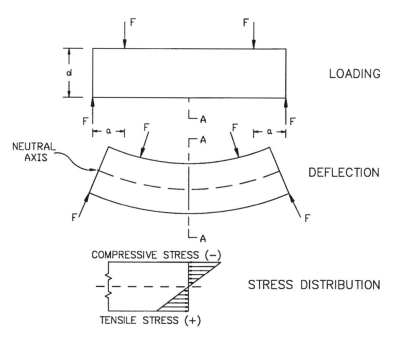

FIG. 4. Stresses associated with flexural loading of beams. Tensile stresses are generated on the convex surface, and compressive stresses on the concave surface. The unstressed central region is referred to as the neutral axis. (From Hayes and Gerhart, ref. 61, with permission.)

surface of the beam is in tension (+) and the other in compression (−).

Because bones are slightly curved and are subjected to compressive loads applied at the joint surfaces, the most common loading situation *in vivo* is a combination of compressive and bending loads. Bending loads arise because the compressive loads do not act through the center of the beam. The resulting stresses on a transverse section through a slightly curved member can be found by summing the stresses caused by the compressive axial forces and by the bending stresses (Fig. 5). As a result of the addition of the compressive stresses from axial loading and the compressive stresses from bending, even higher compressive stresses are created on the concave side of the bar, while the convex side experiences either reduced tensile stresses or even compressive stresses, depending on the magnitude of the axial force and its eccentricity, e, defined as the distance from the center of the beam to the line of action of the applied compressive loads. These stresses can be described with reasonable accuracy by simply combining the stresses caused by axial compression with those from bending:

(combined stress) = (compressive stress) ± (bending stress)

In mathematical terms, this can be written

$$\sigma = -F/A \pm My/I \qquad (5)$$

where, as above, F is the eccentrically applied axial load, A is the cross-sectional area,

M is the bending moment at the cross section, y is the distance from the center of the beam, and I is the moment of inertia. Note that at y = 0 (the neutral axis for pure bending), the bending stress does not contribute to the combined stress. For the case of eccentric axial loading, M is given by eF, and thus, equation 5 becomes

$$\sigma = -F/A \pm eFy/I \qquad (6)$$

where e is the distance from the center of the beam to the line of action of the force F.

Example 2. Neutral axis in combined compression and bending. Note that in Fig. 5, the neutral axis (line of zero stress) is different for combined loading than for pure bending. The compressive load causes a shift in the neutral axis through a distance of, say, y_0. Derive an expression for y_0 and determine the distances from the neutral axis for combined loading to the tensile (c_1) and compressive (c_2) surfaces of the beam. For given values of I and A, find the value of e that would ensure that the combined stresses are completely compressive.

Solution. Noting that the neutral axis is the point at which the combined axial and bending stresses are equal to zero, we have from equation 6 (assuming y to be positive)

$$F/A = eFy/I, \text{ at } y = y_0$$

or

$$y_0 = I/eA$$

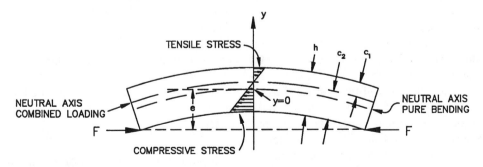

FIG. 5. Stresses caused by eccentric axial compressive loading of a slightly curved beam. Because of the eccentricity of the applied load, stresses related to axial compression and bending are combined, resulting in reduced tensile stresses on the convex surface and increased compressive stresses on the concave surface. (From Hayes, ref. 59, with permission.)

Thus, the location of the neutral axis depends on the ratio of I/A as well as on the eccentricity, e, of the applied load. To determine c_1, we note that the beam depth is h, and thus,

$$c_1 = h/2 - y_0 = h/2 - I/eA$$
$$c_2 = h/2 + I/eA$$

The combined stresses are completely compressive when $c_1 = 0$. Substituting in the above relationship for c_1 gives

$$e = 2I/Ah$$

This relationship indicates that for a beam of given geometry (as defined by the area, moment of inertia, and beam depth), there is a value of load eccentricity that will result in fully compressive axial stresses across the entire beam cross section.

From equation 6 and Example 2, we see that the maximum tensile stress, which occurs on the convex surface of the beam, is

$$\sigma_t = -F/A + eF(h/2)/I \qquad (7a)$$

The maximum compressive stress, which occurs on the concave surface, is given by

$$\sigma_c = -F/A - eF(h/2)/I \qquad (7b)$$

Note particularly that the compressive stresses from axial loading and bending are of the same sign (additive) while the two contributions to stresses on the tensile surface are of opposite sign (Fig. 5). Therefore, the magnitude of the maximum compressive stress is larger than the maximum tensile stress. Also, these relationships for the stresses in an eccentrically loaded beam reflect a number of geometric features that describe the loading and the beam. Such features include both the cross-sectional area and the moment of inertia, the eccentricity of the applied load, and the distances from the center of the beam to the convex and concave surfaces of the beam. Similar situations occur in long bones, and, in general, compressive stresses are higher than tensile stresses throughout the appendicular skeleton.

The moment of inertia I expresses the shape of the cross section and the particular distribution of the cross-sectional area with respect to the neutral axis of bending. This statement is important because it suggests that the moment of inertia must always be expressed with relation to a particular axis. Expressions for the moments of inertia for several regular geometric cross sections (calculated with respect to a transverse axis through the centroid or center of the area) are shown in Fig. 6. Methods for calculating moments of inertia can also be found in any text on elementary strength of materials. Such calculations are equivalent to dividing the cross-sectional area into small elemental areas, multiplying each area by the square of its distance to the axis of interest, and then summing over all elements. Thus, the moment of inertia is highly sensitive to the distribution of area with respect to the axis. An area that is at a greater distance from the neutral axis (i.e., the unstressed axis of the beam) is much more efficient in resisting bending with respect to that axis. These concepts demonstrate why a meterstick turned on edge resists bending more efficiently than a meterstick turned horizontally. The influence of the areal moment of inertia also explains why an I-beam (Fig. 6) is such an efficient section for resisting bending in one direction, because most of the material is located at a distance from the neutral axis.

Example 3. Bending deflection. Consider a wooden meterstick held near its ends so that the thumb and fingers each apply bending forces (Fig. 3) F of 10 N. Calculate the midspan deflection when the meterstick is bent against its strong axis and then against its weak axis. Assume the meterstick is 1.0 m long and that the distance between thumb and fingers is 0.1 m. In cross section the meterstick is 0.5 cm wide and has a depth of 2.5 cm. The modulus of wood is 10,000 MPa.

Solution. From Fig. 3, the midspan deflection for a beam in four-point bending is given by

$$\delta = F/EI \, a(3L^2 - 4a^2)/24$$

From Fig. 6, the moment of inertia I about the neutral axis x–x of a rectangular cross section of width w and depth d is

$$I = wd^3/12$$

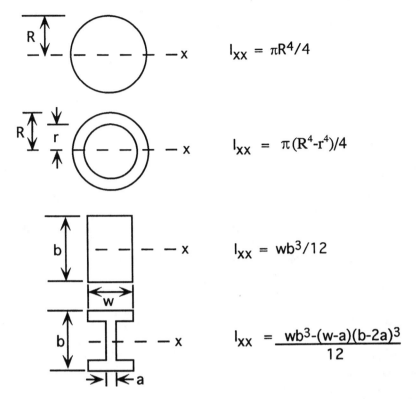

$$I_{xx} = \pi R^4/4$$

$$I_{xx} = \pi(R^4 - r^4)/4$$

$$I_{xx} = wb^3/12$$

$$I_{xx} = \frac{wb^3 - (w-a)(b-2a)^3}{12}$$

FIG. 6. Moments of inertia for some common structural cross sections. (From Hayes, ref. 59, with permission.)

When the meterstick is bent against its strong axis, $d = 2.5$ cm (0.025 m) and $w = 0.5$ cm (0.005 m), and therefore, $I = (0.005)(0.025)^3/12 = 6.5 \times 10^{-9}$ m^4.

When the meterstick is bent against its weak axis, $d = 0.5$ cm and $w = 2.5$ m. In this case, $I = (0.025)(0.005)^3/12 = 2.6 \times 10^{-10}$ m^4.

Substituting the appropriate values into the equation for midspan deflection yields, for the case of bending against the strong axis, $\delta = 0.0019$ m, and for the case of bending against the weak axis, $\delta = 0.0474$ m. Thus, the midspan deflection is nearly 5 cm when the meterstick is bent against its weak axis and less than 2 mm when it is bent against its strong axis, a ratio of about 25:1! This example thus emphasizes the importance of the distribution of cross-sectional area (as reflected by the moment of inertia) when long, thin members (such as bones) are subjected to bending forces.

If bones were subjected to bending loads in only one direction, their cross-sectional shapes would probably have evolved toward something like an I-beam. Instead, long bones are loaded, as suggested above, by axial compression, bending (in multiple directions), and torsion. Under these conditions, the most efficient cross-sectional shape is one that approximates a cylindrical tube. A tubular structure can better distribute the stresses imposed by bending and torsional loading than can a solid bar of the same cross-sectional area because the material is distributed at a greater distance from the center of the beam.

Example 4. Compressive and bending strength: Changes with aging. Consider the case of three cylindrical rods of different cross-sectional geometries, shown on page 82. Bar A is a solid cylinder and has a radius of 0.94 cm. Bar B is a hollow tube of outer radius 1.09 cm and inner radius 0.53 cm. Bar C is

A   **B**   **C**

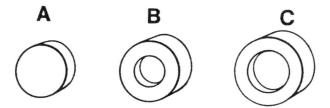

also a hollow tube, but in this instance both the outer radius and the inner radius have been increased to 1.25 cm and 0.76 cm, respectively. What are the areas and moments of inertia of these simple shapes, and how do the compressive and bending strengths of the tubular cross sections compare to those of the solid cylinder? Note that the cross-sectional area is given by $A = \pi r^2$ for the solid cylinder and $A = \pi(r_o^2 - r_i^2)$ for the cylindrical tube. The cross-sectional areas are thus 2.77 cm^2, 2.85 cm^2, and 3.09 cm^2 for A, B, and C, respectively.

Solution. Because the tensile and compressive strengths are inversely proportional to the cross-sectional area ($\sigma = -F/A$), bars A and B exhibit similar compressive and tensile strengths. Bar C is increased in strength, but only by about 11%. The formulas for the moment of inertia of both solid and cylindrical tubes are given in Fig. 6. In this case, the moments of inertia are 0.61 cm^4, 1.06 cm^4, and 1.66 cm^4 for bars A, B, and C, respectively. As noted in equation 3, the flexural formula indicates that the maximum tensile stress on the surface of a beam is given by $\sigma = Fac/I$, where F is the applied force, a is the distance between the two forces applied at each end of the beam, c is the distance from the neutral axis to the surface of the beam, and I is the moment of inertia of the cross section. If Fa is constant for each case, the quantity c/I determines the relative bending strengths for each geometry. The values of c/I are 1.54, 1.03, and 0.75 cm^{-3} for A, B, and C, respectively, indicating that the stresses are highest in the solid bar and are progressively reduced in bars B and C.

Thus, the more favorable distribution of the cross-sectional area results in increases in bending strengths by factors of 1.49 and

2.05 for bars B and C. In particular, the changes in inner and outer radii for tube C in comparison to B result in an increase in bending strength by a factor of about 1.37. These idealized cross-sectional geometries are based on the approximate dimensions of the human femoral midshaft in an archaeologic sample (126–128). The geometries for bars B and C approximate the changes in cross-sectional properties that occur between young adults and the elderly in both ancient and modern populations. These values therefore suggest that, with aging, there are increases in both the periosteal and endosteal geometries of the long bones. Although this age-related remodeling results in only minor changes in cross-sectional area, it is associated with marked increases in moment of inertia and therefore with increases in bending strength (by almost 40% in this simple example). Thus, if age-related changes also result in reductions in the tensile strength of bone tissue (as we will see below), this geometric remodeling process would tend to compensate for those strength reductions and thereby help maintain a bone structure of approximately constant strength.

Torsion: Polar Moment of Inertia

If a bar is subjected to twisting moments (also called torques) applied at its ends (Fig. 7), the cross section at one end rotates with respect to the cross section at the other end. From elementary strength of materials, the total angle of twist, Φ, is given by

$$\Phi = Tl/GJ \qquad (8)$$

where Φ is the angle of twist (in radians; 2π radians = 360°), T is the torque (in Newton-

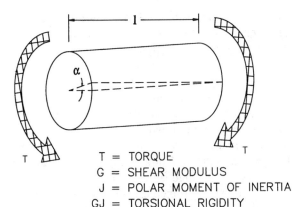

T = TORQUE
G = SHEAR MODULUS
J = POLAR MOMENT OF INERTIA
GJ = TORSIONAL RIGIDITY
α/l = T/GJ

FIG. 7. Variation of strength ratio with stiffness ratio for fractures tested after 5 weeks. The slope of the line indicates that the stiffness of the fracture returns to normal more rapidly than does the strength. (From Hayes, ref. 59, with permission.)

meters), l is the length of the bar (in meters), G is the shear modulus (in Newtons per square meter), and J is the polar moment of inertia. The shear modulus G is a measure of the resistance of a material to shearing deformations and is analogous to the use of Young's modulus to characterize the resistance to tensile or compressive deformations. For most materials, the shear modulus is about one-half the Young's modulus. The polar moment of inertia, like the areal moment of inertia, expresses how the material in a cross-section is distributed with reference to a defined axis. In the case of the areal moment of inertia, the axis (the neutral axis) is in the plane of the cross section (Fig. 6). In the case of torsion, the polar moment of inertia describes the distribution of the cross-sectional area with respect to an axis perpendicular to the cross section (and corresponding to the longitudinal, centroidal axis of the bar). For a solid, cylindrical bar of diameter d, the polar moment of inertia is given by

$$J = \pi d^4/32 \qquad (9)$$

Example 5. Polar moment of inertia of a cylindrical tube. From the known relationship for the polar moment of inertia of a solid cylinder, find the polar moment of inertia J of a cylindrical tube of outer diameter d_o and inner diameter d_i. Assuming $d_o = 2.5$ cm and $d_i = 1.5$ cm, how does J change if both d_o and d_i increase by 10%?

Solution. From equation 7, we have for the polar moment of inertia of a cylindrical tube

$$J = \pi(d_o^4 - d_i^4)/32$$

Substituting $d_o = 2.5$ cm (0.025m) and $d_i = 1.5$ cm (0.015m) gives

$$J_o = 3.34 \times 10^{-8} \text{ m}^4$$

Substituting $d_o = 2.75$ cm and $d_i = 1.65$ cm gives

$$J_i = 4.88 \times 10^{-8} \text{ m}^4$$

Therefore, the percentage increase in J is 46.4%. Thus, a 10% increase in the outer and inner diameter of a cylindrical tube increases the polar moment of inertia by nearly 50%. As we will see below, age-related changes in periosteal and endosteal diameters of long bone diaphyses serve to increase the polar moment of inertia and thereby may serve to help compensate for age-related reductions in the material properties of cortical bone.

MECHANICAL PROPERTIES OF BONE TISSUE

Material Properties of Cortical Bone

The fracture behavior of whole bones is strongly dependent on the material behavior of bone tissue. To determine the mechanical properties of bone tissue, small uniform specimens are loaded under well-defined conditions. As shown in Fig. 2, such testing conditions produce uniform, known stresses throughout the specimen. Specimen deformation can then be measured and the strains calculated using the relationships for stress and strain. The material properties of the tissue can thus be determined for the specific loading conditions imposed. With other modes of loading, this general approach to materials testing has allowed documentation of cortical bone material properties in tension, compression, bending, and torsion (17–19,24,32,40,41,47,48,58,60,89,117,118, 134,154,155).

Several factors influence the material properties of cortical bone. One factor is the rate at which the bone tissue is loaded. A specimen of cortical bone that is loaded very rapidly exhibits increased elastic modulus and ultimate strength compared to a specimen that is loaded more slowly. To quantify the rate of deformation, one can refer to the strain rate (units = sec^{-1}) to which the tissue is exposed during the loading process. In normal activi-

ties, bone is subjected to strain rates that are generally below 0.01 sec^{-1}. Materials such as bone, for which stress–strain characteristics and strength properties depend on the applied strain rate, are said to be *viscoelastic* (or time-dependent) materials. However, this rate dependency is relatively weak (155). The elastic modulus and ultimate strength of bone are approximately proportional to the strain rate raised to the 0.06 power (Fig. 8). Thus, over a very wide range of strain rates, the ultimate tensile strength increases by a factor of three, and the modulus increases by about a factor of two (155).

The stress–strain behavior of cortical bone is also strongly dependent on the orientation of the bone microstructure with respect to the direction of loading. Several investigators have demonstrated that cortical bone is stronger and stiffer in the longitudinal direction (direction of osteon orientation) than in the transverse direction. In addition, bone specimens loaded in a direction perpendicular to the osteons tend to fail in a more brittle manner, with little nonelastic deformation after yielding. Long

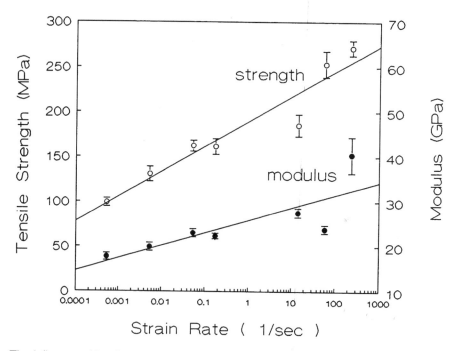

FIG. 8. The influence of loading rate on the tensile strength and modulus of cortical bone. The ultimate tensile strength increases by about a factor of 3, and the modulus by a factor of 2. (From Wright and Hayes, ref. 155, with permission.)

TABLE 1. *Strength of femoral cortical bone*[a]

Loading mode	Ultimate strength (MPa)
Longitudinal	
Tension	133
Compression	193
Shear	68
Transverse	
Tension	51
Compression	133

[a]Age span of population 19–80 years. From Hayes and Gerhart (61), with permission. Mean values from Reilly and Burstein (116b), with permission.

TABLE 2. *Modulus of femoral cortical bone*[a]

Longitudinal	17.0 GPa
Transverse	11.5 GPa
Shear	3.3 GPa

[a]Age span of population 19–80 years.
1GPa (gigapascal) = 1,000 MPa. From Hayes and Gerhart (61), with permission. Mean values from Reilly and Burstein (116b), with permission.

bones are therefore better able to resist stresses *along* the axis of the bone than across the bone axis. Material such as bone, for which elastic and strength properties are dependent on the direction of applied loading, are said to be *anisotropic* materials. The viscoelastic and anisotropic nature of cortical bone distinguish it as a complex material. Because of these characteristics, one must specify the strain rate and the direction of applied loading when describing material behavior.

Ultimate strengths of adult femoral cortical bone under various modes of loading in both the longitudinal and transverse directions (24, 117,118) are summarized in Table 1. These results indicate that the material strength of bone tissue depends on the type of loading as well as on the loading direction. The compressive strength is greater than the tensile strength in both longitudinal and transverse directions. Transverse specimens are weaker than longitudinal specimens in both tension and compression. The shear strength (determined by torsion tests about the longitudinal axis and reflecting shear stresses along transverse and longitudinal planes) is about one-third of the compressive strength. The modulus values for adult femoral cortical bone are shown in Table 2 (24,117,118). The longitudinal elastic modulus is about 50% greater than the transverse elastic modulus. The shear modulus for torsion about the longitudinal axis is about one-fifth the longitudinal modulus.

The material properties of cortical bone also decline with age (18) (Fig. 9). Both tensile strength and modulus decrease about 2%

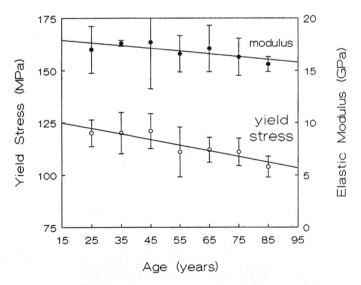

FIG. 9. Ultimate tensile strength and modulus versus age for human femoral cortical bone. (From Burstein et al., ref. 18, with permission.)

per decade over the age range 20 to 90. Thus, the ultimate tensile strength declines from 140 MPa in the third decade to 120 MPa in the ninth decade. Over the same period, the elastic modulus decreases from 17 GPa to 15.6 GPa (18).

Material Properties of Trabecular Bone

The major physical difference between trabecular bone and cortical bone is the increased porosity of trabecular bone. The porosity is reflected by measurements of the apparent density (i.e., the mass of bone tissue divided by the bulk volume of the test specimen, including mineralized bone and bone marrow spaces). In the human skeleton, the apparent density of trabecular bone ranges from approximately 0.1 g/cm³ to 1.0 g/cm³. The apparent density of cortical bone is about 1.8 g/cm³. A trabecular specimen with an apparent density of 0.2 g/cm³ has a porosity of approximately 90%.

Bone apparent density has a profound influence on the compressive stress–strain behavior of trabecular bone (21,22,49–51,66,71, 119,142) (Fig. 10). These stress–strain properties are markedly different from those of cortical bone and are similar to the compres-

sive behavior of many porous engineering materials that can be used to absorb energy on impact (50). The stress–strain curve for trabecular bone exhibits an initial elastic region followed by yield. Yielding occurs as the trabeculae begin to fracture. Yield is then followed by a long plateau region, which is created as progressively more and more trabeculae fracture. The fractured trabeculae begin to fill the marrow spaces, and, at a strain of approximately 0.50, most of the marrow spaces have filled with the debris of fractured trabeculae. Further loading of trabecular bone after pore closure is associated with a marked increase in specimen modulus. Figure 11a shows compressive strength data for trabecular bone from a wide variety of studies plotted against apparent density (50,63). The dependence of compressive strength on apparent density can be described by a power-law function of the form

$$\sigma_c = A\rho^B \qquad (10)$$

The data of Fig. 11A indicate that the compressive strength of trabecular bone is related to the square of the apparent density. Data for compressive modulus (Fig. 11B) indicate that the modulus is also related to apparent density by a power-law function with an exponent

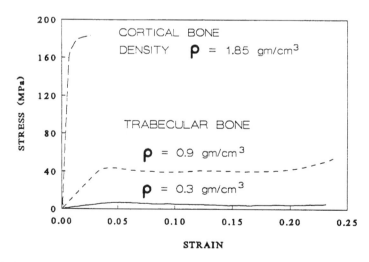

FIG. 10. Typical stress–strain curves for trabecular bone of different apparent densities. (From Hayes and Gerhart, ref. 61, with permission.)

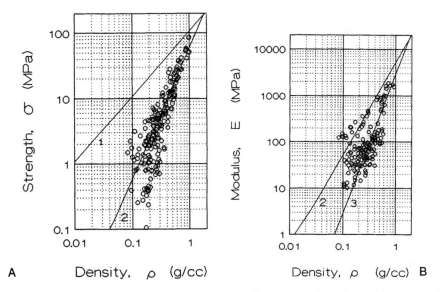

FIG. 11. Compressive strength and modulus of trabecular bone as functions of apparent density: **(A)** compressive strength varies as a power-law function of apparent density with an exponent of approximately 2; **(B)** compressive modulus also varies as a power-law function of apparent density with an exponent ranging between 2 and 3. (From Hayes et al., ref. 63, with permission.)

ranging between 2 and 3 (i.e., between a squared and a cubic relationship with density). Although these relationships were initially derived from compression tests, tensile tests of trabecular bone indicate that its strength in tension is approximately the same as that in compression (23). In addition, the elastic modulus of trabecular bone is approximately the same in both tensile and compressive loading.

These relationships between mechanical properties and the apparent density of bone tissue are of profound physiological and biomechanical importance. First, they indicate that bone tissue can generate large changes in modulus and strength through small changes in bone apparent density. Conversely, subtle changes in bone apparent density result in large differences in strength and modulus, a finding that indicates that order of magnitude reductions in trabecular strength and modulus can occur by the time density reductions of 30% to 50% are apparent radiographically.

Example 6. Trabecular bone properties: Effects of density. The regression lines shown in Fig. 11 indicate that the compressive strength

of trabecular bone is related to its apparent density by a power law of the form

$$\sigma = 60\rho^2$$

where σ is in megapascals and ρ is in grams per cubic centimeter. Similarly, the compressive modulus is approximately related to the apparent density by

$$E = 2915\rho^3$$

where E is in megapascals and ρ is again in grams per cubic centimeter (g/cc). Assuming that the initial apparent density of vertebral trabecular bone is 0.20 g/cc, what is the effect on compressive strength and modulus when the density decreases (as with aging) to 0.15 g/cc?

Solution. The above power-law relations indicate that for $\rho = 0.20$ g/cc, the compressive strength is $\sigma = 2.4$ MPa, and the compressive modulus is 23.3 MPa. A 25% reduction in apparent density to $\rho = 0.15$ g/cc results in a compressive strength of 1.35 MPa and a compressive modulus of 9.8 MPa. Thus, a 25% reduction in density is associated with a 44% reduction in strength and a 58% reduction in modulus. Note that these density values correspond to those measured in elderly cadaveric vertebrae (63,90,99). It is thus not surprising that vertebral compression fractures are common among the elderly and often occur before there is clear radiographic evidence of density reductions.

Material Property Estimates by Computed Tomography

To focus on the material or tissue-level behavior of cortical or trabecular bone, it is necessary to separate those effects related to changes in geometry from those related to changes in material behavior (61). Because of the potential importance of age-related reductions in cortical and trabecular density to the increased risk of fracture among the elderly, it is not surprising that many attempts have been made to use noninvasive radiographic techniques to estimate bone density and thereby predict material properties. In this regard, quantitative computed tomography (QCT) presents a number of significant advantages over other densitometric techniques such as single- or dual-photon absorptiometry, dual-energy x-ray absorptiometry, or conventional radiography. With the information available in QCT scans, it is possible to isolate densitometric and geometric changes in both cortical and trabecular compartments, whereas other radiographic modalities reflect combined densitometric and geometric variations along the scan path in both cortical and trabecular compartments. With QCT, the cross-sectional geometric information is directly available, and, with special calibration phantoms, densitometric data from both cortical and trabecular bone can be obtained in units that can be related directly to bone density and thereby to mechanical properties (74).

Quantitative Computed Tomography Versus Material Properties of Trabecular Bone

To establish correlations between QCT data and the compressive material properties of trabecular bone, scans are taken at defined locations, and then small specimens are removed and tested to determine elastic modulus and strength. Table 3 summarizes literature values for the relationships between modulus and either QCT data or direct measures of trabecular apparent density. Lang et al. (81) found only modest correlations between QCT measures of equivalent mineral density and compressive modulus using either linear ($r^2 = 0.32$) or power-law relations ($r^2 = 0.36$). Their modulus values ranged from 17.4 to 293 MPa (124 ± 76.3, SD, $n = 34$). Lotz et al. (85) found moderate to good power-law relationships in the proximal femur between compressive modulus and both QCT equivalent mineral density ($r^2 = 0.68$) (Fig. 12A) and directly measured apparent density ($r^2 = 0.67$). They reported modulus values for femoral trabecular bone of from 78 to 1530 MPa (441 ± 271, $n = 49$) and directly measured apparent density. Lang et al. (81) found an exponent of 2.44 for their power-law relation with equivalent mineral density, whereas Lotz et al. (85) found exponents of 2.3 and 1.2 for equivalent mineral density and apparent density, respectively. These values compare with the range of expo-

TABLE 3. *Elastic modulus versus QCT and density: femoral and vertebral trabecular bone[a]*

Authors	Location	Dependent variable	n	Relationship[b]	R^2	Relative error (%)
Lang et al. (81)	vert	QCT mg/cc	34	$E = (4.9 \times 10^{-4})\, x^{2.44} + 15.9$	0.36	45.0
Lotz et al. (85)	fem	app den	49	$E = 0.33x^{1.21} - 92$	0.67	36.1
	fem	QCT mg/cc	49	$E = (5.3 \times 10^{-4})x^{2.29} + 221$	0.68	35.5

[a]All significance levels $p < 0.001$. [b]Gives relationship between elastic modulus, *E,* and dependent variable. Abbreviations: app den, apparent density (mg/cc); fem, femur; vert, vertebra. From Hayes et al. (63), with permission.

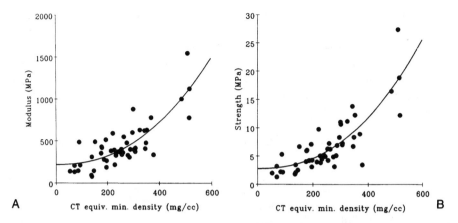

FIG. 12. Quantitative computed tomography versus modulus and strength for femoral trabecular bone: **(A)** compressive modulus, from Lotz et al. (85) ($r^2 = 0.68$, $p < 0.001$, Relative Error = 35.5%) and **(B)** compressive strength, from Lotz et al. (85) ($r^2 = 0.70$, $p < 0.001$, Relative Error = 39.9%). (From Hayes et al., ref. 63, with permission.)

nents for modulus versus density relations of between 2 and 3 shown in Fig. 11B.

Table 4 summarizes literature values for the relationship between trabecular compressive strength and either QCT data or direct measures of trabecular apparent density. Lang et al. (81) found moderate linear ($r^2 = 0.52$) or power-law ($r^2 = 0.58$) relations between compressive strength and QCT equivalent mineral density for vertebral trabecular bone, with strength values ranging from 0.05 to 3.79 MPa (1.49 ± 0.974, SD, $n = 41$). Mosekilde et al. (99) reported moderate linear correlations ($r^2 = 0.66$) between compressive strength and QCT data (in Hounsfield Units, HU) for vertebral trabecular bone, with strength values

ranging from 0.19 to 2.71 MPa (0.844 ± 0.526, $n = 30$). Esses et al. (46) found strong power-law correlations in the proximal femur between compressive strength and both corrected QCT (in HU) ($r^2 = 0.67$) and apparent density ($r^2 = 0.78$). Exponents for their power-law relations were 1.97 for QCT and 1.67 for apparent density. Compressive strength values for trabecular bone from the proximal femur ranged from 0.226 to 15.6 MPa (3.58 ± 3.50, $n = 49$). Comparable findings for trabecular bone of the proximal femur were also reported by Lotz et al. (85). They also found power-law correlations between compressive strength and both QCT equivalent mineral density ($r^2 = 0.70$) and di-

TABLE 4. *Strength vs QCT and density: Femoral and vertebral trabecular bone[a]*

Authors	Location	Dependent variable	n	Relationship[b]	r^2	Relative error (%)
Lang et al. (81)	vert	QCT mg/cc	41	$\sigma = (8.2 \times 10^{-6})x^{2.45} + 0.082$	0.58	46.6
Mosekilde et al. (99)	vert	QCT HU	30	$\sigma = 0.01x + 0.011$	0.66	36.7
Esses et al. (46)	fem	app den	49	$\sigma = (4.7 \times 10^{-5})x^{1.67} + 0.86$	0.78	47.1
	fem	QCT HU	49	$\sigma = (3.3 \times 10^{-5})x^{1.97} + 1.23$	0.67	56.5
Lotz et al. (85)	fem	app den	49	$\sigma = (2.1 \times 10^{-4})x^{1.70} - 0.37$	0.78	34.0
	fem	QCT mg/cc	49	$\sigma = (8.9 \times 10^{-6})x^{2.31} + 2.78$	0.70	39.9

[a] All significance levels $p < 0.001$. [b] Gives relationship between strength σ and dependent variables. Abbreviations: app den, apparent density (mg/cc); fem, femur; vert, vertebra. From Hayes et al. (63), with permission.

rectly measured apparent density ($r^2 = 0.67$). Compressive strength values ranged from 1.31 to 27.3 (6.76 ± 4.84, $n = 49$). The power-law relationship between trabecular compressive strength and QCT equivalent mineral density for the proximal femur from Lotz et al. (85) is shown in Fig. 12B.

Quantitative Computed Tomography Versus Material Properties of Cortical Bone

Comparable correlations between CT measurements and the density and mechanical properties of cortical bone have not been reported, in part because few authors have focused on these relationships and in part because the narrow range of densities exhibited by cortical bone make the determination of such correlations problematic. Recently, Snyder and Schneider (143) measured QCT values (in HU), apparent density, and mechanical properties for cortical bone from the tibial diaphysis for three women and four men ranging in age from 29 to 73 years. Apparent densities ranged from 1.75 to 1.95 mg/cc (1.86 ± 0.57, $n = 45$). By use of linear fits, the coefficients of determination (r^2) between QCT and physical properties were: (a) 0.42 for apparent density; (b) 0.30 for flexural modulus; and (c) 0.25 for flexural strength. As with the trabecular bone data reported above, somewhat better correlations were found between directly measured apparent density and both flexural modulus ($r^2 = 0.55$) and flexural strength ($r^2 = 0.45$). Power-law fits did not result in significant improvements compared to the linear fits.

GEOMETRIC REMODELING OF THE CORTICAL DIAPHYSIS

When the skeleton is exposed to trauma, certain regions can be subjected to large forces. Fracture occurs when the local stresses exceed the ultimate strength of the bone in that region. Bone fracture can therefore be viewed as an event that is initiated at the material level and then affects the load-bearing capacity of the bone at the structural level. As indicated previously, the major difference between be-havior at the material level and at the structural level is the inclusion of geometric properties at the structural level and their exclusion at the material level. Thus, structural behavior includes both the effects of bone geometry and material properties, whereas material behavior reflects only behavior uninfluenced by geometric effects. Any attempt to predict the structural behavior of a skeletal region must therefore reflect both the heterogeneous material properties of the region and the complex geometric arrangement of each type of bone. To focus on this level of behavior and to address the structural consequences of changes in bone geometries and material properties with age and exercise, we summarize research involving changes in the geometric features of long bones with age and exercise.

Geometric Remodeling in Response to Exercise

Although there have been a number of anecdotal reports of bony hypertrophy in response to heavy exercise in human subjects, few studies have provided quantitative measures that might be used to estimate the consequences of chronic exercise on cortical geometry. In one such study, Jones et al. (70) radiographed the upper extremities of 84 active professional tennis players. The mean age of the men was 27 years (range 18 to 50 years), and that of the women 24 years (range 14 to 34 years). The mean length of playing experience of the men was 18 years, and that of the women 14 years. Satisfactory anteroposterior and lateral roentgenograms of both humeri were obtained for 48 men and 30 women. Anteroposterior (A-P) and medial–lateral (M-L) measurements of periosteal and endosteal diameters were made at a site 11 cm proximal to the distal end of the humerus.

Every player showed roentgenographic evidence of cortical hypertrophy on the playing side in all parameters measured. The medullary cavity was usually narrowed as a result of encroachment by the thickened cortex. The combined cortical thickness, defined as the sum of all four thickness values (anterior and posterior cortices in both A-P and M-L planes), showed an increase on the playing side of 34.9% for the men and 28.4% for the women. Data from Jones et al. on the A-P and M-L endosteal and periosteal diameters for the playing and non-playing extremities of both male and female players are shown in Table 5. The results indicate highly significant humeral hypertrophy as a consequence of the chronic stimulus of professional tennis playing. An unanswered question left by this study is if this geometric remodeling occurs with exercise in adults or only during growth and development (all of the players examined began playing during childhood or early adolescence). Despite this open question, it is apparent from these data that dramatic changes in cortical geometry can occur in response to exercise. These geometric changes can also be expected to result in important changes in the structural behavior of the whole bone.

Example 7. Structural consequence of humeral hypertrophy. Assuming that the humeral cross-sectional geometric data of Table 5 can be approximated by a cylindrical tube of uniform thickness, determine the cross-sectional areas and moments of inertia at the measurement site for both the playing and nonplaying side for both men and women. Then, assuming that the same bending forces are applied to the humerus on both playing and nonplaying sides, what is the ratio of maximum bending stresses (nonplaying/playing) for both men and women?

Solution. Averaging the A-P and M-L periosteal and endosteal diameters from Table 5 results in the following values (in centimeters) for inner and outer diameters of the assumed cylindrical cross sections.

	Playing		Nonplaying	
	d_o	d_i	d_o	d_i
Men	2.45	0.975	2.195	1.10
Women	2.07	0.87	1.895	0.96

From Fig. 6, and noting that $r = d/2$, the areas and moments of inertia at the humeral cross section are

	Playing		Nonplaying	
	Men	Women	Men	Women
Area (cm²)	3.97	2.77	2.83	2.10
I (cm⁴)	1.72	0.87	1.07	0.59

If (equation 3) the maximum stress for a beam in four-point bending is

$$\sigma = \pm \, Fac/I$$

and the same bending moment (Fa) is applied to both the playing and the nonplaying side, then the stress ratio (σ_{np}/σ_p) is given by

$$(\sigma_{np}/\sigma_p) = (c_{np}/I_{np})/(c_p/I_p) = c_{np}I_p/c_pI_{np}$$

TABLE 5. *Humeral diameters of tennis players in their playing arm and their nonplaying arm*[a]

Other measurements	Number of subjects	Sex	Playing extremity (cm)	Nonplaying extremity (cm)	Change (%)
Anteroposterior diameter, humerus	43	M	2.47 (0.18)	2.24 (0.16)	9.9 ± 0.02
	23	F	2.11 (0.13)	1.97 (0.14)	7.0 ± 0.01
Anteroposterior diameter, medullary cavity	43	M	1.00 (0.19)	1.18 (0.21)	−14.8 ± 0.02
	23	F	0.92 (0.16)	1.04 (0.15)	−11.2 ± 0.02
Mediolateral diameter, humerus	39	M	2.44 (0.19)	2.15 (0.20)	13.4 ± 0.02
	14	F	2.03 (0.13)	1.82 (0.11)	11.7 ± 0.03
Mediolateral diameter, medullary cavity	39	M	0.95 (0.18)	1.02 (0.20)	−7.0 ± 0.02
	14	F	0.82 (0.16)	0.88 (0.13)	−7.8 ± 0.03 ($p < 0.02$)

[a]Record of measurements made 11 cm proximal to the distal end of the humerus. Changes measured from the lateral view at the 8-cm level were similar to those at the 11-cm level. Probability, calculated using the Fisher two-tailed t test, was $p < 0.001$, except for the single instance noted. The standard error was calculated by matched-pair analysis. From Jones and Priest (70), with permission.

Because c, the maximum distance from the neutral axis to the surface of the beam, is given by $d_o/2$, this may be rewritten as

$$\sigma_{np}/\sigma_p = d_{np}I_p/d_pI_{np}$$

Substituting, we find that the stress ratio for men is $\sigma_{np}/\sigma_p = 1.44$, and that for women is $\sigma_{np}/\sigma_p = 1.35$.

Thus, in the male professional tennis players, the stresses are 44% higher in the humerus of the nonplaying arm when both sides are subjected to the same bending forces. In the female players, the stresses are 35% higher. This is equivalent to saying that the humeri of the playing arms are 44% and 35% stronger than the contralateral nonplaying sides in men and women, respectively.

Age-Related Changes in Cross-Sectional Geometry of the Lower Limb

Age changes in bone mineral mass, volume, and density in the human skeleton have been the subject of intensive investigation over the past 25 years. Changes with age in the histologic and mechanical properties of bone have also been studied by many investigators. The general picture to emerge from these studies is a progressive net loss of bone mass with aging, beginning in the fifth decade and proceeding at a faster rate among women. Concurrent with this overall loss of bone is a change in bone material properties (18), resulting in bone tissue of reduced strength and modulus. The major clinical consequence of these skeletal changes is an age-related increase in fracture incidence.

One structural variable that is not often considered in studies of skeletal aging is the geometry of cortical bone. However, the geometric distribution of bone tissue, together with its material properties, is critical in determining the structural strength and rigidity of the whole bone. The results of various radiographic studies suggest that some geometric remodeling of long bone cortices occurs with aging. In particular, subperiosteal apposition of bone has been observed to occur along with endosteal absorption. This remodeling of the diaphysis to a cylinder of larger diameter is hypothesized to serve a mechanical "compensatory" function by increasing the moment of inertia as the cortex thins with aging.

Ruff and Hayes (129) reported data on cross-sectional geometry of the lower limb bones in a large sample (103 femora and 99 tibiae) of cadaveric skeletal material from American white adults. Changes with age (20 to 100 years) in cross-sectional area and polar moment of inertia were determined at 11 cross sections by sectioning and direct measurement with a semiautomated system (106). Results for the polar moment of inertia J (standardized for body size differences by dividing by the fourth power of bone length) at the middistal tibia are shown in Fig. 13. The data demonstrate that, on average, the polar moment of inertia declines with age in women. In men, the polar moment of inertia increases over the range of 20 to 100 years. For men and women, the rates of change of J with age are significantly different ($p < 0.05$). From this study the key difference in age-related geometric remodeling of the femur and tibia in men and women is that men undergo greater subperiosteal expansion with aging than women. Both sexes exhibit about the same increase in endosteal expansion with age. Because of the parallel changes occurring at both surfaces in men, cortical area remains almost constant, whereas it decreases in women.

As a consequence, age-related changes in bone cross-sectional geometry appear to compensate for age reductions in bone strength in men, but not in women. These data thus confirm earlier findings (88) reporting age-related increases in moment of inertia at the midfemoral diaphysis in men but not in women. The relatively large scatter in the age regressions shown in Fig. 13 is probably caused by random variation in factors other than age and sex that may affect bone remodeling. These include genetic factors, diet, and activity levels and the cross-sectional nature of the population sample. The age-related changes shown in Fig. 13 account for only about 10% to 50% of the total variation in cross-sectional geometric properties. How-

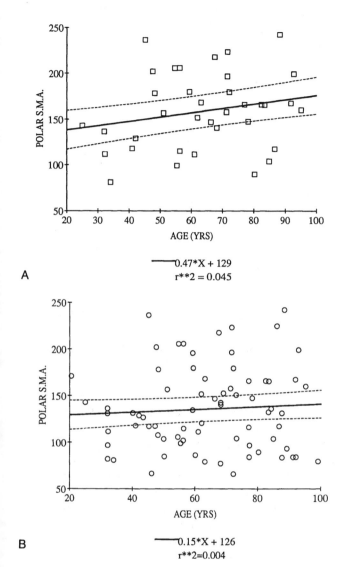

A

0.47*X + 129
r**2 = 0.045

B

0.15*X + 126
r**2=0.004

FIG. 13. Change with age in polar second moment of area of the tibia at the 35% cross section, standardized by dividing by bone length^4/10^8 for: **(A)** men and **(B)** women. Slopes for men and women are significantly different ($p < 0.05$). (From Hayes, ref. 59, with permission.)

ever, because of the number of uncontrolled variables in a cross-sectional study of this type, the findings nevertheless indicate that age alone contributes significantly to biological variation in these geometric properties.

Example 8. Age-related cortical remodeling: Biomechanical homeostasis? On page 94 is a schematic representation of the cortical bone remodeling with age in men and women at the femoral middiaphysis reported by Ruff and Hayes (129). In men, assume that between ages 25 and 85, r_o changes from 1.5 cm to 1.75 cm, and r_i from 0.75 cm to 1.0 cm. In

women, assume r_o stays constant at 1.25 cm as r_i changes from 0.625 to 0.75 cm over the same period. Assume from Fig. 9 that over the same time period the tensile strength of bone changes from 140 to 120 MPa. How does the ratio of tensile bending stress to tensile strength change with age between 25 and 85, and how do the changes differ for men and women? Assume the applied force is about three times body weight (2000 N for a 68-kg man and 1500 N for a 51-kg woman) and that the eccentricity of the applied load is 3.0 cm (0.03 m).

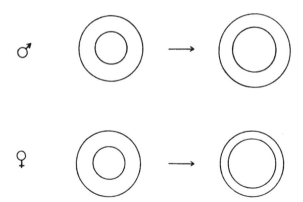

Solution. From equation 7a, the maximum tensile stress in bending is given by

$$\sigma_t = -F/A + eF(h/2)/I$$

Rearranging the terms yields

$$\sigma_t = F(eh/2I - I/A)$$

The cross-sectional area is given by $\pi(r_o^2 - r_i^2)$, the areal moment of inertia by $\pi(r_o^4 - r_i^4)/4$ (Fig. 6), and $r_o = h/2$. Substituting the appropriate values in these equations yields

$$\sigma_t = F(er_o/I - I/A)$$

Thus, σ_t/σ_{ult} has the values 0.15 and 0.11 for men aged 25 and 85, respectively; the corresponding values for women are 0.19 and 0.24. The ratio σ_t/σ_{ult} can be thought of as a kind of fracture risk index that expresses how close the local stresses are to those that could be expected to cause fracture. The tabulated data suggest that for an applied force of three times body weight (approximately equivalent to the force applied during single-legged stance), the maximum tensile stresses at the midfemoral shaft are 0.15 and 0.19, respectively, of the ultimate tensile strength (140 MPa) for men and women of age 25. In men, age-related remodeling of the femoral cortex (i.e., periosteal and endosteal expansion) results in a *decrease* in fracture risk to 0.11 at age 85, even though the ultimate tensile strength of bone decreases from 140 to 120 MPa during that time period. In women, however, the lack of periosteal expansion (while endosteal expansion does occur) results in an increase in fracture risk from 0.19 to 0.24, an increase of about 26%.

FRACTURE RISK PREDICTION

Noninvasive Methods for Predicting the Risk of Age-Related Fractures

In simple terms, a fracture represents a structural failure of the bone whereby the forces applied to the bone exceed its load-bearing capacity. The load-bearing capacity of a skeletal element is determined by its intrinsic material properties as well as the total amount (size) and spatial distribution (shape) of the bone tissue. Thus, the factors that are critical in determining whether a bone will fracture under a given situation include: (a) the direction and magnitude of the applied loads; (b) the size and geometry of the bone; and (c) the material properties of the bone tissue. From this perspective, therefore, factors related both to bone fragility and to the forces applied to the skeleton must be considered in the study of age-related fractures.

Previously, the predominant view of fracture etiology was that bone loss, possibly from estrogen deficiency or age-related changes, was the primary determinant of fracture risk. This view was based on observations of a dramatic age-related increase in fracture incidence as well as a higher fracture incidence in women than men. However, recent clinical data indicate that factors related both to bone fragility and to skeletal loading are important determinants of the risk of fracture (54,108). Insight into the roles of these factors may be gained by using a standard engineering approach for evaluating the risk of structural failure. To design a structure, engineers must consider the size and geometry of the structure, the materials from which it is to be made, and the types of loads to which it will be subjected. With this information, the loads applied to the structure during its normal usage can be compared to the loads known to cause failure. This comparison of applied load versus failure load gives an estimate of how "safely" the structure is designed. If a structure's design appears "unsafe," the engineer may choose to change the geometry of the structure (e.g., increase its size), use stronger materials, or reduce the applied loads. In practice, it is difficult to estimate a structure's strength and the loads applied to it. Therefore, to reduce the likelihood of unexpected failure, structures are often designed with very high safety factors.

These engineering principles can also be applied to skeletal structures. To apply these concepts to study fracture risk and etiology, Hayes and co-workers introduced a parameter called the "factor of risk" (63), Φ, defined as the ratio of the load delivered to a skeletal element (applied load) to the structural capacity of that element (failure load):

$$\Phi = \text{applied load/failure load} \quad (11)$$

Thus, when the factor of risk is low ($\Phi \ll 1$), the forces applied to the skeletal structure are much lower than those required to fracture it, and the structure is at low risk for failure. However, when the factor of risk is high ($\Phi \gg 1$), structural failure is predicted to occur. To apply the factor of risk in studies of hip or vertebral fracture, it is necessary to define the loads applied to the skeletal region of interest and the loads required to cause fracture. For example, most hip fractures are the result of a fall. Therefore, to compute the factor of risk for hip fracture caused by a fall, information is required about the loads applied to the femur during a fall and the structural capacity of the femur in a fall configuration.

Although this approach is relatively straightforward conceptually, in practice it is difficult to apply. Little is known about the magnitude and direction of loads applied to skeletal structures during daily activities and, in particular, during traumatic loading events. In addition, the skeletal structures exhibit markedly more heterogeneity and geometric complexity than many engineering structures, making it difficult to estimate the forces required to fracture the structure. Moreover, because these are "biological structures," both the applied loads and structural capacity can change with aging, pharmacologic intervention, or disease. Despite these uncertainties and limitations, rough estimates of the factor of risk for hip and vertebral fracture can be computed using data from laboratory investigations. These estimates may provide insights into the complex roles of loading severity and skeletal fragility in the etiology of age-related fractures.

In this section we review clinical investigations and laboratory studies related to the biomechanics of age-related fractures. In particular, we discuss factors that are related to the loads applied to the skeleton, either through traumatic events or in everyday activities; the factors that are related to the structural capacity of skeletal elements; and how these factors interact to influence fracture risk.

Estimating Hip Fracture Risk

It has been reported that over 90% of hip fractures in the elderly are associated with a fall (37,55). Thus, studies of the etiology of hip fractures are complicated by the need to examine risk factors for falls as well as risk factors for fracture. In addition, because fewer than 2% of falls in the elderly result in a hip fracture (95,109,146), investigations of hip fracture etiology must also distinguish factors related to "high-risk" falls that result in fracture.

Therefore, studies of the factors related to hip fracture can be grouped into three areas:

(a) factors related to the tendency to fall; (b) factors related to fall severity, including the magnitude and direction of the forces applied to the skeleton as the result of a fall; and (c) factors related to the strength of the proximal femur. Furthermore, as mentioned previously, it is possible to use a "factor of risk" to combine both bone strength and fall severity into a single index that, for a given loading event, compares the load applied to the hip to the load required to fracture the femur. In this section we review clinical and laboratory studies related to the factors influencing fall severity and femoral strength.

Factors That Influence Fall Severity

To investigate the role of fall severity in hip fracture etiology, definitions of a fall itself, as well as of fall severity, are needed. Previously, investigators defined a fall as a sudden, unexpected event that results in a person coming to rest on a horizontal surface (62,133). A fall can be further characterized by several phases: (a) an instability phase resulting in fall initiation; (b) a descent phase; (c) an impact phase; and (d) a postimpact phase during which the faller comes to rest (62). The definition of "fall severity" is more difficult. From a biomechanical perspective, fall severity can be described by the magnitude and direction of the load applied to the hip and the impact site. From a clinical perspective, Cummings and Nevitt (38) suggest that a high-risk fall includes: (a) impact on or near the hip; (b) lack of active protective mechanisms such as an outstretched arm to break the fall; and (c) insufficient energy absorption by local soft tissues. Thus, by these criteria, a high-risk fall could transmit a force to the proximal femur that exceeds the force required to fracture the hip.

A few surveillance studies have been conducted to more fully characterize fall severity as it relates to hip fracture (54,62,108,109). Among nursing home residents, falling to the side and impacting the hip or side of the leg increased the risk of hip fracture approximately 20-fold relative to falling in any other direction (62). An increase in the potential en-

ergy content of the fall, computed from fall height and body mass, was also associated with an increased risk for fracture. Similar results were reported in a nested case-control analysis of the Study of Osteoporotic Fractures cohort, a large, prospective study in community-dwelling women (108). Women who suffered a hip fracture were more likely to have fallen sideways or straight down and to have landed on or near the hip than women who fell and did not suffer a fracture. Furthermore, among women who fell on the hip, compared to those who did not fracture, women who suffered hip fractures were taller, had weaker triceps, were less likely to have landed on a hand or to have broken the fall by grabbing an object, and were more likely to have landed on a hard surface (108). Thus, these surveillance studies have identified several factors that are related to the "severity" of a fall in terms of hip fracture risk. From these data it is clear that a fall to the side represents a particularly risky event.

To further study the characteristics of sideways falls, in particular, the descent and impact phases, our group has conducted several laboratory investigations. In a study of the descent phase of sideways falls, van den Kroonenberg and colleagues (80) provided estimates of the impact velocities and energies that may occur during falls from standing height, the effect of muscle activity on these impact velocities, and insights into the high-risk nature of sideways falls. Six young, healthy adults (age 19 to 30) were asked to fall sideways, as naturally as possible, onto a thick gymnastics mattress. To investigate the effect of muscle activity on fall dynamics, subjects were instructed to fall either as relaxed as they could or to fall naturally, using the musculature of the trunk and upper extremity as they would in a reflex-mediated fall. To investigate potential protective mechanisms, during some falls subjects were instructed to try to break the fall with their arm. The vertical velocity at impact with the floor ranged between 2.1 and 4.8 m/sec. The impact velocity was 7% lower in relaxed than in muscle-active falls, a finding attributed to the observation that hip impact occurs closer to the feet in the muscle-relaxed case. Despite instructions to break the fall with an outstretched arm, only two of six subjects were able to do so (Fig. 14). In the remaining subjects, hip impact occurred first, followed by impact of the arm or hand. Finally, the authors found that, in these young adults, approximately 70% of the total energy available is dissipated during the descent phase of a sideways fall from standing height. This energy dissipation is likely through muscle activity and the stiffness and damping characteristics of the hip and knee joints. It is not known whether elderly fallers are also able to dissipate the same amount of energy during a fall or whether they, in effect, "fall harder than young adults."

The force delivered to the proximal femur during a sideways fall not only depends on the dynamics of the fall but may also be influenced by muscle activity at impact and by the thickness of soft tissue covering the greater trochanter. To study these factors, Robinovitch and colleagues (123) developed the "pelvis release" experiment, in which a small force is applied to the lateral aspect of the hip and the dynamic response of the body is measured. They demonstrated that femoral impact forces are decreased both during muscle-relaxed falls and by increased soft tissue thickness overlying the greater trochanter. In a further study of the force attenuation and energy absorption properties of the trochanteric soft tissue, tissue samples were obtained from nine cadavers, positioned over a surrogate proximal femur and pelvis, and subjected to a typical impact load associated with a sideways fall (122). For a constant impact energy, trochanteric soft tissue thickness was strongly negatively correlated with the peak femoral impact force ($r^2 = 0.91$), such that the force applied to the femur decreased approximately 70 N per 1-mm increase in tissue thickness (Fig. 15).

Finally, Kroonenberg et al. (79) developed a series of biomechanical models to estimate peak impact forces on the greater trochanter in a sideways fall from standing height. The models incorporated stiffness and damping parameters from the "pelvis-release" experiments (123), and the models' behavior was compared with previous observations of the dynamics of voluntary sideways falls (80). According to the most accurate model, peak impact forces applied to the greater trochanter ranged from 2900 to 4260 N for the fifth to 95th percentile woman, based on weight and

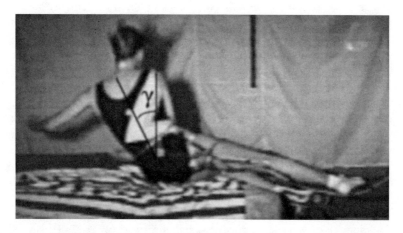

FIG. 14. Example of a sideways fall onto a thick gymnastics mattress. Despite instructions to break the fall with the hand, only two of six subjects were able to do so. In the other subjects, hip impact occurred first, thus providing insight into the high-risk nature of sideways falls. (From Kroonenberg et al., ref. 80, with permission.)

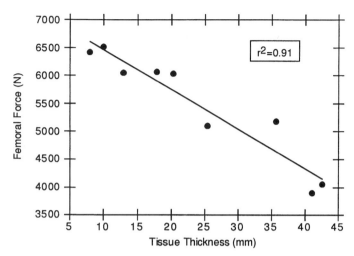

FIG. 15. Effect of trochanteric soft tissue thickness on the force delivered to the femur and for a constant energy impact directed laterally on the hip. (From Robinovitch et al., ref. 122, with permission.)

height. Thus, given an individual's height and weight, these models can be used to estimate femoral impact forces associated with a sideways fall and thereby provide estimates of the numerator of the factor of risk.

Factors That Influence the Strength of the Proximal Femur

Several factors contribute to the load-bearing capacity of the proximal femur, including both its intrinsic material properties as well as the total amount (size) and spatial distribution (shape) of the bone tissue. For bone, as mentioned previously, its intrinsic material properties are strongly related to bone density. This fact has led to the hypothesis that age-related bone loss is a primary contributor to the steep age-related increase in hip fracture incidence. In support of this hypothesis, there is strong evidence, from both clinical as well as laboratory studies, that low bone mineral density is a risk factor for hip fracture. Prospective clinical studies have confirmed that low bone mineral density, measured both at the hip and at other sites, is a risk factor for hip fracture (36,110,125). Furthermore, recent case-control studies have reported that low bone mineral density of the hip is a risk

factor for hip fracture that is independent of fall characteristics (54,108).

The use of noninvasive bone densitometry techniques to predict fracture risk is based on the assumption that bone mineral density directly reflects the mechanical behavior of the bone. Laboratory investigations have confirmed that, under a variety of loading conditions, noninvasive assessments of bone density and bone geometry are strongly related to the failure load of cadaveric femurs (8,14,30, 31,83,84,86,148). Femoral bone mineral density (BMD) correlates strongly with the failure load of cadaveric femurs in loading conditions simulating both single-leg stance (1,8,42,46) and sideways falls (14,30,31,86). For example, in a study by Courtney et al. (30,31), femoral neck BMD, assessed by dual-energy x-ray absorptiometry, explained approximately 80% of the variation in failure loads of cadaveric femurs tested in a configuration designed to simulate a sideways fall with impact to the greater trochanter (Fig. 16).

Other factors that influence the failure load of the proximal femur include the loading rate and direction of applied load. The effect of loading rate on the mechanical behavior of cadaveric proximal femurs has been investigated by comparing the mechanical behavior

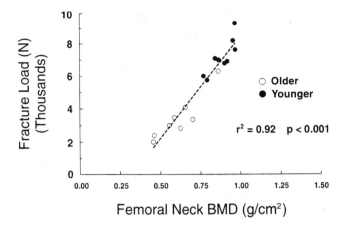

FIG. 16. Graph of the load at fracture and the areal bone mineral density (BMD) of the femoral neck. There was a strong correlation between the load at fracture and the areal bone mineral density of the femoral neck as measured with dual-energy x-ray absorptiometry. (From Courtney et al., ref. 30, with permission.)

of a femur tested at a quasistatic loading rate to the behavior of the contralateral femur tested at a high loading rate (similar to that expected to occur during impact from a fall from standing height) (31,148). In this experimental design, the failure load was 20% to 100% (31,148), and stiffness approximately 100% (31) greater in femurs tested at fast loading rates relative to those tested at quasistatic loading rates. Pinilla and co-workers (116) examined the influence of loading direction on femoral strength for a loading condition simulating a sideways fall with impact to the greater trochanter. They performed failure tests of elderly cadaveric femurs in three different loading configurations: a baseline case representing a typical fall configuration (30) and cases with the femur slightly internally and externally rotated relative to the baseline configuration. After adjustment for femoral BMD, the average failure load of femurs tested with slight internal rotation was 24% ($p < 0.05$) less than those tested with slight external rotation. Thus, subtle changes in the loading direction associated with a sideways fall can influence the femoral failure load to the same extent as approximately 25 years of age-related femoral bone loss (53,144).

In summary, femoral failure loads of elderly cadaveric specimens range from approximately 700 to 10,000 N and 1000 to 13,000 N for specimens tested in a sideways fall and stance configurations, respectively.

These failure loads are influenced, at least in part, by femoral bone mineral density, femoral geometry, loading direction, and loading rate. Although they can change with age or therapeutic intervention, at a given moment, an individual's bone density and geometry are constant. However, other factors, such as loading direction and loading rate, that are influenced by the characteristics of the fall may significantly influence fracture risk.

Interactions Between Fall Severity and Femoral Strength: The Factor of Risk for Hip Fracture

Two case-control studies have demonstrated the importance of both fall severity and bone mineral density as risk factors for hip fracture (54,108). Nevitt and Cummings (108), in a nested case-control analysis of the Study of Osteoporotic Fractures cohort, studied 130 women who fell and suffered a hip fracture and a consecutive sample of 467 women who fell and did not fracture. They reported that among those who fell on or near their hip, those who fell sideways or straight down were at increased risk for hip fracture (odds ratio 4.3), whereas those who fell backwards were less likely to suffer a hip fracture (odds ratio 0.2). Furthermore, low BMD at the femoral neck (odds ratio 2.6 for a 1 SD decrease) or calcaneus (odds ratio 2.4 for a 1 SD decrease) strongly increased the risk of fracture among those who fell on or near the hip. Greenspan and co-workers (54) reported similar findings in a study of 149 community-dwelling men and women, including 72 who fell and suffered a hip fracture and 77 control subjects who fell but did not fracture. They showed that in these elderly fallers, independent risk factors for hip fracture included characteristics related to fall severity, low bone mineral density at the hip, and body habitus (Table 6).

The clinical studies provide valuable information about the independent contributions of fall severity and skeletal fragility to hip fracture risk. However, further insight may be achieved by considering a "factor of risk" for hip fracture. Recall that the factor of risk is defined as the ratio of the force applied to a structure during a given loading condition to the force required to break the structure under the same conditions. Hence, for factors of risk much greater than one, the structure is predicted to fail. Using data from laboratory studies, we can calculate rough estimates of the factor of risk for hip fracture for sideways falls from standing height.

We applied the factor of risk concept in a case-control study of elderly fallers (102). The numerator of the factor of risk, the applied load, was estimated from previous studies of the descent and impact phases of a sideways fall with impact to the lateral aspect of the hip (79,80,123). We used each individual's body height and weight as input parameters for the model to estimate the impact force delivered to the proximal femur during a sideways fall from standing height. The denominator of the factor of risk, or structural capacity of the proximal femur, was determined from linear

regressions between noninvasive bone densitometry and femoral failure loads in a fall configuration (14). For each subject, femoral bone mineral density was assessed by dual-energy x-ray absorptiometry and then used to estimate the femoral failure load. There was a strong association between the factor of risk and hip fracture in these elderly fallers, with the odds of hip fracture increasing by 5.1 for a 1 SD increase in the factor of risk (95% confidence interval 2.9–9.2). In comparison, the odds ratio for a 1 SD decrease in femoral BMD was 2.0 (95% confidence interval 1.4–2.6) (Fig. 17).

It is also possible to make estimates of the factor of risk from literature estimates of hip forces and femoral strength. Early literature investigating correlations between densitometric measures and femoral fracture has focused exclusively on gait loads. Reported ranges of failure loads for the proximal femur are: (a) 1000 to 9750 N (42); (b) 1597 to 12,740 N (83); (c) 1600 to 12,750 N (97); (d) 1764 to 8820 N (132); and (e) 2750 to 9610 N (1). To estimate factors of risk for the hip, these ranges and the data provided by Esses et al. (46) must be compared against estimates of *in vivo* loading on the proximal femur. A variety of mathematical models for single-legged stance have predicted forces that range from as low as 1.8 times body weight (BW) (93) to 6 BW (150). During normal gait, predictions are from about 3 BW to 8 BW (33,34,57,114,124). Hip joint forces of 7 or 8 BW have been predicted for stair ascent and descent (34,113) and of 3 BW for rising from a chair (34). *In vivo* forces at the hip joint

TABLE 6. *Multiple logistic regression analysis of factors associated with hip fracture in community-dwelling men and women who fell*

Factor	Adjusted odds ratio	95% confidence interval	p
Fall to the side	5.7	2.3–14	<0.001
Femoral neck BMD (g/cm²)[a]	2.7	1.6–4.6	<0.001
Potential energy of fall (Joules)[b]	2.8	1.5–5.2	<0.001
Body mass index (kg/m²)[a]	2.2	1.2–3.8	0.003

[a]Calculated for a decrease of 1 SD.
[b]Calculated for an increase of 1 SD.
From Bouxsein et al. (15), with permission; data from Greenspan et al. (54), with permission.

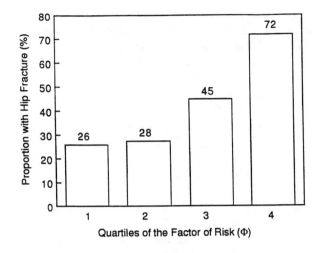

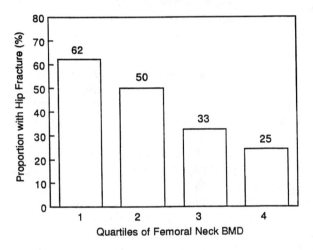

FIG. 17. Proportion of subjects with hip fracture in each quartile of the factor of risk for hip fracture **(top)** and femoral neck BMD **(bottom).** (From Bouxsein et al., ref. 15, with permission; data from Myers et al., ref. 102.)

have also been measured directly using instrumented implants (43,44,77,130). For normal, quiet gait, all of these studies have reported hip joint forces of about 3 BW. Kotzar et al. (77) reported forces as high as 5.5 BW for dynamic loading associated with periods of instability during single-legged stance.

For the 55-kg individual typical of elderly populations at high risk of hip fracture, forces of 3 BW for single-legged stance correspond to values of about 1620 N. Forces of 6 BW (representative of stair climbing and more dynamic activities) correspond to values of about 3240 N. The mean value of *in vitro* failure load (5250) from Esses et al. (46) would then indicate a factor of risk of about 0.31 for single-legged stance and about 0.62 for more

dynamic activities. The entire range of *in vitro* failure loads reported in the recent literature (1000 to 12,750 N) suggest a range of factors of risk of between 0.13 and 1.6 for single-legged stance and between 0.25 and 3.2 for stair climbing.

Example 9. Hip fracture risk. What is the factor of risk associated with normal gait in a 55-kg individual with a subcapital QCT value of 250 HU?

Solution. To estimate a factor of risk for spontaneous fracture of the hip, patient QCT data at the subcapital site can be used in the relationship between femoral failure load and QCT established by Esses et al. (46):

$$F = 14.9 \, (QCT) + 1750$$

where F is in Newtons and QCT is in HU. To estimate a factor of risk for normal gait, the *in vivo* force estimate for this activity ($3 \times BW$ or 1620 N for a 55-kg individual) is divided by the predicted failure force (Eq. 5)

$$\Phi = 1620/[14.9 \, (QCT) + 1750]$$

For a patient with a subcapital QCT value of 250 HU (near the midrange of the subcapital QCT data of Esses et al.), this corresponds to a factor of risk of about 0.3 for normal gait. For stair climbing and more dynamic loading associated with single-legged stance, the factor of risk doubles to a value of 0.6.

Estimating Vertebral Fracture Risk

Investigations of the etiology and biomechanics of vertebral fractures are particularly difficult, as the precise definition of a vertebral fracture remains controversial (76,111). In addition, many fractures that are identified by radiographic review are asymptomatic (29), further complicating the interpretation of many studies.

In contrast to the growing recognition of the importance of bone fragility and fall severity in the etiology of hip fractures, the role of spinal loading in the etiology of age-related vertebral fractures has received relatively little attention (107). Although no clinical study has yet examined the relative roles of bone fragility and load severity as risk factors for vertebral fracture, several investigators have reviewed medical records or interviewed patients to assess the "degree of trauma" associated with vertebral fractures (11,29,112,131). In a comprehensive account of the circumstances associated with "clinically diagnosed" vertebral fractures in 341 Rochester, Minnesota, residents (29), a specific loading event was reported for approximately 50% of the total fractures (Table 7). Contrary to the presumption that lifting plays a major role in the development of vertebral fractures, few of the fractures were associated with lifting. Outside of fractures that were diagnosed incidentally, only 10% of fractures were associated with "lifting a heavy object," whereas nearly 40% were associated with falling. Thus, fall incidence and severity may not only be important factors in hip fracture etiology but may also play a significant role in the development of vertebral fractures.

Factors That Influence the Loads Applied to the Spine

Although it is impossible to measure the loads on the vertebral bodies *in vivo,* several investigators have used kinematic analysis, electromyographic measurements, and biomechanical modeling to estimate the loads on the lumbar spine during various activities. In these analyses, static or dynamic equilibrium conditions are used to define the resultant forces and moments at a particular spinal level for a given activity. These resultant forces are then balanced by internal reactions comprised of muscle forces, ligament forces, intraabdominal pressure, and a compressive force on the vertebral body. The biomechanical models vary in

TABLE 7. *Circumstances associated with clinically diagnosed vertebral fractures*

Reported activity/ circumstance	Number of persons	Percentage of symptomatic fractures	Percentage of total fractures
Pathologic fracture	12	4	3.5
Traffic accident	20	7	6
Fall from more than standing height	27	9	8
Fall from standing height or less	86	30	25
Lifting a heavy object	29	10	8.5
"Spontaneous"	113	39	33
Diagnosed incidentally (asymptomatic)	54	NA	16

From Bouxsein et al. (15), with permission; data from Cooper et al. (29), with permission.

sophistication, ranging from planar, static, single-muscle-force models (9,135,141) to complex two- and three-dimensional static and dynamic analyses with optimization routines for determining muscle forces (5,26,52,91,92, 137–140). The biomechanical models have been verified by comparing predicted compressive spine loads and muscle activity with direct measurements of intradiscal pressure (67,104,105,138) and myoelectric trunk muscle activity (2,26,136–138,156).

These models were originally developed to study the potential mechanisms of low-back pain and injury in working adults. Therefore, they are generally based on anthropometric data from young, healthy adults and are limited to estimating the vertebral forces in the lumbar region. However, Wilson (151) has recently extended these models to include the mid- and lower thoracic spine by incorporating the rib cage and muscles of the thoracic region. Although the biomechanical models have been validated for young, healthy adults, little is known regarding their ability to estimate spinal loading in the elderly. It is likely that the anthropometric data, such as body segment weights, muscle cross-sectional areas, and muscle moment arms, used in the models depend on both age and sex. Therefore, to examine the etiology of vertebral fractures, future models should incorporate anthropometric data from studies of elderly men and women.

Despite these limitations in the current models, they are still useful for providing estimates of spinal loading during various activities. We used the model developed by Wilson to estimate compressive loads on the T11 and L2 vertebrae during common activities (Table 8). For example, rising from a chair without the use of one's hands results in compressive forces equal to 60% and 173% of body weight on the T11 and L2 vertebrae, respectively. These estimates also reinforce the concept that subtle changes in body position can dramatically alter spinal loading. Standing straight and holding an 8-kg mass with the arms slightly extended creates a compressive load on L2 equal to 230% of body weight, whereas flexing the trunk forward 30° and holding the same weight generates a compressive force on L2 of over 320% of body weight. From these estimates, it is clear that everyday activities, such as rising from a chair or bending over and picking up a full grocery bag, can generate high forces on the spine.

Factors That Influence Vertebral Strength

The use of noninvasive assessments of skeletal status to predict vertebral strength *in vivo* is based on the assumption that much of the variability in the strength of whole vertebrae can be explained by variations in bone density. In this regard, there are strong correlations ($r = 0.7$ to 0.9) between the strength of

TABLE 8. *Predicted compressive loads on the L2 and T11 vertebrae during various activities*[a]

Activity	Predicted load on T11		Predicted load on L2	
	n	Percentage of body weight	*n*	Percentage of body weight
Relaxed standing	240	41	290	51
Rising from a chair without use of hands	340	60	980	173
Standing, holding 8-kg weight close to body	320	57	420	74
Standing, holding 8-kg weight with arms extended	660	117	1302	230
Standing, trunk flexed 30°, arms extended	370	65	830	146
Standing, trunk flexed 30°, holding 8 kg with arms extended	760	135	1830	323
Lift 15 kg from floor, knees bent, arms straight down	593	104	1810	319

[a] The loads were computed from the model developed by Wilson (151) for a woman who weighs 58 kg and is 162 cm tall. From Bouxsein et al. (15), with permission.

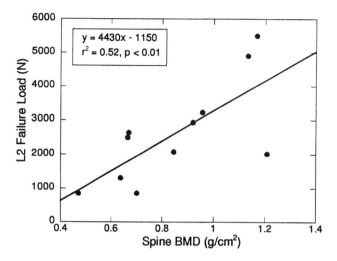

FIG. 18. Lumbar BMD versus ultimate load of the second lumbar (L2) vertebral body. (Data from Moro et al., ref. 98, with permission.)

whole vertebrae and either direct or non-invasive measures of bone mass and bone density (4,10,12,13,16,28,45,56,90,98,100, 101,147). For example, Moro et al. (98) recently demonstrated that lumbar bone mineral density assessed by DXA correlates strongly with the compressive failure load and energy to failure of both the L2 and T11 vertebrae (Fig. 18). The standard error of the estimate for predicting vertebral failure load from lumbar BMD was 527 N (25% of the mean failure load) for T11 and 733 N (28% of the mean failure load) for L2. These data confirm that clinical BMD measurements may be used to predict the structural capacity of lumbar vertebrae. Depending on the specimen characteristics and mechanical testing protocol, the compressive failure loads of lum-bar and thoracic vertebrae range approximately from 1000 to 7000 N (28,90,98,99,103) and 800 to 5000 N (98,103), respectively.

Interactions Between Spinal Loads and Vertebral Strength: The Factor of Risk for Vertebral Fracture

Although it has not been clearly demonstrated by clinical surveillance studies, it seems reasonable to suggest that, in common with hip fractures, both bone fragility and skeletal loading are important factors in the etiology of vertebral fractures (59). To investigate the potential roles of bone fragility and spinal loading, we estimated a factor of risk for vertebral fractures for various activities (Table 9). As before, the factor of risk was de-

TABLE 9. *Estimated factor of risk for fracture of T11 and L2 for various activities and levels of spinal osteopenia from age-related bone loss[a]*

	Factor of risk (Φ) for T11		Factor of risk (Φ) for L2	
Activity	30 yr old	75 yr old	30 yr old	75 yr old
Rising from a chair without use of hands	0.09	0.20	0.22	0.43
Standing, arms extended, holding 8-kg weight	0.17	0.38	0.29	0.57
Standing, trunk flexed 30°, holding 8-kg weight with arms extended	0.19	0.44	0.41	0.80
Lifting 15 kg from the floor, knees straight	0.15	0.34	0.42	0.81

[a]Age-adjusted L2 BMD from the lateral view taken from the data base supplied by Hologic, Inc. For ages 30 and 75, lateral L2 BMDs were 0.797 and 0.518 g/cm², respectively. From Bouxsein et al. (15), with permission.

fined as the ratio between load applied to the bone and the failure load for a given loading event. We estimated the numerator of the factor of risk (i.e., the applied load) using predictions of compressive loading in the spine from the model developed by Wilson (151). The denominator of the factor of risk (i.e., the failure load) was estimated from linear regressions between lumbar BMD and the compressive failure load of cadaveric vertebrae (98). We computed the factor of risk using the mean lateral L2 BMD for a 30- and a 75-year-old woman (65). For even the most strenuous activities, the factor of risk for the 30-year-old was well below one, indicating that fracture was unlikely. For the 75-year-old, however, more strenuous activities, such as lifting a grandchild or removing a turkey from the oven, may generate forces in the spine that are dangerously close to the vertebral failure load. These data reinforce the concept that loading conditions and bone strength are important factors in determining vertebral fracture risk.

To further investigate the role of bone fragility in the risk of vertebral fractures, we estimated the factor of risk for a range of lumbar BMD values (Fig. 19). We found that a woman who bends over to pick up a 15-kg object is predicted to be at great risk for vertebral fracture (i.e., $\Phi > 1$) when her lateral L2 BMD is less than 0.57 g/cm^2. To put this in context, the mean lateral L2 BMD for a 65-year-old woman is 0.58 ± 0.10 g/cm^2 (65). Hence, for the same lifting activity as above, a 65-year-old woman whose spine BMD is 1 SD below the mean for her age would have a factor of risk equal to 1.4 and would be at high risk for fracture. To reduce her factor of risk below 1 without altering the applied load from lifting, the osteopenic woman would have to increase her spine BMD by 20%, an increase much greater than is currently achieved through the use of pharmacologic agents (27,75). This example illustrates the need for alternative strategies to prevent vertebral fractures, such as reducing spinal loading by avoiding certain "high-risk" activities.

Example 10. Vertebral fracture risk. An elderly woman bends forward at the waist to pick up a 20-kg child. Assuming that a DXA scan is available, that her lumbar BMD (L2–L4) is 0.8 g/cm^2, and that her L2 vertebra is subjected to a force of 1850 N when lifting the child, estimate the factor of risk, Φ.

Solution. To estimate the factor of risk, the relationship between vertebral failure load and BMD established by Moro et al. can be used. From Fig. 18, $F = 4430$ (BMD) $- 1150$, where F is in Newtons and BMD is in grams per square centimeter. To estimate a factor of risk Φ for forward flexion of 20° with a 10-kg weight in each hand, the *in vivo* force estimate for that activity (1850 N) is divided by the predicted failure force (eq. 4) for the patient,

$$\Phi = 1850/[6800 \text{ (BMD)} - 2175]$$

For a patient with a lumbar BMD value of 0.8 g/cm^2, this corresponds to a factor of risk of 0.57.

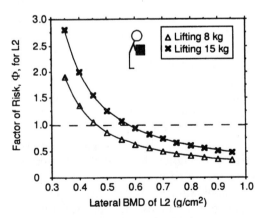

FIG. 19. Factor of risk, Φ, for L2 fracture as a function of L2 BMD for standing with the trunk flexed 30° and lifting either an 8- or 15-kg weight with arms extended. The *horizontal dashed line* is drawn at $\Phi = 1$, where the applied load equals the vertebral strength. For $\Phi > 1$, fracture is likely. (From Bouxsein et al., ref. 15, with permission.)

SUMMARY AND CLINICAL IMPLICATIONS

In this chapter, we have emphasized the concept that age-related fractures represent a structural failure whereby the forces applied to a bone exceed its load-bearing capacity. Viewing fractures in this manner makes it clear that studies of their etiology must include both factors that influence skeletal fragility or its load-bearing capacity, as well as those that influence the forces that are applied to the skeleton.

The load-bearing capacity of a skeletal structure is determined by both its intrinsic material properties as well as the total amount (size) and spatial distribution (shape) of the bone tissue. There is considerable evidence indicating that the material properties, in particular the elastic modulus and ultimate strength, of both cortical and trabecular bone decrease with increasing age in both men and women. This decrease in material properties is likely related, in part, to age-related reductions in bone mass, as the elastic modulus and strength of trabecular bone are related to density by a squared relationship. Therefore, small changes in bone density can dramatically influence bone material properties. These decrements in bone density and material properties may be partially offset by geometric rearrangement of the bone tissue, particularly in the long bones, that helps to preserve the bone's ability to resist bending and torsional loads.

Recent investigations confirm that skeletal status and fall severity are both significant and independent risk factors for hip fracture (54,108). Estimates of the forces applied to the proximal femur during a sideways fall range from 2900 to 4260 N for the 5th to 95th percentile woman based on height and weight. Factors that influence the load applied to the femur include, but are not limited to, fall height, fall direction, body habitus, muscle activity, trochanteric soft tissue thickness, and the intrinsic stiffness of the hip and knee joints. In comparison, estimates of the load required to fracture the elderly cadaveric femur in a configuration simulating a sideways fall range from 800 to 10,000 N. This femoral failure load is influenced by femoral bone mineral content and density, femoral geometry, and the direction and rate of the applied load. In particular, it appears that subtle changes in the direction of the load applied to the femur during a fall can influence femoral

failure loads as much as nearly 25 year's worth of age-related bone loss. Many of these factors that influence fall severity and femoral strength are independent of femoral bone mineral density and thus may prove useful in improving current estimates of fracture risk that are based on bone densitometry alone.

In contrast to hip fractures, little is known about the combined roles of spinal loading and skeletal fragility in the etiology of vertebral fractures. Contrary to previously held beliefs that vertebral fractures are caused primarily by bending and lifting activities, there is evidence that falls may play a significant role in the etiology of vertebral fractures. In one study, nearly 40% of clinically diagnosed, symptomatic fractures were associated with falls, whereas 10% were attributed to lifting a heavy object (29). Moreover, preliminary findings from a surveillance study currently being conducted in our laboratory indicate that approximately one-half of acute vertebral fractures are associated with falls. Thus, future studies should incorporate assessments of fall severity in order to determine the characteristics of falls associated with vertebral fracture. In addition, models to estimate the loads applied to the spine during a fall should be developed.

Activities of daily living may also place the elderly, osteopenic person at high risk for vertebral fracture. Mathematical models used to estimate the forces generated in the spine during bending and lifting activities indicate that compressive forces generated in the lower thoracic and upper lumbar spine range from approximately 200 N for relaxed standing to nearly 2000 N for bending forward slightly and lifting 8 kg. These forces can be compared to the failure loads of elderly cadaveric vertebrae tested in compression, which range from approximately 800 to 7000 N. Thus, it is apparent that for most individuals, daily activities do not present a great risk for vertebral fracture. However, among persons with substantial bone loss, common activities such as lifting a child or removing groceries from the trunk of the car may place the person at increased risk for vertebral fracture.

To date investigators have focused primarily on methods to prevent bone loss and to restore bone to the osteopenic skeleton. However, alternative approaches for fracture prevention that are directed at reducing the loads applied to the skeleton may prove to be both effective and cost-efficient. For example, trochanteric padding systems designed to reduce the load applied to the hip during a fall have shown great potential for reducing fracture risk (82,121). In one study, analyzed on an intention-to-treat basis, hip fracture incidence was reduced 53% in the group assigned to wear the hip pads (82). In addition, energy-absorbing floors, particularly in institutional environments, may help lower the risk of fractures from falls (25,87). Vertebral fracture incidence may be reduced by teaching high-risk patients to avoid activities that generate high loads on the spine and thereby put them at increased risk for fracture. Clearly, identification of these high-risk activities is critical to the success of this approach for preventing fractures. Ultimately, fracture prevention may be best achieved by an educational program designed to limit high-risk activities in conjunction with interventions targeted at increasing bone mass and reducing loads applied to the skeleton during traumatic events.

Acknowledgments

We gratefully acknowledge the support of grants from the National Institutes of Health (CA41295 and CCR103605), the Centers for Disease Control (CR102550), from the National Cancer Institute (CA40211), and the Maurice E. Mueller Professorship in Biomechanics at Harvard Medical School. We thank Jeanine Dulong for her assistance in manuscript preparation.

REFERENCES

1. Alho, A., Husby, T., and Hoiseth, A. (1988): Bone mineral content and mechanical strength. An *ex-vivo* study of human femora at autopsy. *Clin. Orthop.*, 227: 292–297.
2. Andersson, G. B. J., Ortengren, R., and Schultz, A. B. (1980): Analysis and measurement of the loads on the lumbar spine during work at a table. *J. Biomech.*, 13: 513–520.
3. Ashman, R. B., Rho, J. Y., and Turner, C. H. (1989): Anatomical variation of orthotropic elastic moduli of the proximal human tibia. *J. Biomech.*, 22:895–900.
4. Bartley, M. H., Arnold, J. S., Haslam, R. K., and Jee, W. S. S. (1966): The relationship of bone strength and bone quantity in health, disease, and aging. *J. Gerontol.*, 21:517–521.
5. Bean, J. C., and Chaffin, D. B. (1988): Biomechanical model calculation of muscle contraction forces: A double linear programming method. *J. Biomech.*, 21:59–66
6. Beaupre, G. S., Orr, T. E., and Carter, D. R. (1990): An approach for time-dependent bone modeling and remodeling. Theoretical development. *J. Orthop. Res.*, 8: 651–661.
7. Beaupre, G. S., Orr, T. E., and Carter, D. R. (1990): An approach for time-dependent bone modeling and remodeling. Application: A preliminary remodeling situation. *J. Orthop. Res.*, 8:662–670.
8. Beck, T. J., Ruff, C. B., Warden, K. E., Scott, W. W., and Rao, G. U. (1990): Predicting femoral neck strength from bone mineral data. *Invest. Radiol.*, 25:6–18.
9. Bejjani, F. J., Gross, C. M., and Pugh, J. W. (1984): Model for static lifting: Relationship of loads on the spine and the knee. *J. Biomech.*, 17:281–286.
10. Bell, G. H., Dunbar, O., and Beck, J. S. (1967): Variations in strength of vertebrae with age and their relation to osteoporosis. *Calcif. Tissue Int.*, 1:75–86.
11. Bengner, U., Johnell, O., and Redlund-Johnell, I. (1988): Changes in incidence and prevalence of vertebral fractures during 30 years. *Calcif. Tissue Int.*, 42:293–296.
12. Biggemann, M., Hilweg, D., and Brinckmann, P. (1988): Prediction of the compressive strength of vertebral bodies of the lumbar spine by quantitative computed tomography. *Skeletal Radiol.*, 17:264–269.
13. Biggemann, M., Hilweg, D., Seidel, S., Horst, M., and Brinckmann, P. (1991): Risk of vertebral insufficiency fractures in relation to compressive strength predicted by quantitative computed tomography. *Eur. J. Radiol.*, 13:6–10.
14. Bouxsein, M. L., Courtney, A. C., and Hayes, W. C. (1995): Ultrasound and densitometry of the calcaneus correlate with the failure loads of cadaveric femurs. *Calcif. Tissue Int.*, 56:99–103.
15. Bouxsein, M. L., Myers, E. R., and Hayes, W. C. (1996): Biomechanics of age-related fractures. In: *Osteoporosis*, edited by R. Marcus, D. Feldman, and J. Kelsey, pp. 373–393. Academic Press, San Diego.
16. Brinckmann, P., Biggemann, M., and Hilweg, D. (1989): Prediction of the compressive strength of human lumbar vertebrae. *Clin. Biomech.*, 4:S1–S27.
17. Burstein, A. H., Currey, J. D., Frankel, V. H., and Reilly, D. T. (1972): The ultimate properties of bone tissue: The effects of yielding. *J. Biomech.*, 5:35–44.
18. Burstein, A. H., Reilly, D. T., and Martens, M. (1976): Aging of bone tissue: Mechanical properties. *J. Bone Joint Surg. [Am.]*, 58:82–86.
19. Burstein, A. H., Zika, J. M., Heiple, K. G., and Klein, L. (1975): Contribution of collagen and mineral to the elastic–plastic properties of bone. *J. Bone Joint Surg. [Am.]*, 57:956–961.
20. Carter, D. R. (1987): Mechanical loading histories and skeletal biology. *J. Biomech.*, 12:1095–1109.

21. Carter, D. R., and Hayes, W. C. (1976): Bone compressive strength: The influence of density and strain rate. *Science,* 194:1174–1176.

22. Carter, D. R., and Hayes, W. C. (1977): The compressive behavior of bone as a two-phase porous structure. *J. Bone Joint Surg. [Am.],* 59:954–962.

23. Carter, D. R., Schwab, G. H., and Spangler, D. M. (1980): Tensile fracture of cancellous bone. *Acta Orthop. Scand.,* 51:733–741.

24. Carter, D. R., and Spengler, D. M. (1978): Mechanical properties and composition of cortical bone. *Clin. Orthop.,* 135:192–217.

25. Casalena, J., Streit, D., and Cavanaugh, P. (1993): Preliminary design of a dual stiffness floor for injury prevention. In: *Injury Prevention Through Biomechanics,* edited by K. Yang, p. 155. Wayne State University, Detroit.

26. Cholewicki, J., McGill, S., and Norman, R. (1995): Comparison of muscle forces and joint load from an optimization and EMG assisted lumbar spine model: Towards development of a hybrid approach. *J. Biomech.,* 28:321–331.

27. Christiansen, C. (1992): Prevention and treatment of osteoporosis: A review of current modalities. *Bone,* 13: S35–S39.

28. Cody, D., Goldstein, S., Flynn, M., and Brown, E. (1991): Correlations between vertebral regional bone mineral density (rBMD) and whole bone fracture load. *Spine,* 16:146–154.

29. Cooper, C., Atkinson, E., O'Fallon, W., and Melton, L. J. (1992): Incidence of clinically diagnosed vertebral fracture: A population-based study in Rochester, Minnesota, 1985–1989. *J. Bone Miner. Res.,* 7:221– 227.

30. Courtney, A. C., Wachtel, E. F., Myers, E. R., and Hayes, W. C. (1995): Age-related reductions in the strength of the femur tested in a fall loading configuration. *J. Bone Joint Surg. [Am.],* 77:387–395.

31. Courtney, A. C., Wachtel, E. F., Myers, E. R., and Hayes, W. C. (1994): Effects of loading rate on the strength of the proximal femur. *Calcif Tissue Int.,* 55:53–58.

32. Cowin, S. C. (1989): *Bone Mechanics.* CRC Press, Boca Raton, FL.

33. Crowninshield, R. D. (1978): Use of optimization techniques to predict muscle forces. *J. Biomech. Eng.,* 100: 88.

34. Crowninshield, R. D., Johnston, R. C., Andrews, J. G., and Brand, R. A. (1978): A biomechanical investigation of the human hip. *J. Biomech.,* 11:75–85.

35. Cummings, S. R. (1987): Epidemiology of hip fractures. In: *Osteoporosis: Proceedings of the International Symposium on Osteoporosis,* edited by J. Jensen, B. Riis, and C. Christiansen, pp. 40–43. Norhaven A/S, Viborg Denmark.

36. Cummings, S. R., Black, D., Nevitt, M. C., Browner, W., Cauley, J., Ensrud, C., Genant, H. K., Palermo, L., Scott, J., and Vogt, T. M. (1993): Bone density at various sites for prediction of hip fractures. *Lancet,* 341: 72–75.

37. Cummings, S., Black, D., Nevitt, M., Browner, W., Cauley, J., Genant, H., Mascioli, S., and Scott, J. (1990): Appendicular bone density and age predict hip fractures in women. *JAMA,* 263:665–668.

38. Cummings, S., and Nevitt, M. (1989): A hypothesis: The causes of hip fracture. *J. Gerontol.,* 44:M107–M111.

39. Currey, J. D. (1984): *The Mechanical Adaptations of Bones.* Princeton University Press, Princeton.

40. Currey, J. D. (1988): The effect of porosity and mineral content on the Young's modulus of elasticity of compact bone. *J. Biomech.,* 21:131–139.

41. Currey, J. D. (1988): The effects of drying and re-wetting on some mechanical properties of cortical bone. *J. Biomech.,* 21:439–441.

42. Dalen, N., Hellstrom, L. G., and Jacobson, B. (1976): Bone mineral content and mechanical strength of the femoral neck. *Acta Orthop. Scand.,* 47:503–508.

43. Davy, D. T., Kotzar, G. M., Brown, R. H., Heiple, K. G., Goldberg, V. M., Heiple, K. G., Jr., Reilla, J., and Burstein, A. H. (1988): Telemetric force measurements across the hip after total arthroplasty. *J. Bone Joint Surg. [Am.],* 70:45–50.

44. English, T. A., and Kilvington, M. (1979): *In vivo* records of hip loads using a femoral implant with telemetric output (a preliminary report). *J. Biomed. Eng.,* 1:111–115.

45. Eriksson, S. A., Isberg, B. O., and Lindgren, J. U. (1989): Prediction of vertebral strength by dual photon absorptiometry and quantitative computed tomography. *Calcif. Tissue Int.,* 44:243–250.

46. Esses, S. I., Lotz, J. C., and Hayes, W. C. (1989): Biomechanical properties of the proximal femur determined *in-vitro* by single-energy quantitative computed tomography. *J. Bone Miner. Res.,* 4:715–722.

47. Evans, F. G. (1957): *Stress and Strain in Bones.* Charles C. Thomas, Springfield, IL.

48. Evans, F. G. (1973): *Mechanical Properties of Bone.* Charles C. Thomas, Springfield, IL.

49. Gibson, L. J. (1985): The mechanical behaviour of cancellous bone. *J. Biomech.,* 18:317–328.

50. Gibson, L. J. (1988): Cancellous bone. In: *Cellular Solids,* pp. 316–331. Pergamon Press, New York.

51. Goldstein, S. A. (1987): The mechanical properties of trabecular bone: Dependence on anatomic location and function. *J. Biomech.,* 20:1055–1061.

52. Gracovetsky, S., Farfan, H. F., and Lamy, C. (1981): The mechanism of the lumbar spine. *Spine,* 6:249–261.

53. Greenspan, S. L., Maitland, L. A., Myers, E., Krasnow, M., and Kido, T. (1994): Femoral bone loss progresses with age: A longitudinal study in women over age 65. *J. Bone Miner. Res.,* 9:1959–1965.

54. Greenspan, S. L., Myers, E. R., Maitland, L. A., Resnick, N. M., and Hayes, W. C. (1994): Fall severity and bone mineral density as risk factors for hip fracture in ambulatory elderly. *JAMA,* 217:128–133.

55. Grisso, J. A., Kelsey, J. L., Strom, B. L., Chiu, G. Y., Maislin, G., O'Brien, L. A., Hoffman, S., and Kaplan, F. (1991): Risk factors for falls as a cause of hip fracture in women. *N. Engl. J. Med.,* 324:1326–1331.

56. Hansson, T., Roos, B., and Nachemson, A. (1980): The bone mineral content and ultimate compressive strength of lumbar vertebrae. *Spine,* 5:46–55.

57. Hardt, D. E. (1978): Determining muscle forces in the leg during normal human walking—An application and evaluation of optimization methods. *J. Biomech. Eng.,* 100:72–82.

58. Hayes, W. C. (1978): Biomechanical measurements of bone. In: *CRC Handbook of Engineering in Medicine and Biology: Section B. Instruments and Measurements,* edited by A. Burstein, pp. 333–372. CRC Press, Cleveland.

59. Hayes, W. C. (1991): Biomechanics of cortical and trabecular bone: Implications for assessment of fracture risk. In: *Basic Orthopedic Biomechanics,* edited by V.

C. Mow and W. C. Hayes, pp. 93–142. Raven Press, New York.

60. Hayes, W. C., and Carter, D. R. (1979): Biomechanics of bone. In: *Skeletal Research: An Experimental Approach*, edited by D. J. Simmons, pp. 263–300. Academic Press, New York.

61. Hayes, W. C., and Gerhart, T. N. (1985): Biomechanics of bone: Applications for assessment of bone strength. In: *bone and Mineral Research*, edited by W. A. Peck, pp. 259–294. Elsevier Science Publishers, Amsterdam.

62. Hayes, W. C., Myers, E. R., Morris, J. N., Yett, H. S., and Lipsitz, L. A. (1993): Impact near the hip dominates fracture risk in elderly nursing home residents who fall. *Calcif. Tissue Int.*, 52:192–198.

63. Hayes, W. C., Piazza, S. J., and Zysset, P. K. (1991): Biomechanics of fracture risk prediction of the hip and spine by quantitative computed tomography. *Radiol. Clin. North Am.*, 29:1–18.

64. Holbrook, T. L., Grazier, K., Kelsey, J. L., and Stauffer, R. N. (1984): *The frequency of occurence, impact and cost of selected musculoskeletal conditions in the United States.* American Academy of Orthopedic Surgeons, Chicago.

65. Hologic I (1994): Hologic reference data base. Hologic, Inc., Waltham, MA.

66. Hvid, I. (1988): *Mechanical Strength of Trabecular Bone at the Knee.* University of Aarhus, Aarhus, Denmark.

67. Jager, M., and Luttmann, A. (1989): Biomechanical analysis and assessment of lumbar stress during load lifting using a dynamic 19-segment human model. *Ergonomics*, 32:93–112.

68. Jensen, J. S. (1984): Determining factors for the mortality following hip fractures. *Injury*, 15:411–414.

69. Jensen, J. S., and Tondevold, E. (1979): Mortality after hip fractures. *Acta Orthop. Scand.*, 50:161–167.

70. Jones, H. H., Priest, J. D., Hayes, W. C., Tichenor, C. C., and Nagel, D. A. (1977): Humeral hypertrophy in response to exercise. *J. Bone Joint Surg. [Am.]*, 59: 204–208.

71. Keaveny, T. M., and Hayes, W. C. (1992): Mechanical properties of cortical and trabecular bone. In: *Bone, Volume VII: Bone Growth–B*, edited by B. K. Hall, pp. 285–344. CRC Press, Boca Raton, FL.

72. Kelsey, J. L., and Hoffman, S. (1987): Risk factors for hip fracture. *N. Engl. J. Med.*, 316:404–406.

73. Kenzora, J. E., McCarthy, R. E., Lowell, J. D., and Sledge, C. B. (1984): Hip fracture mortality. *Clin. Orthop.*, 186:45–56.

74. Keyak, J., Lee, I., and Skinner, H. (1994): Correlations between orthogonal mechanical properties and density of trabecular bone: Use of different densitometric measures. *J. Biomed. Mater. Res.*, 28:1329–1336.

75. Kimmel, D., Slovik, D., and Lane, N. (1994): Current and investigational approaches for reversing established osteoporosis. In: *Rheumatic Disease Clinics of North America*, edited by N. Lane, pp. 735–758. W. B. Saunders, Philadelphia.

76. Kleerekoper, M., and Nelson, D. (1992): Vertebral fracture or vertebral deformity? *Calcif. Tissue Int.*, 50:5–6.

77. Kotzar, G. M., Davy, D. T., Goldberg, V. M., Heiple, K. G., Berilla, J., Heiple, K. G., Jr., Brown, R. H., and Burstein, A. H. (1991): Telemeterized *in vivo* hip joint force data: A report on two patients after total hip surgery. *J. Orthop. Res.*, 9:621–633.

78. Kreutzeldt, J., Haim, M., and Bach, E. (1984): Hip fracture among the elderly in a mixed urban and rural population. *Age Ageing*, 13:111–119.

79. Kroonenberg, A. J., Hayes, W. C., and McMahon, T. A. (1995): Dynamic models for sideways falls from standing height. *J. Biomech. Eng.*, 117:309–318.

80. Kroonenberg, A. J., Hayes, W. C., and McMahon, T. A. (1996): Hip impact velocities and body configurations for voluntary falls from standing height. *J. Biomech.*, 29:807–811.

81. Lang, S. M., Moyle, D. D., Berg, E. W., Detoria, N., Gilpin, A. T., Pappas, N. J., Reynolds, J. C., and Tkacik, M. (1988): Correlation of mechanical properties of vertebral trabecular bone with equivalent mineral density as measured by computed tomography. *J. Bone Joint Surg. [Am.]*, 70:1531–1538.

82. Lauritzen, J., Petersen, M., and Lund, B. (1993): Effect of external hip protectors on hip fractures. *Lancet*, 341: 11–13.

83. Leichter, I., Margulies, J. Y., Weinreb, A., Mizrahi, J., Robin, G. C., Conforty, B., Makin, M., and Bloch, B. (1982): The relationship between bone density, mineral content, and mechanical strength in the femoral neck. *Clin. Orthop.*, 163:272–281.

84. Leichter, I., Simkin, A., Margulies, J. Y., Bivas, A., Roman, I., Deutsch, D., and Weinreb, A. (1988): Can the weight-bearing capacity of the femoral neck be estimated by physical measurements on the greater trochanter? *Eng. Med.*, 17:59–62.

85. Lotz, J. C., Gerhart, T. N., and Hayes, W. C. (1990): Mechanical properties of trabecular bone from the proximal femur: A quantitative CT study. *J. Comput. Assist. Tomogr.*, 14:107–114.

86. Lotz, J. C., and Hayes, W. C. (1990): Estimates of hip fracture risk from falls using quantitative computed tomography. *J. Bone Joint Surg. [Am.]*, 72:689–700.

87. Maki, B., and Fernie, G. (1990): Impact attenuation of floor coverings in simulated falling accidents. *Appl. Ergonomics*, 21:107–114.

88. Martin, R. B., and Atkinson, P. J. (1977): Age and sex-related changes in the structure and strength of the human femoral shaft. *J. Biomech.*, 10:223–231.

89. Martin, R. B., and Burr, D. B. (1989): *Structure, Function, and Adaptation of Compact Bone.* Raven Press, New York.

90. McBroom, R. J., Hayes, W. C., Edwards, W. T., Goldberg, R. P., and White, A. A. III (1985): Prediction of vertebral body compressive fracture using quantitative computed tomography. *J. Bone Joint Surg. [Am.]*, 67:1206–1214.

91. McGill, S. M. (1992): A myoelectrically based dynamic three-dimensional model to predict loads on lumbar spine tissues during lateral bending. *J. Biomech.*, 25:395–414.

92. McGill, S. M., and Norman, R. W. (1985): Dynamically and statically determined low back moments during lifting. *J. Biomech.*, 18:877–885.

93. McLeish, R. D., and Charnley, J. (1970): Abduction forces in the one-legged stance. *J. Biomech.*, 3:191–209.

94. Melton, L. J. III, and Riggs, B. L. (1986): Hip fracture: A disease and an accident. In: *Current Concepts of Bone Fragility*, edited by H. K. Uhthoff and E. Stahl, pp. 385–389. Springer-Verlag, Berlin.

95. Michelson, J., Myers, A., Jinnah, R., Cox, Q., and Van Natta, M. (1995): Epidemiology of hip fractures among the elderly. Risk factors for fracture type. *Clin. Orthop.*, 311:129–135.

96. Miller, C. W. (1978): Survival and ambulation following hip fracture. *J. Bone Joint Surg. [Am.],* 60:930–933.

97. Mizrahi, J., Margulies, J. Y., Leichter, I., and Deutsch, D. (1984): Fracture of the human femoral neck: Effect of density of the cancellous core. *J. Biomed. Eng.,* 6:56–62.

98. Moro, M., Hecker, A. T., Bouxsein, M. L., and Myers, E. R. (1995): Failure load of thoracic vertebrae correlates with lumbar bone mineral density measured by DXA. *Calcif. Tissue Int.,* 56:206–209.

99. Mosekilde, L., Bentzen, S. M., Ortoft, G., and Jorgensen, J. (1989): The predictive value of quantitative computed tomography for vertebral body compressive strength and ash density. *Bone,* 10:465–470.

100. Mosekilde, L., Viidik, A., and Mosekilde, L. (1985): Correlation between the compressive strength of iliac and vertebral trabecular bone in normal individuals. *Bone,* 6:291–291.

101. Myers, B., Arbogast, K., Lobaugh, B., Harper, K., Richardson, W., and Drezner, M. (1994): Improved assessment of lumbar vertebral body strength using supine lateral dual-energy x-ray absorptiometry. *J. Bone Miner. Res.,* 9:687–693.

102. Myers, E. R., Robinovitch, S. N., Greenspan, S. L., and Hayes, W. C. (1994): Factor of risk is associated with frequency of hip fracture in a case-control study. *Trans. 40th ORS,* 19:526.

103. Myers, E. R., Yang, K. A., Moro, M., Silva, M. J., and Hayes, W. C. (1996): Lumbar bone mineral density predicts thoracolumbar failure load in compression and flexion. *Trans. 42nd ORS,* 21:645.

104. Nachemson, A. L. (1976): The lumbar spine: An orthopaedic challenge. *Spine,* 1:59–71.

105. Nachemson, A. L., and Elfstrom, G. (1970): Intravital dynamic pressure measurements in lumbar discs. *Scand. J. Rehab. Med. [Suppl.],* 1:3–40.

106. Nagurka, M. L., and Hayes, W. C. (1980): Technical note: An interactive graphics package for calculating cross-sectional properties of complex shapes. *J. Biomech.,* 13:59–64.

107. Nevitt, M. C. (1994): Epidemiology of osteoporosis. In: *Rheumatic Disease Clinics of North America: Osteoporosis,* edited by N. E. Lane, pp. 535–560. W. B. Saunders, Philadelphia.

108. Nevitt, M. C., and Cummings, S. R. (1993): Type of fall and risk of hip and wrist fractures: The study of osteoporotic fractures. *J. Am. Geriatr. Soc.,* 41:1226–1234.

109. Nevitt, M. C., Cummings, S. R., and Hudes, E. S. (1991): Risk factors for injurious falls: A prospective study. *J. Gerontol.,* 46:M164–170.

110. Nevitt, M., Johnell, O., Black, D., Ensrud, K., Genant, H., and Cummings, S. (1994): Bone mineral density predicts non-spine fractures in very elderly women. *Osteoporosis Int.,* 4:325–331.

111. O'Neill, T., Varlow, J., Felsenberg, D., Johnell, O., Weber, K., Marchant, F., Delmas, P., Cooper, C., Kanis, J., and Silman, A. (1994): Variation in vertebral height ratios in population studies. *J. Bone Miner. Res.,* 9: 1895–1907.

112. Patel, U., Skingle, S., Campbell, G., Crisp, A., and Boyle, I. (1991): Clinical profile of acute vertebral compression fractures in osteoporosis. *Br. J. Rheumatol.,* 30:418–421.

113. Paul, J. P. (1967): Forces transmitted by joints in the human body. *Proc. Inst. Mechan. Eng.,* 181:8–15.

114. Paul, J. P. (1976): Approaches to design. *Proc. R. Soc. Lond.,* 192:163–172.

115. Phillips, S., Fox, N., Jacobs, J., and Wright, W. (1988): The direct medical costs of osteoporosis for American women aged 45 and older. *Bone,* 9:271–279.

116. Pinilla, T. P., Boardman, K., Bouxsein, M. L., Myers, E. R., and Hayes, W. C. (1995): Differences in loading direction from a fall can reduce the failure load of the proximal femur as much as age-related bone loss. *Trans. 41st ORS,* 20:239.

116a. Praemer, A., Furner, S., Rice, D. (1992): Musculoskeletal conditions in the U.S. AAOS, Park Ridge, IL.

116b. Reilly, D. T., and Burstein, A. H. (1975): The elastic and ultimate properties of compact bone tissue. *J. Biomech.,* 8:393–405.

117. Reilly, D. T., and Burstein, A. H. (1974): The mechanical properties of cortical bone. *J. Bone Joint Surg. [Am.],* 56:1001–1022.

118. Reilly, D. T., Burstein, A. H., and Frankel, V. H. (1974): The elastic modulus for bone. *J. Biomech.,* 7:271–275.

119. Rice, J. C., Cowin, S. C., and Bowman, J. A. (1988): On the dependence of the elasticity and strength of cancellous bone on apparent density. *J. Biomech.,* 21:155–168.

120. Riggs, B. L., and Melton, L. J. III (1988): *Osteoporosis: Etiology, Diagnosis and Management.* Raven Press, New York.

121. Robinovitch, S. N., McMahon, T. A., and Hayes, W. C. (1995): Energy shunting hip padding system attenuates femoral impact force in a simulated fall. *J. Biomech. Eng.,* 117:409–413.

122. Robinovitch, S. N., McMahon, T. A., and Hayes, W. C. (1995): Force attenuation in trochanteric soft tissues during impact from a fall. *J. Orthop. Res.,* 13:956–962.

123. Robinovitch, S. N., McMahon, T. A., and Hayes, W. C. (1991): Prediction of femoral impact forces in falls on the hip. *J. Biomech. Eng.,* 113:366–374.

124. Rohrle, H., Scholten, R., Sigolotto, C., Sollbach, W., and Kellner, H. (1984): Joint forces in the human pelvis–leg skeleton during walking. *J. Biomech.,* 17: 409–424.

125. Ross, P. D., Davis, J. W., Vogel, J. M., and Wasnich, R. D. (1990): A critical review of bone mass and the risk of fractures in osteoporosis. *Calcif. Tissue Int.,* 46: 149–161.

126. Ruff, C. B., and Hayes, W. C. (1983): Cross-sectional geometry of Pecos Pueblo femora and tibiae—a biomechanical investigation: II. Sex, age and size differences. *Am. J. Phys. Anthropol.,* 60:383–400.

127. Ruff, C. B., and Hayes, W. C. (1983): Cross-sectional geometry of Pecos Pueblo femora and tibiae: A biomechanical investigation. I. Method and general patterns of variation. *Am. J. Phys. Anthropol.,* 60:359–381.

128. Ruff, C. B., and Hayes, W. C. (1984): Age changes in geometry and mineral content of the lower limb bones. *Ann. Biomed. Eng.,* 12:573–584.

129. Ruff, C. B., and Hayes, W. C. (1988): Sex differences in age-related remodeling of the femur and tibia. *J. Orthop. Res.,* 6:886–896.

130. Rydell, N. W. (1966): Forces acting on the femoral head-prosthesis. A study on strain gauge supplied prostheses in living persons. *Acta Orthop. Scand.,* 37: 1–132.

131. Santavirta, S., Konttinen, Y., Heliovaara, M., Knekt, P., Luthje, P., and Aromaa, A. (1992): Determinants of osteoporotic thoracic vertebral fracture. *Acta Orthop. Scand.,* 63:198–202.

132. Sartoris, D. J., Andre, M., Resnick, C., and Resnick, D. (1986): Trabecular bone density in the proximal femur: Quantitative CT assessment. *Radiology,* 160:707–712.

133. Sattin, R. (1992): Falls among older persons. *Annu. Rev. Public Health,* 13:489–508.

134. Schaffler, M. B., and Burr, D. B. (1988): Stiffness of compact bone: Effects of porosity and density. *J. Biomech.,* 21:13–16.

135. Schultz, A. B., and Andersson, G. B. J. (1981): Analysis of loads on the lumbar spine. *Spine,* 6:76–82.

136. Schultz, A. B., Andersson, G. B. J., Haderspeck, K., Ortengren, R., Nordin, M., and Bjork, R. (1982): Analysis and measurement of lumbar trunk loads in tasks involving bends and twists. *J. Biomech.,* 15:669–675.

137. Schultz, A. B., Andersson, G. B. J., Ortengren, R., Bjork, R., and Nordin, M. (1982): Analysis and quantitative myoelectric measurements of loads on the lumbar spine when holding weights in standing postures. *Spine,* 7:390–397.

138. Schultz, A. B., Andersson, G. B. J., Ortengren, R., Haderspeck, K., and Nachemson, A. (1982): Loads on the lumbar spine. Validation of a biomechanical analysis by measurements of intradiscal pressures and myoelectric signals. *J. Bone Joint Surg. [Am.],* 64:713–720.

139. Schultz, A. B., Cromwell, R., Warwick, D., and Andersson, G. B. J. (1987): Lumbar trunk muscle use in standing isometric heavy exertions. *J. Orthop. Res.,* 5:320–329.

140. Schultz, A. B., Haderspeck, K., Warwick, D., and Portillo, D. (1983): Use of lumbar trunk muscles in isometric performance of mechanically complex standing tasks. *J. Orthop. Res.,* 1:77–91.

141. Smidt, G. L., and Blanpied, P. R. (1987): Analysis of strength tests and resistive exercises commonly used for low-back disorders. *Spine,* 12:1025–1034.

142. Snyder, B. D., and Hayes, W. C. (1990): Multiaxial structure–property relations in trabecular bone. In: *Biomechanics of Diarthrodial Joints,* edited by V. C. Mow, A. Ratcliffe, and S. L.–Y. Woo, pp. 31–59. Springer-Verlag, New York.

143. Snyder, S. M., and Schneider, E. (1991): Estimation of mechanical properties of cortical bone by computed tomography. *J. Orthop. Res.,* 9:422–431.

144. Steiger, P., Cummings, S., Black, D., Spencer, N., and Genant, H. (1992): Age-related decrements in bone mineral density in women over 65. *J. Bone Miner. Res.,* 7:625–632.

145. Thompson, D. W. (1961): *On Growth and Form.* Cambridge University Press, Cambridge.

146. Tinetti, M. (1987): Factors associated with serious injury during falls among elderly persons living in the community. *J. Am. Geriatr. Soc.,* 35:644–648.

147. Vesterby, A., Mosekilde, L., Gundersen, H., Melsen, F., Mosekilde, L., Holme, K., and Sorensen, S. (1991): Biologically meaningful determinants of the *in vitro* strength of lumbar vertebrae. *Bone,* 12:219–224.

148. Weber, T., Yang, K., Woo, R., and Fitzgerald, R. (1992): Proximal femur strength: Correlation of the rate of loading and bone mineral density. *Adv. Bioeng.,* 22:111–114.

149. Weiss, N. S., Liff, J. M., Ure, C. L., Ballard, J. H., Abbott, G. H., and Daling, J. R. (1983): Mortality in women following hip fracture. *J. Chron. Dis.,* 36:879–882.

150. Williams, J. F., and Svensson, J. L. (1968): A force analysis of the hip joint. *Biomed. Eng.,* 3:365–371.

151. Wilson, S. (1994): *Development of a model to predict the compressive forces on the spine associated with age-related vertebral fractures.* Master's Thesis, Massachusetts Institute of Technology, Cambridge.

152. Wolff, J. (1892). The law of bone remodeling. Trans. by P. Maquet and R. Furlong. Springer-Verlag.

153. Woo, S. L.-Y., Kuei, S. C., Amiel, D., Gomez, M. A., Hayes, W. C., White, F. C., and Akeson, W. H. (1981): The effect of prolonged physical training on the properties of long bone: A study of Wolff's Law. *J. Bone Joint Surg. [Am.],* 63:780–787.

154. Wright, T. M. (1980): Mechanics of fracture and fracture propagation. In: *Scientific Foundations of Orthopaedics,* edited by O. Goodfellow, pp. 252–258. William Heinemann Medical Books, London.

155. Wright, T. M., and Hayes, W. C. (1976): Tensile testing of bone over a wide range of strain rates: Effects of strain rate, micro-structure and density. *Med. Biol. Eng. Comput.,* 14:671–680.

156. Yettram, A., and Jackman, M. (1980): Equilibrium analysis for the forces in the human spinal column and its musculature. *Spine,* 5:402–411.

Basic Orthopaedic Biomechanics, 2nd ed.,
edited by Van C. Mow and Wilson C. Hayes.
Lippincott–Raven Publishers, Philadelphia © 1997.

4

Structure and Function of Articular Cartilage and Meniscus

Van C. Mow and *Anthony Ratcliffe

*Departments of Mechanical Engineering and Orthopaedic Surgery,
Center for Biomedical Engineering, Columbia University, New York, New York 10032;
and *Department of Orthopaedic Biochemistry, Biochemistry Section,
New York Orthopaedic Hospital Research Laboratory, and Department of Orthopaedic Surgery,
Columbia University, New York, New York 10032.*

There are three broad classes of cartilaginous tissues present in the body: hyaline cartilage, elastic cartilage, and fibrocartilage (324). These tissues are distinguished by their biochemical composition, their molecular microstructure, and their biomechanical properties and functions. Hyaline cartilage, as the name implies, is glassy smooth, glistening, and bluish-white in appearance (although older tissues tend to lose this appearance). The most common hyaline cartilage, and the most studied, is articular cartilage (178,212, 252). This tissue covers the articulating surfaces of long bones and sesamoid bones within synovial joints, e.g., the surfaces of the tibia, the femur, and the patella of the knee joint. Another example of hyaline cartilage is the growth plate, which controls, for example, the growth of all bones during skeletal maturation (51,307,324). Other tissues include the larynx, the support structures of the tracheal tube, rib and costal cartilage, and the nasal septum (105,106,324). Examples of elastic cartilage are the epiglottis, the external auditory canal, and the eustachian tube. These tissues are generally yellowish and opaque in appearance and are more flexible than hyaline cartilage (324). Two fibrocartilages are the annulus fibrosus of the intervertebral disk, which provides the flexible junctions between the vertebral bodies in the spine (1,25,101, 282,287,308,309,324; see Chapter 10 for more details on the spine) and the meniscus of the knee (2,3,13,78,83,155,194,214,239,243, 259,286,333). Articular cartilage and meniscus are vital to maintain normal joint motion, and both are involved in degenerative disease of the knee such as osteoarthritis (also called osteoarthrosis or simply designated as OA). Therefore, they have been the focus of much research over the past several decades. In this chapter, we describe the biochemical composition and ultrastructural organization of these two tissues and relate these to their mechanical properties in order to provide an understanding of the structure–function relationships of these tissues.

Articular cartilages in freely movable joints, such as hip and knee, can withstand very large loads (4,5,96,129; also see Chapters 1 and 2 of this text) while providing a smooth, lubricating bearing material with minimal wear (see Chapter 8 on joint lubrication). The major motivation for the study of articular cartilage and meniscus has been the development of an understanding of the OA disease processes that can afflict most of the load-bearing joints (e.g., 9,31,136,157,178, 245,290). The reader is referred to the recent excellent text by Moskowitz and co-workers (201) for a complete description of OA and other degenerative joint diseases. More recently, tissue engineering as it pertains to cartilage repair has become another motivating factor for innovative studies of cartilage biol-

ogy (e.g., 215,321; also see Chapter 5 for more details on chondrocyte function).

The breakdown of cartilage leading to OA can result from a multitude of factors, mechanical and humoral, and can occur in an acute and traumatic form or in a chronic fashion, occurring over many years. These changes ultimately result in alterations of the biomechanical properties of the tissue and a reduction in its ability to function in the highly stressed environment of the joint (e.g., 4,5,40,136,178,212,216,299,316). Therefore, it is important to understand (a) the mechanical properties of normal cartilage; (b) the manner by which biochemical and structural factors contribute to the material properties of cartilage; and (c) the manner by which changes in tissue composition affect the mechanical properties of cartilage. Furthermore, in order to understand how knees, hips, and other diarthrodial joints carry and support load and provide lubrication and protection against wear, one must know, in a quantitative manner, the exact shape of each of these joints (see Chapter 7 for a description of a quantitative determination of joint anatomy and Chapter 8 for details of diarthrodial joint tribology).

STRUCTURE OF A DIARTHRODIAL JOINT

All diarthrodial joints have common structural features. First, all diarthrodial joints are enclosed in a strong fibrous capsule (top left, Fig. 1) (212). Second, the inner surfaces of the joint capsules are lined with the synovium, which secretes the synovial fluid and provides the nutrients required by the tissues within the joint (297). It has long been thought that the synovial fluid also serves as the lubricant for diarthrodial joints (257). Third, each articulating bone end within the joint is lined with a thin layer of hydrated soft tissue, i.e., the articular cartilage. These linings, i.e., the synovium and the two articular cartilage layers, form the joint cavity, which contains the synovial fluid. Thus, the synovial fluid, articular

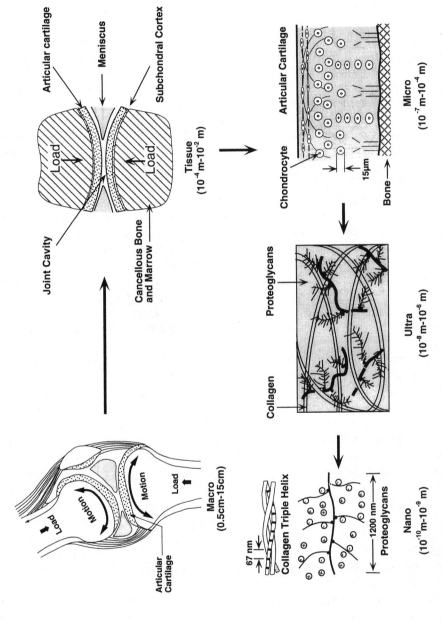

FIG. 1. Some of the important structural features of a typical diarthrodial joint at different levels of scale: macro (0.5 to 15 cm); tissue (10^{-4} to 10^{-2} m); micro (10^{-7} to 10^{-4} m); ultra (10^{-8} to 10^{-6} m); and nano (10^{-10} to 10^{-9} m) (212).

cartilage, and supporting bone form a "closed" biomechanical bearing system that provides the smooth, nearly frictionless bearing system of the body. Although diarthrodial joints are subjected to an enormous range of loading conditions, slow cyclical conditions, and high loads (e.g., 4,5,96,236), the cartilage surfaces have the potential to remain unimpaired and functionally normal for the lifetime of an individual.

Two geometric features of diarthrodial joints are most important for their biomechancial function: (a) the anatomic forms of the articulating surfaces and (b) the thickness contours of the cartilage layers (e.g., 14,16,17,61–63,168,197,238,291,292). The overall anatomic form largely dictates the types of motion (rolling and/or sliding) that a joint may have, and the thickness contours of the articular cartilage layers (along with their material properties and loadings) dictate the types of stresses and their magnitudes existing within the tissue. The hip, for example, is a close-fitting ball-and-socket joint that is nearly spherical, and because the acetabulum (socket) is a deep cup, this is a very stable joint. However, at times, congenital childhood abnormalities of acetabulum shape (shallow cup) lead to severe hip diseases. Also, deviations from sphericity of the articular and subchondral bone surfaces on the acetabulum and femoral head (ball) have been noted, and hypothesized as being an important factor in the etiology of OA (42,266). In severe arthritis, both sides of the hip become grossly distorted by the formation of bony spurs (osteophytes), which, in their advanced stages, severely restrict the motion of the hip (31,136). The glenohumeral joint of the shoulder is also a close-fitting, spherical, ball-and-socket joint, though here the glenoid surface on the scapula is a very shallow spherical sector covering only one-third of the spherical humeral head (291). This is necessary because of all the joints in the body, the shoulder must provide the largest range of motion required by the activities of daily living. Because of this, however, the shoulder is very susceptible to instability and dislocation, i.e., shifting of

contact region within the joint (292), which could often lead to the development of severe arthritis. For both the hip and the shoulder, under normal conditions, the articulation is characterized by a sliding motion of one articular surface over the other (96,146). These close-fitting sliding articulations also provide the necessary geometric forms for the formation of fluid-film lubrication in these joints (for more details on joint lubrication, see Chapter 8).

Other joint surfaces have more complex geometric forms. For example, the knee is actually comprised of two joints: the patellofemoral joint and the femorotibial joint. This anatomic arrangement (lever) can produce the large moments required for knee function (e.g., the extension moments required to rise from deep knee bends). To produce these moments, very large forces must be generated by the surrounding muscles, thus creating very large joint reaction forces (see Chapters 1 and 2 for more information on joint reaction forces). These large joint reaction forces significantly deform and stress the articular cartilage layers.

Factors affecting the magnitude and type of stresses and strains in articular cartilage are its form, thickness contour, loading, and material properties (15–18,212). Recently, there has been much interest in developing MRI methods to quantitatively assess articular cartilage thickness contours *in vivo*, in normal subjects and in patients with OA (e.g., 14,61–63,168,197,238). To date, however, the accuracies of these MRI methods for determining the articular surface contours, using commercially available MRI, are between 1 and 2 mm. These methods, along with further refinements of MRI technology, offer opportunities for researchers to develop realistic joint models to calculate the stresses and strains in the cartilaginous layers *in vivo*. Recently, accurate *in vitro* methods (<100 μm) for assessing joint anatomy and cartilage thickness maps have also been developed using stereophotogrammetry (16,17,26,137, 291,292; Chapter 7). These results of studies are very accurate (<90 μm for knees and <25 μm for wrist joints), and they have shown that the articular cartilage layer thicknesses are, in general, not uniform and that the surfaces have high curvatures with regular patterns of ridges and grooves running across them. Obviously, these features will have pronounced effects on the stresses and strains developed in the cartilage layer during joint loading.

COMPOSITION AND STRUCTURE OF ARTICULAR CARTILAGE AND MENISCUS

Articular cartilage and meniscus, in their young, normal, and healthy state, are glistening, smooth, intact, and substantial tissues. In older individuals and in preclinical disease states, the tissues lose this appearence and often look dull and roughened. Menisci degenerate in the form of tears and fraying. Articular cartilage fibrillates, forms deep fissures, and, in advanced OA, is entirely lost at weight-bearing sites over the joint surface. These readily evident macroscopic manifestations of pathologies (often simplistically referred to as "wear and tear") have not yet been fully explained in mechanical, molecular, and cellular terms. However, to provide a basis for understanding this disease process, it is necessary first to understand the structure–function relationships existing for articular cartilage and menisci. This necessarily means knowing the stress–strain behaviors of these materials. Thus, in the following sections, the biochemical composition and organization of articular cartilage and menisci are described, and these are related to the mechanical properties of the tissue.

Articular cartilage and menisci can be regarded as multiphasic materials with two major phases: a fluid phase composed of water and electrolytes and a solid phase composed of collagen, proteoglycans, and other proteins, glycoproteins, and the chondrocytes (e.g., 184,205,207,212) (see Table 1). For an understanding of cartilage swelling, the dissolved electrolytes (Na^+, Ca^{2+}, Cl^-, etc.)

TABLE 1. *Composition of articular cartilage and meniscus*

Tissue	Water	Collagen (wet wt.)	Proteoglycan (wet wt.)
Articular cartilage	68–85%	10–20% (type II)	5–10%
Meniscus	60–70%	15–25% (type I)	1–2%

within the interstitial fluid must be considered as a separate third phase (160–162), and the solid phase must be charged. Indeed, each phase of the tissue contributes significantly to its known mechanical and physicochemical properties. Table 2 provides a summary of the biochemical components of cartilage and menisci. Of the organic components, the collagens (e.g., 72,196,227–229,312) provide the quantitatively major organic component, followed by aggrecans and proteoglycan aggregates (e.g., 39,41,87,109,110,115–118,123–125,177,219,220,240,241,249,310). Quantitatively minor components include link protein (59,108), the smaller proteoglycans versican (98), biglycan, decorin (54,81,315), and perlican (140), fibromodulin and thrombospondin (124), and COMP (cartilage oligomeric matrix protein) (122). Although

TABLE 2. *A summary of the components of articular cartilage and/or menisci*

Component	Wet weight
Quantitatively major	
Water	60–85%
Collagen, type II	15–22%
Aggrecan	4–7%
Quantitatively minor (<5%)	
Link protein	
Hyaluronan	
Biglycan	
Collagen type I	
Collagen type V	
Collagen type VI	
Collagen type IX	
Collagen type XI	
COMP	
Decorin	
Fibromodulin	
Perlican	
Thrombospondin	

these are not major components in terms of the absolute mass of the solid phase, they may approach the molar concentrations of collagen and aggrecan and serve important biological regulating functions. It should be noted that much of the noncollagenous component of articular cartilage and menisci is yet to be accounted for, and it is likely that only when these, as yet undescribed, molecules are characterized, and their biological and mechanical functions are defined, will a comprehensive understanding of the structure–function relations for articular cartilage and menisci be developed.

Interstitial Water

By far, water is the most abundant component of articular cartilage, (e.g., 28,64,65,170, 179,182,187,192,205,304,313). It is believed that in normal cartilage, a portion of this water (approximately 30%) resides within the intrafibrillar space of collagen, and for normal tissue this proportion appears not to vary with age (144,145,189,191,303,320). The diameter of collagen fibers, and thus the amount of water within the intrafibrillar compartment, is modulated by the swelling pressure generated by the "fixed charge density" (FCD) of the surrounding proteoglycans (145,189,320). In the native tissue, it appears that most of this intrafibrillar water is not available for transport under mechanical loading and is excluded from the proteoglycans. This exclusion effectively raises the density of the fixed charges within the tissue, thus raising the interstitial osmotic pressure (by the Donnan osmotic pressure law) and charge–charge repulsion (for more details, see discussions below in the section on Swelling of Articular Cartilage). In contrast, there is a significant increase of water content in degenerating articular cartilages (e.g., 10,28,32,179,186,190,205,212,313,314). It is not known, however, whether the same proportion of water exists in the intrafibrillar space within these degenerating cartilages. Scanning electron microscopic examinations of some canine articular cartilages subsequent

to high-impact loading have shown the collagen fibers in the traumatized tissue to be highly swollen (58,299), but no information exists about whether the water in these swollen fibers is free to flow and be available for proteoglycan solvation. If both occur, then there will be an increased permeability (which is biomechanically highly detrimental) and a decrease of FCD (which decreases the swelling pressure and its concomitant load support). It is known, phenomenologically, that changes in the total water content have strong influences in the mechanical, swelling, and fluid-transport properties exhibited by the tissue (e.g., 6,7,10,99,103, 183–185,209,212,283). From the recently developed triphasic theory, mathematical relationships have now been derived for the dependence of hydraulic permeability, electric conductivity, swelling pressure, streaming potential, and other physicochemical and electromechanical phenomena on the water content in articular cartilage (99,162). Details of these functional relationships are described below.

The amount of water present depends largely on several factors: (a) the concentration of the proteoglycans, i.e., FCD, and the resultant swelling pressure exerted by the negative charge groups on the proteoglycans and the ions dissolved in the interstitial fluid; (b) the organization of the collagen network; and (c) the strength and stiffness of this network, which surrounds the proteoglycan molecules and resists the swelling pressure (e.g., 7,97,162,183,184,223,225). The predominant ions within the interstitial fluid are sodium, chloride, potassium, and calcium (170). In cartilage from osteoarthritic joints, disruption of the collagen network can cause the water content of the tissue to increase by more than 10% (28,179,183,190,193). This increase greatly affects the mechanical properties of the tissue (9,10,31,128,141,142,205,212,283).

Most of the fluid and ions within the tissue are freely exchangeable by diffusion with the bathing solution surrounding the tissue (170,179,182,184,303,304). The interstitial fluid may also be extruded from the tissue by applying a pressure gradient across the tissue (180,181,192) or by simply compressing the tissue (e.g., 10,20,64,65,70,170,192,203,209, 212,288). As the interstitial fluid flows through the pores of the collagen–proteoglycan solid matrix, significant frictional drag forces are exerted on the walls of the pores of the solid matrix, thus causing compaction (130–132,163,212). This nonlinear flow-induced compression effect (sometimes known as the strain-dependent permeability) is very important in the physiology of articular cartilage because it means that it becomes more difficult to squeeze fluid from such tissues with prolonged compression. For both cartilage and meniscus, the frictional drag force not only dominates their compressive viscoelastic behaviors, e.g., creep and stress relaxation, but also provides the mechanism for energy dissipation (163,192,205–208,243). A major focus of this chapter is the description of this flow-dependent, i.e., biphasic, viscoelastic phenomenon.

Collagen

In articular cartilage and meniscus, the primary function of the collagen appears to be to provide the tensile properties to the tissues. However, because there are an array of different collagens present, most in quantitatively minor amounts, it is likely that other, as yet undefined, functions exist. The importance of the collagens in contributing to tissue function is easily demonstrated by the evidence of collagen mutations contributing to heritable disorders, including precocious OA (8, 227–229,231).

Collagen Types

There are now at least 18 different types of collagen that have been described (298,312). Of these, articular cartilage contains primarily type II, with smaller amounts of types V, VI, IX, and XI. Type X collagen exists in the hypertrophic zone of the growth plate. Ninety percent of collagen in the meniscus is type I, with small amounts (1% to 2%) of types II, V, and VI. The major collagen types (I and II) are

what distinguish the fibrocartilaginous meniscus from articular cartilage (72,78). They all have a basic structure of three chains forming a triple helix, but within this there is much variation, presumably to provide for extensive differences in function (Table 3). Types I, II, X, and XI are fibrillar collagens, whereas types VI and IX are nonfibrillar collagens, in a group termed FACITs (fibril-associated collagens with interrupted triple helices). Type I collagen molecules are composed of two $\alpha1(I)$ and one $\alpha2(I)$ polypeptide chains, and type II contains three $\alpha1(II)$ polypeptide chains (72,227). Type IX contains three distinct α chains, $\alpha1(IX)$, $\alpha2(IX)$, and $\alpha3(IX)$, and it is unusual in the collagen family in that it is also a proteoglycan because it contains a glycosaminoglycan (GAG) chain attached to the $\alpha2$ chain (311). Type X is a low-molecular-weight collagen and has three identical $\alpha1(X)$ chains. Type I collagen is the most abundant collagen of the body and is distributed widely throughout the body; it is found in many tissues including meniscus, intervertebral disk, bone, skin, tendons, and ligaments. Type II collagen is present primarily in articular cartilage, nasal septum, and the sternal cartilage as well as in the intervertebral disk. Type X is typically present in the hypertrophic cartilage (196,227–229).

Collagen Structure

Collagen has a high degree of structural organization (Fig. 2). The basic triple helical structural unit of collagen is formed from

TABLE 3. *A summary of the fibrillar organization of the genetically distinct collagens in cartilage and meniscus*

Collagen type	Chain organization
Type I	$[\alpha1(I)]_2\alpha2(I)$
Type II	$[\alpha1(II)]_3$
Type V	$[\alpha1(V)]_2\alpha2(V)$
Type VI	$\alpha1(VI)\alpha2(VI)\alpha3(VI)$
Type IX	$\alpha1(IX)\alpha2(IX)\alpha3(IX)$
Type X	$[\alpha1(X)]_3$
Type XI	$\alpha1(XI)\alpha2(XI)\alpha3(XI)$

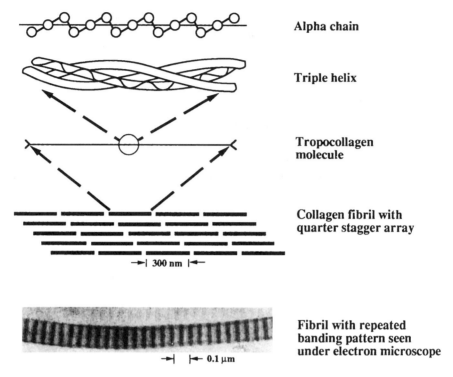

Alpha chain

Triple helix

Tropocollagen molecule

Collagen fibril with quarter stagger array

300 nm

Fibril with repeated banding pattern seen under electron microscope

0.1 μm

FIG. 2. Schematic representation and photomicrograph of the collagen fibril structure.

three polypeptide chains (α chains), each of which has a natural left-handed helix, that together form a right-handed helix (Fig. 2). Each α chain is composed of glycine/proline/X, where X could be either hydroxyproline or another amino acid. This highly organized structure appears to have been specifically designed to resist tension (6,91,147–150,258,263,275,317,318,325–327). Type I collagen, the major collagen of meniscus, is a heterotrimer consisting of two α1(I) and one α2(I) chains. Type II collagen, the primary collagen of articular cartilage, is a homotrimer and, as such, contains three α1(II) polypeptide chains, although alternative splicing at the transcription of the gene can alter the final synthetic product in a tissue-specific and developmentally regulated manner (271).

In articular cartilage, type II tropocollagen molecules are polymerized extracellularly to form collagen fibrils. Small-diameter (10 to 25 nm) fibrils are formed in the pericellular region, and much larger diameter fibrils (up to 300 nm diameter) are formed in the territo-

rial and interterritorial matrix (33–36,48,49, 139). However, these are still much smaller than the collagen fibers present in menisci or ligaments and tendons, where large-diameter fibers are formed by the type I collagen (45, 82,331). Type IX collagen contributes only 1% of the total collagen in mature articular cartilage, although it is present at a much higher concentration in fetal tissues. It contains three distinct α chains, α1(IX), α2(IX), and α3(IX), and is regarded as a FACIT collagen (Fig. 3). It is present on the surface of type II collagen fibrils in an antiparallel fashion, and each type IX collagen is covalently linked to at least one type II collagen molecule (74,311,329). These are similar to the intramolecular and intermolecular covalent crosslinks of type II collagen, the trifunctional hydroxypyridinium crosslink (75–77, 226,330). Type IX collagen therefore appears to have an important role in stabilizing the three-dimensional organization of the collagen network (75,311,329) and thus contributes to the ability of collagen to resist the

CS
COL3
COL2
COL1
C
NC3
NC2
NC1
A
N
NC4
type IX molecule
C
N
N
C
type II fibril
B

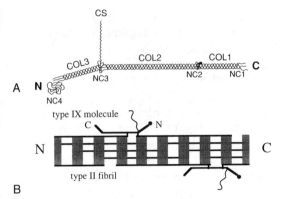

FIG. 3. The structure of type IX collagen and its association with type II collagen. **(A)** Type IX collagen consists of three triple helical domains (COL1, COL2, COL3) with four nonhelical domains (NC1–NC4), and the molecule is stabilized by interchain disulfide bridges. The single chondroitin sulfate chain is attached at the NC3 domain. **(B)** The majority of type IX collagen molecules exist in the extracellular matrix covalently bound to the surface of type II collagen fibrils in an antiparallel manner.

swelling pressure of the proteoglycans and the tensile stresses developed within the tissue when it is loaded *in situ* (153,183,212,274).

Recently, it has been shown that a reduction in function of type IX collagen has the potential to contribute to degeneration of articular cartilage (79). For a comprehensive description of collagen synthesis, biochemistry, molecular structure, and organization, the reader is referred to review volumes (227–229).

Proteoglycans

Proteoglycans are large complex biomolecules and are composed of a protein core to which one or more GAG chains are covalently attached. The major proteoglycan in articular cartilage is aggrecan, and it has been studied extensively because of its role in skeletal growth, joint function, and the development of OA (Fig. 4) (e.g., 39,110–112,115–118, 124,220,240). Other more recently described proteoglycans in articular cartilage include versican, biglycan, and decorin. In meniscus, the proteoglycans aggrecan, biglycan, and decorin are also present. In cartilage, the large aggregating proteoglycans (aggrecan and versican) contribute 50% to 85% of the proteoglycans, while the small proteoglycans (e.g., biglycan and decorin) probably contribute less than 10%. As aggregates, the aggrecan

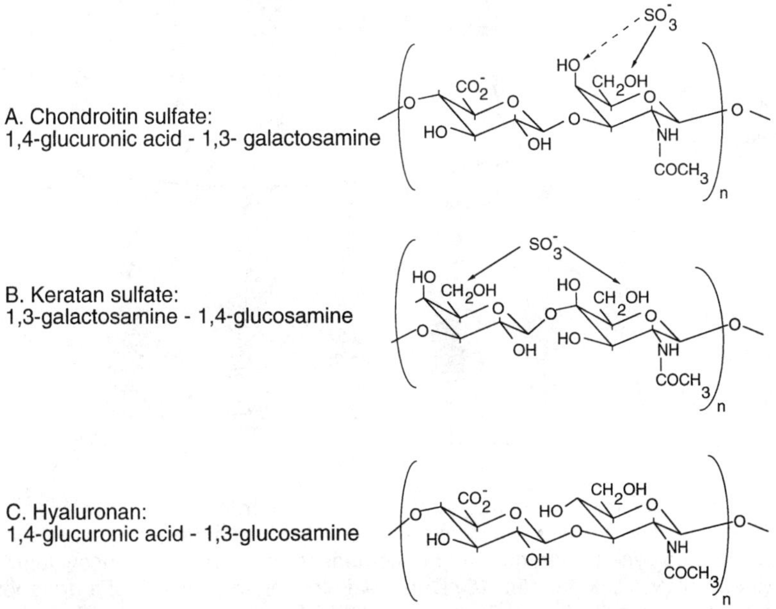

A. Chondroitin sulfate:
1,4-glucuronic acid - 1,3- galactosamine
B. Keratan sulfate:
1,3-galactosamine - 1,4-glucosamine
C. Hyaluronan:
1,4-glucuronic acid - 1,3-glucosamine

FIG. 4. The disaccharide units of the three primary glycosaminoglycan chains in cartilage (178).

molecules can form macromolecular complexes of $300–400 \times 10^6$ Da and make major contributions to the mechanical and physicochemical properties of cartilage (e.g., 99,162,181,184,209,212). Aggrecan has an overall mass of $1–4 \times 10^6$ Da and consists of an extended protein core (220,000 to 250,000 Da) with up to 50 keratan sulfate chains and 100 chondroitin sulfate chains attached (Fig. 5) (e.g., 39,55,56,109,110,115,124,310).

The protein core is organized into several distinct domains. The N-terminal G1 domain interacts with both link protein (in a 1:1 stoichiometry) and a monofilament chain of hyaluronan (a decamer is a minimal length for binding), and when these three components come together, they form a complex that is extremely stable (108,111,112,237,250,254). Link protein is a separate globular protein (40,000 to 48,000 Da) (59,108,250) and shares structural similarities with the G1 and G2 domains of aggrecan. The G1 domain is separated from the adjacent G2 domain by a short extended region, and the C-terminal of

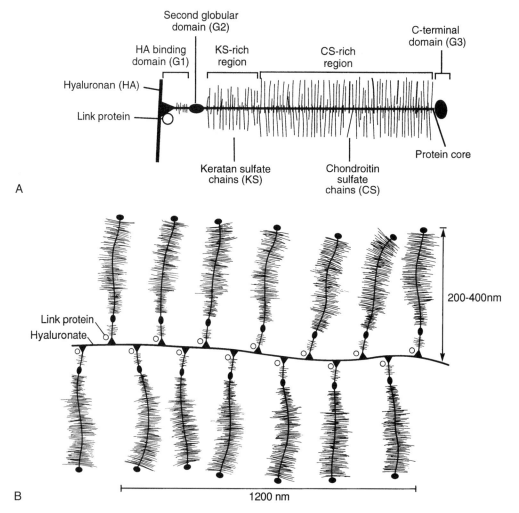

FIG. 5. (A) Schematic depiction of an aggregating proteoglycan molecule (aggrecan) composed of keratan sulfate and chondroitin sulfate chains bound covalently to a protein core molecule. **(B)** A representation of a proteoglycan aggregate that is composed of aggrecans noncovalently attached to hyaluronan with stabilizing link proteins. **(C)** Dark-field electron micrograph of a proteoglycan aggregate from bovine humeral articular cartilage (×120,000). (Courtesy of Dr. Joseph A. Buckwalter.)

the G2 domain is the GAG-binding region of the protein core. The keratan sulfate-rich region is composed of two distinct zones (KSI and KSII) and is adjacent to the chondroitin sulfate attachment region, which also is present as two zones (CSI and CSII). At the C-terminal end, the protein has a final globular region, which is in fact made up of several small domains. Because the protein core constitutes only approximately 10% of the total mass (the rest being the GAG and oligosaccharides), there is a large potential for post-translational modifications. This can be by the addition of more, or fewer, of the chondroitin and keratan sulfate chains or by variation in the length of the chains, and can contribute considerably to the heterogeneity of the proteoglycan population in the cartilage. The other aggregating proteoglycan in cartilage, versican, is expressed at much lower levels (98).

Two important nonaggregating proteoglycans are biglycan (81,262,270) and decorin (54,315). Biglycan in cartilage has a molecular mass of approximately 100,000 Da, with a protein core of 38,000 Da and two GAG chains, 40% to 50% being dermatan sulfate and the remainder being chondroitin sulfate. Decorin is present in cartilage in molar amounts similar to aggrecan and is the dominant proteoglycan in meniscus (259). It has a protein core similar (55% homology) to biglycan, with a single GAG chain that can be dermatan sulfate or chondroitin sulfate. Although functions for these small proteoglycans are still being described, it seems clear that they are able to interact with collagen (see below).

The function of hyaluronan, sometimes referred to as an "honorary proteoglycan" (although hyaluronan is not covalently associated with protein and therefore is not a proteoglycan), is well described in its interactions with aggrecan and link protein (e.g., 108,111,112,220). In this role, its function is to form macromolecular aggregates with aggrecan that are immobilized within the collagen network. A further function still being defined is linking the extracellular matrix (ECM) with the chondrocytes. The cells have hyaluronan receptors (CD44) on their surfaces that specifically bind extracellular hyaluronan (156). This forms a direct linkage between the cells and their surrounding matrix and, as such, may provide an important mechanism by which the chondrocyte can detect changes in the ECM (composition, mechanical deformation) and respond accordingly.

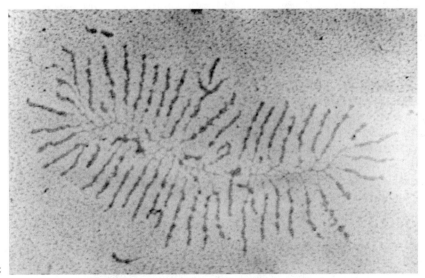

C

FIG. 5. *Continued.*

The GAG chains of the proteoglycan impart many of the physical properties to the molecule (Fig. 4). Chondroitin sulfate is composed of repeating disaccharide units of glucuronic acid and galactosamine with a sulfate group per disaccharide and may reach a molecular mass of 20,000 Da. Keratan sulfate consists of repeating disaccharide units of glucosamine and galactose, again averaging approximately one sulfate group per disaccharide. The sulfate (SO_4) and carboxyl ($COOH$) groups on the chondroitin sulfate and keratan sulfate chains become charged in solution and *in situ*. The total FCD in cartilage ranges from 0.05 to 0.3 mEq/g wet weight of tissue (181,184,188). Briefly, these charges provide the swelling properties of the tissue in the following way (a more detailed explanation is given later in this chapter). First, the fixed negative charges are placed close together in the dense solid matrix and so create charge–charge repulsion forces. At the same time, to maintain electroneutrality, counterions, e.g., Na^+, will be present, and these will cause a Donnan osmotic pressure (see below) (57,143,162,181,184). These two phenomena define the swelling pressure (162), which has been measured and calculated to be less than 0.25 MPa. The swelling pressure contributes compressive stiffness to cartilage, which usually ranges from 0.5 to 1.0 MPa, depending on the type of tissue (e.g., 19, 20,203,207,208). The FCD also largely determines the transport of electrolytes and electrokinetic properties of cartilage (67,68,84–86, 99–101). Finally, the bulk properties of the proteoglycans will contribute to the flow-dependent viscoelastic properties that occur when cartilage or meniscus is loaded.

The size, structural rigidity, and complex molecular conformation of normal proteoglycan aggregates make important contributions to the mechanical behavior of articular cartilage. In dilute aqueous solution of pure proteoglycans, it has been shown that these molecules will occupy a large solvation domain, five to ten times larger than that available within the interfibrillar space of native cartilage (116,220,235,260,261). Their sheer size, reduced in their compacted state *in situ*, act to retard their movement by diffusion and by hy-

drodynamic convective transport through the fine interfibrillar space by steric exclusion and by frictional drag (53,99,114,163,182,184, 211,212,241). All these proteoglycan characteristics undoubtedly will promote PG–PG networking and PG–collagen interactions *in situ* (113,139,200,213,218,220,334,336,337, 339), which are important in stabilizing the collagen–proteoglycan solid matrix (33,34), thus enabling it to function in the highly loaded environment of diarthrodial joints.

Collagen–Proteoglycan Interactions

In articular cartilage and meniscus, important molecular interactions exist not only between the proteoglycans and between the collagens, but also between the networks formed by the collagens and the proteoglycan aggregates (Fig. 6). These interactions, along with forces acting within the tissue (e.g., swelling pressure) and those applied on the tissue (i.e., external loading), can affect chondrocyte metabolism, collagen fibrillogenesis, and collagen network organization (220). The interactions existing between the collagen network and the proteoglycan aggregates are mainly frictional in nature (153,275). In addition, these studies showed that proteoglycans do not contribute to the tensile stiffness and strength of the collagen network; these properties are altered only when a collagenase is used to disrupt the collagen fibers (148,274).

There are molecular networks formed by proteoglycans in solution at physiological con-

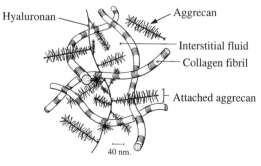

FIG. 6. A schematic diagram indicating the collagen–proteoglycan matrix in cartilage (213).

centrations *in vitro* (113,211,218,336,339), and the potential exists for proteoglycan–collagen (type II) network formation at similar concentrations (334). The proteoglycan networks and the proteoglycan–collagen composite matrix formed *in vitro* are capable of storing elastic energy, but their shear stiffnesses ($\approx$10 Pa) are far (less than 10^{-5} times) lower than that for normal articular cartilage. Therefore, other factors (e.g., collagen crosslinking, interactions with type IX collagen) must have strong influences on the shear properties of cartilage and meniscus (294, 333,338). Another factor arises from the physicochemical interactions existing between the collagen network and the proteoglycan network. The swelling pressure exerted by FCD (162,183,184) serves to inflate the collagen network and thus helps to maintain the ECM organization. This inflated state also allows the collagen network to sustain tensile loads and thus provide shear stiffness to the ECM (338).

Interactions between collagen and proteoglycan are also required in the biology of tissue maintenance. First, biochemical evidence exists indicating that collagen and proteoglycan synthesis, although largely independent, are nevertheless related. For example, the small proteoglycan decorin has been characterized as binding to fibril-forming collagens and inhibits collagen fibrillogenesis *in vitro* and *in vivo* (38). Also, it is known that aggrecan molecules can accelerate fibril formation whereas aggrecan aggregates have little influence on fibril formation (145,276,277). Thus, it is possible that different proteoglycans in the matrix affect fibril formation differently, giving rise to the possibility of biologically controlled collagen fiber architecture throughout the tissue.

Cartilage Ultrastructure

From the material standpoint, the ECM of cartilage is a fiber-reinforced composite solid consisting of a dense stable network of collagen fibers embedded in a very high concentration of proteoglycan gel, which itself is also a viscoelastic network. The content and structure of collagen and proteoglycan within the tissue vary with depth from the articulating surface. The collagen content is highest in the surface zone ($\approx$85% by dry weight), and it decreases to approximately 68% in the middle zone (171,184,221). Electron microscopy studies have shown that the tissue can be regarded as having three separate structural zones (Fig. 7). In the superficial tangential zone (10% to 20%

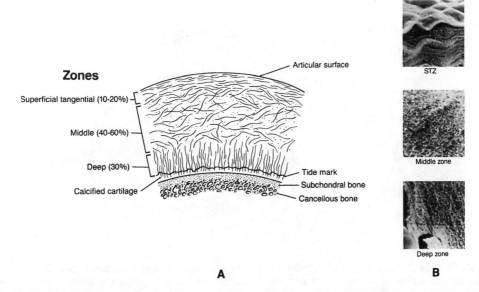

FIG. 7. (A) Layered structure of cartilage collagen network showing three distinct regions, and **(B)** corresponding SEM collagen fibrillar arrangement (SEMs are courtesy of Dr. T. Takei; 213).

of the total tissue thickness), fine collagen fibrils are organized parallel to the articular surface (48,49,167,210,323). In the middle zone (40% to 60% of the total thickness), the collagen fibrils have a larger diameter and appear to be oriented either randomly or in vertical columns (e.g., 12,24,33–36,48,49,167,210, 323). Studies by Broom and associates have suggested that in normal cartilage, the collagen ultrastructure in the middle zone is random, whereas in traumatized cartilage, the interfibrillar connections between the random collagen fibrils are disrupted, thus allowing the swelling pressure to expand the collagen network to form the vertical arcades suggested by Benninghoff and others (24,33–36,48). In the deep zone (about 30% of the total thickness), the fibers appear to be woven together to form large fiber bundles organized perpendicular to the surface (35,48,256). These bundles cross the "tidemark" to insert into the calcified cartilage and subchondral bone, thus securely anchoring the uncalcified tissue onto the bone ends (44,49,167,256).

On the articular surface, a specific collagen orientation in the joint can be demonstrated by the split-line pattern generated when the surface is punctured with a pointed round instrument, though controversy exists as to whether these split-line patterns actually do represent a preferred collagen fiber orientation at the articular surface (24,43,138,210). Many biomechanical tensile tests, however, have used this split-line pattern to provide the appropriate orientation for harvesting specimens (147–150,223,263,325,326). In a later section, we provide the tensile data for specimens obtained parallel and perpendicular to the split-line directions. Finally, it is noted that the concentration of proteoglycan in cartilage is lowest in the surface zone and highest in the middle zone (87,171,184,186,249, 296); this produces pronounced variations in the tensile stiffness and swelling behaviors of samples harvested from various zones of the tissue and causes swelling when the tissue is removed from the bone (278,280). The composition of the proteoglycans may also vary with depth, with the proteoglycans of the upper zone containing less keratan sulfate (332).

Meniscus Ultrastructure

The fibrous structure of the meniscus also has a layered appearance, but it differs from that of articular cartilage. The menisci are semilunar in shape and are situated between the femoral condyles and tibial plateau of the knee (Fig. 8). The articulating surface of the

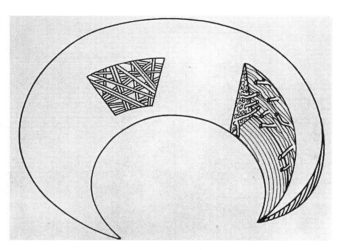

FIG. 8. Collagen ultrastructure of the meniscus, showing the surface and deep zone fiber orientations. The surface zone fibers are arranged in a random fashion, whereas the deep zone fibers are large and arranged predominantly in a circumferential manner. Radial fibers are also shown (82).

meniscus is composed of fine fibrils in a random mesh-like woven matrix (13,45,331), though split lines are also present. Approximately 100 μm from the surface layers are large rope-like collagen fiber bundles that are principally arranged circumferentially around the semilunar meniscus. Smaller radial fibers appear to reinforce the structure of the meniscus by tying the large circumferential fiber bundles together (45,155,243,286). This fibrillar organization predominates throughout the peripheral two-thirds of the tissue, while the inner region appears to contain more randomly arranged smaller collagen fibers and proteoglycans, resembling hyaline cartilage (93,226,331).

Inhomogeneous and Anisotropic Material Properties

The layered morphology of the collagen network (inhomogeneity) and the preferred orientation of collagen fibers (anisotropy) of both articular and meniscal cartilages provide a convenient means to examine how the collagen content and organization influence their strengths and stiffnesses. Anisotropic properties have been assessed by simply cutting test specimens oriented in a specific direction relative to the split-line pattern, whereas tissue inhomogeneity has been measured by testing tissue from different layers (Fig. 7). Anisotropic and inhomogeneous tensile and shear properties of articular cartilage and the meniscus have been demonstrated (82,148, 212,243,263,275,286,325,326,333). Details of various tensile tests and results are provided below.

METABOLIC ACTIVITIES OF ARTICULAR CARTILAGE

Articular cartilage and meniscus, like all soft connective tissues, are metabolically active and are synthesized and maintained by their own cell population, which in cartilage are the chondrocytes, and in menisci, cells termed fibrochondrocytes (195,297). In these tissues (in contrast to tissues contained in organs such as liver, kidney, brain) the extracellular matrix contributes the vast majority ($\geq 90\%$) of the tissue volume, and in skeletally matured tissue, the cells occupy only a small proportion of the total volume ($\leq 10\%$). The metabolic activities involve both anabolic (synthetic) and catabolic (degradative) events, which include (a) the synthesis of matrix components, (b) the incorporation and organization of these components into the matrix, and (c) their degradation and loss from the matrix (Fig. 9). The cells are responsible for the orchestration of these events, and the balance between these will result in a maintenance of the extracellular matrix and its biological function throughout life. However, this balance can be disturbed during disease processes, resulting in a remodeling of the extracellular matrix or a degradation of that matrix, as occurs in articular cartilage during OA. The descriptions below are based primarily on the metabolic events that have been described for articular cartilage. It is assumed, although not proven, that similar processes are ongoing in meniscus, the major obvious difference being the molecules being synthesized.

Synthesis of Proteoglycans

The synthesis of aggrecan, the major proteoglycan of articular cartilage, is well studied and serves as an example for all of the proteoglycans synthesized in other cartilaginous tissues. Proteoglycans are synthesized by the chondrocytes along intracellular pathways in common with other secreted GAG, and these cells are a specific phenotype of chondrocytes. Although tissues have usually been shown to express aggrecan at low levels (255), high levels of expression can occur in other cartilaginous tissues, for example, intervertebral disk. Meniscus has low levels of aggrecan, and ligaments and tendons usually have low levels except in areas that are regularly subjected to compression (71).

The synthesis of proteoglycan involves a number of important and distinct steps, which

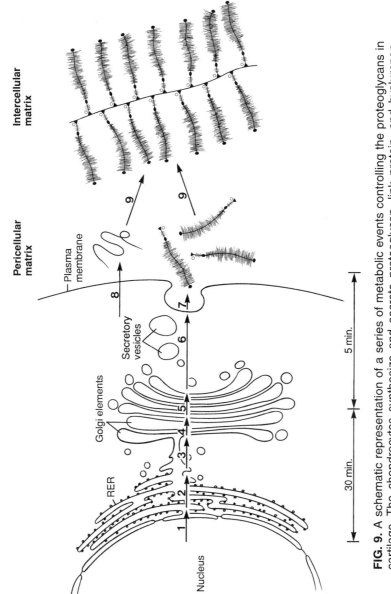

FIG. 9. A schematic representation of a series of metabolic events controlling the proteoglycans in cartilage. The chondrocytes synthesize and secrete proteoglycan, link protein, and hyaluronan, which become incorporated into the matrix as functional aggregates. Enzymes released by the cells break down these aggregates into fragments, which are released from the matrix into the synovial fluid. The fragments are then taken up by the lymphatics and moved to the circulating blood (178).

include (a) *transcription* of the gene to form a specific mRNA, (b) *translation* of that specific mRNA to generate a protein core, and (c) *posttranslational modifications*, where the GAG chains and smaller oligosaccharides are added during processing before secretion into the extracellular matrix. Because the protein core of aggrecan can have more than ten times its weight of carbohydrate attached to it (Fig. 5), there is considerable scope for "modulation" of structure during the posttranslational stages of processing (110). The control of the synthesis and processing of the proteoglycan involves the selection and expression of the protein core, followed by the determination of the number, size, and type of GAG chains that are added.

The specific gene of aggrecan (310) is transcribed in the nucleus of the chondrocyte to produce mRNA (although what regulates this is as yet unknown), and this is transported to the endoplasmic reticulum of the cell, where the specific mRNA is transcribed to generate the protein core. The protein core is then transported to the Golgi complex, where the GAG chains are added (249). This involves a complicated and highly organized sequence of enzymatic events, finally resulting in the sulfation of the disaccharide units (Fig. 4). Addition of the sulfate groups is rapidly followed by secretion of the completed proteoglycan from the cell into the pericellular matrix.

The formation extracellularly of the aggrecan aggregate also depends on the synthesis of two other molecules, link protein and hyaluronan (Fig. 5). Link protein is a separate gene product and is synthesized at a rate that gives a final ratio of aggrecan to link protein in cartilage close to 1:1. Link protein plays a major role in contributing to the material properties exhibited by the proteoglycan networks in solution (218,336), and therefore, the control of the synthesis of link protein and proteoglycan is vital. Although the aggrecan and link protein are separate gene products, they are often synthesized together and at similar rates (251). However, it has been shown that the chondrocyte has the ability to control the biosynthesis of these two molecules independently, although they use the same intracellular pathways (251). It remains to be determined what regulation mechanisms are used by the cells at the DNA level to dictate the rates of production of these two molecules. Indeed, cell biology studies yet to be performed will define those mechanisms that are common in the synthesis of aggrecan and link protein and those mechanisms that are independent.

The third component of the proteoglycan aggregate is hyaluronan, and it is synthesized outside the pathways used by proteoglycan and link protein, at the plasma membrane (242). Thus, the association of aggrecan with hyaluronan and its stabilization by link protein can occur only after secretion, in the extracellular matrix, probably including sites distant from the pericellular matrix (339). Portions of unattached hyaluronan at the pericellular region are free to bind to hyaluronan receptors on the surface of the chondrocytes, thus forming a defined and specific linkage between the cell and its extracellular matrix (156). There is, therefore, the potential for the cells to receive information from the proteoglycans of the extracellular matrix. This may be one of the mechanisms used by the chondrocytes to detect its extracellular matrix.

Synthesis of Collagen

All collagens are complexes of three polypeptides, and the gene organization of these is complex; to date, of the at least 18 distinct collagens described, the peptides are coded by 30 distinct genes. Types II and X collagen are each derived from one single gene, whereas types VI, IX, and XI collagens are each formed from the gene products of three different genes (see Fig. 2 and Table 3). The synthesis of collagen proceeds as that of other secreted glycoproteins, that is, the transcription of the specific mRNAs, translation to the α chains, which contain the signal peptide, the collagenous domain, and the noncollagenous domains at the N- and C-terminal ends. In the endoplasmic reticulum, the signal peptide is removed, and because hydroxyproline and hydroxylysine are not incorporated directly into protein, they are generated by hydroxylation of proline and lysine after peptide formation. Triple helix formation then occurs, starting at the carboxy-terminal end, where disulfide bonds are formed (for type II collagen, this would be an $\alpha1[II]_3$ complex), and it is only then that the procollagen molecule is allowed to progress into the secretory pathway. The procollagen molecule passes into the Golgi apparatus where further carbohydrate additions may occur. Only after secretion, as the molecules reach the extracellular space, are the nonhelical domains at the ends of the molecule cleaved from the helical domain.

Assembly of Macromolecules in the Extracellular Matrix

Aggrecan, link protein, and hyaluronan are secreted independently from the cell and then assembled as aggregates within the extracellular matrix (Fig. 9): a) transcription of the aggrecan and link protein genes to mRNA; b) translation of the mRNA in the rough endoplasmic reticulum (RER) to form the protein core of the aggrecan; c) transport of the newly formed protein from the RER to d) the *cis* and e) medial *trans* Golgi compartments, where the GAG chains are added to the protein core. f) On completion of the glycosylation and sulfation, the molecules are transported via secretory vesicles to the plasma membrane, and g) they are released into the extracellular matrix. h) Hyaluronan is synthesized separately at the plasma membrane. i) Only in the extracellular matrix can aggrecan, link protein, and hyaluronan come together to form proteoglycan aggregates. The formation of a stable proteoglycan aggregate requires the presence of all three individual components and for each of them to be functional.

Experimental evidence suggests that in some cartilage, the G1 domain of aggrecan may not be functional on secretion and may only become functional after extracellular processing. This delayed aggregation may allow the aggrecan molecules to move away from the cell before forming aggregates in the interterritorial matrix at a distance from the chondrocyte, thus allowing the newly synthesized proteoglycans to be incorporated into both the territorial matrix and the interterritorial matrix. A phenomenon of rapid polymeric transport through gels has been proposed to describe the movement of proteoglycan components through the extracellular matrix (114).

The secretion of the collagen molecules into the extracellular matrix is followed by an orderly sequence of events that results in the incorporation of the new collagen into the existing matrix. At the time of secretion, the nonhelical regions are enzymatically removed so that the resultant tropocollagen molecules are able to become organized in a quaterstaggered array to form fibrils (Fig. 2). During the event of secretion from the cell, the microfibrils of collagen are enzymatically modified to allow initiation of the formation of intrafibrillar covalent crosslinks between the molecules. The process of aggregation of these fibrils, both in the lateral direction and end to end, is known as fibrillogenesis. The fibril/fiber diameter, orientation, network formation, and ultrastructural organization vary at all levels of tissue organization. There may be variations in size at the same site of cartilage, between zones of the same tissue, and between different types of cartilage. They also vary in age, disease, and in repair. Although the precise mechanisms that control fibril formation are still to be precisely determined (227,319), it is believed that contributing factors include the presence of large and small proteoglycans and other types of collagen (e.g., type IX and XI collagens).

A major contributor to the structural organization of the collagen is the formation of covalent crosslinks. In cartilage, the major crosslink is the trivalent 3-hydroxypyridinium residue, which is present in articular cartilage at a ratio of 1.5:1 (mole:mole collagen) (76). These crosslinks are vital for maintaining tissue stiffness and strength (148,274). Also, quantitative analysis indicates that, in cartilage, every type IX collagen molecule is co-valently crosslinked to a type II collagen fiber (74). Thus, type IX collagen may play a pivotal role in providing interfibrillar stabilization between the type II collagen fibers.

Proteoglycan Catabolism

During the processes of normal maintenance of cartilage, in its synthesis, repair, and degradation, the proteoglycans of cartilage are continually being broken down and released from the matrix (Fig. 9). The current understanding of proteoglycan catabolism comes from studies of aggrecan. Major and specific proteolytic cleavage sites on aggrecan are between the G1 and G2 domains (254,273). This action separates the part of the proteoglycan involved in aggregation (the G1 domain) from the GAG-containing regions. This now nonaggregating GAG-containing fragment, although large, is able to pass through the matrix and is lost to the synovial fluid (172,173,246–248). This appears to be an efficient mechanism of catabolism of aggrecan. Further degradation of the G1 domain and link protein results in their release (247). From the synovial fluid these fragments are taken up by the synovium, pass through the lymphatic system to the blood, and are cleared by the liver and kidneys (Fig. 9). Thus, the level of proteoglycan fragments in the synovial fluid can be used to indicate rates of proteoglycan degradation in cartilage diseases. The enzymes responsible for this degradative activity are thought to include a group called metalloproteinases (e.g., stromelysin), although the specific enzyme responsible (presently termed aggrecanase) has not yet been discovered.

Collagen Catabolism

Collagen of articular cartilage is much more resistant to degradation, although it is subject to catabolism, probably at accelerated rates during cartilage degeneration. The mechanism of breakdown of type II collagen is likely to be first by the metalloproteinase collagenase, which cleaves the fibrillar structure three-fourths of the way along from the N terminus. This then allows further degradation by other proteolytic enzymes, for example, gelatinase and stromelysin (328). Type IX collagen is also susceptible to proteolytic cleavage by stromelysin (328).

Metabolic Maintenance of Cartilage

Articular cartilage maintenance and degradation are dependent on the activities of the chondrocytes. Because cartilage also lacks a blood supply, the survival of the chondrocytes must depend on the diffusion and convective transport of nutrients through the matrix. Chondrocytes are metabolically active, and they respond to their environment, which can include soluble mediators (e.g., cytokines, growth factors, hormones, pharmaceutical agents) and the mechanical environment (e.g., stresses, strains, flow velocities, osmotic and hydraulic pressures, electric currents and potentials, and other physicochemical events) (e.g., 23,47,95,102,230,232,246,268; also see Chapter 5 for more details on cell–matrix interactions). In some cases, the response of the cells may lead to matrix degradation, and this can be induced by changing the mechanical environment of the cells. For example, transection of the anterior cruciate ligament of the knee in dogs results in an increase in proteoglycan and collagen synthesis and an increase in matrix breakdown (46,73,246,272). Moreover, alterations to joint loading by immobilization create very different chondrocyte responses (23,142,246,253). *In vitro* explant studies have also shown that compression of cartilage and hydrostatic pressure can alter matrix component synthesis and breakdown (95,102,107,232,268). The pathway(s) by which the cells perceive these mechanical signals is (are) unknown. The stimulus may be changes in cell shape and volume (104) or fluid flow (21,204,217) and could involve interaction of the extracellular matrix with the cell surface integrins and the intracellular cytoskeleton (269,285,297) or stretch-activated ion channels (267).

The other important influences on chondrocyte activity come from the cytokines and growth factors. One of the most important cytokines for cartilage, at least in pathology, is interleukin 1 (IL-1). It has the ability to accelerate proteoglycan degradation (254) and suppress proteoglycan synthesis (306). However, IL-1 does not seem to degrade the collagen network until proteoglycan degradation is advanced. Growth factors have been shown to have influence on the regulation of chondrocyte activities. They are known to play a major role in cartilage development, and they may have major roles in the OA process (198). Growth factors that have significant effects on chondrocytes include basic fibroblast growth factor (b-FGF), insulin-like growth factor 1 (IGF-1), transforming growth factor-β, and some of the bone morphogenetic proteins (BMPs) (174).

In summary, the cartilage extracellular matrix can be viewed as a tissue in which a continuous set of metabolic events are occurring. As degradation products are released from the cartilage, they are replaced by newly synthesized components. To replace the degraded matrix components, the chondrocytes must synthesize the complex and specific molecules at the appropriate rate, and the newly synthesized molecules must then be incorporated into the macromolecular framework of the extracellular matrix. This carefully coordinated process is controlled by the chondrocytes, which respond in a variety of ways to a multitude of biochemical and biomechanical factors. Any disturbance of this carefully coordinated process may well lead to deterioration of the extracellular matrix.

BASIC CONCEPTS OF MATERIAL BEHAVIOR

Material Versus Structural Properties

When an object is subjected to an external load, it will move and deform. If all the exter-nal forces acting on the object sum up to zero, it will deform, but its center of mass will not move. The load and deformation responses of any material or structure depend on many factors, including the magnitude and direction of the applied load, the materials that constitute the body, and the size and shape of the body. Structural properties reflect the mechanical behavior of the body as a whole, including both material and geometric contributions to the load–deformation response (e.g., a bridge, an airplane wing, a femur or tibia, a knee or hip is a structure). The mechanical properties describe the intrinsic characteristics of the material itself and depend on its composition, molecular structure, and ultrastructure (e.g., steel, aluminum, bone tissue, and cartilage tissue are materials). Consequently, studies on the intrinsic mechanical properties of cartilage and meniscus have focused on the relationships between these properties and biochemical components and molecular organization (e.g., 6,10,82,153,162,205,243). These intrinsic material properties reflect the compositional and ultrastructural characteristics of the tissue during its normal development and during aging and disease such as OA.

Stresses, Strains, and Constitutive Equations

Two types of physical quantities are necessary to determine the deformational response of a material body: stress and strain. Stress acting on or within an object is defined as force per unit area. Six components are required to completely define the state of stress at any point. There are three normal stress components, each of which could be tensile (positive) or compressive (negative), and three shear stress components. For the beginner, it is important to emphasize that stress can never be measured; i.e., there is no "stress gauge." Stress must be calculated. Strain is the local deformation at any point inside or on the object. There are also six components of strain: three lineal strains (change in length per original length) and three shear strains (change of angle between two mutually perpendicular line elements emanating from a material point). Strain on the surface of an object *can* be measured. There are *strain* gauges, and there are many techniques, mechanical, electronic, and optical, that are readily available for use in measuring strains on the surface of an object. For more details, the reader is referred to standard engineering mechanics textbooks (89,166,300).[1]

In general, when an object is under load, theoretical models and mathematical (or numerical) analyses are required to determine the states of stress (six components) and strain (six components) within the object. These analyses are based on Cauchy's equations (ca. 1830), which are derived from Newton's second and third laws of motion (ca. 1680), and on an assumed stress–strain relationship for the material. For each material (steel, wood, glass, PMMA, cartilage, meniscus, tendon, ligament, etc.), its stress–strain relationship must be individually measured in the laboratory. There is no exception to this rule. The mathematical expression used to describe the experimentally determined stress–strain response is known as the constitutive equation. Each constitutive equation is an idealization, or mathematical abstraction, of a measured stress–strain response of a real material. However, one cannot arbitrarily use any mathematical expression for the stress–strain law. Each stress–strain law must satisfy a set of fundamental and rigorous restrictions such as the laws of thermodynamics and observer independence (305).

The isotropic, linearly elastic constitutive law has often been used to describe such material as steel, titanium, and bone. This mathematical relationship assumes that, for these materials, their stress and strain responses are related in a linear manner and that the stress–strain response is not directionally dependent (isotropy). (For bone, however, the

assumption of isotropy is dubious.) This constitutive equation is the simplest stress–strain law possible and is known as the generalized Hooke's law (ca. 1680). Two independent material coefficients are necessary to describe such materials: Young's modulus (E) (ca. 1810) and shear modulus (μ). In engineering textbooks, the shear modulus is often referred to as the modulus of rigidity. For isotropic materials, these material coefficients are related to other coefficients such as the Poisson's ratio (ν) (ca. 1835), bulk modulus (k), aggregate modulus (H_A), and Lame's coefficients (λ,μ) (ca. 1850) (89,166,300). Depending on the convenience of the problem, these alternative material coefficients are often preferred. In other words, for isotropic, linearly elastic materials, there are only two independent material coefficients. Table 4 provides the relationships for these various commonly used isotropic elastic coefficients.

To begin analyzing the deformational behavior of any material, one must first assume a constitutive law for the material and then use it to mathematically analyze its response in a laboratory experiment. If the mathematical predictions can accurately describe the experimentally measured strain or deformation, then the coefficients of the constitutive law for the material can be determined. This is usually done by a curve-fitting procedure using a numerical optimization algorithm, e.g., least square. Such curve-fitting procedures, however, do not provide a unique solution. Therefore, it is always prudent to verify the validity of the calculated material coefficients with another independent experiment and by using the material coefficients calculated from the first experiment to predict the results of a second experiment. For example, if the material coefficients are obtained from a creep experiment, then the response of an independent stress relaxation experiment should be predicted using these coefficients. This validation procedure is very important, especially in biomechanics, where the material stress–strain responses are often nonlinear and anisotropic. If an incorrect constitutive law has been assumed at the outset, this vali-

---

[1]For birefringent photoelastic materials, polarized light is refracted as it passes through the strained material. In such cases, the strain field inside the object becomes visible via the pattern of color light. There have been photoelasticity studies of stress and strain fields in bone.

TABLE 4. *Conversion of constants for isotropic linearly elastic material*

Basic pairs	λ	μ	B	E	ν	H_A
λ,μ	λ	μ	$\lambda + (2/3)\mu$	$\mu(3\lambda + 2\mu)/(\lambda + \mu)$	$\lambda/2(\lambda + \mu)$	$\lambda + 2\mu$
E,ν	$\nu E/(1 + \nu)(1 - 2\nu)$	$E/2(1 + \nu)$	$E/3(1 - 2\nu)$	E	ν	$E(1 - \nu)/(1 + \nu)(1 - 2\nu)$
μ,ν	$2\mu\nu/(1 - 2\nu)$	μ	$2\mu(1 + \nu)/3(1 - 2\nu)$	$2\mu(1 + \nu)$	ν	$2\mu(1 - \nu)/(1 - 2\nu)$

λ, Lame constant; μ, shear modulus; B, bulk modulus; E, Young's modulus; ν, Poisson's ratio; H_A, aggregate modulus.

dation procedure will fail, and the analysis would render incorrect interpretations of the data. This situation is well recognized, and indeed, Fung (1968) has gently advised that: "If no agreement is obtained, new analyses based on a different starting point would become necessary" (90).

History of Constitutive Modeling for Articular Cartilage

Various constitutive models have been used to describe cartilage. Some of the earliest models assumed the tissue to be isotropic and linearly elastic (e.g., 22,94,120,127,133,151, 152,289). This model can describe the mechanical behavior of soft hydrated tissues such as articular cartilage under static or equilibrium conditions but lacks the ability to describe the time-dependent creep and stress-relaxation behaviors exhibited by the tissue. Later, various viscoelastic models composed of springs and dashpots were proposed for cartilage to account for its creep and stress-relaxation behaviors (e.g., 52,121,233,234). Although these viscoelasticity models are able to describe those behaviors successfully, they cannot describe the known effects of interstitial fluid flow. Studies by McCutchen (192), Sokoloff (288), Linn and Sokoloff (170), Edwards (64,65), and Maroudas (181,182) have demonstrated that when the tissue is compressed, it will lose water, and when soaked in fluid, it will absorb water. Further, the time rate of change of tissue hydration was shown to follow a pattern similar to that of compressive creep, suggesting that the compressive mechanical response of articular cartilage may be related to the fluid movement in the tissue (64,121,170,182,202). Thus, various poroelastic and biphasic models have been developed and used to account for interstitial

fluid flow and its influence on the creep and stress-relaxation behaviors of cartilage (64, 192,205,207,208).

To date, the most successful theories for cartilage compressional behaviors are the biphasic theories developed by Mow and co-workers (e.g., 132,205,207,208,293). These mixture theories model soft hydrated tissues as composite materials consisting of two intrinsically incompressible phases (a solid phase and a fluid phase) (29,30,207). The porous solid phase is elastic and permeable to fluid flow. It may be isotropic or anisotropic, linear or nonlinear. In this theory, the frictional drag associated with the interstitial fluid flow through the porous solid matrix is responsible for the compressive viscoelastic behavior of the tissue. The intrinsic viscoelastic nature of the solid matrix becomes important when interstitial fluid drag effects are not significant. A biphasic porovis-coelastic theory has also been developed to describe the compressive behavior of cartilage by incorporating the intrinsic viscoelasticity of the solid matrix and the biphasic nature of the tissue (175). This theory has been shown to be successful in describing tissues with high permeabilities (281,282). Recently, a triphasic theory has been developed by Lai and co-workers (160–162,165) that accounts for the observed Donnan osmotic pressure effect (57,182,184, 302,308,309), the ion-induced chemical expansion effect (67,68,225), ion transport through the tissue (99,143), and other streaming potential and electrokinetic effects (84–86, 99–101). The biphasic and triphasic constitutive equations are discussed in greater details in later sections of this chapter.

Throughout the maze of equations and complexities, it is important to remember that each constitutive equation is only a model adopted to describe the most salient and idealized mechanical behavior of the material. It represents a simplification of the real stress–strain behavior of the specific material and has significant restrictions and limitations for its general applicability.

Elastic Solids, Viscous Fluids, and Viscoelastic Materials

A material is linear if the stress and strain are related in a linear manner and is elastic if the material always returns to its original shape when the applied stress is removed. The latter concept implies that all the energy stored in the material as a result of deformation is entirely recoverable, and the material response is insensitive to the rate of the applied stress or strain. In other words, there is no internal energy dissipation within an elastic material. The mechanical behavior of an elastic material such as a metal spring can be entirely determined by a graph showing a linear load–deformation, $F = kX$, or stress–strain relationship, $\sigma = E\varepsilon$ (Fig. 10A). The slope of the linear region of the $F–X$ graph is the structural stiffness k (N/m), and that of the $\sigma–\varepsilon$ graph is the Young's modulus of elasticity E (N/m²). For a straight prismatic elastic bar of cross-sectional area A and length L, the re-

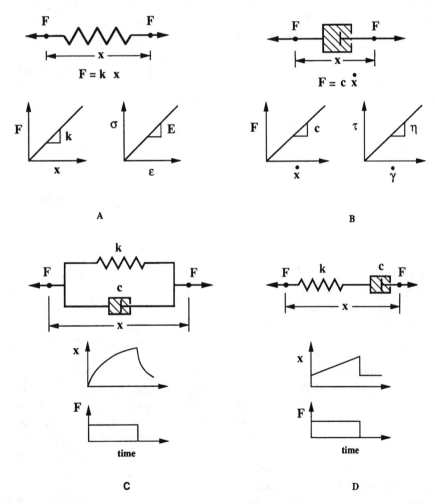

FIG. 10. Linear elastic, viscous, and viscoelastic responses: **(A)** an elastic spring, **(B)** a viscous dashpot, **(C)** a Kelvin-Voigt body, and **(D)** a Maxwell body. Under constant load or stretch, the elastic solid responses are independent of time. Under constant stretching, the viscous dashpot response is independent of time. Viscoelastic materials show time-dependent responses.

lationship between structural stiffness k and Young's modulus E is given by

$$k = EA/L. \qquad (1)$$

We see that the structural stiffness k depends directly on A and inversely on L and hence is not an intrinsic property of the structure. The ranges of the Young's modulus for stainless steel, titanium, polymethylmethacrylate (PMMA), and bone are 193 to 207 GPa ($1\ \text{GPa} = 10^9$ Pa), 106 to 114 GPa, 2.4 to 3.5 GPa, and 0.1 to 15 GPa, respectively. The shear modulus for steel and titanium are 73 GPa and 41 GPa, respectively. As will be seen below, the Young's modulus of the solid matrix of cartilage in compression ranges from 0.3 to 1.0 MPa ($1\ \text{MPa} = 10^6$ Pa), and that of the meniscus ranges from 0.1 to 0.6 MPa (10,19,20,69,205,207,243,283).

A dashpot is a piston moving through a viscous fluid contained in a closed cylinder (Fig. 10B). The registered force F is linearly related to the piston's rate of displacement $\dot{x}$; i.e., $F = c\dot{x}$. Here, the constant of proportionality c (N-s/m) is called the viscous damping coefficient of the dashpot. For a linear, purely viscous material the shear stress (τ) and shear rate ($\dot{\gamma}$) are linearly related; i.e., $\tau = \eta\dot{\gamma}$. This is known as a Newtonian fluid (see Chapter 8 on synovial fluid for discussions on more complex fluid flow behaviors). The slope of this linear graph is the viscosity coefficient η (Ns/m^2) of the fluid. The viscosity coefficient η describes an intrinsic property of the viscous fluid. A viscous fluid does not exhibit any tendency to recover its original shape when the applied stress is removed. This means no energy is stored in the material, and all the energy required to cause the flow is dissipated as heat by internal friction. Common viscous fluids are water, air, and low-molecular-weight oils. The viscosity coefficients of air and water at 20°C are 1.8×10^{-4} poise and 1.0×10^{-2} poise, respectively.[2]

Simple elastic or viscous responses are time-independent when subject to constant stress, constant strain, or constant strain rate. Most biological materials, however, exhibit time-dependent creep (i.e., deformation will increase with a constant applied stress) and stress relaxation (i.e., stress will decrease at constant applied strain) until an equilibrium is reached. Liquids that exhibit a shear stress response that decreases with time at a constant shear rate are known as thixotropic liquids.[3] Consequently, it is often necessary to use viscoelastic models to describe a material whose response to a constant applied load or constant deformation is time dependent.

A viscoelastic material, as the name suggests, combines the properties of both elastic and viscous substances. Using the elastic and viscous models described above, a viscoelastic material may be conceptualized as elastic springs and dashpots linked together. The Kelvin-Voigt body is defined by a spring and a dashpot connected in parallel (Fig. 10C), and a Maxwell body is one where a spring and dashpot are connected in series (Fig. 10D). The equation governing the force–displacement relation for a Kelvin-Voigt body is

$$F = kx + c\dot{x}, \quad x = 0 \quad \text{at} \quad t = 0 \qquad (2)$$

and for a Maxwell body, it is given by

$$(F/c) + (\dot{F}/k) = \dot{x}, \quad x = F/k \quad \text{at} \quad t = 0. \quad (3)$$

When these equations are written in terms of stress and strain, they represent the intrinsic stress–strain response of the viscoelastic material.

The initial conditions are also given in equations 2 and 3. When a load is applied to the Kelvin-Voigt body, its initial response is given by that of the dashpot, i.e., $x(0)$ is zero, and when a load is applied to the Maxwell body, its initial response is the sudden formation of the spring, i.e., $x(0)= F/k$. The creep is defined as the deformation produced by a sudden application at $t = 0$ of a constant force F. Equations 4 and 5 below give the creep re-

---

[2]Poise is used as a measure of viscosity; 1.0 poise = 0.1 Pa-sec = 0.1 Ns/m^2.

[3]Thixotropic liquids are polymeric solutions that have a molecular network that breaks down during shearing. A common example is tomato catsup; it flows more easily after being shaken.

sponse of the Kelvin-Voigt and Maxwell bodies, respectively:

$$x(t) = [F/k][1 - e^{-(k/c)t}], \quad t > 0 \qquad (4)$$

$$x(t) = F[(1/k) + (t/c)], \quad t > 0. \qquad (5)$$

The creep and recovery curves of these two idealized viscoelastic bodies are also depicted in Fig. 10C,D. The reader is referred to standard engineering references on viscoelasticity for models in which more springs and dashpots are connected in series and parallel (27,80,89). Whether or not any real material behaves in accord with the patterns predicted by these idealized viscoelastic laws can be ascertained by matching these predictions with the experimental data (305). If the patterns of these load-deformation responses are similar to a specific material, then the elastic and viscous coefficients of the assumed constitutive law can be calculated for the material.

For single-phase materials such as polymeric plastics, the mechanisms responsible for their viscoelastic behaviors may include intermolecular friction, stretching and uncoiling of molecules, and random vibration (from thermal excitation) of the long-chain polymers comprising the material (27,80,89). However, by virtue of composition, molecular structure, and water content, the viscoelastic behavior of cartilage and meniscus has another dimension. For example, in compression, their viscoelastic behaviors are dominated by the frictional drag of interstitial fluid flow through the porous collagen–proteoglycan solid matrix, thus causing viscous dissipation (132,192,205,207,281,283,288). Because viscous dissipation associated with interstitial fluid flow dominates the creep and stress-relaxation behaviors, the degree of hydration of these tissues and tissue permeability are important parameters governing their deformational behaviors. In fact, the earliest compositional change in articular cartilage that occurs during OA is an increase in hydration (28,179,190), which has been shown to affect the intrinsic properties of articular cartilage (10,128,281,283).

Biphasic Materials and Permeation Experiments

Permeation studies have demonstrated that water is capable of flowing through the porous-permeable solid matrix of cartilage and meniscus under an imposed pressure gradient (64,163,180–182,192,222,243). In this experiment, a specimen is subjected to an applied pressure gradient ΔP across the thickness h of the specimen. The rate of volume discharge Q across an area A is related to the hydraulic permeability coefficient k by Darcy's law:

$$Q = kA\Delta P/h. \qquad (6)$$

The permeation speed V is related to Q by the expression $V = Q/A\phi^f$ where the parameter ϕ^f is the porosity of the tissue defined as the ratio of the interstitial fluid volume (V^f) to the total tissue volume (V^T). Results from this permeation experiment showed that for normal cartilage and meniscus, k ranges from 10^{-15} to 10^{-16} m^4/Ns. The diffusive drag coefficient K is inversely related to the permeability coefficient k and is given by (163):

$$K = (\phi^f)^2/k. \qquad (7)$$

Because the porosity ϕ^f for cartilage and meniscus is approximately 0.75, the K ranges from 10^{14} to 10^{15} Ns/m^4. The very large drag coefficient indicates that interstitial fluid flow will cause large drag forces to be generated in these tissues.

Water is also capable of flowing through the porous permeable solid matrix as the tissue is compressed (10,20,64,170,192,203, 205,207,283). In this case, the compressive stress causes the solid matrix to be compacted, thus raising the pressure in the interstitium and forcing the fluid out of the tissue. The rate of efflux is controlled by the drag force generated during flow. In general, the manner with which an applied load is shared between the fluid phase (fluid pressure) and the solid phase (stress in the solid matrix) is determined, among other things, by the volumetric ratios of the tissue, i.e., the porosity ϕ^f and solidity $\phi^s(=V^s/V^T)$, the loading rates and the type of loading (tension, compression and shear), and load partition at the surface (130,131,134,135,164,205,207,209). The load-carrying capacity of each phase is determined by balancing the viscous drag forces against the elastic forces at each point within the tissue. For example, flow of fluid through a very permeable solid matrix would cause little frictional drag or fluid pressurization. A compressive stress acting on very permeable materials would be predominantly supported by the stress developed within the solid matrix, e.g., highly porous rigid steel filters. Conversely, flow of fluid through a solid matrix with very low permeability would cause high frictional drag forces, thus requiring high hydrodynamic pressures or large compressive loads to maintain the flow. In this case, fluid pressure can provide a significant component of total load support, thus minimizing the stress acting on the solid matrix. Such is the case for cartilage and meniscus.

The biphasic theory was developed by Mow and co-workers (e.g., 132,205,207,208) to describe the flow and deformational behaviors of cartilage and meniscus under a variety of conditions. The theory may be conceptually understood by the following simplified constitutive assumptions:

1. The solid matrix may be linearly elastic or hyperelastic, and isotropic or anisotropic.
2. The solid matrix and interstitial fluid are intrinsically incompressible; i.e., compression of the tissue as a whole is possible only if there is fluid exudation.
3. Viscous dissipation is a result of interstitial fluid flow relative to the solid matrix.
4. Frictional drag is directly proportional to the relative velocity—the proportionality factor is known as the diffusive drag coefficient (K), and this may be strain dependent.

This general biphasic theory takes its simplest form under the condition of infinitesimal strain, where the stress–strain law of the solid matrix may be described by the generalized Hooke's law, and where the diffusive

drag coefficient is a constant. These constitutive assumptions embody what is generally known as the linear biphasic theory for cartilage and meniscus (205,207,209,243,326). Under strict laboratory testing conditions, the isotropic form of the linear biphasic theory has been shown to provide a very accurate description of the compressive creep and stress-relaxation behaviors of these tissues (e.g., 10,19,20,25,131,203,205,243,283,326).

It should be emphasized that these simple constitutive assumptions are not generally valid to describe the nonhomogeneous and anisotropic nature of articular cartilage and meniscus. There are many obvious areas for improving the sophistication of these assumptions. For example, a material symmetry could be introduced into the constitutive equations in order to describe the transversely isotropic or orthotropic material properties of articular cartilage and meniscus (50,148,212, 243,244,263,325). However, to solve such problems is mathematically very challenging, and to perform the experiments to extract the material coefficients is nearly impossible. Further, if the material is subject to heavy loads, large deformations, and rapid loading rates, nonlinear finite deformational effects occur, and more advanced theories may be required (131,132,159,208,322). Because these types of biological tissues are soft and generally have high water contents, care must always be exercised to choose the correct form of the biphasic theory for the specific loading and deformational conditions (37,208,212). In this chapter, we discuss only the linear biphasic theory for articular cartilage and meniscus for the purpose of material property determinations.

Tension, Compression, and Shear

Uniaxial stress and uniaxial strain tests are often used to determine the mechanical response of a material. In these experiments, the loads or deformations are applied in only one direction. In general, an experiment with an applied uniaxial stress will yield multiaxial

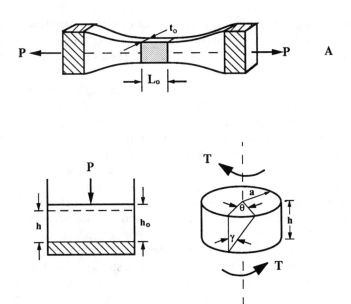

FIG. 11. (A) Tensile testing of a specimen with gauge length L_o, thickness t_o, and cross-sectional area A. **(B)** Confined compression test of a specimen of thickness h_o. **(C)** Shear test of a circular specimen of radius a; γ is the shear strain.

strains, and conversely, an experiment with uniaxial strain will generate multiaxial stresses in the tissue. These types of experiments greatly simplify the theoretical analyses required to describe the data.

In a uniaxial tension or compression test, a cylindrical specimen of known cross-sectional area (A) is placed in a testing machine and subjected to a tensile load (P) along one axis (Fig. 11A). The uniaxial stress σ acting in the specimen is P/A. With time, the specimen elongates along the direction of the applied tension. The stretch, $\lambda(t) = L(t)/L_o$, of the specimen is measured as the tensile test proceeds. Here, $L(t)$ is the deformed gauge length of the cylindrical specimen at time t, and L_o is the original undeformed gauge length. The tensile strain ε is calculated by the relation $\varepsilon = (L - L_o)/L_o$.[4] For linearly

elastic materials, the Young's modulus E is given by the expression:

$$E = \sigma/\varepsilon = (P/A)/[(L - L_o)/L_o]. \qquad (8)$$

For all materials, tension would cause a lateral contraction, whereas compression would cause a lateral expansion. To be consistent with the laws of thermodynamics, tension must always produce an increase in volume. The Poisson's ratio ν is used as a measure of the lateral strain (ε_d) relative to the axial strain and is defined as:

$$\nu = -\varepsilon_d/\varepsilon = -[(d - d_o)/d_o]/[(L - L_o)/L_o]. (9)$$

Here, d is the deformed lateral dimension, and d_o is the original lateral dimension. For isotropic materials, the Poisson's ratio ranges from 0 to 0.5. A Poisson's ratio of 0.5 means the material is incompressible, and a Poisson's ratio of zero means the material is maximally compressible. The values of ν for some common isotropic materials are: stainless steel, 0.30; titanium, 0.34; adult articular cartilage,

---

[4]For large deformation, the ε along the direction of applied stress is given by $(\lambda^2 - 1)/2$. See references 89 and 166 for more details.

0.10 to 0.40; cork, 0; and rubber, 0.5. For anisotropic materials, there are no such restrictions on the Poisson's ratio.

Another type of uniaxial experiment is the confined compression experiment (Fig. 11B). In this experiment, the deformation is maintained in one direction. This is done by restricting the material from expanding in the lateral direction by placing the test sample in a confining chamber. The confining wall serves to exert a normal compressive force onto the lateral surface of the cylinder in order to maintain one-dimensional motion. Thus, the uniaxial confined compression experiment is actually a multiaxial stress experiment; the stress acting on the lateral surface has the effect of increasing the compressive modulus. This modulus is known as the compressive aggregate modulus. For isotropic materials (207), the Young's modulus (E), Poisson's ratio (v), and aggregate modulus (H_A) are related by the expression $H_A = E(1 - v)/(1 + v)(1 - 2v)$.

The third common experiment utilizes torsion to determine the shear properties of a material. Torsion of a circular cylinder of a homogeneous material yields a state of pure shear in the material, which experiences no volume change (Fig. 11C). The shear strain γ is related to the total angle of twist θ, the thickness h, and the radius of the disk a by $\gamma = \theta a/h$. The shear stress τ at a circumferential position is determined from the resulting torque T as $\tau = Ta/I_p$ where I_p is the polar area moment of inertia given by $\pi a^4/2$. These quantities can be used to calculate the shear modulus of an isotropic, linearly elastic material as

$$\mu = \tau/\gamma = Th/I_p. \qquad (10)$$

See Table 4 for the relationships among the elastic constants (E, v, H_A, μ, λ) in terms of any of the basic pairs. With these general concepts, it is now possible to develop an understanding of the material properties of articular cartilage and meniscus. These topics occupy the remainder of this chapter.

MATERIAL PROPERTIES OF THE EXTRACELLULAR MATRIX OF CARTILAGINOUS TISSUES

The material coefficients most commonly used to describe the intrinsic or "flow-independent" properties of the porous-permeable solid matrix of cartilage and meniscus are Young's modulus, the compressive aggregate modulus, the shear modulus, and Poisson's ratio. The experiments used to determine these coefficients are (a) creep or stress-relaxation equilibrium measurements in confined compression or indentation; (b) slow, constant-strain-rate or equilibrium tensile tests; and (c) shear tests with infinitesimal shear strains. The specific choice of test depends on the size, shape, and amount of tissue available for study and the objectives of the study.

Tensile Properties of the Solid Matrix

Equilibrium Tensile Measurements

The tensile modulus of the solid matrix of cartilage has been determined using the equilibrium data from the tensile stress-relaxation experiment (6,103,225,283). For normal cartilage, the equilibrium stress–strain relationship is linear for strains up to 15%, from which the equilibrium tensile modulus is determined. Various studies showed that the tensile modulus of articular cartilage may vary from less than 1 MPa to over 30 MPa. This variation arises from a number of factors: (a) type of tissue (e.g., human, bovine, canine); (b) age of the animal; (c) type of joint in the body; (d) sample location in the joint, i.e., weight-bearing characteristics; (e) depth of sample from the articular surface; (f) relative orientation with respect to the split-line; (g) biochemical composition and molecular structure; and (h) state of degeneration (6,60, 103,147,150,153,263,283,325). For example, Table 5A shows the variation of this equilibrium tensile modulus for normal articular cartilage from bovine, canine, and human knee

TABLE 5A. *Equilibrium tensile modulus (MPa) of normal human, bovine, and canine articular cartilage: Inhomogeneous variations through the depth of the cartilage layer[a]*

	Bovine		Canine		Human	
	Glenoid	Humerus	Femoral groove	Femoral condyle	Femoral groove	Femoral condyle
Surface	5.9 (2.4)	13.4 (4.6)	27.4 (8.4)	23.3 (8.5)	13.9 (2.4)	7.8 (1.7)
Middle	0.9 (0.5)	2.7 (1.6)			3.4 (1.4)	4.0 (1.1)
Deep	0.2 (0.2)	1.7 (0.8)			1.0 (0.5)	

[a]All samples harvested in a direction parallel to the local split-line direction. Data are expressed as mean (SD). From Akizuki et al. (6) and Setton et al. (283), with permission. Data on bovine cartilage from Ebara et al. (60) with permission.

and shoulder joints (6,60,283), and Table 5B fibrillated and osteoarthritic human knee cartilage (6). Further, recent studies on canine knee joint cartilage from the surface zone, in which OA was experimentally induced by sectioning the anterior cruciate ligament, show dramatic decreases of the tensile modulus (Table 6) (103,224,283).

Some general conclusions may be drawn: (a) the tensile modulus of cartilage from the surface zone is larger than that of the middle zone in the skeletally mature animal; (b) the tensile modulus of specimens aligned parallel to the split-line direction is larger than that of specimens aligned perpendicular to the split-line direction (148,150,212,263,326,327), and this is true regardless of the state of tissue degeneration; (c) the tensile modulus of normal cartilage is larger than that of fibrillated and OA cartilage. The presence of fibrillation and OA, whether occurring naturally in hu-mans (Table 5B) or induced experimentally in animals (Table 6), greatly reduces the tensile modulus near the articular surface; and (d) the tensile modulus is not affected by the proteoglycan content (275). The first general conclusion is consistent with the idea that the surface zone of cartilage is rich in collagen (see above). The second is consistent with the observation that there is a subtle preferred alignment of collagen fibers at the articular surface, though often not observable by scanning electron microscopy (12,33–36,49,210,323). The third conclusion is consistent with the preponderant microscopic data on the morphology of tissue disruption occurring during OA. Finally, the last conclusion indicates that the bonding between collagen and proteoglycan in the solid matrix is not covalent.

These studies showed that there is a highly significant correlation between the tensile modulus and the ratio of collagen to proteoglycan in normal human articular cartilage (r

TABLE 5B. *Equilibrium tensile modulus (MPa) of normal, fibrillated, and osteoarthritic human articular cartilage: Inhomogeneous variations through the depth of the cartilage layer[a]*

	Normal	Fibrillated	Osteoarthritic
Surface	7.79	7.15	1.36
	(1.73)	(1.89)	(0.09)
Subsurface	4.85	7.47	0.85
	(1.37)	(0.65)	(0.81)
Middle	4.00	4.90	2.11
	(1.05)	(1.03)	(0.30)

[a]All samples were harvested from the femoral condyle in an orientation parallel to the local split-line direction. Data are expressed as mean (SD). From Akizuki et al. (6), with permission.

TABLE 6. *Equilibrium tensile modulus (MPa) of surface-zone canine articular cartilage in an animal model of osteoarthritis[a]*

	Greyhound femoral groove	Greyhound femoral condyle	Beagle femoral condyle
Control	27.4 (8.4)	23.3 (8.5)	15.5 (4.5)
6 Weeks	23.3 (8.7)	13.2 (4.4)	
12 Weeks	12.5 (2.9)	6.7 (2.5)	
16 Weeks			8.6 (5.0)

[a]All cartilage is harvested from the surface and subsurface zones parallel to the split-line direction. Data are expressed as mean (SD). From Guilak et al. (102) and Setton et al. (283), with permission.

= 0.714, $p < 0.001$) (Fig. 12). Clearly, specimens from the surface are stiffer than those from the midzone, and surface-zone specimens from high-weight-bearing (HWA) areas are less stiff than those from the low-weight-bearing areas (LWA). This is at least in part a result of the lower collagen/proteoglycan ratio in the HWA than in the LWA. This physiological phenomenon seems to be true for other soft hydrated tissues, such as tendons (71, 319). When tendons are under compressive load, they remodel by producing higher concentrations of aggrecan, proteoglycan aggregates, byglycan, and decorin.

Constant-Strain-Rate Tensile Measurements

When a strip of cartilage is stretched under a constant strain rate, the tensile stress–strain behavior is nonlinear. A typical nonlinear stress–strain (σ–ε) curve for cartilage, meniscus, and other soft tissues is depicted in Fig. 13. This figure also shows the cause of the nonlinear behavior; i.e., the initial toe region of the σ–ε curve results from the straightening of the coiled collagen structure, and the

linear region of the σ–ε curve represents the stretching of the straightened parallel array of collagen fibers (e.g., 91,147,148,258,263, 317,318,325). It is thought that the linear region reflects the stiffness of the collagen fibers as they are pulled in uniaxial tension (see also Chapter 6 on tendons and ligaments), and the slope of this curve gives a tensile modulus (E) of the specimen. Beyond the linear region, the collagen fibrils will fracture, and the tensile failure stress is the measure of the strength of the collagen fibrils.

A number of investigators have shown that the nonlinear stress–strain data can be described by a two-parameter (A,B) exponential stress–strain relationship (e.g., 91,154,199, 258,263,327):

$$\sigma = A[\exp(B\varepsilon) - 1]. \qquad (11)$$

It can be shown from this representation that the derivative or tangent modulus is directly related to the stress:

$$d\sigma/d\varepsilon = B\sigma + C. \qquad (12)$$

This means that the increase in the stiffness of the specimen is directly related to the applied stress σ. The concept of fiber recruitment has

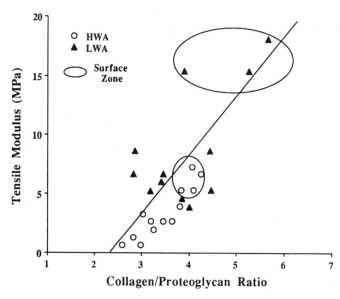

FIG. 12. Relationship between intrinsic tensile modulus and collagen/proteoglycan ratio for normal human knee joint cartilage ($r = 0.714$, $p < 0.001$) (6).

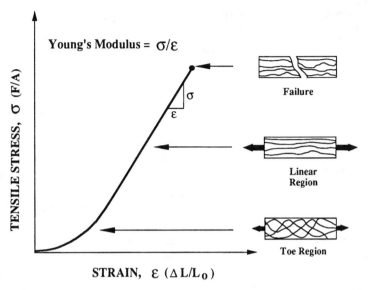

FIG. 13. Typical stress–strain curve for articular cartilage in a uniaxial and uniform strain rate experiment. The toe region is marked by an increasing slope, whereas the linear region appears to be a straight line with a slope of σ/ε (213).

long been proposed as an explanation for this stiffening effect (317). As illustrated in Fig. 13, as tension proceeds, and more of the coiled or slack fibers are straightened and stretched, the number of fibers actively resisting the applied load will increase, resulting in an increased tensile stiffness. The concept of fiber recruitment as the specimens are stretched is commonly used in tensile studies of tendons and ligaments (see Chapter 6 for more details on tendons and ligaments).

In equation 12, the tangent modulus ($d\sigma/d\varepsilon$) is proportional to the factor B, and C is the product AB and represents the tangent modulus as $\sigma \to 0$. Table 7 provides the coefficients A, B, and C and the tensile Young's modulus E determined from the linear portion of the tensile stress–strain curve for bovine cartilage. As expected, these coefficients vary with the depth from the articular surface and the split-line direction. Specimens taken from the articular surface and parallel to the split-line direction have the greatest tensile modulus.

The uniaxial constant strain-rate experiments have also been used to determine the tensile stress–strain relationship for human and bovine meniscal tissues (82,83,214,243). As with cartilage, these tensile properties vary with respect to location (anterior, central, and posterior) and specimen orientation relative to the predominant collagen fiber direction (circumferential and radial). The regional variation in tensile modulus (E), as shown in Table 8, indicates that specimens from the posterior half of the medial meniscus are significantly less stiff and less strong in tension than specimens from all other regions. The

TABLE 7. *Parameters A, B, and C (= AB) and Young's Modulus, E, of bovine articular cartilage: Dependence on depth and split-line orientation*

	Slice	A (MPa)	B	C	E (MPa)
Group ‖					
	1	2.1	5.0	10.6	43.2
	2	1.0	3.2	3.3	13.0
	3	0.6	1.6	0.9	2.6
Group ⊥					
	1	0.9	3.6	3.2	15.6
	2	0.5	2.2	1.0	4.7
	3	0.3	1.3	0.3	1.1

‖ and ⊥ represent parallel and perpendicular specimens, respectively, and 1, 2, and 3 represent the first three layers of tissue. Data from Roth and Mow (263).

TABLE 8. *Parameters* A, B, *and* C *(= AB) and tensile modulus, E, of human meniscus: Dependence on location*[a]

Location	A	B	C	E (MPa)
MA	1.6	28.4	42.4	159.6
MC	0.9	27.3	23.7	93.2
MP	1.4	20.1	25.2	110.2
LA	1.4	28.8	30.2	159.1
LC	2.1	31.9	55.7	228.8
LP	3.2	27.5	67.5	294.1

[a]MA, medial anterior; MC, medial central; MP, medial posterior; LA, lateral anterior; LC, lateral central; LP, lateral posterior. Data from Fithian et al. (83).

rate of change (B) of the tangent modulus ($d\sigma/d\varepsilon$) is uniform throughout the meniscus, indicating the relative uniformity of collagen and proteoglycan content present in normal human meniscus. On the other hand, the tangent modulus at very low stresses, C, varies in a manner similar to that seen for tangent modulus beyond the toe region.

Ultrastructural studies using polarized light (83) showed that in lateral meniscus, large type I collagen fiber bundles are highly oriented and are arranged parallel to the periphery of the tissue. However, in the posterior half of the medial meniscus, collagen fiber bundles have significantly reduced circumferential organization, i.e., they are not highly aligned in the circumferential direction. This observation appears to explain the lower measured tensile modulus of the medial posterior specimens. This site has a high frequency of clinically observed tears, which may result from the inferior tensile properties of the meniscus in this region.

Although the collagen fibers of the meniscus are arranged predominantly in the circumferential direction, there is evidence of large radially oriented fibers within human and bovine menisci (Fig. 8). It has long been conjectured that these radial fibers act to "tie" the large circumferentially oriented collagen fibers together, thus providing the tissue with greater strength in the radial direction (45). This hypothesis was examined by Skaggs and co-workers (286), who harvested tensile specimens of meniscal tissue oriented in the radial direction. From their histologic observations, it was noted that the size and density of radial fibers in bovine meniscus gradually increased from the anterior region to the posterior region of the meniscus (Fig. 14). This gradual decrease also manifested in the tensile modulus and ultimate tensile stress of radial specimens, those specimens containing full radial fibers being the stiffest (Fig. 15A,B).

The tensile stress–strain relationship for articular cartilage and the resulting tensile modulus are also dependent on the rate of

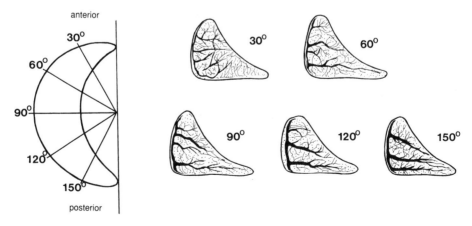

FIG. 14. Schematic representations of the regional variation in the architecture of the radial tie fibers. The anterior region contains no radial tie fibers, and the posterior region often contained large multiple radial tie fibers (286).

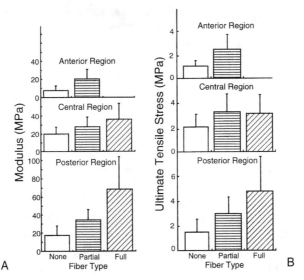

FIG. 15. (A) Variation of mean tensile modulus (±SD) for specimens by region and by presence of the radial tie fibers. **(B)** Variation of mean tensile ultimate stress (±SD) for specimens by region and by presence of the radial tie fibers.

strain. It has been shown that substantial quantities of fluid are expressed from cartilage specimens during the stretching process (263). This fluid movement must necessarily cause fluid pressurization in the interstitium and frictional drag to be exerted onto the solid matrix. These effects increase as the rate of strain increases. Thus, the specimens would appear to stiffen with increasing strain rate. Conversely, as the strain rate becomes very low, the tensile modulus would decrease and would approach the equilibrium tensile modulus measured from stress relaxation.

This hypothesis was examined and verified experimentally (169).

Compressive Properties of the Solid Matrix

The equilibrium compressive properties of the solid matrix have been most extensively studied in confined compression and indentation tests (e.g., 10,22,67–69,94,121,127,128, 151,152,159,176,203,207,322) (see description of the indentation test below). In the confined compression experiment, a small cylin-

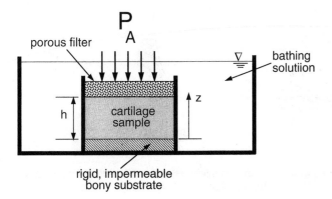

FIG. 16. Confined compression test. Load (P_A) is applied to the cartilage surface with a rigid-porous filter, allowing free escape of the interstitial fluid (h is cartilage thickness, z is displacement coordinate). Lateral extension of the specimen is prevented by the confining test chamber.

TABLE 9. *Equilibrium aggregate modulus (MPa) of lateral condyle and patellar groove cartilage and meniscus*

	Human[a]	Bovine[b]	Canine[c]	Monkey[d]	Rabbit[e]
Lateral condyle	0.70	0.89	0.60	0.78	0.54
Patellar groove	0.53	0.47	0.55	0.52	0.51
Meniscus	NA[f]	0.41	NA	NA	NA

[a]Young normal.
[b]18 months to 2 years old.
[c]Mature beagles and greyhounds.
[d]Mature cynomologus monkeys.
[e]Mature New Zealand white rabbits.
[f]Not Available. Data shown were obtained from indentation creep tests.

drical cartilage–bone plug is placed in a cylindrical confining chamber, schematically shown in Fig. 16. Ideally, the lateral expansion of cartilage is prevented. A constant compressive load is applied to the specimen through a rigid porous filter. Creep deformation occurs as the fluid is forced to flow from the tissue. The aggregate modulus is determined at creep equilibrium. Just as in tension, for small strains (<20%), human and bovine cartilage tissues demonstrate a linear stress–strain relationship (69,159,207,208,322). The average aggregate modulus for the lateral condyle and femoral groove cartilages of nor-

mal human, canine, cynomolgus monkey, and rabbit knees, and bovine meniscus are given in Table 9 (20,243). These data indicate significant species and site variations of the aggregate modulus. To illustrate the site variations on a specific joint, Fig. 17 provides a map of the aggregate modulus and cartilage thickness on a normal 21-year-old male human tibial plateau.

Besides variations related to tissue location and species, other factors such as tissue composition, ultrastructure, and pathology also have strong influences on tissue properties. The equilibrium aggregate modulus for hu-

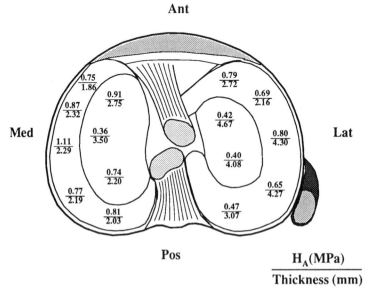

FIG. 17. Variation of equilibrium compressive modulus and thickness of cartilage with joint location on a tibial plateau (Courtesy of Dr. Shaw Akizuki; normal, human, 21-year-old specimen).

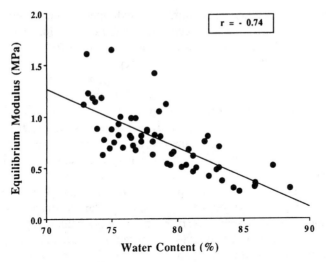

FIG. 18. Variation of the confined compression equilibrium modulus with water content for articular cartilage from the lateral facet of human patellae (10).

man articular cartilage correlates in an inverse manner with water content ($r = -0.74$) (Fig. 18) and in a direct manner with proteoglycan content per wet weight ($r = 0.69$) (Fig. 19) (216,264). No correlation exists between the compressive stiffness and collagen content. Thus, these correlations suggest that proteoglycans are responsible for providing compressive stiffness of the tissue. Recent investigations have revealed that the highly loaded

regions of articular cartilage generally have a greater proteoglycan content (6,141). These results are consistent with the fact that highly loaded regions of articular cartilages are stiffer in compression than the less-loaded regions, as mentioned above (Fig. 17) (4,47). Degenerative changes of the extracellular matrix during OA often include loss of proteoglycan and thus have a profound influence on cartilage material properties and joint func-

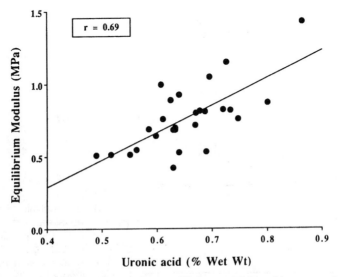

FIG. 19. Variation of the confined compression equilibrium modulus of human patellar articular cartilage specimens with uronic acid content (216).

tion. Indeed, removal of proteoglycans from articular cartilage samples *in vitro* has been shown to result in a tenfold decrease of tissue compressive modulus (148,295).

Shear Properties of the Solid Matrix

The intrinsic viscoelastic properties of the solid matrix of cartilage can be determined in a pure shear experiment and under small strain conditions. When these two conditions exist, no volumetric change or hydrodynamic pressures are produced in the tissue; thus, no interstitial fluid flow can occur (119,265,284, 294,335,338). The intrinsic or flow-independent viscoelastic behavior of the cartilage matrix has been measured under these two conditions, and both stress-relaxation and dynamic oscillatory shear behaviors have been characterized.

In the pure shear experiment, a circular specimen is subjected to a torsional shear deformation. The mechanical response of a cartilage specimen to a sudden change of angular displacement is an instantaneous increase in shear stress followed by a rapid decay until an equilibrium is reached. This stress-relaxation behavior is the basic manifestation of the intrinsic viscoelastic behavior of the solid ma-

trix exhibited in shear. Figure 20 shows a typical mean of a normalized shear stress-relaxation function $G(t)$ calculated from ten levels of step shear strain (0.002 to 9.02 rads) for normal human patellar cartilage specimens (335). Using the quasilinear viscoelastic theory (91), this normalized stress-relaxation function yields the spectrum parameters: $C = 0.13$, $\tau_1 = 0.0004$ sec, and $\tau_2 = 36.2$ sec. Clearly, the quasilinear viscoelastic theory provides an excellent description of the intrinsic stress-relaxation behavior of normal human patellar cartilage. Equilibrium stress–strain relationships from this shear stress-relaxation test are linear for shear strains up to 0.03 rad. The average equilibrium shear modulus for human patellar cartilage is 0.23 MPa (335,338), although patellar cartilage is known to be particularly soft when compared to other cartilages in the knee. For canine femoral condylar cartilage at 6 or 12 weeks following anterior cruciate ligament transection, the equilibrium shear modulus was found to decrease from 0.22 MPa to 0.07 MPa and 0.06 MPa, respectively (284).

The dynamic viscoelastic shear behaviors of the solid matrix of cartilage and meniscus have also been determined using the pure shear experiment. In this test, the specimen is subjected to a steady sinusoidal torsional strain of small

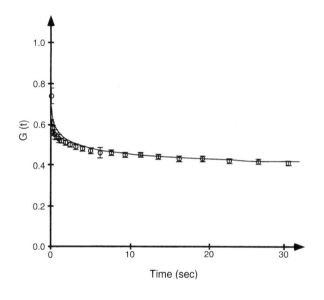

FIG. 20. Analysis of articular cartilage reduced shear stress-relaxation function using the quasilinear viscoelastic (QLV) theory proposed by Fung (91). The three material parameters of the QLV theory for this specimen are: $C = 0.13$, $\tau_1 = 0.0004$ sec, and $\tau_2 = 36.2$ sec (335).

amplitude over a range of frequencies (265, 284,335,338). A sinusoidal angular displacement $\theta = \theta_o e^{i\omega t}$ is applied to the specimen, and the torque response $T = T_o \exp(i\omega t + \delta)$ is registered. Here, ω is the circular frequency in radians per second (frequency $f = \omega/2\pi$ in hertz; the period $p = 2\pi/\omega = 1/f$ in seconds), and δ is the phase-shift angle between the sinusoidal displacement input and torque output. To calculate the dynamic shear modulus (G^*), the following formula is used:

$$G^* = G' + iG'' = \frac{T_o h}{I_p \theta_o}(\cos \delta + i \sin \delta) \quad (13)$$

where $i = \sqrt{-1}$. The storage modulus G' is proportional to elastically stored strain energy, and the loss modulus G'' is proportional to dissipated strain energy in the material over one cycle of periodic oscillation. Often, it is convenient to calculate the magnitude of dynamic shear modulus $|G'|$ and phase-shift angle δ. They are related to G' and G'' by

$$|G^*| = \sqrt{G'^2 + G''^2} = \frac{T_o h}{I_p \theta_o}, \; \delta = \tan^{-1}\left(\frac{G''}{G'}\right). \quad (14)$$

The magnitude of the shear modulus $|G^*|$ reflects the overall stiffness of the tissue in shear. The phase-shift angle characterizes the energy dissipation relative to energy storage within the tissue. For more details, the reader is referred to standard engineering texts on continuum mechanics or viscoelasticity (e.g., 27,80,89,166).

The values of $|G^*|$ vary from 0.2 MPa to 2.5 MPa for bovine articular cartilage (265) under infinitesimal strain (<0.001 rad). We note that a material is purely elastic when $\delta = 0°$ and purely viscous when $\delta = 90°$, whereas δ lies somewhere between $0°$ and $90°$ for a general viscoelastic material. The solid matrix of both normal human and bovine articular cartilage exhibits a slightly viscoelastic behavior (119,265,284,335,338). The phase-shift angle δ lies between $9°$ and $20°$ over a frequency range of 0.01 to 20 Hz.

The collagen network plays an active mechanical role in contributing to the shear stiffness and energy storage in cartilage. Conceptually, the role played by collagen

when the specimen is in shear may be visualized as shown in Fig. 21. The tension in the diagonally oriented collagen acts to increase the shear stiffness of the solid matrix. This effect is confirmed by the result shown in Fig. 22, where $|G^*|$ is directly and significantly related to the collagen content of articular cartilage.

In the recent canine OA studies of Setton and co-workers (284), the $|G^*|$ of the tissue at the femoral condyle decreased from 0.8 MPa at 10 rad/s for controls to 0.25 MPa at 6 and 12 weeks following anterior cruciate ligament transection, and tan δ increased from 0.22 for controls to 0.31 at 12 weeks postoperative. These findings are consistent with the major drop in tensile modulus and loss of collagen cross-linking of the superficial tangential zone in this canine OA model (103) and a general disorganization of the collagen–proteoglycan solid matrix.

For the most part, collagen stores energy like an elastic material. Based on the work of Woo and co-workers (326,327) on canine medial collateral ligaments (composed mainly of collagen), the energy dissipation of these tissues in tension is very slight, with a phase shift angle δ of about $3.6°$. The energy dissipation of pure proteoglycan solutions at high concentrations (10 to 50 mg/ml) has also been determined. These phase-shift angles range from $50°$ to $75°$ (113,211,218,

Pure Shear

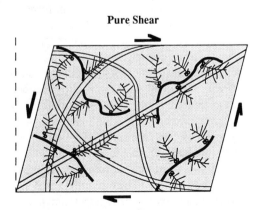

FIG. 21. A schematic representation of cartilage in pure shear. The tension of collagen provides shear stiffness (205).

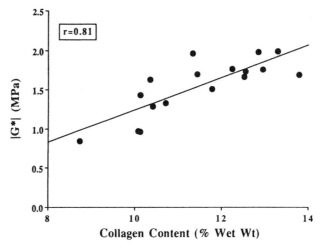

FIG. 22. A direct correlation between the collagen content (by wet weight) and magnitude of dynamic modulus |G^*| for bovine articular cartilage. The compressive clamping strain is 20%, and frequency $f = 1.0$ Hz.

336). Thus, from these results, we may conclude that the ability of collagen to resist tension provides the strength of solid matrix in shear, and energy dissipation in collagen fibrils is minimal when it is stretched. Furthermore, the interaction of proteoglycans with collagen fibrils functions to maintain collagen fibrils in proper spatial orientations, thus providing cartilage with its strength and stiffness in shear (275,338). Note that the magnitude of the dynamic shear modulus is significantly greater than the equilibrium shear modulus. This situation is similar to any viscoelastic material where stiffness increases with increasing rates of deformation.

The viscoelasticity of meniscus in response to shear is qualitatively similar to that exhibited by articular cartilage, although the magnitudes of the material coefficients of these tissues are significantly different. First, meniscus shear properties exhibited an orthotropic symmetry, i.e., the three planes of symmetry defined by its fibrous architecture dominate the shear properties of the meniscus. The equilibrium shear moduli are 36.8 KPa, 29.8 KPa, and 21.4 KPa in the circumferential, axial, and radial directions, respectively. The circumferential, perpendicular, and radial specimens relative to the collagen fiber orientation for these shear tests are defined in Fig. 23. It is to be noted that these shear values are ten times less than those observed for articular cartilage. For these tests,

the |G^*| and δ for circumferential, axial, and radial specimens reflect orthotropic symmetry as well (Fig. 24). As with tension, the dynamic shear modulus is stiffer than the equilibrium shear modulus.

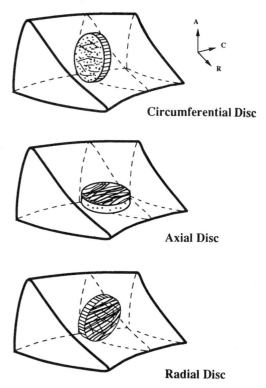

FIG. 23. Orientation of meniscal test specimens for anisotropic shear studies (333).

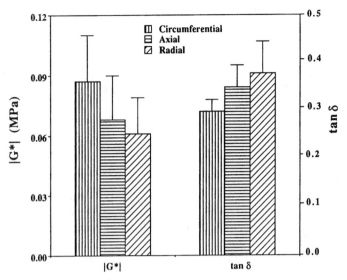

FIG. 24. The magnitude of dynamic shear modulus |G*| and tan δ for circumferentially, axially, and radially oriented meniscal specimens at 1 rad/sec.

In summary, the collagen–proteoglycan solid matrix of articular cartilage and meniscus are viscoelastic. However, the contribution of the intrinsic viscoelasticity appears to be minor when one examines the mechanical response of these tissues in compression (175,281). Thus, in compression, the predominant loading mode, the creep and stress-relaxation responses of normal cartilage and meniscus are dominated by the frictional drag of interstitial fluid flow. For pathologic tissues, where the permeability is increased (reduced frictional drag force), the intrinsic viscoelasticity of the solid matrix becomes important.

BIPHASIC VISCOELASTIC PROPERTIES OF ARTICULAR CARTILAGE IN COMPRESSION

In this section, the transient compressive creep and stress-relaxation behaviors of cartilage and meniscus are discussed. We have shown that the dominant physical mechanism affecting these time-dependent responses is the frictional drag caused by interstitial fluid flow through the porous-permeable solid matrix. These are the *flow-dependent* properties of the tissue, and they

are best described and understood using the biphasic theory.

Strain-Dependent Permeability

As described above, the permeability coefficient of the soft-hydrated tissue can be determined from the permeation experiment using Darcy's law (eq. 6). The values of permeability for cartilage and meniscus obtained were very low (10^{-15} to 10^{-16} m⁴/N-sec), and by equation 7, the diffusive drag coefficients were very high (10^{15} to 10^{16} N-sec/m⁴). Thus, very large drag forces are exerted by interstitial fluid as it flows through the porous-permeable solid matrix. These large drag forces can cause significant compaction of the porous-permeable solid matrix (131,132,163); this phenomenon is known as flow-induced compaction of the solid matrix. Indeed, for articular cartilage, the permeability is highly dependent on the compressive strain and applied pressures. As can be seen in Fig. 25, the permeation measurements show the dramatic effects of compressive strain ε_c and pressure gradient ΔP on the permeability coefficient k of the tissue (132,163,180,207).

These experimental observations indicate that a reduction in the dimensions of the car-

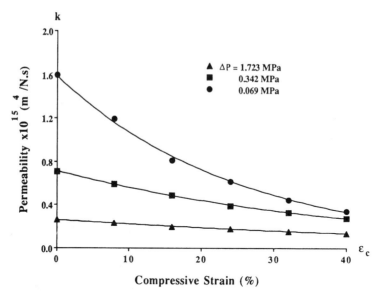

FIG. 25. Variation of the apparent permeability *k* with compressive clamping strain (ε_c) and pressure gradient ΔP. This is known as the strain-dependent permeability effect (163,207).

tilage would lead to a reduction of fluid content and thus in the porosity and permeability of the solid matrix. This nonlinear strain-dependent permeability effect plays an important physiological role in regulating the transient compressive responses of cartilage and in dissipating energy. It serves to prevent rapid and excessive fluid exudation from the tissue by compression (131,132,163,207,208, 322).

The Mechanism of Biphasic Creep and Stress Relaxation

Confined Compression Experiment and Analysis

The observed creep and stress-relaxation behaviors of articular cartilage and meniscus result from the balance of stresses between that carried by the drag force of interstitial fluid flow and that supported by the solid matrix. An estimate of the drag force can be made using data on cartilage permeability and the diffusive drag coefficient relationship (eq. 7). Consider the case of a cartilage specimen

with permeability coefficient of 1.5×10^{-15} m^4/Ns and porosity of 0.75, then the diffusive drag coefficient is 0.375×10^{15} Ns/m^4. For a fluid filtration velocity of 15 µm/sec, according to equation 6, this drag force would require a pressure differential of 7.5 MPa to move a 1-mm column of fluid through the tissue at that speed (163). Thus, even for this very low flow speed, very large drag forces and hydraulic pressures are exerted on the solid matrix. Further, we note that for normal cartilage with a compressive modulus less than 1.0 MPa (Table 9), a compressive stress of approximately 0.25 MPa is required to compress the tissue by 25% (a normal occurrence *in vivo*). In this example, the ratio of the stress from fluid drag to the stress required to compress the tissue is about 30:1. Thus, the drag force of interstitial fluid flow and the associated fluid pressure appear to be the major mechanisms for load support in the joint. This is the most important fact in understanding how cartilage and meniscus support load in the joint.

The compressive creep behaviors of articular cartilage and meniscus have been studied extensively in the confined compression test

(20,69,130,131,158,164,203,205,207,208,243, 326). In the creep experiment, a cartilage surface of a small cylindrical plug is loaded against a free-draining, rigid, porous-permeable filter (Fig. 16). The pressure in the pores of the filter is at ambient; thus, a free-draining condition is maintained that allows fluid exudation from the tissue to occur in an unimpeded manner. A load is suddenly applied to, and constantly maintained on, the specimen. Exudation of the interstitial fluid begins immediately. As fluid leaves the tissue, compressive creep deformation occurs. A typical creep curve, on a log scale, for intervertebral disk is shown in Fig. 26. The rate of creep is controlled by the rate of fluid exudation and thus by tissue permeability. In the confined compression experiment, the fluid movement and solid matrix deformation occur only in the axial direction. From the linear biphasic formulation for cartilage (207), the principle of conservation of mass yields an explicit relationship between fluid exudation velocity $v^f(0,t)$ and surface creep velocity $v^s(0,t)$. This is given by:

$$\phi^s v^s(0,t) = -\phi^f v^f(0,t), \qquad (15)$$

where $z = 0$ defines the position of the articular surface. The negative sign means com-

pression of the solid matrix that would yield fluid exudation. From this expression, it is clear that creep will reach equilibrium when fluid exudation ceases. Thus, at creep equilibrium (i.e., no interstitial fluid flow), the load applied via the rigid-porous filter is entirely borne by the solid matrix. This result also shows that the kinetics of creep may be used as a convenient way to determine tissue permeability.

According to the biphasic constitutive law, the total stress σ^T acting on the tissue is given by:

$$\sigma^T = \sigma^s + \sigma^f, \qquad (16)$$

where σ^s is the stress acting on the elastic collagen–proteoglycan solid matrix, and σ^f is the stress acting on the interstitial fluid. The stress differential on σ^T is balanced by the frictional drag force acting on the solid and fluid phases, which are given respectively by

$$f^s = -f^f = K(v^s - v^f) + p\nabla\phi^f \qquad (17)$$

These fundamental concepts provide the basis for understanding the creep and stress-relaxation behaviors of hydrated soft tissues. For creep, the analytic solution for the surface displacement $u(0,t)$ in the axial direction is obtained:

$$(u(0,t)/h) = (F_0/H_A) \left\{ 1 - 2 \sum_{n=0}^{\infty} \right.$$

$$\left. (\exp[-(n+1/2)^2\pi^2 H_A kt/h^2]/(n+1/2)^2\pi^2) \right\} \qquad (18)$$

where h is the thickness of the specimen, F_0 is the applied compressive stress, and H_A is the aggregate modulus. Equation 18 predicts that at time $t = 0$, the surface displacement $u(0,0) = 0$; i.e., there is no instantaneous displacement of cartilage at the surface under confined compression conditions (Fig. 26). Physically, this is because fluid flux (volume/time) through the interstitium can not occur instantaneously because of the frictional drag. This situation is analogous to the viscous dashpot (Fig. 10B), which can not respond instantaneously. Equation 18 also shows that the kinetics of creep from $t = 0^+$ (shortly after load-

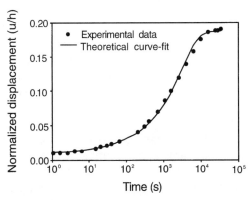

FIG. 26. Predicted and experimental results of the biphasic viscoelastic creep in confined compression for a plug of intervertebral disk. The solid line represents the creep response predicted by the linear biphasic model, equation 18. The results for the curve fit yielded a confined compression modulus of 0.52 MPa and an average hydraulic permeability of 0.17×10^{-15} m^4/N-sec (25).

ing) to $t \to \infty$ is governed by the time constant T defined by

$$T = \frac{h^2}{H_A k} = \frac{h^2 K}{(\phi^f)^2 H_A}. \qquad (19)$$

This constant is known as the characteristic time for a biphasic material. It is proportional to the ratio of the frictional drag coefficient K to the compressive aggregate modulus H_A. Theoretically, it has been shown that this time constant T is the most important parameter governing the kinetics of creep and stress relaxation in compression (130,209). With material coefficients for normal and osteoarthritic cartilages, their characteristic times (≈ 1500 sec versus 500 sec) differ considerably, as does the manner of their load support (Problem 14). This means that normal cartilage would take more than three times longer to reach creep equilibrium than does degenerative cartilage; i.e., the fluid pressurization effect is more important in load carriage for normal tissue than for OA tissue. This characteristic time also shows that a tissue that is twice as thick will take four times as long to reach creep equilibrium. An increase of permeability would decrease creep time, and a decrease of compressive modulus would increase creep time.

The solution given by equation 18 provides the explicit expression to determine the properties of the test specimens under the uniaxial confined compression creep condition. Note that as time approaches infinity, the specimen would reach a compressive equilibrium strain given by $u/h = F_o/H_A$. Therefore, the compressive aggregate modulus H_A can be determined from the equilibrium displacement, the thickness of the tissue, and the applied compressive stress.[5] The permeability coefficient of the specimen may be determined from the kinetics of the confined compression creep data. This is done by analyzing the experimental data with equation 18 and by using a least-squares numerical curve-fitting procedure (10,25,209,243). As shown in Fig. 26, the experimental creep data are compared

with the predictions of equation 18. To check the accuracy of this curve-fitting procedure, the calculated value of k may be compared with the values of k determined from the uniaxial permeation experiment (see above). Indeed, the average permeability coefficient k determined from the confined compression experiment is consistent with those obtained from the direct permeation experiment (163, 180,203). The permeability coefficients determined from this creep test for various tissues are presented in Table 10A. The corresponding thickness of the articular cartilage is presented in Table 10B. The average value of permeability of normal bovine meniscus is 0.81×10^{-15} m^4/Ns) (243). The variations with time of the aggregate modulus, shear modulus, Poisson's ratio, permeability, and thickness of greyhound tibial plateau cartilage following anterior cruciate ligament (ACL) transection (control, 6 weeks, 12 weeks) are shown in Table 10C (283). Clearly, injuries of this type have significant detrimental effects on knee joint cartilage.

The compressive stress-relaxation test has the same experimental setup as the uniaxial confined compression creep test. In this test, a displacement function $u(0,t)$ is imposed at the specimen surface via the rigid porous-permeable platen. During the ramp phase ($0 < t < t_o$), the tissue is compressed at a constant rate, $u(0,t) = Rt$, where R is the rate of compression. Fluid exudation occurs across the surface (see Fig. 27) (points A and B). Because of the large frictional drag associated with fluid flow through the solid matrix, large loads are needed to compress the tissue. Figure 27 (bottom right) depicts the stress rising during the ramp phase. During the relaxation phase ($t > t_o$), the compressive strain is held constant. Thus, by equation 15, no fluid exudation occurs (Fig. 27C,D,E). The compressive stress at the surface decays with time as solid compaction at the surface is relieved. This results in a transfer of stress away from the compacted regions. This phenomenon also indicates that it is difficult to maintain high stresses in the solid matrix of normal cartilage. It has been shown that the rate of

---

[5]From the expresssion $u/h = F_o/H_A$, it can be seen that for the linear biphasic theory to be valid, F_o must be $\ll H_A$.

TABLE 10A. *Permeability coefficient (10^{-15} m⁴/Ns) of lateral condyle and patellar groove cartilage*

	Human[a]	Bovine[b]	Canine[c]	Monkey[d]	Rabbit[e]
Lateral condyle	1.18	0.43	0.77	4.19	1.81
Patellar groove	2.17	1.42	0.93	4.74	3.84

[a]Young normal.
[b]18 months to 2 years old.
[c]Mature beagles and greyhounds.
[d]Mature cynomologus monkeys.
[e]Mature New Zealand white rabbits.
Data shown were obtained from indentation creep tests.

TABLE 10B. *Average cartilage thickness (mm) of lateral condyle and patellar groove*

	Human[a]	Bovine[b]	Canine[c]	Monkey[d]	Rabbit[e]
Lateral condyle	2.31	0.94	0.58	0.57	0.25
Patellar groove	3.57	1.38	0.52	0.41	0.20

[a]Young normal.
[b]18 months to 2 years old.
[c]Mature beagles and greyhounds.
[d]Mature cynomolgus monkeys.
[e]Mature New Zealand white rabbits.
Data shown were obtained from indentation creep tests.

TABLE 10C. *Properties of greyhound tibial plateau cartilage at two time periods following ACL transection[a]*

Mean (SD)	Control	6 weeks post-ACLT	12 weeks post-ACLT
k ($\times 10^{-15}$ m⁴/Ns)	2.4 (1.3)	2.6 (0.4)	4.1 (1.0)*
H_A (MPa)	0.56 (0.19)	0.31 (0.10)*	0.42 (0.10)*
μ_s (MPa)	0.25 (0.08)	0.14 (0.03)*	0.19 (0.05)*
v_s	0.07 (0.10)	0.08 (0.07)	0.09 (0.06)
Thickness (mm)	0.85 (0.17)	0.85 (0.11)	0.94 (0.24)

*Results of biphasic indentation testing of cartilage sites on the tibial plateau covered by the meniscus significantly different from control ($p < 0.05$).
[a]Data from Setton et al. (283).

stress relaxation in such a material occurs four times faster than the rate of creep (131,209). At equilibrium, the compressive aggregate modulus computed from the stress-relaxation experiment reflects the intrinsic material stiffness and is therefore equal to that determined from the compressive creep experiment.

It is important to emphasize that during the creep and stress-relaxation processes, a severely nonhomogeneous compressive strain field is developed in the solid matrix, and because of the porous-permeable loading platen, the surface region will experience the most severe compaction. This nonhomogeneous strain field has three important physiological consequences: (a) the permeability at the surface is significantly reduced as a result of the strain-dependent permeability effect; (b) the frictional drag force caused by fluid exudation is exerted most severely at the surface; and (c) the nominal strain in an experiment (e.g., grip-to-grip strain measurement) does not provide an accurate assessment of the actual nonhomogeneous compressive strains experienced by the tissue. However, as the compacted region gradually diffuses into the deeper zones of the tissue, the creep and stress-relaxation processes eventually cease; at equilibrium, a homogeneous state of compression is reached. Thus, in measuring the intrinsic material properties of soft hydrated tissues,

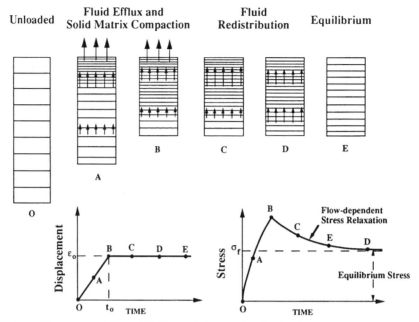

FIG. 27. Schematic representation of fluid exudation and redistribution within cartilage during a rate-controlled compression stress-relaxation experiment **(lower left)**. The horizontal bars in the upper figures indicate the distribution of strain in the tissue. The lower graph **(right)** shows the stress response during the compression phase (O,A,B) and the relaxation phase (B,C,D,E).

grip-to-grip motion may only be used at equilibrium.

Indentation Creep Experiment

The indentation experiment is the most frequently used method for studying the biomechanical properties of articular cartilage (e.g., 9,22,52,70,94,127,128,133,141,151,152,203, 233,234,288,289). A schematic diagram of an articular cartilage indentation experiment, where the tissue is compressed by a circular rigid, smooth, porous, free-draining indenter of radius a, is shown in Fig. 28. This experiment is attractive because it does not require special specimen preparation techniques such as microtoming precise strips required for the tensile tests or preparing precise cartilage–bone plugs for the confined compression tests. Further, the indentation test has the added advantage that the material properties of cartilage are determined *in situ* on the bone, a condition more closely resembling the physiological situation. It also provides a method to determine the variation of cartilage properties over the joint surface (19,20,52,88, 128,151,152,283) and does not affect the ultrastructure or composition of the tissue. It is this relative simplicity that has led many investigators to adopt the indentation test.

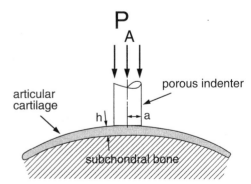

FIG. 28. A schematic diagram showing a layer of articular cartilage of thickness h being indented by a circular, rigid, smooth, porous, free-draining indenter of radius a.

The mathematics of modeling the indentation experiment of cartilage-on-bone configuration is very complex because of the multidimensional deformations in the layer of tissue as well as the biphasic nature of the tissue (176,203). Because of the mathematical difficulties involved with modeling the indentation test, early investigators used linear elastic constitutive law to analyze and interpret the experimental viscoelastic creep data without accounting for the interstitial fluid flow in the tissue (120,127,151,288,289). Because elastic analyses cannot predict time-dependent behavior, these models necessarily cannot describe the creep and stress-relaxation behaviors exhibited by cartilage. Hence, researchers introduced the use of elastic modulus determined at a specific time, for example, Kempson's 2-sec creep modulus (151,152). For a detailed discussion of the history of the indentation experiment, the reader is referred to reviews by Mow and co-workers (212) and Mak and co-workers (176) on this subject.

As discussed above, in the specific case of uniaxial confined compression, two material coefficients (H_A and k) can be determined using the linear biphasic theory. In general, however, the biphasic theory contains three material coefficients (H_A, v, k); these three coefficients are equivalent to any other set, e.g., (E, v, k) or (E, μ, k) (see Table 4). In the application of the early model such as the mathematical solutions of *elastic* theory for indentation (120), *a priori* assumptions for Poisson's ratio must be made. Various investigators have chosen the Poisson's ratio to be between 0.4 to 0.5 (e.g., 128,151,289). The indentation creep test, analyzed using the linear biphasic theory, provides the determination of all three material coefficients simultaneously (e.g., 19,20,203). The mathematics of modeling the indentation experiment is very complex and is beyond the scope of this chapter. The reader is referred to published references (120,176,203) for a complete mathematical description of the problem.

The nature of the mathematical solution showing the dependence of biphasic indentation creep on the aggregate modulus, Poisson's ratio, and permeability is shown in Fig. 29A. From this result, we now know that: (a) the equilibrium displacement value, $u(\infty)$, defines a relationship for the intrinsic compressive modulus (H_A) and the Poisson's ratio (v); (b) the shape of the creep curve is also defined by the Poisson's ratio; and (c) the rate of the creep curve (i.e., the kinetics of creep) is defined by the shift factor $S = \log_{10}(H_A k/a^2)$, where a is the radius of the indenter tip. This shift factor provides the third necessary relationship to determine the permeability (k) of the tissue from the creep data. These three relationships have been used to determine the three intrinsic properties of articular cartilage (H_A, v, k) (176,203). This problem has been solved numerically. To determine these three coefficients for the indentation site, the numerical solutions are curve-fitted using a least-square procedure. Typical curve-fitting results are shown in Fig. 29B on a $\log_{10}(t)$ scale. Tables 9 and 10A,C provide the aggregate modulus and permeability determined by this method. Table 11 provides the Poisson's ratio for the same population of animals.

The available data on Poisson's ratio reflects some important characteristics of cartilage: (a) it varies with species and location; (b) it almost always falls outside of the 0.4 to 0.5 range, the commonly *assumed* range; (c) *a priori* estimates of Poisson's ratio in the range 0.4 to 0.5 may lead to significant errors in calculating the aggregate modulus. For example, errors as large as 200% can occur if one assumes $v = 0.4$ in the calculation for H_A and the actual Poisson's ratio is zero (203). For an isotropic porous-permeable solid matrix, Poisson's ratio is a measure of the compressibility of its pores: $v = 0$ means the pores are maximally compressible, and $v = 0.5$ means the pores are incompressible. For isotropic biphasic materials, a measure of the volume efflux of fluid through the tissue when it is compressed is Poisson's ratio. For a biphasic material with $v = 0.5$, no fluid flow can occur, and thus no creep and stress-relaxation behaviors are possible. The species and anatomic site variation of Poisson's ratio over the joint surface may in fact reflect the fluid efflux requirement at a specific loca-

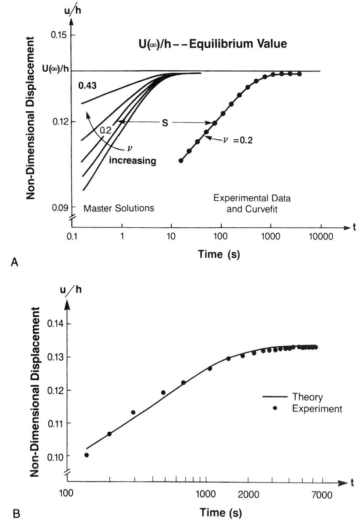

FIG. 29. (A) Representation of the time-shift method in which a master solution is shifted by an amount S along the logarithmic time axis. Diagram illustrates how the shape of the displacement curve is controlled by the Poisson's ratio v. **(B)** A typical nonlinear regression curve fit using the bicubic spline interpolation for biphasic creep indentation solution in logarithmic time scale.

TABLE 11. *Average Poisson's ratio (v) of lateral condyle and patellar groove cartilage*

	Human[a]	Bovine[b]	Canine[c]	Monkey[d]	Rabbit[e]
Lateral condyle	0.10	0.40	0.30	0.24	0.34
Patellar groove	0.00	0.25	0.09	0.20	0.21

[a]Young normal.
[b]18 months to 2 years old.
[c]Mature beagles.
[d]Mature cynomologus monkeys.
[e]Mature New Zealand white rabbits.

tion on the joint surface, say for purposes of joint lubrication (see Chapter 8 for more details on lubrication).

SWELLING OF ARTICULAR CARTILAGE

Mechanism of Swelling: Change of Hydration and Dimensions

In cartilage, proteoglycan aggregates are immobilized and restrained in the collagen meshwork. They contain a large number of negatively charged groups (SO_3^- and COO^-) along their GAG chains. For normal and degenerate femoral head cartilage, the fixed charge density (FCD) ranges from 0.04 to 0.18 mEq/g wet tissue at physiological pH (181,184,188). Each negative charge requires a counter-ion to be nearby to maintain electroneutrality. Thus, the total ion concentration inside the tissue is greater than the ion concentration in the external bathing solution. This imbalance of ions gives rise to a pressure in the interstitial fluid that is higher than the ambient pressure in the external bath. This is known as the Donnan osmotic pressure (57). This osmotic pressure is one of the causes of cartilage swelling.

In the extracellular matrix, it is estimated that the proteoglycans are restrained to one-fifth of their volume in free solution (115,220). Thus, the charge groups fixed along the GAG chains of the solid matrix are very close to each other, causing large charge–charge repulsive forces to be exerted against each other. These forces also cause the extracellular matrix to swell. The charge–charge electrostatic forces are modulated by the counter- and co-ions swarming around the proteoglycan molecules in solution. With increasing ion concentration within the tissue, the equivalent Debye length between the ion cloud and the fixed charges is decreased. This results in charge shielding, which decreases the net charge–charge repulsive force (92,162). Decrease of the size of the PG molecule in solution with charge shielding has been measured (235). Changes in the di-

mensions and shape of the tissue specimen and isometric stress caused by NaCl concentration changes in the external bathing solution have also been measured (7,67,68,97,212,223,225, 278–280,283,301).

Maroudas and co-workers were the first to provide significant amounts of data on changing tissue hydration and interstitial ion concentration (c) with changing external bathing solution c^* (181,182,188). In those studies the cartilage swelling is measured by weight. Later, Mow and co-workers (225,279) measured the tendency for cartilage to swell dimensionally or curl when c^* is changed. The results of these dimensional swelling studies show that swelling of articular cartilage is nonhomogeneous (Fig. 30A) and anisotropic (Fig. 30B), which would produce curling when the tissue is excised from the bone. The length and width directions correspond to directions parallel and perpendicular to the split-line directions. The magnitude of contraction is largest along the thickness direction and in the deep zone of the tissue. Further, as can be seen in Fig. 30A, the ion-induced contractions of cartilage under free swelling conditions vary linearly with c^*. This result is described by the relationship $\varepsilon_s = -\alpha_c c^*$, where α_c is known as the coefficient of chemical contraction, and ε_s is the ion-induced contraction (223,225). For articular cartilage, the value α_c ranges from 0.05 M^{-1} to 0.3 M^{-1}.

Donnan Equilibrium, Ion Distribution, and Osmotic Pressure

If the tissue is bathed in deionized water, the total internal counter-ion concentration c^F would equal the total FCD. If the tissue is bathed in an external solution containing ions at concentration c^*, the total internal ion concentration would be determined by the Donnan equilibrium ion distribution equation:

$$c(c + c^F) = (c^*)^2. \qquad (20)$$

This equation was derived by Donnan in 1924 (57) and governs the ion concentration in an

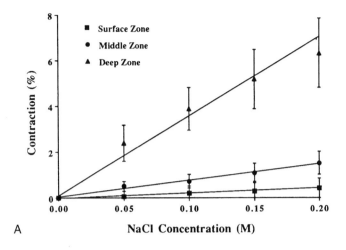

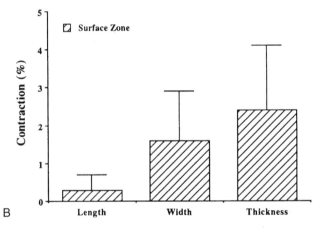

FIG. 30. Free swelling of articular cartilage strips: **(A)** along the length axis as a function of depth (surface, middle, and deep zones); **(B)** in the directions of length, width, and thickness of the specimen (225).

ideal polyelectrolyte solution. However, it has been used extensively for articular cartilage (181,182,184).[6] The total internal ion concentration in cartilage as a function of the fixed charge density c^F at an external concentration $c^* = 0.15$ M NaCl is shown in Fig. 31. If the tissue is bathed in a very high-concentration solution, i.e., $c^* \gg c^F$, the difference between the total number of ions in the tissue $(2c + c^F)$ and the total number of ions outside $(2c^*)$ is given by (162):

$$(2c + c^F) - 2c^* = (c^F)^2/(4c^*). \quad (21)$$

Thus, the difference approaches zero as the external concentration $c^* \to \infty$. From the classical relationship for osmotic pressure, the Donnan osmotic pressure (π) that results from the excess of ion particles inside the tissue (see Fig. 31) is given by:

$$\pi = RT[\Phi(2c + c^F) - 2\Phi^*c^*] + P_\infty. \quad (22)$$

---

[6]Cartilage, by virtue of its solid matrix, is not an ideal polyelectrolyte solution. However, predictions of total ion concentrations using equation 20 seem to be accurate.

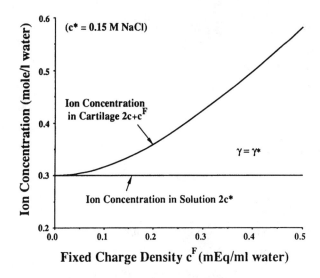

FIG. 31. Ion concentration in the interstitium versus fixed charge density (FCD).

where R is the universal gas constant, T is the absolute temperature, Φ and Φ^* are osmotic coefficients, and P_∞ is the osmotic pressure attributable to the concentration of proteoglycan particles in the tissue (66,302). Usually, because of the size of proteoglycan molecules, P_∞ is negligibly small. We emphasize that this expression is for polyelectrolyte solutions, where there is no solid matrix. However, it has nevertheless been used extensively to describe the swelling pressures of cartilage and the intervertebral disk (181,182, 184,308).

Triphasic Swelling Theory

A triphasic theory (comprising a miscible ion phase along with the two immiscible fluid and solid phases of the biphasic theory) has been developed to account for the ion-induced swelling effects and the biphasic deformational effects (160–162). This theory describes a) all biphasic viscoelastic effects, b) the Donnan equilibrium ion distributions (c^F, c), c) the dimensional swelling effect (ε_s), d) the Donnan osmotic pressures (π), e) kinetics of swelling (i.e., transient effects), and f) all electrokinetic effects (e.g., streaming potentials).

Typical experimental or theoretical swelling studies of cartilage are performed under

either confined compression (e.g., 158,205, 207), unconfined compression (e.g., 11,182, 184,268), or the free (unloaded and unconstrained) condition (223,279). For the confined-compression swelling experiment, the tissue specimen is held at a fixed compressive strain by a rigid, free-draining loading platen. Under these conditions, the triphasic theory predicts that the total axial stress σ^T at the loading platen will have three components:

$$\sigma^T = \sigma^s + \sigma^c + \pi. \qquad (23)$$

Here, σ^s is the stress in the elastic solid matrix caused by the imposed uniaxial compression (i.e., from the biphasic theory), σ^c is the stress caused by the chemical expansion ε_s resulting from charge–charge repulsion, which depends on both c^F and c, and π is the Donnan osmotic swelling pressure (i.e., equation 22). From existing experimental data on the compressive aggregate modulus, $H_A = 1.0$ MPa, chemical expansion data (225), physicochemical data, $c^F = 0.1$ and $\phi^f = 1.0$ (184), and assuming $P_\infty = 0$ and an external bathing solution of 0.15 M NaCl, the equilibrium response of cartilage to increasing compressive strains is shown in Fig. 32. In this figure, the total swelling pressure P^s is defined as $\sigma^c + \pi$. With these results for the stress–strain relationships, the contribution to cartilage stiffness (slope of the curve) from the three mechanisms may be

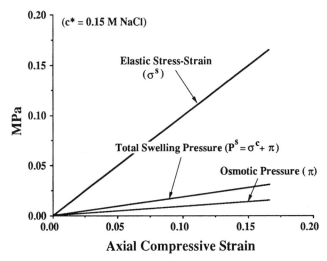

FIG. 32. Stress–strain curve as well as the predicted total swelling pressure P^s ($= \sigma^c + \pi$) and Donnan osmotic pressure (π) in 0.15 M NaCl bathing solution and as functions of the compressive strain.

calculated. It is seen that the largest portion of the compressive stiffness is derived from the elastic solid matrix. Donnan osmotic pressure π and stress from chemical expansion σ^c contribute in approximately equal proportions to the overall compressive stiffness, but their slopes are much less than 1.0 MPa for normal articular cartilage.

Fluid and Ion Transport, Kinetic Effects, and Streaming Potentials

The previous section focused on equilibrium events (i.e., Donnan equilibrium ion distribution, Donnan osmotic pressure, and swelling pressure) in cartilage when bathed in a solution of electrolytes (e.g., NaCl) at concentration c^*. In this section we present results from the triphasic theory for kinetic events that are related to the transport of fluid and ions through charged hydrated tissues (99–101).

From an analysis of the one-dimensional permeation experiment (Fig. 33), Gu and coworkers (99) were able to derive some fundamental relations between some extrinsic parameters (e.g., hydraulic permeability k, electric conductivity κ_o, and streaming potential $\Delta\psi$)

and intrinsic tissue variables defining the tissue. For example, it was found that the hydraulic permeability k is governed by the following equation:

$$k = \phi^f/[K_1 + RT(c^F)^2/(c^+D^+ + c^-D^-)]. \quad (24)$$

where K_1 is proportional to the frictional coefficient between the porous-permeable solid matrix and interstitial fluid ($= f_{ws}/\phi^f$; f_{ws} is the friction between the interstitial water and the porous-permeable solid matrix), R and T are the universal gas constant and absolute temperature, respectively, and $c^\pm$ and $D^\pm$ are the concentration and diffusion coefficients of the cation ($+$) and anion ($-$), respectively.

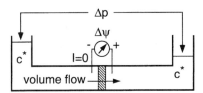

FIG. 33. A one-dimensional permeation experiment on a permeable charged hydrated tissue specimen under an open-circuit condition to determine the streaming potential $\Delta\psi$. Here, Δp is the pressure differential, I is the current ($= 0$), and c^* is the concentration of a neutral salt (e.g., NaCl) in the permeating fluid (99).

These are all intrinsic tissue parameters.[7] It is clear from equation 24 that tissues with higher c^F and lower ϕ^f will have lower permeability, as experimentally observed (e.g., 10,184,205,283). Note also that for large c^F or $c^F/c^* \gg 1$, equations 21 and 24 simplify to:

$$k = \phi^f/(K_1 + RTc^F/D^+).\qquad(25)$$

This equation states that when c^F is large, only the resistance between the counter-ion (e.g., Na^+) and water, expressed as D^+, and that between water and solid, expressed as K_1, are significant factors governing the hydraulic permeability. Clearly, these results can provide significant insights into electrokinetic phenomena in cartilage. An expression for the conductivity κ_o and the intrinsic variables was also derived:

$$\kappa_o = (F_c)^2\phi^f(c^+D^+ + c^-D^-)/RT\qquad(26)$$

where F_c is the Faraday constant. Again, for $c^F \gg c^*$, $c^+/c^F \to 1$ and $c^-/c^+ \ll 1$, equation 26 reduces to the form:

$$\kappa_o = (F_c)^2c^FD^+/RT.\qquad(27)$$

This expression for the conductivity of charged-hydrated tissues may be found in the classical book of nonequilibrium thermodynamics by Katchalsky and Curran (143); again, it provides insight into the basic electrokinetic processes involved during conduction.

Finally, it is well known that all charged hydrated tissues exhibit a phenomenon known as streaming potential (e.g., 126,143). This streaming potential effect results from the macroscopic requirement for electroneutrality within the tissue when there are no currents. To visualize how a streaming potential may be created, consider the one-dimensional permeation experiment again (Fig. 33). As the fluid is forced through a porous-permeable, charged, hydrated matrix of a tissue specimen, it will tend to convect the dissolved ions downstream, thus tending to cause a separation of charges. This cannot occur by virtue of the electroneutrality condition and open circuit condition. Thus, an electrical potential is required to drive the ions back, preventing charge separation, and this potential is known as the streaming potential. Again, from the triphasic theory, the expression for the streaming potential $\Delta\psi$ across the specimen is given by:

$$\Delta\psi = -c^FF_ck\Delta p/\kappa_o\qquad(28)$$

where Δp is the pressure differential applied across the specimen (99). This is the well-known streaming-potential equation (e.g., 126). Typical values of $\Delta\psi/\Delta p$ for articular cartilage and intervertebral disk material have been determined. It ranges from 4 to 6 mV/MPa (1 mV = 10^{-3} V) at a pressure differential $\Delta p = 0.1$ MPa. It has also been shown experimentally that $\Delta\psi/\Delta p$ depends on the FCD, i.e., tissue pathology (100,101,184, 188). Clearly, these five fundamental relationships, i.e., equations 24 to 28, among the measurable extrinsic variables (k, κ_o, and $\Delta\psi/\Delta p$) and the intrinsic tissue parameters (K_1, c^F, $D^\pm$, and $c^\pm$) provide alternative means for their determinations for tissue characterization. Future studies will determine their eventual usefulness.

SUMMARY

Articular cartilage and meniscus are two specialized, charged, hydrated soft tissues of the body. Each tissue possesses a specific biochemical composition, molecular conformation, and ultrastructure. The biomechanical properties of articular cartilage and meniscus are different and are dependent on their own specific biochemical composition and architectural arrangement. These features are altered during disease or when the tissues are injured. Both tissues exhibit biphasic mechanical properties, with the frictional drag force of interstitial fluid flow being the dominant factor controlling their compressive viscoelastic creep and stress-relaxation behav-

---

[7]Note that equations 24 and 25 have an identical form to equation 7; i.e., they both relate the frictional drag K (or f_{ws}) with the inverse of permeability ($1/k$) by the square of the porosity ϕ^f.

iors. The aggregate modulus and permeability of normal cartilage are on the order of 1.0 MPa and 1 to 10×10^{-15} m⁴/N-sec, and for degenerate cartilage, they are 0.35 MPa and 10^{-14} m⁴/Ns, respectively. There are significant variations in these material properties with sites on the joint surface as well as with species. For the meniscus, the aggregate modulus and permeability are 0.4 MPa and 0.5 to 1.0×10^{-15} m⁴/Ns, respectively. These differences have strong implications for the manner in which loads are supported by cartilage and meniscus in the joint. The permeability is strain dependent; i.e., it decreases with compressive strain. This effect serves to restrict excessive fluid exudation when prolonged compression occurs.

Both cartilage and meniscus have anisotropic and nonhomogeneous properties. The intrinsic tensile properties of the collagen–proteoglycan solid matrix of both tissues are nonlinear, and their shear properties are viscoelastic. The magnitude of the complex shear modulus of normal cartilage is of the order of 0.5 MPa whereas, for the meniscus, this is less than 0.15 MPa. Viscoelastic dissipation in shear is slight; the phase shift angle is approximately $15°$ for both tissues. These viscoelastic shear properties appear to be of little significance unless the permeability of the solid matrix becomes large, i.e., when the frictional drag effects are minimized. The Poisson's ratio of the solid matrix of articular cartilage may range anywhere from 0 to 0.4.

Donnan osmotic pressure is due to the difference of total ion concentration in the interstitium and the ion concentration in the external bathing solution. The Donnan equilibrium ion distribution in the interstitium depends on the fixed charge density of the negative charge groups on the proteoglycans and on the external ion concentration of bathing solution. Strictly speaking, these two concepts are valid only for charged polymeric *liquids,* though they have been widely adopted for cartilage, a solid. In cartilage, the swelling pressure is the sum of chemical expansion stress and the Donnan osmotic pressure. The contribution of the swelling pressure to the overall

stiffness of articular cartilage appears to be small relative to the aggregate modulus of the elastic solid matrix.

Results from one-dimensional permeation experiments for electrokinetic phenomena give important fundamental relationships between the extrinsic tissue variables such as permeability, conductivity, and streaming potential and the intrinsic tissue parameters such as fixed charge density and diffusion coefficients. These relationships offer new methods to characterize the physicochemical properties of any porous-permeable, charged, hydrated tissues. Articular cartilage and meniscus are two examples of charged, hydrated soft tissues exhibiting multiphasic properties that depend on the nature of the tissues' biochemical composition, molecular structure, and fibrous architecture. Other important connective tissues such as the intervertebral disks offer new opportunities for future investigation for advances in the understanding of degenerative disk disease. Some examples of recent results from the biomechanics literature on this complex and intriguing tissue have been introduced in this chapter as well.

Acknowledgment

The materials and data presented in this chapter are based on studies sponsored by grants from the National Science Foundation, the National Institutes of Health, and the Orthopaedic Research and Education Foundation.

PROBLEMS

1. A. Read reference 220 and write a three-page summary of this paper.
   B. Sketch and describe the molecular architecture of a proteoglycan aggrecan and aggregate (a 1996 version).
2. A. Read reference 196 and write a three-page summary of this paper.
   B. Sketch and describe the molecular architecture of a collagen fibril.
3. A. Read reference 49 and write a three-page summary of this paper.

B. Sketch the collagen ultrastructure of adult articular cartilage.

4. Derive equations 2 and 3 governing the force–displacement relationship of the Kelvin-Voigt and Maxwell bodies. Explain why the Kelvin-Voigt body behaves as a solid and why the Maxwell body behaves as a fluid.

5. Given equations 2 and 3 for Kelvin-Voigt and Maxwell bodies, derive the solutions for their stress-relaxation behaviors for $t > 0$ if the applied initial displacement is $x(0) = 1$.

6. Given equations 2 and 3 for Kelvin-Voigt and Maxwell bodies, derive the solutions for their creep behaviors for $t > 0$, if the applied initial load is $F(0)=1$.

7. A standard three-element linear viscoelastic body is one for which a spring is connected in series with the Kelvin-Voigt body.
   a. Sketch a spring–dashpot arrangement for the standard body.
   b. Derive the force–displacement relationship for this material.
   c. Show that this arrangement is equivalent to a spring connected in parallel with a Maxwell body.
   d. Does the standard three-element body behave as a solid or a fluid? Explain why.

8. The fluid transport Q (volume discharge per unit time, m^3/sec) is given by Darcy's linear relationship $Q = kA\Delta P/h$, where ΔP is the applied pressure differential, A is the area of perfusion, and h is the thickness of the tissue.
   a. For a cartilage tissue with the thickness $h = 1.75$ mm and the perfusion area $A = 6.25$ mm^2, and the permeability $k = 4.6 \times 10^{-15}$ m^4/Ns, calculate the volume flux across the tissue if $\Delta P = 0.5$ MPa and 1.0 MPa. (Ans. 8.2×10^{-12} m^3/sec; 16.4×10^{-12} m^3/sec)
   b. For a meniscus tissue with $h = 10$ mm, $A = 15$ mm^2, and the permeability $k = 0.8 \times 10^{-15}$ m^4/Ns calculate the volume flux across the tissue. (Ans. 0.6×10^{-12} m^3/sec; 1.2×10^{-12} m^3/sec)
   c. How long will it take for a fluid particle to travel across the cartilage and the meniscus at $\Delta P = 1.0$ MPa, assuming $\phi^f = 0.75$? (Ans. 500 sec; 9.4×10^4 sec)

9. If normal cartilage and meniscus have water contents of 80% and 74%, respectively, calculate the diffusive drag coefficient for these two tissues. Water content, defined as the ratio of water weight to total weight, is equivalent to porosity. (Ans. 0.14×10^{15} Ns/m^4, 0.69×10^{15} Ns/m^4)

10. The Poiseuille's law for volume discharge per unit time (Q) of a fluid with viscosity η through a cylindrical circular tube of radius a and length l is given by $Q = \pi a^4(\Delta p)/8\eta l$. If cartilage and meniscus are modeled by uniform collections of identical cylindrical circular tubes, given the permeabilities of cartilage and meniscus, calculate the average pore size for these tissues. Use the viscosity of water for this calculation. (Hint: The ratio l/h is known as the tortuosity. It is the actual path traveled by a fluid particle as it flows through the tissue of thickness h. Assume this value to be no more than 2.) (Ans. 68 to 86 Å; 29 to 42 Å)

11. Rubber is an incompressible material. Its Young's modulus is 1.5 MPa, and its Poisson's ratio is 0.5. Using Table 4, determine the aggregate modulus of rubber. Explain your result.

12. Using Table 4, calculate the aggregate modulus for steel and cork. Give a physical explanation of your result for cork. (Ans. $1.35E$, E)

13. From the data given in Table 7 for bovine articular cartilage, calculate the tangent modulus for slices 1 and 3, ∥ specimens at 5%, 10%, and 15% tensile strains. Compare this result with the Young's modulus E. Explain similarities and differences. (Ans. Slice 1: 13.6, 17.4, 22.3 MPa; Slice 3: 0.98, 1.07, 1.16 MPa).

14. Assume normal human tibial plateau cartilage has an equilibrium aggregate modulus of 0.79 MPa. If the average *in situ* compression of cartilage in the medial

compartment of the tibial plateau cartilage is 15%, using equation 8, calculate the size of the total contact area required to support a joint load of 375 N (75 lb) in this knee. Is this a reasonable answer? Explain.

15. If, as in Problem 14, the individual had the medial meniscus removed during surgery, causing the contact area to be reduced by a factor of 3, calculate the average compressive strain acting in the collagen–proteoglycan solid matrix of cartilage. Is this a reasonable answer? Explain.

16. Use the equation in Problem 10 for calculating the average pore size and the permeability results in Fig. 25, and assume a tortuosity of 2.
    a. Find the change in pore size in cartilage at 8% compressive strain between $\Delta P = 0.069$ MPa and 1.723 MPa. (Ans. 69 Å and 28 Å)
    b. Find the change in pore size in cartilage at $\Delta p = 0.069$ MPa between clamping strains $\varepsilon_c = 0\%$ and 31%. (Ans. 80 Å and 45 Å)

17. The permeability, porosity, and compressive modulus of cartilage are changed during osteoarthrosis. If, for a diseased tissue, the permeability is increased by a factor of 10 to 1.5×10^{-14} m^4/Ns, the porosity increased to 85%, and the compressive aggregate modulus decreased to 0.35 MPa:
    a. Calculate the pressure differential required to cause 1 mm of fluid to flow through this diseased tissue at 15 μm/sec. (Ans. 0.85 MPa) How does this compare to a normal tissue when $\phi^f = 0.75$ and $k = 1.5 \times 10^{-15}$ m^4/Ns?
    b. Calculate the stress required to produce 25% compression of this diseased tissue. (Ans. 0.0875 MPa)
    c. What is the ratio of stress from fluid drag to stress required to deform the solid matrix? How does this compare to normal cartilage? (Ans. 10:1)

18. The surface of cartilage in a joint is covered by synovial fluid, and during joint motion a pressure of $P = 4$ MPa is generated in this fluid. From theoretical considerations, it can be shown that the pressure at the articular surface is partitioned according to the porosity ϕ^f; i.e., the pressure acting on the interstitial fluid at the articular surface is $\phi^f P$, and the pressure acting on the solid matrix at the articular surface is $(1 - \phi^f)P$.
    a. For normal cartilage, the porosity ϕ^f is 75%, the permeability is 1.5×10^{-15} m^4/Ns, and aggregate modulus is 1.0 MPa. How much pressure is acting on the interstitial fluid at the articular surface? What is the filtration speed of the interstitial fluid across a layer of cartilage of thickness $h = 1.5$ mm (assuming the downstream pressure is zero)? At equilibrium, how much compressive strain exists in the solid matrix? Comment on this result. (Ans. 3 MPa; 5.3 μm/sec; 1.)
    b. For abnormal cartilage, the porosity ϕ^f is 85%, the permeability is 1.5×10^{-14} m^4/N-sec, and the aggregate modulus is 0.35 MPa. Repeat the questions of part a. All other variables remain the same. Compare the results of parts a and b. (Ans. 3.4 MPa; 0.47 μm/sec; 1.7)

19. Show that $T = h^2/H_A k$ has the dimension of time.

20. Calculate the characteristic time T for human, bovine, and rabbit lateral condyle and patellar groove cartilage. From equation 18, explain which tissue will creep the fastest and which will creep the slowest?

21. Describe some circumstances by which the composition and structure of articular cartilage might change. How would the biphasic properties (H_A, ν, k, ϕ^f) of the tissue be changed with these changes in composition and tissue structure? How would these changes affect the creep behavior of the tissue?

22. If the fixed charge density of cartilage c^F = 0.2 mEq/ml (i.e., 0.2 mole/liter), and the external NaCl concentration is 0.15 mole/liter, using equation 20, calculate

the total concentration of NaCl within the tissue. Hint: First determine c from data given and that sodium and chlorine are both monovalent ions. (Ans. $c = 0.216$ mole/liter)

23. For a cartilage specimen with $c^F = 0.2$ mEq/ml, bathed in an external electrolyte solution of $c^* = 0.3$ mole/liter, calculate the Donnan osmotic pressure π at room temperature ($T = 24°C$). In this calculation, assume the osmotic coefficients $\Phi = \Phi^* = 0.8$, $P_\infty = 0$, R (universal gas constant) = 8.314 mN/mole-K, and K = 273°C. (Ans. $\pi = 0.063$ MPa) Describe justification for the assumption $P_\infty = 0$.

24. Using equation 25, calculate the frictional coefficient between water and the solid matrix (f_{ws}) if $\phi^f = 0.8$, $k = 1.5 \times 10^{-15}$ m^4/Ns, $c^F = 0.2$ mEq/ml, $D^+ = 0.5 \times 10^{-9}$ m^2/sec. Use data in problem 23.

25. Using equation 27, calculate the conductivity κ_o of cartilage using the data in problem 24. If the inequality $c^F \gg c^*$ holds true, use equation 26 to calculate κ_o. Hint: First determine c^+ and c^- in cartilage. The diffusion coefficient of chlorine in cartilage is $D^- = 0.9 \times 10^{-9}$ m^2/sec, and the Faraday constant $F_c = 9.648 \times 10^4$ amp-sec/mole. Use data in problems 22 and 23.

26. The measured streaming potential for a cartilage specimen is 5 mV at an applied pressure $\Delta p = 0.15$ MPa. Use equation 28 to calculate the electrical conductivity κ_o. Use data in problems 22–25. (Ans. 0.87/ohm-m).

REFERENCES

1. Acaroglu, E. R., Iatridis, J. C., Setton, L. A., Foster, R. J., Mow, V. C., and Weidenbaum, M. (1995): Degeneration and aging affect the tensile behavior of human lumbar anulus fibrosus. *Spine*, 20:2690–2701.
2. Adams, M. E., and Muir, H. (1981): The glycosaminoglycans of canine meniscus. *Biochem. J.*, 197:385–389.
3. Adams, M. E., and Ho, Y. A. (1987): Localization of glycosaminoglycans in human and canine menisci and their attachments. *Connect. Tissue Res.*, 16:269–279.
4. Ahmed, A. M., and Burke, D. L. (1983): *In-vitro* measurement of static pressure distribution in synovial joints—part I: Tibial surface of the knee. *J. Biomech. Eng.*, 105:216–225.
5. Ahmed, A. M., and Burke, D. L. (1983): In-vitro measurement of static pressure distribution in synovial joints—part II: Retropatellar surface. *J. Biomech. Eng.*, 105:226–236.
6. Akizuki, S., Mow, V. C., Muller, F., Pita, J. C., Howell, D. S., and Manicourt, D. H. (1986): Tensile properties of human knee joint cartilage: I. Influence of ionic concentrations, weight bearing, and fibrillation on the tensile modulus. *J. Orthop. Res.*, 4:379–392.
7. Akizuki, S., Mow, V. C., Muller. F., et al. (1987): Tensile properties of knee joint cartilage: II. Correlations between weight bearing and tissue pathology and the kinetics of swelling. *J. Orthop. Res.*, 5:173–186.
8. Ala-Kokko, L., Baldwin, C. T., Moskowitz, R. W., and Prockop, D. J. (1990): Single base mutation in the type II procollagen gene (COL2A1) as a cause of primary osteoarthritis associated with a mild chondrodysplasia. *Proc. Natl. Acad. Sci. USA*, 87:6565–6568.
9. Altman, R. D., Tenenbaum, J., Latta, L., Riskin, W., Blanco, L. N., and Howell, D. S. (1984): Biomechanical and biochemical properties of dog cartilage in experimentally induced osteoarthritis. *Ann. Rheum. Dis.*, 43:83–90.
10. Armstrong, C. G., and Mow, V. C. (1982): Variations in the intrinsic mechanical properties of human articular cartilage with age, degeneration and water content. *J. Bone Joint Surg.*, 64A:88–94.
11. Armstrong, C. G., Mow, V. C., and Lai, W. M. (1984): An analysis of unconfined compression of articular cartilage. *J. Biomech. Eng.*, 106:165–173.
12. Aspden, R. M., and Hukins, D. W. L. (1981): Collagen organization in articular cartilage, determined by X-ray diffraction, and its relationship to tissue function. *Proc. R. Soc. Lond.*, B212:299–304.
13. Aspden, R. M., Yarker, Y. E., and Hukins, D. W. L. (1985): Collagen orientations in the meniscus of the knee joint. *J. Anat.*, 140:371–380.
14. Ateshian, G. A., Cohen, Z. A., Kwak, S. D., et al. (1995): Determination of *in-situ* contact in diarthrodial joints by MRI. *Adv. Bioeng. Trans. ASME*, BED31:225–226.
15. Ateshian, G. A., Lai, W. M., Zhu, W. B., and Mow, V. C. (1994): An asymptotic solution for two contacting biphasic cartilage layers. *J. Biomechanics*, 27:1347–1360.
16. Ateshian, G. A., Rosenwasser, M. P., and Mow, V. C. (1992): Curvature characteristics and congruence of the thumb carpometacarpal joint. *J. Biomechanics*, 25:591–607.
17. Ateshian, G. A., Soslowsky, L. J., and Mow, V. C. (1991). Quantitation of articular surface topography and cartilage thickness in knee joints using stereophotogrammetry. *J. Biomechanics*, 24:761–776.
18. Ateshian, G. A., and Wang, H. (1995): A theoretical solution for the frictionless rolling contact of cylindrical biphasic articular layers. *J. Biomechanics*, 28:1341–1355.
19. Athanasiou, K. A., Agarwal, A., Muffoletto, A., Dzida, F. J., Constantinides, G., and Clem, M. (1995): Biomechanical properties of hip cartilage in experimental animal models. *Clin. Orthop. Rel. Res.*, 316:254–266.
20. Athanasiou, K. A., Rosenwasser, M. P., Buckwalter, J. A., Malinin, T. I., and Mow, V. C. (1991): Interspecies comparison of *in situ* intrinsic mechanical properties of distal femoral cartilage. *J. Orthop. Res.*, 9:330–340.

21. Bachrach, N. M., Valhmu, W. B., Stazzone, E., Ratcliffe, A., Lai, W. M., and Mow, V. C. (1995): Changes in proteoglycan synthesis rates of chondrocytes in articular cartilage are associated with the time dependent changes in their mechanical environment. *J. Biomechanics,* 28:1561–1569.

22. Bar, E. (1926): Elasticitatsprufungen der gelenkknorpel. *Arch. Entwicklungsmech. Organ,* 108:739–760.

23. Behrens, F., Kraft, E. L., and Oegema, T. R. (1989): Biochemical changes in articular cartilage after joint immobilization by casting or external fixation. *J. Orthop. Res.,* 7:335–343.

24. Benninghoff, A. (1925). Form und Bau der Gelenkknorpel in ihren Beziehungen zu Funktion. II: Der Aufbau des Gelenkknorpel in seinen Beziehungen zu Funktion. *Z. Zellforsch.,* 2:783–862.

25. Best, B. A., Guilak, F., Setton, L. A., Zhu, W. B., Saed-Nejad, F., Ratcliffe, A., Weidenbaum, M., and Mow, V. C. (1994): Compressive mechanical properties of the human annulus fibrosus and their relationship to biochemical composition. *Spine,* 19:212–221.

26. Blankevoort, L., Kuiper, J. H., Huiskes, R., and Grootenboer, H. J. (1991): Articular contact in a three-dimensional model of the knee. *J. Biomech. Eng.,* 24:1019–1031.

27. Bland, D. R. (1960): *The Theory of Linear Viscoelasticity.* Pergamon Press, Oxford.

28. Bollet, A. J., and Nance, J. L. (1966): Biochemical findings in normal and osteoarthritic articular cartilage II chondroitin sulfate concentration and chain length, water and ash content. *J. Clin. Invest.,* 45:1170–1177.

29. Bowen, R. M. (1971): *Continuum Theory of Mixtures. Nat. Tech. Inf. Ser.,* BRL45:1–170.

30. Bowen, R. M. (1980): Incompressible porous media models by use of the theories of mixtures. *Int. J. Eng. Sci.,* 18:1129–1148.

31. Brandt, K. D. (1990): *Cartilage Changes in Osteoarthritis.* Indiana University School of Medicine Press, Indianapolis, pp. 1–144.

32. Brocklehurst, R., Bayliss, M. T., Maroudas, A., Coysh, H. L., Freeman, M. A., Revell, P. A., and Ali, S. Y. (1984): The composition of normal and osteoarthritic articular cartilage from human knee joints. *J. Bone Joint Surg.,* 66A:95–106.

33. Broom, N. D. (1986): Structure consequences of traumatising articular cartilage. *Ann. Rheum. Dis.,* 45:225–234.

34. Broom, N. D., and Marra, D. L. (1986): Ultrastructural evidence for the fibril-to-fibril association in articular cartilage and their functional implication. *J. Anat.,* 146:185–200.

35. Broom, N. D. (1988): The collagen framework of articular cartilage: Its profound influence on normal and abnormal load-bearing function. In: *Collagen: Chemistry, Biology and Biotechnology,* Vol. II, edited by M. E. Nimni, pp. 243–265. CRC Press, Boca Raton, FL.

36. Broom, N. D., and Silyn-Roberts, H. (1990): Collagen–collagen versus collagen–proteoglycan interactions in the determination of cartilage strength. *Arthritis Rheum.,* 33:1512–1517.

37. Brown, T. D., and Singerman, R. J. (1987): Experimental determination of the linear biphasic constitutive coefficients of human fetal proximal femoral chondroepiphysis. *J. Biomechanics,* 19:597–605.

38. Brown, D. C., and Vogel, K. G. (1989): Characteristics of the *in vivo* interaction of a small proteoglycan (PGII) of bovine tendon with type I collagen. *Matrix,* 9:468–478.

39. Buckwalter, J. A., Kuettner, K. E., and Thonar, E. J.-M. (1985): Age-related changes in articular cartilage proteoglycans: Electron microscopic studies. *J. Orthop. Res.,* 3:251–257.

40. Buckwalter, J. A., Mow, V. C., and Ratcliffe, A. (1994): Restoration of injured or degenerated articular cartilage. *J. Am. Acad. Orthop. Surg.,* 2:192–201.

41. Buckwalter, J. A., and Rosenberg, L. C. (1982): Electron microscopic studies of cartilage proteoglycans: Direct evidence for the variable length of the chondroitin sulfate rich region of the proteoglycan subunit core protein. *J. Biol. Chem.,* 257:9830–9839.

42. Bullough, P. G. (1981): The geometry of diarthrodial joints, its physiological maintenance, and the possible significance of age-related changes in geometry-to-load distribution and the development of osteoarthritis. *Clin. Orthop. Rel. Res.,* 156:61–66.

43. Bullough, P. G., and Goodfellow, J. (1968): The significance of the fine structure of articular cartilage. *J. Bone Joint Surg.,* 50B:852–857.

44. Bullough, P. G., and Jasannath, P. (1983): The morphology of the calcification front in articular cartilage: Its significance in joint function. *J. Bone Joint Surg.,* 65B:72–78.

45. Bullough, P. G., Munuera, L., Murphy, J., and Weinstein, A. M. (1970): The strength of the menisci of the knee as it related to their fine structure. *J. Bone Joint Surg.,* 52B:564–570.

46. Carney, S. L., Billingham, M. E. J., and Muir, H. (1984): Demonstration of increase proteoglycan turnover in cartilage explants from dogs with experimental arthritis. *J. Orthop. Res.,* 2:201–206.

47. Caterson, B., and Lowther, D. A. (1978): Change in the metabolism of the proteoglycans from sheep articular cartilage in response to mechanical stress. *Biochim. Biophys. Acta,* 540:412–422.

48. Clark, J. M. (1985): The organization of collagen in cryofractured rabbit articular cartilage: a scanning electron microscopic study. *J. Orthop. Res.,* 3:17–29.

49. Clarke, I. C. (1971): Articular cartilage: a review and scanning electron microscope study—1. The interterritorial fibrillar architecture. *J. Bone Joint Surg.,* 53B:732–750.

50. Cohen, B., Lai, W. M., Chorney, G. S., Dick H. M., and Mow, V. C. (1992): Unconfined compression of transversely-isotropic biphasic tissue. *Adv. Bioeng. Trans. ASME,* BED19:187–190.

51. Cohen, B., Chorney, G. S., Phillips, D. P., Dick, H. M., and Mow, V. C. (1994): Compressive stress-relaxation behavior of bovine growth plate may be described by the nonlinear-biphasic theory. *J. Orthop. Res.,* 12:804–813.

52. Coletti, J. M., Akeson, W. H., and Woo, S. L.-Y. (1972): A comparison of the physical behavior of normal articular cartilage and the arthroplasty surface. *J. Bone Joint Surg.,* 54A:147–160.

53. Comper, W. D., Williams, R. P. W., and Zamparo, O. (1990): Water transport in extracellular matrices. *Connect. Tissue Res.,* 25:89–102.

54. Danielson, K. G., Fazzio, A., Cohen, I., Cannizzaro, L. A., Eichstetter, I., and Iozzo, R. V. (1993): The human decorin gene: intron–exon organization, discovery of

two alternatively spliced exons in the 5' untranslated region, and mapping of the gene to chromosome 12q23. *Genomics,* 15:146–160.

55. Doege, K. J., Sasaki, M., Kimura, T., and Yamada, Y . (1991): Complete coding sequence and deduced primary structure of the human cartilage large aggregating proteoglycan, aggrecan. *J. Biol. Chem.,* 266: 894–902.

56. Doege, K. J., Garrison, K., Coulter, S. N., and Yamada, Y. (1994): The structure of the rat aggrecan gene and preliminary characterization of its promoter. *J. Biol. Chem.,* 269:29232–29240.

57. Donnan, F. G. (1924): The theory of membrane equilibria. *Chem. Rev.,* 1:73–90.

58. Donohue, J. M., Buss, D., Oegema, T. R., and Thompson, R. C. (1983): The effects of indirect blunt trauma on adult canine articular cartilage. *J. Bone Joint Surg.,* 61A:948–957.

59. Dudhia, J., Bayliss, M. T., and Hardingham, T. E. (1994): Human link protein structure and transcription pattern in chondrocytes. *Biochem. J.,* 303:329–333.

60. Ebara, S., Kelkar, R., Bigliani, L. U., Pollock, R. G., Pawluk, R. P., Flatow, E. L., Ratcliffe, A., and Mow, V. C. (1994): Bovine glenoid cartilage is less stiff than humeral head cartilage in tension. *Trans. Orthop. Res. Soc.,* 19:146.

61. Eckstein, F., Muller-Gerbl, M., and Putz, R. (1992): Distribution of subchondral bone density and cartilage thickness in the human patella. *J. Anat.,* 180:425–433.

62. Eckstein, F. Sittek, H., Gavazzeni, A., Schulte, E., Milz, S., Kiefer, B., Reiser, M., and Putz, R. (1996): Magnetic resonance chondro-crassometry (MR-CCM): A method for accurate determination of articular cartilage thickness. *Mag. Res. Med.,* 35:89–96.

63. Eckstein, F., Sittek, H., Milz, S., Putz, R., and Reiser, M. (1994): The morphology of articular cartilage assessed by magnetic resonance imaging (MRI)—reproducibility and anatomical correlation. *Surg. Radiol. Anat.,* 16:429–438.

64. Edwards, J. (1967): Physical characteristics of articular cartilage. *Proc. Inst. Mech. Engrs.,* 181-3J:16–24.

65. Edwards, J., and Smith, A. U. (1966): The uptake of fluid by living cartilage after compression. *J. Physiol.,* 183:5P–6P.

66. Edmond, E., and Ogston, A. G. (1968): An approach to the study of phase separation in ternary aqueous systems. *Biochem. J.,* 109:569–576.

67. Eisenberg, S. R., and Grodzinsky, A. J. (1985): Swelling of articular cartilage and other connective tissues: Electromechanochemical forces. *J. Orthop. Res.,* 3:148–159.

68. Eisenberg, S. R,. and Grodzinsky, A. J. (1987): The kinetics of chemically induced nonequilibrium swelling of articular cartilage and corneal stroma. *J. Biomech. Eng.,* 109:79–89.

69. Eisenfeld, J., Mow, V. C., and Lipshitz, H. (1978): Mathematical analysis of stress relaxation in articular cartilage during compression. *J. Math. Biosci.,* 39:97–112.

70. Elmore, S. M., Sokoloff, L., Norris, G., and Carmeci, P. (1962): Nature of "imperfect" elasticity of articular cartilage. *J. Appl. Physiol.,* 18:393–396.

71. Evanko, S. P., and Vogel, K. G. (1993): Proteoglycan synthesis in fetal tendon is differentially regulated by cyclic compression *in vitro. Arch. Biochem. Biophys.,* 307:153–164.

72. Eyre, D. R. (1980): Collagen: Molecular diversity in the body's protein scaffold. *Science,* 207:1315–1322.

73. Eyre, D. R., McDevitt, C. A., Billingham, M. E. J., and Muir, H. (1980): Biosynthesis of collagen and other matrix components by articular cartilage in experimental osteoarthritis. *Biochem. J.,* 188:823–837.

74. Eyre, D. R., Apone, S., Wu, J. J., Ericsson, L. H., and Walsh, K. A. (1987): Collagen type IX: evidence for covalent linkages to type II collagen in cartilage. *FEBS Lett.,* 220:337–341.

75. Eyre, D. R., Dickson, I. R., and Van Ness, K. P. (1988): Collagen cross-linking in human bone and articular cartilage. Age related changes in the content of mature hydroxypyridinium residues. *Biochem. J.,* 252: 495–500.

76. Eyre, D. R., Koob, T. J., and Van Ness, K. P. (1984): Quantitation of hydroxypyridinium crosslinks in collagen by high-performance liquid chromatography. *Anal. Biochem.,* 137:308–388.

77. Eyre, D. R., and Oguchi, H. (1980): The hydroxypyridinium crosslinks of skeletal collagens: Their measurement, properties and a proposed pathway of formation. *Biochem. Biophys. Res. Commun.,* 92:402–410.

78. Eyre, D. R., and Wu, J. J. (1983): Collagen of fibrocartilage: a distinctive molecular phenotype in bovine meniscus. *FEBS Lett.,* 158:265–270.

79. Fassler, R., Schnegelsberg, P. N., Dausman, J., Shinya, T., Muragaki, Y., McCarthy, M. T., Olsen, B. R., and Jaenisch, R. (1994): Mice lacking alpha 1(IX) collagen develop noninflammatory degenerative joint disease. *Proc. Natl. Acad. Sci. USA,* 91:5070–5074.

80. Ferry, J. D. (1970): *Viscoelastic Properties of Polymers.* John Wiley & Sons, New York.

81. Fisher, L. W., Heegarard, A.-M., Vetter, U., Vogel , W., Just, W., Termine, J. D., and Young, M. F. (1991): Human biglycan gene; putative promoter, intron–exon junctions, and chromosomal localization. *J. Biol. Chem.,* 266:14371–14377.

82. Fithian, D. C., Kelly, M. A., and Mow, V. C. (1990) : Material properties and sturcture–function relationships in the menisci. *Clin. Orthop. Rel. Res.,* 252:19–31.

83. Fithian, D. C., Zhu, W. B., Ratcliffe, A., Kelly, M. A., and Mow, V. C. (1989): Exponential law representation of tensile properties of human meniscus. *Proc. Inst. Mech. Eng.,* c384/058:85–90.

84. Frank, E. H., and Grodzinsky, A. J. (1987): Cartilage electromechanics—I. Electrokinetic transduction and the effects of electrolyte pH and ionic strength. *J. Biomechanics,* 20:615–627.

85. Frank, E. H., and Grodzinsky, A. J. (1987): Cartilage electromechanics—II. A continuum model of cartilage electrokinetics and correlation with experiments. *J. Biomechanics,* 20:629–639.

86. Frank, E. H., Grodzinsky, A. J., Koob, T. J., and Eyre, D. R. (1987): Streaming potentials: a sensitive index of enzymatic degradation in articular cartilage. *J. Orthop. Res.,* 5:497–508.

87. Franzen, A., Inerot, S., Hejderup, S.-O., and Heinegard, D. (1981): Variation in the composition of bovine hip articular cartilage with distance from the articular surface. *Biochem. J.,* 195:535–566.

88. Froimson, M. I., Ratcliffe, A., and Mow, V. C. (1989): Patellar cartilage mechanical properties vary with site and biochemical composition. *Trans. Orthop. Res. Soc.,* 14:150

89. Fung, Y. C. (1965): *Foundations of Solid Mechanics.* Prentice-Hall, Englewood Cliffs, NJ.
90. Fung, Y. C. (1968): Biomechanics: Its scope, history, and some problems of continuum mechanics in physiology. *Appl. Mech. Rev.,* 21(1):1–20.
91. Fung, Y. C. (1981): *Mechanical Properties of Living Tissues.* Springer-Verlag, New York.
92. Gabler, R. (1978): *Electrical Interactions in Molecular Biophysics: An Introduction.* Academic Press, New York.
93. Ghosh, P., Taylor, T. K. F., Pettit, G. D., Horsburgh, B. A., and Bellenger, C. R. (1983): Effect of postoperative immobilization on the regrowth of the knee joint semilunar cartilage: An experimental study. *J. Orthop. Res.,* 1:153–164.
94. Gocke, E. (1927): Elastizitasstudien an jungen und alten gelenkknorpel. *Verh. Dtsch. Orthop. Ges.,* 22:130–147.
95. Gray, M. L., Pizzanelli, A. M., Grodzinsky, A. J., and Lee, R. C. (1988): Mechanical and physicochemical determinants of the chondrocyte biosynthetic response. *J. Orthop. Res.,* 6:777–792.
96. Greenwald, A. S., and O'Connor, J. J. (1971): The transmission of load through the human hip joint. *J. Biomechanics,* 4:507–528.
97. Grodzinsky, A. J., Roth, V., Myers, E. R., Grossman, W. D., and Mow, V. C. (1981): The significance of electromechanical and osmotic forces in the nonequilibrium swelling behavior of articular cartilage in tension. *J. Biomech. Eng.,* 103:221–231.
98. Grover, J., and Roughley, P. G. (1993): Versican gene expression in human articular cartilage and comparison of mRNA splicing variation. *Biochem. J.,* 291:361–367.
99. Gu, W. Y., Lai, W. M., and Mow, V. C. (1993): Transport of fluid and ions through a porous-permeable charged–hydrated tissue, and streaming potential data on normal bovine articular cartilage. *J. Biomechanics,* 26:709–723.
100. Gu, W. Y., Rabin, J., Lai, W. M., and Mow, V. C. (1995): Measurement of streaming potential of bovine articular and nasal cartilage in 1-D permeation experiments. *Adv. Bioeng. Trans. ASME,* BED31:49–50
101. Gu, W. Y., Rabin, J., Iatridis, J. C., Rawlins, B. A., and Mow, V. C. (1996): Streaming potential of human lumbar anulus fibrosus. *Trans. Orthop. Res. Soc.,* 22(1):192.
102. Guilak, F., Meyer, B. C., Ratcliffe, A., and Mow, V. C. (1994): Quantitation of the effects of matrix compression on proteoglycan metabolism in articular cartilage explants. *Osteoarth. Cartilage,* 2:91–101.
103. Guilak, F., Ratcliffe, A., Lane, N., Rosenwasser M. P., and Mow, V. C. (1994): Mechanical and biochemical changes in the superficial zone of articular cartilage in a canine model of osteoarthritis. *J. Orthop. Res.,* 12:474–484.
104. Guilak, F., Ratcliffe, A., and Mow, V. C. (1995): Chondrocyte deformation and local tissue strain in articular cartilage: A confocal microscopy study. *J. Orthop. Res.,* 13:410–421.
105. Hall, B. K. (1983): *Cartilage: Structure Function and Biochemstry,* Vol. 1. Academic Press, New York.
106. Hall, B. K. (1983): *Cartilage: Development, Differentiation and Growth,* Vol. 2. Academic Press, New York.
107. Hall, A. C., Urban, J. P. G., and Gehl, K. A. (1991): The effect of hydrostatic pressure on matrix synthesis in articular cartilage. *J. Orthop. Res.,* 9:1–10.
108. Hardingham, T. E. (1979): The role of link protein in the structure of cartilage proteoglycan aggregates. *Biochem. J.,* 177:237–247.
109. Hardingham, T. E. (1981): Proteoglycans: Their structure, interactions and molecular organization in cartilage. *Biochem. Soc. Trans.,* 9:489–497.
110. Hardingham, T. E., and Fosang, A. (1992): Proteoglycans: many forms and many functions. *FASEB J.,* 6:861–870.
111. Hardingham, T. E., and Muir, H. (1972): The specific interaction of hyaluronic acid with cartilage proteoglycans. *Biochim. Biophys. Acta,* 279:401–405.
112. Hardingham, T. E., and Muir, H. (1974): Hyaluronic acid in cartilage and proteoglycan aggregation. *Biochem. J.,* 139:565–581.
113. Hardingham, T. E., Muir, H., Kwan, M. K., Lai, W. M., and Mow, V. C. (1987): Viscoelastic properties of proteoglycan solutions with varying proportion present as aggregate. *J. Orthop. Res.,* 5:36–46.
114. Harper, G. S., Comper, W. D., and Preston, B. N. (1984) Dissapative structures in proteoglycan solutions. *J. Biol. Chem.,* 259:10582–10589.
115. Hascall, V. C. (1977): Interactions of cartilage proteoglycans with hyaluronic acid. *J. Supramol. Struct.,* 7:101–120.
116. Hascall, V. C., and Hascall, G. K. (1981): Proteoglycans. In: *Cell Biology of Extracelullar Matrix,* edited by E. D. Hay, pp. 39–63. Plenum Press, New York.
117. Hascall, J. R., Kimura, J. H., and Hascall, V. C. (1986): Proteoglycan core protein families. *Annu. Rev. Biochem.,* 55:539–567.
118. Hascall, V. C., and Sajdera, S. W. (1969): Protein–polysaccharide complex from bovine nasal cartilage: The function of glycoprotein in the formation of aggregates. *J. Biol. Chem.,* 244:2384–2396.
119. Hayes, W. C., and Bodine, A. J. (1978): Flow-independent viscoelastic properties of articular cartilage matrix. *J. Biomechanics,* 11:407–419.
120. Hayes, W. C., Keer, L. M., Herrman, G., and Mockros, L. F. (1972): A mathematical analysis for indentation tests of articular cartilage. *J. Biomechanics,* 5:541–551.
121. Hayes, W. C., and Mockros, L. F. (1971): Viscoelastic properties of human articular cartilage. *J. Appl. Physiol.,* 31:562–568.
122. Hedbom, E., Antonsson, P., Hjerpe, A., Aeschlimann, D., Paulsson, M., Rosa-Pilentel, E., Sommarin, Y., Wendel, M., Oldberg, A., and Heinegard, D. (1992): Cartilage matrix proteins. An acidic oligomeric protein (COMP) detected only in cartilage. *J. Biol. Chem.,* 267:6132–6136.
123. Heinegard, D. K., and Axelsson, I. (1977): Distribution of keratan sulfate in cartilage proteoglycans. *J. Biol. Chem.,* 252:1971–1979.
124. Heinegard, D., and Oldberg, A. (1989): Structure and biology of cartilage and bone noncollagenous macromolecules. *FASEB J.,* 3:2042–2051.
125. Heinegard, D., Paulsson, M., Inerot, S., and Carlstrom, C. (1981): A novel, low molecular weight chondroitin sulfate proteoglycan isolated from cartilage. *Biochem J.,* 197:355–366.
126. Helfferich, F. (1962): *Ion Exchange.* McGraw-Hill, New York.

127. Hirsch, C. (1944): The pathogenesis of chondromalacia of the patella. *Acta Chir. Scand.,* 83(Suppl):1–106.
128. Hoch, D. H., Grodzinsky, A. J., Koob, T. J., Albert, M. L., and Eyre, D. R. (1983): Early changes in material properties of rabbit articular cartilage after meniscectomy. *J. Orthop. Res.,* 1:4–12.
129. Hodge, W. A., Fijan, R. S., Carlson, K. L., Burgess, R. G., Harris, W. H., and Mann, R. W. (1986): Contact pressure in the human hip joint measured *in vivo. Proc. Natl. Acad. Sci. USA,* 83:2879–2883.
130. Holmes, M. H., Lai, W. M., and Mow, V. C. (1985): Compression effects on cartilage permeability. In: *Tissue Nutrition and Viability,* edited by A. R. Hargins, pp. 73–100. Springer-Verlag, New York.
131. Holmes, M. H., Lai, W. M., and Mow, V. C. (1985): Singular perturbation analysis of the nonlinear flow dependent compressive stress relaxation behavior of articular cartilage. *J. Biomech. Eng.,* 107:206–218.
132. Holmes, M. H., and Mow, V. C. (1990): The nonlinear characteristics of soft gels and hydrated connective tissues in ultrafiltration. *J. Biomechanics,* 23:1145–1156.
133. Hori, R. Y., and Mockros, L. F. (1976): Indentation tests of human articular cartilage. *J. Biomechanics,* 9:259–268.
134. Hou, J. S., Holmes, M. H., Lai, W. M., and Mow, V. C. (1989): Boundary conditions at the cartilage–synovial fluid interface for joint lubrication and theoretical verfications. *J. Biomech. Eng.,* 111:78–87.
135. Hou, J. S., Mow, V. C., Lai, W. M., and Holmes, M. H. (1992): An analysis of the squeeze film lubrication mechanism for articular cartilage. *J. Biomechanics,* 25:247–259.
136. Howell, D. S., Treadwell, B. V., and Trippel, S. B. (1992): Etiopathogenesis of osteoarthritis. In: *Osteoarthritis, Diagnosis and Medical/Surgical Management,* 2nd ed., edited by R. W. Moskowitz, D. S. Howell, V. M. Goldberg, and H. J. Mankin, pp. 233–252. W. B. Saunders, Philadelphia.
137. Huiskes, R., Kremers, J., Lange, A. de, Woltring, H. J., Selvik, G., and van Rens, T. J. (1985): Analytical stereophotogrammetric determination of three-dimensional knee-joint anatomy. *J. Biomechanics,* 18:559–570.
138. Hulkrantz, W. (1898): Ueber die spaltrichtungen der gelenkknorpel. *Verh. D. Anat. Ges.,* 12:248–256.
139. Hunziker, E. B., and Schenk, R. K. (1987): Structural organization of proteoglycans in cartilage. In: *Biology of Proteoglycans,* edited by T. W. Wight and R. P. Mecham, pp. 155–183. Academic Press, New York.
140. Iozzo, R. V., Cohen, I. R., Grassel, S., and Murdoch, A. D. (1994): The biology of perlican: the multifaceted heparan sulfate proteoglycan of basement membranes and pericellular matrices. *Biochem. J.,* 302:625–639.
141. Jurvelin, J., Kiviranta, I., Aronkoski, J., Tammi, M., and Helminen, H. J. (1987): Indentation study of the biomechanical properties of articular cartilage in canine knee. *Eng. Med.,* 16:16–22.
142. Jurvelin, J., Kiviranta, I., Tammi, M., and Helminen, H. J. (1986): Softening of canine cartilage after immobilization of the knee joint. *Clin. Orthop. Rel. Res.,* 207:246–252.
143. Katchalsky, A., and Curran, P. F. (1975): *Non-equilibrium Thermodynamics in Biophysics,* Chapters 11, 12. Harvard University Press, Cambridge, MA.
144. Katz, E. P., and Li, S.-T. (1973): The intermolecular space of reconstituted collagen fibrils. *J. Mol. Biol.,* 73:351–369.
145. Katz, E. P., Wachtel, E. J., and Maroudas, A. (1986): Extrafibrillar proteoglycans osmotically regulate the molecular packing of collagen in cartilage. *Biochim. Biophys. Acta,* 882:136–139.
146. Kelkar, R., Flatow, E. L., Bigliani, L. U., and Mow, V. C. (1994): The effect of articular congruence and humeral head rotation on glenohumeral kinematics. *Adv. Bioeng. Trans. ASME,* BED28:19–20.
147. Kempson, G. E. (1975): Mechanical properties of articular cartilage and their relationship to matrix degradation and age. *Ann. Rheum. Dis.,* 34:111–113.
148. Kempson, G. E. (1979): Mechanical properties of articular cartilage, In: *Adult Articular Cartilage,* edited by M. A. R. Freeman, pp. 333–414. Pitman Medical, Kent, England.
149. Kempson, G. E. (1982): Relationship between the tensile properties of articular cartilage from the human knee and age. *Ann. Rheum. Dis.,* 41:508–511.
150. Kempson, G. E. (1991): Age-related changes in the tensile properties of human articular cartilage: a comparative study between the femoral head of the hip joint and the talus of the ankle joint. *Biochim. Biophys. Acta,* 1075:223–230.
151. Kempson, G. E., Freeman, M. A. R., and Swanson, S. A. V. (1971): The determination of a creep modulus for articular cartilage from indentation tests on the human femoral head. *J. Biomechanics,* 4:239–250.
152. Kempson, G. E., Spivey, C. J., Swanson, S. A. V., and Freeman, M. A. R. (1971): Patterns of cartilage stiffness on normal and degenerate femoral heads. *J. Biomechanics,* 4:597–609.
153. Kempson, G. E., Tuke, M. A., Dingle, J. T., Barrett, A. J., and Horsfield, P. H. (1976): The effects of proteolytic enzymes on the mechanical properties of adult human articular cartilage. *Biochim. Biophys. Acta,* 428:741–760.
154. Kenedi, R. M., Gibson, T., and Daly, C. H. (1964): Bioengineering studies of the human skin, the effects of unidirectional tension. In: *Structure and Function of Connective and Skeletal Tissues,* edited by S. F. Jackson, S. M. Harkness, and G. R. Tristrain, pp. 388–395. Scientific Committee, St. Andrews, Scotland.
155. Kelly, M. A., Fithian, D. C., Chern, K. Y., and Mow, V. C. (1990): Structure and function of the meniscus: Basic and clinical implications. In: *Biomechanics of Diarthrodial Joints,* Vol. I, edited by V. C. Mow, A. Ratcliffe, and S. L.-Y. Woo, pp. 191–211. Springer-Verlag, New York.
156. Knudson, W., and Knudson, C. B. (1991): Assembly of a chondrocyte-like pericellular matrix on non-chondrogenic cells. Role of the cell surface hyaluronan receptors in the assembly of a pericellular matrix. *J. Cell Sci.,* 99:227–235.
157. Kuettner, K. E., Schleyerbach, R., Peyron, J. G., and Hascall, V. C., eds. (1991): *Articular Cartilage and Osteoarthritis.* Raven Press, New York.
158. Kwan, M. K., Wayne, J. S., Woo, S. L–Y., Field, F. P., Hoover, J., and Meyers, W. (1989): Histological and biomechanical assessment of articular cartilage from stored osteochondral shell allografts. *J. Orthop. Res.,* 7:637–644.
159. Kwan, M. K., Lai, W. M., and Mow, V. C. (1990): A finite deformation theory for cartilage and other soft hy-

drated connective tissues: I. Equilibrium results. *J. Biomechanics,* 23:145–155.

160. Lai, W. M., Hou, J. S., and Mow, V. C. (1989): Triphasic theory for articular cartilage swelling. *Proc. Biomech. Symp. Trans. ASME,* AMD98:33–36.

161. Lai, W. M., Hou, J. S., and Mow, V. C. (1989): Application of triphasic theory to the study of transient behavior of cartilage. *Adv. Bioeng. Trans. ASME,* BED15:101–102.

162. Lai, W. M., Hou, J. S., and Mow, V. C. (1991): A triphasic theory for the swelling and deformational behaviors of articular cartilage. *J. Biomech. Eng.,* 113:245–258.

163. Lai, W. M., and Mow, V. C. (1980): Drag-induced compression of articular cartilage during a permeation experiment. *Biorheology,* 17:111–123.

164. Lai, W. M., Mow, V. C., and Roth, V. (1981): Effects of a nonlinear strain-dependent permeability and rate of compression on the stress behavior of articular cartilage. *J. Biomech. Eng.,* 103:61–66.

165. Lai, W. M., Mow, V. C., and Zhu, W. B. (1993): Constitutive modelling of articular cartilage and biomacromolecular solutions. *J. Biomech. Eng.,* 115:474–480.

166. Lai, W. M., Rubin, D., and Krempl, E. (1993): *Introduction to Continuum Mechanics,* 3rd ed. Pergamon Press, London.

167. Lane, J. M., and Weiss, C. (1975): Review of articular cartilage collagen research. *Arthritis Rheum.,* 18: 553–562.

168. Lehner, K. B., Rechl, H. P., Gmeinwiesser, J. K., Heuck, A. F., Lukas, H. P., and Kohn, H. K. (1989): Structure, function, and degeneration of bovine hyaline cartilage: assessment with MR imaging *in vitro. Radiology,* 170:495–499.

169. Li, J. T., Armstrong, C. G., and Mow, V. C. (1983): The effect of strain rate on mechanical properties of articular cartilage in tension. *Proc. Biomech. Symp. Trans. ASME,* AMD56:117–120.

170. Linn, F. C., and Sokoloff, L. (1965): Movement and composition of interstitial fluid of cartilage. *Arthritis Rheum.,* 8:481–494.

171. Lipshitz, H., Etheredge, R., and Glimcher, M. J. (1976): Changes in the hexosamine content and swelling ratio of articular cartilage as functions of depth from the surface. *J. Bone Joint Surg.,* 58A: 1149–1153.

172. Lohmander, S. L., Dahlberg, L., Ryd, L., and Heinegard, D. (1989): Increased levels of proteoglycan fragments in knee joint fluid after injury. *Arthritis Rheum.,* 32:1434–1442.

173. Lohmander, L. S., Roos, H., Dahlberg L., Hoerrner L. A., and Lark, M. W. (1994): Temporal patterns of stromelysin-1, tissue inhibitor, and proteoglycan fragments in human knee joint fluid after injury to the cruciate ligament or meniscus. *J. Orthop. Res.,* 12:21–28.

174. Luyten, F. P., Yu, Y. M., Yanagishita, M., Vukicevic, S., Hammonds, R. G., and Reddi, A. H. (1992): Natural bovine osteogenin and recombinant human bone morphogenetic protein-2B are equipotent in the maintenance of proteoglycans in bovine articular cartilage explant cultures. *J. Biol. Chem.,* 267:3691–3695.

175. Mak, A. F. (1986): The apparent viscoelastic behavior of articular cartilage—The contributions from the intrinsic matrix viscoelasticity and interstitial fluid flows. *J. Biomech. Eng.,* 108:123–130.

176. Mak, A. F., Lai, W. M., and Mow, V. C. (1987): Biphasic indentation of articular cartilage: I. Theoretical analysis. *J. Biomechanics,* 20:703–714.

177. Manicourt, D. H., Pita, J. C., Pezon, C. F., and Howell, D. S. (1986): Characterization of the proteoglycans recovered under nondissociative conditions from normal articular cartilage of rabbits and dogs. *J. Biol. Chem.,* 261:5426–5433.

178. Mankin H. J., Mow V. C., Buckwalter, J. A., Ianotti, J. P., and Ratcliffe, A. (1994): Structure and function of articular cartilage. In: *Orthopaedic Basic Science,* edited by S. R. Simon, pp. 1–44. American Academy of Orthopaedic Surgeons, Rosemont, IL.

179. Mankin, H. J., and Thrasher, A. Z. (1975): Water content and binding in normal and osteoarthritic human cartilage. *J. Bone Joint Surg.,* 57A:76–79.

180. Mansour, J. M., and Mow, V. C. (1976): The permeability of articular cartilage under compressive strain and at high pressures. *J. Bone Joint Surg.,* 58A:509–516.

181. Maroudas, A. (1968): Physicochemical properties of cartilage in the light of ion–exchange theory. *Biophys. J.,* 8:575–595.

182. Maroudas, A. (1975): Biophysical chemistry of cartilaginous tissues with special reference to solute and fluid transport. *Biorheology,* 12:233–248.

183. Maroudas, A. (1976): Balance between swelling pressure and collagen tension in normal and degenerate cartilage. *Nature,* 260:808–809.

184. Maroudas, A. (1979): Physicochemical properties of articular cartilage. In: *Adult Articular Cartilage,* edited by M. A. R. Freeman, pp. 215–290. Pitman Medical Publishing, Kent, England.

185. Maroudas, A., and Bannon, C. (1981): Measurements of swelling pressure in cartilage and comparison with the osmotic pressure of constituent proteoglycans. *Biorheology,* 18:619–632.

186. Maroudas, A., Bayliss, M. T., and Venn, M. F. (1980): Further studies on the composition of human femoral head cartilage. *Ann. Rheum. Dis.,* 39:514–523.

187. Maroudas, A., and Grushko, G. (1990): Measurement of swelling pressure of cartilage. In: *Methods in Cartilage Research,* edited by A. Maroudas and K. Kuettner, pp. 298–302. Academic Press, San Diego.

188. Maroudas, A., Muir, H., and Wingham, J. (1969): The correlation of fixed negative charge with glycosaminoglycan content of human articular cartilage. *Biochim. Biophys. Acta,* 177:492.

189. Maroudas, A., and Schneiderman, R. (1987): Free and exchangeable or trapped and non-exchangeable water in cartilage. *J. Orthop. Res.,* 5:133–138.

190. Maroudas, A., and Venn, M. (1977): Chemical composition and swelling of normal and osteoarthrotic femoral head cartilage. *Ann. Rheum. Dis.,* 36:399–406.

191. Maroudas, A., Wachtel, E., Grushko, G., Katz, E. P., and Weinberg, P. (1991): The effect of osmotic and mechanical pressures on water partitioning in articular cartilage. *Biochim. Biophys. Acta,* 1073:285–294.

192. McCutchen, C. W. (1962): The frictional properties of animal joints. *Wear,* 5:1–17.

193. McDevitt, C. A., and Muir, H. (1976): Biochemical changes in the cartilage of the knee in experimental and natural osteoarthritis in the dog. *J. Bone Joint Surg.,* 58B:94–101.

194. McDevitt, C. A., and Webber, R. J. (1990): The ultrastructure and biochemistry of meniscal cartilage. *Clin. Orthop. Rel. Res.,* 252:8–18.

195. McDevitt, C. A., Miller, R. R., and Spindler, K. P . (1992): The cells and cell matrix interaction of the meniscus. In: *Knee Meniscus: Basic and Clinical Foundations,* edited by V. C. Mow, S. P. Arnoczky, and D. W. Jackson, pp. 29–36. Raven Press, New York.

196. Miller, E. J. (1988): Collagen types: structure, distribution and functions. In: *Collagen: Biochemistry,* Vol. I, edited by M. E. Nimni, pp. 139–156. CRC Press, Boca Raton, FL.

197. Modl, J. M., Sether, L. A., Houghton, V. M., and Kneeland, J. B. (1991): Articular cartilage: correlation of histologic zones with signal intensity at MR imaging. *Radiology,* 181:853–855.

198. Morales, T. I. (1992): Polypeptide regulators of matrix homeostasis in articular cartilage. In: *Articular Cartilage and Osteoarthritis,* edited by K. E. Kuettner, R. Schleyerbach, J. G. Peyron, and V. C. Hascall, pp. 265–280. Raven Press, New York.

199. Morgan, F. R. (1960): The mechanical properties of collagen fibers: stress–strain curves. *J. Soc. Leather Trades Chem.,* 44:171–182.

200. Montes, G. S., and Jungueira, L. C. U. (1988): Histochemical localization of collagen and proteoglycans in tissues. In: *Collagen: Biochemistry and Biomechanics,* Vol. II, edited by M. E. Nimni, pp. 41–72. CRC Press, Boca Raton, FL.

201. Moskowitz, R. W. (1992): Osteoarthritis—symptoms and signs. In: *Osteoarthritis, Diagnosis and Medical/Surgical Management,* 2nd ed., edited by R. W. Moskowitz, et al., pp. 255–261. W. B. Saunders, Philadelphia.

202. Mow, V. C. (1969): The role of lubrication in biomechanical joints. *J. Lubr. Tech. Trans. ASME,* 91: 320–329.

203. Mow, V. C., Gibbs, M. C., Lai, W. M., Zhu, W. B., and Athanasiou, K. A. (1989): Biphasic indentation of articular cartilage—Part II. A numerical algorithm and an experimental study. *J. Biomechanics,* 22:853–861.

204. Mow, V. C., and Guilak, F. (1993): Deformation of chondrocytes within the extracellular matrix of articular cartilage. In: *Tissue Engineering: Current Perspectives,* edited by E. Bell, pp. 128–145. Birkhauser, Boston.

205. Mow, V. C., Holmes, M. H., and Lai, W. M. (1984): Fluid transport and mechanical properties of articular cartilage; A review. *J. Biomechanics,* 102:73–84.

206. Mow, V. C., Holmes, M. H., and Lai, W. M. (1986): Energy dissipation in articular cartilage under finite deformation. *Adv. Bioeng. Trans. ASME,* BED2:160–161.

207. Mow, V. C., Kuei, S. C., Lai, W. M., and Armstrong, C. G . (1980): Biphasic creep and stress relaxation of articular cartilage in compression: theory and experiment. *J. Biomech. Eng.,* 102:73–84.

208. Mow, V. C., Kwan, M. K., Lai, W. M., and Holmes, M. H. (1986): A finite deformation theory for nonlinearly permeable soft hydrated biological tissues. In: *Frontiers in Biomechanics,* edited by G. Schmid-Schonbein, S. L.-Y. Woo, and B. Zweifach, pp. 153–179. Springer-Verlag, New York.

209. Mow, V. C., and Lai, W. M. (1980): Recent developments in synovial joint biomechanics. *SIAM Rev.,* 22:275–317.

210. Mow, V. C., Lai, W. M., and Redler, I. (1974): Some surface characteristics of articular cartilage, part I: A scanning electron microscopy study and a theoretical

211. model for the dynamic interaction of synovial fluid and articular cartilage. *J. Biomechanics,* 7:449–456.

211. Mow, V. C., Mak, A. F., Lai, W. M., Rosenberg, L. C., and Tang, L. T. (1984): Viscoelastic properties of proteoglycan subunits and aggregates in varying solution concentrations. *J. Biomechanics,* 17:325–338.

212. Mow, V. C., Ratcliffe, A., and Poole, A. R. (1992): Cartilage and diarthrodial joints as paradigms for hierarchical materials and structures. *Biomaterials,* 13: 67–97.

213. Mow, V. C., Proctor, C. S., and Kelly, M. A. (1989): Biomechanics of articular cartilage. In: *Basic Biomechanics of the Locomotor System,* edited by M. Nordin and V. H. Frankel, pp. 31–58. Lea and Febiger, Philadelphia.

214. Mow, V. C., Proctor, C. S., Schmidt, M. B., and Kelly, M. A. (1988): Tensile and compressive properties of normal meniscus. In: *Progress and New Directions of Biomechanics,* edited by Y. C. Fung, K. Hayashi, and Y. Seguchi, pp. 107–122. Mita Press, Tokyo.

215. Mow, V. C., Ratcliffe, A., Rosenwasser, M. P., and Buckwalter, J. A. (1991): Experimental studies on repair of large osteochondral defects at a high weight bearing area of the knee joint: A tissue engineering study. *J. Biomech. Eng.,* 113:198–207.

216. Mow, V. C., Setton, L. A., Ratcliffe, A., Buckwalter, J. A., and Howell, D. S. (1990): Structure–function relationships for articular cartilage and effects of joint instability and trauma on cartilage function. In: *Cartilage Changes in Osteoarthritis,* edited by K. D. Brandt, pp. 22–42. Indiana University School of Medicine Press, Indiana,

217. Mow, V. C., Setton, L. A., Bachrach, N. M., and Guilak, F. (1994): Stress, strain, pressure and flow fields in articular cartilage and chondrocytes. In: *Cell Mechanics and Cellular Engineering,* edited by V. C. Mow, R. Tran-Son-Tay, F. Guilak, and R. M. Hochmuth, pp. 345–379. Springer Verlag, New York.

218. Mow, V. C., Zhu, W. B., Lai, W. M., Hardingham, T. E., Hughes, C., and Muir, H. (1989): The influence of link protein stabilization on the viscometric properties of proteoglycan aggregate solutions. *Biochim. Biophys. Acta,* 992:201–208.

219. Muir, H. (1979): Biochemistry. In: *Adult Articular Cartilage,* edited by M. A. R. Freeman, pp. 145–214. Pitman Medical, Kent, England.

220. Muir, H. (1983): Proteoglycans as organizers of the extracellular matrix. *Biochem. Soc. Trans.,* 11:613–622.

221. Muir, H., Bullough, P. G., and Maroudas, A. (1970): The distribution of collagen in human articular cartilage with some of its physiological implications. *J. Bone Joint Surg.,* 52B:554–563.

222. Mulholland, R., Millington, P. F., and Manners, J. (1975): Some aspects of the mechanical behavior of articular cartilage. *Ann. Rheum. Dis.,* 34:104–107.

223. Myers, E. R., Armstrong, C. G., and Mow V. C. (1984): Swelling pressure and collagen tension. In: *Connective Tissue Matrix,* D. W. L. Hukins, ed., MacMillan Press Ltd, London, pp. 161–186.

224. Myers, E. R., Hardingham, T. E., Billingham, M. E. J., and Muir, H. (1986): Changes in the tensile and compressive properties of cartilage in a canine model of osteoarthritis. *Trans. Orthop. Res. Soc.,* 11:231.

225. Myers, E. R., Lai, W. M., and Mow, V. C. (1984): A continuum theory and an experiment for the ion-

induced swelling behavior of articular cartilage. *J. Biomech. Eng.,* 106:151–158.

226. Nakano, T., Thompson, J. R., and Aherne, F. X. (1986): Distribution of glycosaminoglycans and the nonreducible collagen crosslink, pyridinoline in porcine menisci. *Can. J. Vet. Res.,* 50:532–536.

227. Nimni, M. E. (1988): *Collagen: Biochemistry,* Vol. 1, M. E. Nimni, ed., CRC Press, Boca Raton, Florida.

228. Nimni, M. E. (1988): *Collagen: Biochemistry and Biomechanics,* Vol. 2, M. E. Nimni, ed., CRC Press, Boca Raton, Florida.

229. Nimni, M. E. (1988): *Collagen: Biotechnology*, Vol. 3, M. E. Nimni, ed., CRC Press, Boca Raton, Florida.

230. Palmoski, M. J., and Brandt, K. D. (1981): Running inhibits reversal of atrophic changes in canine knee cartilage after removal of a leg cast. *Arthritis Rheum.,* 24:1329–1337.

231. Palotie, A., Vaisanen, P., Ott, J., Ryhanen, L., Elima, K., Vikkula, M., Cheah, K., Vuorio, E., and Peltonen, L. (1989): Predisposition to familial osteoarthrosis linked to type II collagen gene. *Lancet* 1:924–927.

232. Parkkinen, J. J., Ikonen, J., Lammi, M. J., Laakkonen, J., Tammi, M., and Helminen, H. J. (1993): Effects of cyclic hydrostatic pressure on proteoglycan synthesis in cultured chondrocytes and articular cartilage explants. *Arch. Biochem. Biophys.,* 300:458–465.

233. Parsons, J. R., and Black, J. (1977): The viscoelastic shear behavior of normal rabbit articular cartilage. *J. Biomechanics,* 10:21–29.

234. Parsons, J. R., and Black, J. (1979): Mechanical behavior of articular cartilage: Quantitative changes with alteration of ionic environment. *J. Biomechanics,* 12:765–773.

235. Pasternack, S. G., Veis, A., and Breen, M. (1974): Solvent–dependent changes in proteoglycan subunit conformation in aqueous guanidine hydrochloride solutions. *J. Biol. Chem.,* 239:2206–2211.

236. Paul, J. P. (1980): Joint kinetics. In: *The Joints and Synovial Fluid,* L. Sokoloff, ed., Vol. II, Academic Press, New York, pp. 139–176.

237. Perkins, S. J., Miller, A., Hardingham, T. E., and Muir, H. (1981): Physical properties of the hyaluronate binding region of proteoglycan from pig laryngeal cartilage. *J. Mol. Biol.,* 150:69–95.

238. Peterfy, C. G., van Dijke, C. F., Janzen, D. L., Gluer, C. C., Namba, R., Majumdar, S., Lang, P., and Genant, H. K. (1994): Quantification of articular cartilage in the knee with pulsed saturation transfer subtraction and fat-suppressed MR imaging: optimization and validation. *Radiology,* 192:485–491.

239. Peters, T. J., and Smillie, I. S. (1972): Studies on the chemical composition of the menisci of the knee joint with special reference to the horizontal cleavage lesion. *Clin. Orthop. Rel. Res.,* 86:245–252.

240. Poole, A. R., (1986): Proteoglycans in health and disease: structure and functions. *Biochem. J.,* 236:1–14.

241. Pottenger, L. A., Lyon, N. B., Hecht, J. D., Neustadt, P. M., and Robinson, R. A. (1982): Influence of cartilage particle size and proteoglycan aggregation on immobilization of proteoglycans. *J. Biol. Chem.,* 257:11479–11485.

242. Prehm, P. (1983): Synthesis of hyaluronate in differentiated teratocarcinoma cells. *Biochem. J.,* 211:191–198.

243. Proctor, C. S., Schmidt, M. B., Whipple, R. R., Kelly, M. A., and Mow, V. C. (1989): Material properties of normal medial bovine meniscus. *J. Orthop. Res.,* 7:771–782.

244. Puso, M. A., Weiss, J. A., Maker, B. N., and Schauer, D. A. (1995): A transversely isotropic hyperelastic shell finite element. *Adv. Bioeng. Trans. ASME,* BED29:103–104.

245. Radin, E. L., and Rose, R. M. (1986): Role of subchondral bone in the initiation and progression of cartilage damage. *Clin. Orthop. Rel. Res.,* 213:34–40.

246. Ratcliffe, A., Beauvais, P. J., and Saed–Nejad, F. (1994): Differential levels of aggrecan aggregate components in synovial fluids from canine knee joints with experimental osteoarthritis and disuse. *J. Orthop. Res.,* 12:464–473.

247. Ratcliffe, A., Billingham, M. E. J., Saed–Nejad, F., Muir, H., and Hardingham, T. E. (1992): Increased release of matrix components from articular cartilage in experimental canine osteoarthritis. *J. Orthop. Res.,* 10:350–358.

248. Ratcliffe, A., Doherty, M., Maini, R. N., and Hardingham, T. E. (1988): Increased concentrations of proteoglycan components in the synovial fluids of patients with acute but not chronic joint disease. *Ann. Rheum. Dis.,* 47:826–832.

249. Ratcliffe, A., Fryer, P. R., and Hardingham, T. E. (1984): The distribution of aggregating proteoglycans in articular cartilage: Comparison of quantitative immunoelectron microscopy with radioimmunoassay and biochemical analysis. *J. Histochem. Cytochem.,* 32:193–201.

250. Ratcliffe, A., and Hardingham, T. E. (1983): Cartilage proteoglycan binding region and link protein. Radioimmunoassays and the detection of masked determinants in aggregates. *Biochem. J.,* 213:371–378.

251. Ratcliffe, A., Hughes, C., Fryer, P. R., Saed-Nejad, F., and Hardingham, T. E. (1987): Immunochemical studies on the synthesis and secretion of link protein and aggregating proteoglycan by chondrocytes. *Coll. Rel. Res.,* 7:409–421.

252. Ratcliffe, A., and Mow, V. C. (1996): The structure and function of articular cartilage. In: *Structure and Function of Connective Tissues,* edited by W. D. Comper-Harwood Academic Press, Amsterdam, the Netherlands, pp. 234–302.

253. Ratcliffe, A., Shurety, W., and Caterson, B. (1993): The quantitation of a native chondroitin sulfate epitope in synovial fluid and articular cartilage from canine experimental osteoarthritis and disuse atrophy. *Arthritis Rheum.,* 36:543–551.

254. Ratcliffe, A., Tyler, J., and Hardingham, T. E. (1986): Articular cartilage cultured with interleukin 1: Increased release of link protein, hyaluronate–binding region and other proteoglycan fragments. *Biochem. J.,* 238:571–580.

255. Re, P., Valhmu, W. B., Vostrejs, M., Howell, D. S., Fischer, S. G., and Ratcliffe, A. (1995): Quantitative PCR assay for aggrecan and link protein gene expression in cartilage. *Anal. Biochem.,* 225:356–360.

256. Redler, I., Zimny, M. L., Mansell, J., and Mow, V. C. (1975): The ultrastructure and biomechanical significance of the tidemark of articular cartilage. *Clin. Orthop. Rel. Res.,* 112:357–362.

257. Reynolds, O. (1886): On the theory of lubrication and

its application to Mr. Beauchamp Tower's experiment, including an experimental determination of the viscosity of olive oil. *Proc. Phil. Trans. R. Soc.,* 177: 157–234.

258. Ridge, M. D., and Wright, V. (1964): The description of skin stiffness. *Biorheology,* 2:67–74.

259. Roughley, P. J., and White, R. J. (1992): The dermatan sulfate proteoglycans of the adult human meniscus. *J. Orthop. Res.,* 10:631–637.

260. Rosenberg, L. C. (1974): Structure of cartilage proteoglycans. In: *Dynamics of Connective Tissue Macromolecules,* edited by P. M. C. Burleigh and A. R. Poole, pp. 105–128. North-Holland, Amsterdam.

261. Rosenberg, L. C., Hellmann, W., and Kleinschmidt, A. K. (1975): Electron microscopic studies of proteoglycan aggregates from bovine articular cartilage. *J. Biol. Chem.,* 250:1877–1883.

262. Rosenberg, L. C., Choi, H. U., Tang, L. H., Johnson, T. L., and Pal, S. (1985): Isolation of dermatan sulfate proteoglycans from mature bovine articular cartilages. *J. Biol. Chem.,* 260:6304–6313.

263. Roth, V., and Mow, V. C. (1980): The intrinsic tensile behavior of the matrix of bovine articular cartilage and its variation with age. *J. Bone Joint Surg.,* 62A: 1102–1117.

264. Roth, V., Mow, V. C., Lai, W. M., and Eyre, D. R. (1981): Correlation of intrinsic compressive properties of bovine articular cartilage with its uronic acid and water content. *Trans. Orthop. Res. Soc.,* 6:21.

265. Roth, V., Schoonbeck, J. M., and Mow, V. C. (1982): Low frequency dynamic behavior of articular cartilage under torsional shear. *Trans. Orthop. Res. Soc.,* 7:150.

266. Rushfeldt, P. D., Mann, R. W., and Harris, W. H. (1981): Improved techniques for measuring *in vitro* the geometry and pressure distribution in the human acetabulum—I. Ultrasonic measurement of acetabular surfaces, sphericity and cartilage thickness. *J. Biomechanics,* 14:253–260.

267. Sachs, F. (1991): Mechanical transduction by membrane ion channels; a mini review. *Mol. Cell. Biochem.,* 104:20–29.

268. Sah, R. L.-Y., Doong, J.-Y. H., Grodzinsky, A. J., Plaas, A. H. K., and Sandy, J. D. (1991): Effects of compression on the loss of newly synthesized proteoglycans and proteins from cartilage explants. *Arch. Biochem. Biophys.,* 286:20–29.

269. Salter, D. M., Godolphin, J. L., and Gourlay, M. S. (1995): Chondrocyte heterogeneity: immunohistologically defined variation of integrin expression at different sites in human fetal knees. *J. Histochem. Cytochem.,* 43:447–457.

270. Sampaio, L. de O., Bayliss, M. T., Hardingham, T. E., and Muir, H. (1988): Dermatan sulfate proteoglycan from human articular cartilage: Variation in its content with age and its structural comparison with a small chondroitin sulfate proteoglycan from pig laryngeal cartilage. *Biochem. J.,* 254:757–764.

271. Sandell, L. J., Morris, N., Robbins, J. R., and Goldring, M. B. (1991): Alternatively spliced type II procollagen mRNAs define distinct populations of cells during vertebral development; differential expression of the amino-propeptide. *J. Cell Biol.,* 114:1307–1319.

272. Sandy, J. D., Adams, M. E., Billingham, M. E. J., Plaas, A. H. K., and Muir, H. (1984): *In vivo* and *in vitro* stimulation of chondrocyte biosynthetic activity in

early experimental osteoarthritis. *Arthritis Rheum.,* 27:388–397.

273. Sandy, J. D., Flannery, C. R., Neame, P. J., and Lohmander, S. L. (1992): The structure of aggrecan fragments in human synovial fluid: evidence for the involvement in osteoarthritis of a novel proteinase which cleaves the Glu 373-Ala 374 bond of the interglobulin domain. *J. Clin. Invest.,* 89:1512–1516.

274. Schmidt, M. B., Chun, L. E., Eyre, D. R., and Mow, V. C. (1987): The relationship between collagen cross-linking and tensile properties of articular cartilage. *Trans. Orthop. Res. Soc.,* 12:134.

275. Schmidt, M. B., Mow, V. C., Chun, L. E., and Eyre, D. R. (1990): Effects of proteoglycan extraction on the tensile behavior of articular cartilage. *J. Orthop. Res.,* 8:353–363.

276. Scott, J. E. (1988): Proteoglycan–fibrillar collagen interactions. *Biochem. J.,* 253:313–323.

277. Scott, J. E. (1990): Proteoglycan–collagen interactions and subfibrillar structure in collagen fibrils. Implications in the development and ageing of connective tissues. *J. Anat.,* 169:23–35.

278. Setton, L. A., Gu, W. Y., Lai, W. M., and Mow, V. C. (1992): Pre-stress in articular cartilage due to internal swelling pressures. *Adv. Bioeng. Trans. ASME,* BED19: 485–492.

279. Setton, L. A., Lai, W. M., and Mow, V. C. (1993): Swelling-induced residual stress and the mechanism of curling in articular cartilage *in vitro. Adv. Bioeng. Trans. ASME,* BED26:59–62.

280. Setton, L. A., Tohyama, H., Lai, W. M., Guilak, F., and Mow, V. C. (1994): Experimental measurement of the in vitro curling behavior of articular cartilage. *Adv. Bioeng. Trans. ASME,* BED28:135–136.

281. Setton, L. A., Zhu, W. B., and Mow, V. C. (1993): The biphasic poroviscoelastic behavior of articular cartilage in compression: Role of the surface zone. *J. Biomechanics,* 26:581–592.

282. Setton, L. A., Zhu, W. B., Weidenbaum, M., Ratcliffe, A., and Mow, V. C. (1993): Compressive properties of the cartilaginous endplates of the baboon lumbar spine. *J. Orthop. Res.,* 11:228–239.

283. Setton, L. A., Mow, V. C., Muller, F. J., Pita, J. C., and Howell, D. S. (1994): Mechanical properties of canine articular cartilage are significantly altered following transection of the anterior cruciate ligament. *J. Orthop. Res.,* 12:451–463.

284. Setton, L. A., Mow, V. C., and Howell, D. S. (1995): The mechanical behavior of articular cartilage in shear is altered by transection of the anterior cruciate ligament. *J. Orthop. Res.,* 13:473–482.

285. Singhvi, R., Kumar, A., Lopez, G. P., Stephanopoulos, G. N., Wang, D. I., Whitesides, G. M., and Ingber, D. E. (1994): Engineer cell shape and function. *Science,* 264:696–698.

286. Skaggs, D. L., Warden, W. H., and Mow, V. C. (1994): Radial tie fibers influence the tensile properties of the bovine medial meniscus. *J. Orthop. Res.,* 12:176–185.

287. Skaggs, D. L., Weidenbaum, M., Iatridis, J. C., Ratcliffe, A., and Mow, V. C. (1994): Regional variation in tensile properties and biochemical composition of the human lumbar anulus fibrosus. *Spine,* 12:1310–1319.

288. Sokoloff, L. (1963): Elasticity of articular cartilage: Effect of ions and viscous solutions. *Science,* 141: 1055–1057.

289. Sokoloff, L. (1966): Elasticity of aging cartilage. *Fed. Proc.,* 25:1089–1095.
290. Sokoloff, L. (1969): *The Biology of Degenerative Joint Disease,* pp. 69–93. University of Chicago Press, Chicago.
291. Soslowsky, L. J., Flatow, E. L., Bigliani, L. U., and Mow, V. C. (1992): Articular geometry of the glenohumeral joint. *Clin. Orthop. Rel. Res.,* 285:181–190.
292. Soslowsky, L. J., Flatow, E. L., Bigliani, L. U., Pawluk, R. J., Ateshian, G. A., and Mow, V. C. (1992): Quantitation of *in situ* contact areas at the glenohumeral joint: A biomechanical study. *J. Orthop. Res.,* 10:524–534.
293. Spilker, R. L., Suh, J. K., and Mow, V. C. (1992): A finite element analysis of the indentation stress-relaxation response of linear biphasic articular cartilage. *J. Biomech. Eng.,* 114:191–201.
294. Spirt, A. A., Mak, A. F., and Wassell, R. P. (1989): Nonlinear viscoelastic properties of articular cartilage in shear. *J. Orthop. Res.,* 7:43–49.
295. Stahurski, T. M., Armstrong, C. G., and Mow, V. C. (1981): Variation of the intrinsic aggregate modulus and permeability of articular cartilage with trypsin digestion. *Proc. Biomech. Symp. Trans. ASME,* AMD43: 137–140.
296. Stockwell, R. A., and Scott, J. E., (1967): Distribution of glycosaminoglycans in human articular cartilage. *Nature,* 215:1376–1378.
297. Stockwell, R. A. (1979): *Biology of Cartilage Cells,* pp. 7–31. Cambridge University Press, Cambridge.
298. Thomas, J. T., Ayad, S., and Grant, M. E. (1994): Cartilage collagens; strategies for the study of their organization and expression in the extracellular matrix. *Ann. Rheum. Dis.,* 53:488–496.
299. Thompson, R. C., Oegema, T. R., Lewis, J. L., and Wallace, L. (1991): Osteoarthrotic changes after acute transarticular load, an animal model. *J. Bone Joint Surg.,* 73A:990–1001.
300. Timoshenko, S. P., and Goodier, J. N. (1970): *Theory of Elasticity.* McGraw-Hill, New York.
301. Tohyama, H., Gu, W. Y., Setton, L. A., Lai, W. M., and Mow, V. C. (1995): Ion-induced swelling behavior of articular cartilage in tension. *Trans. Orthop. Res. Soc.,* 20:702.
302. Tombs, M. P., and Peacocke, A. R. (1974): *The Osmotic Pressure of Biological Macromolecules.* Clarendon Press, Oxford.
303. Torzilli, P. A. (1985): The influence of cartilage conformation on its equilibrium water partition. *J. Orthop. Res.,* 3:473–483.
304. Torzilli, P. A. (1988): Water content and equilibrium water partition in immature cartilage. *J. Orthop. Res.,* 6:766–769.
305. Truesdell, C. T., and Noll, W. (1965): *The Nonlinear Field Theories of Mechanics, Handbuck der Physik,* Vol. III/3, edited by S. Flugge. Springer-Verlag, Berlin.
306. Tyler, J. A. (1985): Articular cartilage cultured with catabolin (pig interleukin 1) synthesises a decreased number of normal proteoglycan molecules. *Biochem. J.,* 227:869–878.
307. Uhthoff, H. K., and Wiley, J. J. (1988): *Behavior of the Growth Plate.* Raven Press, New York.
308. Urban, J. P. G., and Maroudas, A. (1981): Swelling of the intervertebral disc *in vivo. Connect. Tissue Res.,* 9:1–10.
309. Urban, J. P. G., and McMullin, J. F. (1985): Swelling pressure of the intervertebral disc: Influence of collagen and proteoglycan contents. *Biorheology,* 22: 145–157.
310. Valhmu, W. B., Palmer, G. D., Rivers, P. A., Ebara, S., Cheng, J.-F., Fischer, S. G., and Ratcliffe A. (1995): Structure of the human aggrecan gene: exon–intron organization and association with the protein domains. *Biochem. J.,* 309:535–542.
311. van der Rest, M., and Mayne, R. (1988): Type IX collagen proteoglycan from cartilage is covalently cross-linked to type II collagen. *J. Biol. Chem.,* 263: 1615–1618.
312. van der Rest, M., and Garrone, R. (1991): Collagen family of proteins. *FASEB J.,* 5:2814–2823.
313. Venn, M., and Maroudas, A. (1977): Chemical composition and swelling of normal and osteoarthrotic femoral head cartilage: I. Chemical composition. *Ann. Rheum. Dis.,* 36:121–129.
314. Venn, M. F. (1978): Variation of chemical composition with age in human femoral head cartilage. *Ann. Rheum. Dis.,* 37:168–173.
315. Vetter, U., Vogel, W., Just, W., Young, M. F., and Fisher, L. W. (1993): Human decorin gene: intron–exon junctions and chromosomal localization. *Genomics,* 15: 161–168.
316. Vener, J. M., Thompson, R. C., Oegema, T. R., Lewis, J. L., and Wallace, L. (1992): Subchondral damage after acute transarticular loading: an *in vitro* model of joint injury. *J. Orthop. Res.,* 10:759–765.
317. Viidik, A. (1968): An ideological model for uncalcified parallel fibered collagenous tissue. *J. Biomechanics,* 1:3–11.
318. Viidik, A. (1980): Mechanical properties of parallel fibered collagenous tissues. In: *Biology of Collagen,* edited by A. Viidik and J. Vuust, pp. 237–255. Academic Press, New York.
319. Vogel, K. G., Paulsson, M., and Heinegard D. (1984) : Specific inhibition of type I and type II collagen fibrillogenesis by the small proteoglycan of tendon. *Biochem. J.,* 223:587–597.
320. Wachtel, E., Maroudas, A., and Schneiderman, R. (1995): Age-related changes in collagen packing of human articular cartilage. *Biochim. Biophys. Acta.,* 1243:239–243.
321. Wakitani, S., Goto, T., Pineda, S. J., Young, R. G., Mansour, J. M., and Caplan, A. I. (1994): Mesenchymal cell-based repair of large, full thickness defects of articular cartilage. *J. Bone Joint Surg.,* 76A:579–592.
322. Warden, W. H., Ateshian, G. A., Grelsamer, R. P., and Mow, V. C. (1994): Biphasic finite deformation material properties of bovine articular cartilage. *Trans. Orthop. Res. Soc.,* 19:413.
323. Weiss, C., Rosenberg, L. C., and Helfet, A. J. (1968): An ultrastructural study of normal young adult human articular cartilage. *J. Bone Joint Surg.,* 50A:663–674.
324. Williams, P. L. (1995): *Gray's Anatomy,* 38th ed. Churchhill and Livingston, New York.
325. Woo, S. L.-Y., Akeson, W. H., and Jemmott, G. F. (1976): Measurements of nonhomogeneous directional mechanical properties of articular cartilage in tension. *J. Biomechanics,* 9:785–791.
326. Woo, S. L.-Y., Mow, V. C., and Lai, W. M. (1987): Biomechanical properties of articular cartilage. In: *Handbook of Bioengineering,* edited by R. Skalak and S. Chien, pp. 4.1–4.44. McGraw-Hill, New York,
327. Woo, S. L.-Y., Simon, B. R., Kuei, S. C., and Akeson, W. H. (1980): Quasilinear viscoelastic properties of

normal articular cartilage. *J. Biomech. Eng.,* 102: 85–90.

328. Wu, J.-J., Lark, M. W., Chun, L. E., and Eyre, D. R. (1991): Sites of stromelysin cleavage in collagen types II, IX, and XI of cartilage. *J. Biol. Chem.,* 266: 5625–5628.

329. Wu, J.-J., Woods, P. E., and Eyre, D. R. (1992): Identification of cross-linking sites in bovine cartilage type IX collagen reveals an antiparallel type II–type IX molecular relationshop and type IX to type IX bonding. *J. Biol. Chem.,* 267:23007–23014.

330. Yamauchi, M., and Mechanic, G. (1988): Cross-linking of collagen. In: *Collagen: Biochemistry,* Vol. I, edited by M. E. Nimne, pp. 157–172. CRC Press, Boca Raton, FL.

331. Yasui, K. (1978): Three-dimensional architecture of human normal menisci. *J. Jpn. Orthop. Assoc.,* 52:391–399.

332. Zanetti, M., Ratcliffe, A., and Watt, F. M. (1985): Two subpopulations of differentiated chondrocytes identified with a monoclonal antibody to keratan sulfate. *J. Cell. Biol.,* 101:53–59.

333. Zhu, W. B., Chern, K. Y., and Mow, V. C. (1994): Anisotropic viscoelastic shear properties of bovine meniscus. *Clin. Orthop. Rel. Res.,* 306:34–45.

334. Zhu W. B., Iatridis J. C., Hlibczuk V., Ratcliffe A., and Mow, V. C. (1996): Determination of collagen–proteoglycan interactions *in vitro. J. Biomechanics,* 29: 773–784.

335. Zhu, W. B., Lai, W. M., and Mow, V. C. (1986): Intrinsic quasilinear viscoelastic behavior of the extracellular matrix of cartilage. *Trans. Orthop. Res. Soc.,* 11:407.

336. Zhu W. B., Lai W. M., and Mow, V. C. (1991): The density and strength of proteoglycan–proteoglycan interaction sites in concentrated solutions. *J. Biomechanics,* 24:1007–1018.

337. Zhu, W. B., Lai, W. M., Mow, V. C., Tang, L. H., Rosenberg, L. C., Hughes, C., Hardingham, T. E., and Muir, H. (1988): Influence of composition, size and structure of cartilage proteoglycans on the strength of molecular network formed in solution. *Trans. Orthop. Res. Soc.,* 13:67.

338. Zhu, W. B., Mow, V. C., Koob, T. J., and Eyre, D. R. (1993): Viscoelastic shear properties of articular cartilage and the effects of glycosidase treatment. *J. Orthop. Res.,* 11:771–781.

339. Zhu, W. B., Mow, V. C., Rosenberg, L. C., and Tang L. H. (1994): Determinations of kinetic changes of aggrecan–hyaluronan interaction in solutions from its rheological properties. *J. Biomechanics,* 27:571–579.

Basic Orthopaedic Biomechanics, 2nd ed.,
edited by Van C. Mow and Wilson C. Hayes.
Lippincott–Raven Publishers, Philadelphia © 1997.

5

Physical Regulation of Cartilage Metabolism

Farshid Guilak, *Robert Sah, and †Lori A. Setton

*Department of Surgery, Division of Orthopaedic Surgery, Duke University Medical Center,
Durham, North Carolina 27710; *Department of Bioengineering, University of California,
San Diego, La Jolla, California 92093; and †Department of Biomedical Engineering,
Duke University, Durham, North Carolina 27708*

Under normal physiological conditions, articular cartilage provides a nearly frictionless surface for the transmission and distribution of joint loads, exhibiting little or no wear over decades of use (146). These unique properties of cartilage are determined by the structure and composition of the fluid-filled extracellular matrix. The fluid component consists primarily of water with dissolved solutes and mobile ions (119). The solid material of the extracellular matrix is composed largely of collagen (mainly type II) and polyanionic glycosaminoglycans that are covalently attached to a core protein to form aggrecan, which in turn is stabilized as proteoglycan aggregates (74,127,147). The remainder of the solid matrix includes smaller amounts of other collagens, proteoglycans, proteins, and glycoproteins.

The composition and structure of articular cartilage are maintained through a balance of the anabolic and catabolic activities of the chondrocyte cell population, which comprises a small fraction of the tissue volume (200, 203). Chondrocyte activity is controlled not only by biochemical factors (e.g., growth factors, cytokines, and hormones) but also by physical factors such as joint loading. Chondrocytes are able to perceive and respond to signals generated by the normal load-bearing activities of daily living, such as walking and running (77). The physical mechanisms involved in this transduction process potentially involve mechanical, chemical, and electric signals. Joint loading produces deformation of the cartilage layer and associated changes in the mechanical environment of the cell within the extracellular matrix, such as spatially varying tensile, compressive, and shear stresses and strains (146). In addition, the presence of a large fluid phase containing mobile ions as well as a high density of negatively charged proteoglycans in the solid matrix (i.e., fixed charge density) gives rise to coupled electric and chemical phenomena during joint loading (47,55,107). The ability of the chondrocytes to regulate their metabolic activity in response to the mechanical, electric, or chemical signals of their physical environment provides a means by which articular cartilage can alter its structure and composition to meet the physical demands of the body. In this sense, the mechanical environment of the chondrocytes plays a major role in the health and function of the diarthrodial joint.

A number of different approaches have been used to decipher the role of physical stimuli in regulating cartilage and chondrocyte activity and range from *in vivo* studies to experiments at the cell and molecular level (77,201,216). Each level of study provides specific advantages and disadvantages. *In vivo* animal studies based on emulating physiologically relevant loading conditions provide a means to study long-term (i.e., weeks to years) tissue changes associated with growth, remodeling, or aging (142,168). These studies are limited, however, by the difficulties in determining the precise loading history of the articular cartilage. Further, such studies may be complicated by the effects of systemic factors or local soluble mediators (e.g., hormones, cytokines, enzymes) that are difficult to control *in vivo*. These confounding effects make it difficult to relate specific mechanical stimuli directly to the biological response within the joint.

At the next level, *in vitro* studies on the regulation of chondrocyte metabolism provide a system in which both the applied loading and the biochemical environment of the chondrocyte can be better controlled over time periods generally ranging from hours up to several months. These studies have used a variety of model systems (216), including cartilage explants and isolated chondrocytes grown in three-dimensional matrices. In explant cultures, the chondrocytes maintain their differentiated phenotype, and interactions between the cells and the extracellular

matrix that are naturally present in articular cartilage are also maintained (13,198,204). These studies have provided information on the relationships between matrix loading and chondrocyte anabolic and catabolic activities. However, the presence of the dense extracellular matrix generates physical signals associated with applied stress or strain which vary markedly in space and time. Chondrocytes that are cultured in a three-dimensional matrix such as agarose also tend to retain their phenotype in terms of aggrecan and collagen synthesis (13,204) and provide a means to assess the role of the extracellular matrix in transducing physical stimuli and inducing metabolic responses. However, the loading of an explant or artificial matrix in a controlled and isolated manner *in vitro* (e.g., uniaxial compression) will not completely reproduce the *in vivo* environment of the chondrocytes. It is difficult, therefore, to extrapolate information to physiologically relevant situations characteristic of daily living in an intact joint. Furthermore, many of the biophysical phenomena that the chondrocytes are exposed to, and to which they respond, cannot be uncoupled in most *in situ* configurations.

Studies at the cellular level are particularly useful for examining involvement of single pathways of signal transduction (201) or for isolating the effects of a single biophysical stimulus (e.g., osmotic or hydrostatic pressure, pH, deformation). Studies of isolated chondrocytes in monolayer culture allow for direct stimulation of cells as well as rapid isolation of cells for analysis. However, in such cultures, chondrocytes tend to dedifferentiate and lose the chondrocyte phenotype (13,81). As with explant studies, single-cell systems are further removed from the *in vivo* situation and present difficulties in extrapolating results to a physiologically relevant condition.

It is important to take into account the strengths and limitations associated with experimental models at each level and to evaluate the implications of the results from each of these different systems. Taken together, these culture systems have allowed various studies of the mechanisms by which physical forces may regulate chondrocyte metabolism at the molecular, cellular, tissue, and organ levels.

In this chapter, we present a review of the effects of physical factors on articular cartilage chondrocytes in three model systems: *in vivo* human and animal studies, *in vitro* three-dimensional culture systems, and *in vitro* two-dimensional cell culture systems. The primary mechanism for altering the physical environment of cartilage *in vivo* is through loading of the diarthrodial joint. Therefore, studies of chondrocyte response to physical stimulus seek to examine the role of mechanical strains, stresses, pressures, electric fields, and altered solute transport properties, individually or in combination, as these aspects relate to the natural loading condition in the joint. Together, these studies present us with an understanding of the chondrocyte and its interactions with its native environment. This information, in turn, provides the basis for ongoing and future studies of cell-based repair and remodeling mechanisms for maintaining the healthy and normal function of articular cartilage.

IN VIVO STUDIES OF CARTILAGE RESPONSE TO LOAD

In the 19th century, it was generally believed that articular cartilage was inert and without structure (31,220). However, by the turn of the century, many investigators had hypothesized not only that articular cartilage had form and structure but that changes in the normal physical environment of the joint could alter the composition and morphology of the tissue (77). By the mid-1900s, it was suggested that specific relationships existed between the structural characteristics and functional history of articular cartilage, and with increased knowledge of the composition and structure of cartilage, investigators began to hypothesize how these properties may be affected by alterations in the mechanical envi-

ronment *in vivo*. Further, it was suggested that physiological loading was necessary for the proper maintenance of the joint and that deviations from normal loading patterns could be a source of significant joint degeneration (44,99,185,207).

A number of more recent *in vivo* investigations have been undertaken to examine the effects of altering the normal pattern of joint loading using models of disuse and immobilization, overuse, impact loading, and joint "instability" (e.g., 142,168). These studies have provided strong evidence that "abnormal" joint loading can significantly affect the composition, structure, metabolic activity, and mechanical properties of articular cartilage and other joint tissues.

For example, disuse of the joint, achieved through immobilization, casting, or muscle transection, may result in changes in cartilage composition and mechanical behavior that are characteristic of degeneration. Important changes observed in the cartilage include a loss of proteoglycans and changes in proteoglycan conformation, a decrease in cartilage thickness, and material property changes including a decreased compressive stiffness and increased tensile stiffness (11,26,90,92,148,157, 159,160,176,177,194,206,222). In addition, there is direct evidence of decreased proteoglycan and collagen biosynthesis and elevated levels of metalloproteinases, suggesting an altered metabolic balance following periods of unloading and disuse in both human and experimental animal tissue (26,57,160,205,206,222). Many of these changes are localized to specific sites and depths in the cartilage layer, and some of these changes have been shown to be partly reversible with remobilization of the joint (90,101,160).

In contrast to studies of joint disuse, moderate exercise seems to have few deleterious effects on the cartilage and has been shown to increase proteoglycan content, reduce the extractability of proteoglycans, and increase the cartilage thickness (89,92,102,111). More strenuous exercise has been shown to cause site-specific changes in proteoglycan content and cartilage stiffness, although it is not clear that these changes affect cartilage function (91,100).

Experimental models of altered joint loading have been developed for studies of cartilage degeneration following observations of natural degeneration in the human joint following traumatic loading, joint instability, or isolated injury. These studies have provided a means for tracking the time sequence of events that occur in cartilage with degeneration and also provide an important tool for isolating aging changes from the degenerative process of osteoarthritis. In one experimental model of joint degeneration, an impact load delivered to the joint (i.e., a rapid increase of force across the joint) has been shown to cause both immediate and progressive damage to the articular cartilage (5,36,154,170,171,208,221). These studies have utilized single or repetitive impact loading to emulate different loading conditions in the human related to injury or repetitious daily activity, respectively. In studies of the canine or porcine patellofemoral joint cartilage changes following isolated impact, included altered cellular activity and histologic appearance, and increased hydration and proteoglycan content within 2 weeks after loading (5,36). Subfracture impact loads also caused a significant decrease in the tensile stiffness of the surface zone cartilage but no detectable changes in either the compressive modulus or hydraulic permeability of the full-thickness cartilage (5). Impact loading to the articular surface can be expected to produce a combination of tensile, compressive, and shear stresses and strains as well as very high hydrostatic pressure (5). The mechanical environment during and following impact can be expected to vary significantly with depth in the cartilage layer, although there is little information on the local chondrocyte response to these changes except for one report of increased cellular activities in the deep zone of cartilage (36). These studies suggest that changes in the mechanical environment caused by impact loads delivered to the cartilage layer may serve as a cellular signal that alters biosynthetic activities in a manner that will modify tissue composition and mechanical behavior.

Damage to the pericapsular and intracapsular soft tissues, such as ligaments and menisci, has often been observed to produce degenerative changes in the knee joint under both clinical and experimental conditions. Alterations in the mechanisms of force attenuation in the joint, occur with meniscal or ligamentous injuries, will alter the magnitude and distribution of forces applied to the cartilage layers *in vivo*. It has been well documented that the clinical phenomena of "joint laxity" and "joint instability" lead to alterations in contact areas and stresses (105,118), and therefore surgical destabilization of the joint has been used as an animal model to study the effects of altered joint loading on cartilage degeneration. (2,20,25, 38,45,52,67,78,112,136,137,143,155,167,192, 193,195,202).

Transection of the anterior cruciate ligament has been the most widely used model for studying degenerative changes in articular cartilage that occur following "destabilization" of the joint (2,20,25,38,52,67,136,137, 143,155,167,192,193,202). This model has been studied by Brandt and co-workers over an extended time course of 54 months and has been found to produce degenerative changes in the joint similar to those of human osteoarthritis (20). Morphologic and histologic changes include fibrillation of the articular surface, loss of proteoglycan content and collagen fibril organization, increased cellularity, meniscal changes, and joint capsule thickening. Compositional and metabolic changes include an increase in water content, increased rates of proteoglycan and collagen synthesis, decreased concentration of collagen crosslinks, decreased content of hyaluronic acid, and alterations in the number and size of proteoglycan aggregates (25,38,43,67, 126,136,148,173,186). These structural and compositional changes are accompanied by distinct changes in the biomechanical properties of the articular cartilage, including a decrease in the tensile, compressive, and shear moduli, increased evidence of swelling behavior, and increased hydraulic permeability of the tissue (2,67,192,193) (Fig. 1).

Surgical resection of the meniscus has also proved to be a valuable experimental system for studying altered joint loading and cartilage degeneration in a number of animal models (6,45,78,87,143,195). Degenerative changes following meniscectomy are observed in the articular cartilage, including signs of cartilage fibrillation (i.e., a roughening of the cartilage surface as collagen fiber bundles become frayed), increased hydration and decreased proteoglycan content of the extracellular matrix, and elevated collagen and proteoglycan synthesis rates (14,45,78,123,195). In addition, changes in the mechanical behavior of the cartilage layer have been observed, including alterations in the magnitude of streaming potentials and changes in both the compressive and tensile properties (42,78,112). As with the experimental models of impact loading or ligament transection, it is unclear what specific role is played by the chondrocytes in eliciting these changes in the composition and mechanical behavior of the extracellular matrix. The changes in biosynthetic rates provide indirect evidence that altered physical and/or biological factors following meniscectomy influence chondrocyte activity.

Recent studies suggest that changes in the mechanical loading history of the cartilage caused by loss of joint congruity as a result of a "step-off" defect may also lead to progressive joint degeneration. Twenty weeks after the creation of 3-mm-wide sagittal defect displaced 5 mm from the joint surface, rabbit knee joints exhibited progressive osteoarthritic changes such as osteophytes, carti-

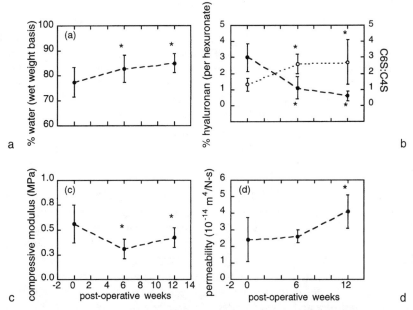

FIG. 1. The effect of transection of the anterior cruciate ligament on the composition and properties of canine articular cartilage. Data are shown for changes in **(a)** water content, **(b)** hyaluronate (*closed circles*) and GAG composition (ratio of chondroitin 6-sulfate to chondroitin 4-sulfate; *open circles*), **(c)** compressive modulus, and **(d)** hydraulic permeability of canine cartilage following transection of the anterior cruciate ligament. Data are expressed as mean ± SD ($n = 6$–11 per group); *significantly different from control by a Student Neuman-Keul's test. All data were measured in full-thickness cartilage from covered regions of the tibial plateau of the operated knee. Increased hydration and changes in proteoglycan content and structure are known to contribute to the observed changes in the compressive behavior of articular cartilage. Data adapted from Muller et al. (148) and Setton et al. (193).

lage fibrillation, hypocellularity, and severe loss of safranin-O staining (116). A similar defect displaced 2 mm from the joint surface, showed cartilaginous and bony repair, and resulted in closure of the surgical defect with restoration of femoral congruity that did not lead to progressive degeneration (117).

In all of these experimental *in vivo* models, the observed changes suggest that the articular cartilage chondrocytes exhibit altered biological activity following changes in the joint-loading history. These *in vivo* studies emphasize the relationship between joint loading and the function of articular cartilage and suggest that the chondrocyte population plays an active role in maintaining this relationship. It appears that a critical level and manner of joint loading is required to send physical signals to the chondrocyte, which will, in turn, maintain the composition, material properties, and mechanical function of the cartilage extracellular matrix. Although these studies demonstrate important characteristics of chondrocyte function *in vivo,* they also point to the many unknowns in the chondrocyte–matrix relationship. Related studies are needed to determine the nature of the chondrocyte's metabolic response to physical signals as well as the precise relationships between isolated factors of mechanical loading and specific physical signaling mechanisms.

AGGRECAN METABOLISM IN CARTILAGE EXPLANTS AND CHONDROCYTE CULTURES

With the knowledge that the loading history of the joint has an important influence on the health of articular cartilage, considerable research effort has been directed toward understanding the processes by which physical signals are converted to a biochemical signal by the chondrocyte population. Clarification of the specific signaling mechanisms in cartilage would not only provide a better understanding of the processes that regulate cartilage physiology but would also be expected to yield new insights on the pathogenesis of joint disease.

Studies of cartilage in an *in vitro* system allow for control of sample geometry, physical environment, and biochemical environment, so that changes in metabolic activity can be correlated with physical phenomena that can be either measured directly or predicted by theoretical models. Because load-induced physical phenomena in cartilage consist of time-averaged and time-varying components, studies are naturally divided into those that examine the metabolic responses during one or a combination of the following conditions: (a) prolonged static loading; (b) the onset or release of a load; and (c) cyclic or intermittent ("dynamic") loading. The use of alternative mechanical, electrical, and physicochemical test protocols such as imposed displacements or hydrostatic pressures, or application of electric fields or current densities have been used to assess the regulatory effects of specific static or cyclic physical signals on chondrocyte metabolism.

Experimental studies of the physical regulation of cartilage matrix metabolism have focused primarily on the large aggregating proteoglycan aggrecan (74,147). The regulation of aggrecan metabolism is of particular interest because of the contribution of aggrecan to the critical load-bearing functions of articular cartilage, including compressive and shear behaviors, hydraulic permeability, and hydration of the extracellular matrix (93,132,146). The maintenance of aggrecan in the extracellular matrix is a dynamic process and dependent on the coordinated synthesis, assembly, and degradation of this molecule. This is in contrast to the relatively slow turnover of the collagen macromolecule *in vivo* (127,134). In the following sections, the regulation of aggrecan biosynthesis by physical factors is reviewed as one measure of chondrocyte activity in *in vitro* culture systems.

The effects of physical factors on aggrecan metabolism have been studied extensively by examining the incorporation and release of radiolabeled sulfate using pulse-chase techniques (133). In such studies, ^{35}S-sulfate is included in the culture medium before, during, or following application of the physical stimulus.

Because sulfate is a relatively small anion, it diffuses quickly through the matrix, where it rapidly equilibrates with intracellular sulfate pools and is incorporated primarily into the glycosaminoglycans of newly synthesized aggrecan (75,132). Although aggrecan turnover does occur, the quantity of sulfate reutilized from degraded glycosaminoglycan is small compared with the utilization of sulfate from the extracellular medium. Therefore, the kinetics of ^{35}S-sulfate incorporation into macromolecules and the subsequent release of ^{35}S-sulfate are highly indicative of aggrecan metabolism. To examine the effects of various physical factors on aggrecan metabolism, radiolabel incorporation studies have been performed in each of the *in vitro* culture systems discussed above: explant cultures, chondrocytes in three-dimensional matrices, and chondrocytes in isolated cell culture systems.

Static Compression

In studies of cartilage explants, static compression has been shown to produce a dose-dependent inhibition of proteoglycan synthesis (22,53,54,65,88,97,183,189,213) (Figs. 2 and 3). In studies in which tissue compression is maintained for at least several hours and as long as several days, the magnitude of the biosynthetic inhibition is relatively stable. Furthermore, the inhibition of aggrecan synthesis within different zones of immature articular cartilage appears to be similarly affected by various levels of applied stress (65). Static compression of cylindrical cartilage explants will generate stresses and strains in the solid matrix of articular cartilage and a decrease in cartilage hydration or an increase in the solid volume fraction of the extracellular matrix (119,145). These changes are associ-

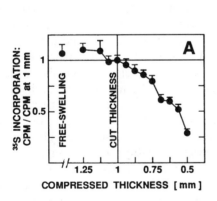
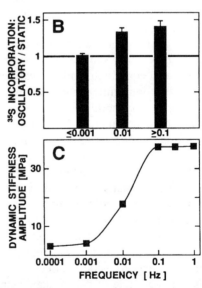

FIG. 2. Effect of static and oscillatory compression on ^{35}S-sulfate incorporation (as a measure of aggrecan synthesis rates) into disks of articular cartilage. **(A)** Disks were radiolabeled during 12 hr of static compression. Incorporation is expressed relative to disks held at 1 mm (the original cartilage thickness). Static compression showed a dose-dependent decrease in the rate of ^{35}S-sulfate incorporation. Data are expressed as mean ± SEM (*n* = 9–12). **(B)** Disks were radiolabeled during the last 8 hr of 23-hr oscillatory compression protocols. Experimental disks were statically compressed to a thickness of 1 mm with a superimposed oscillatory strain of 1–2% at frequencies of 0.0001–1.0 Hz; controls were statically compressed at 1 mm. A significant increase in the rate of ^{35}S-sulfate incorporation was observed at frequencies of 0.01 Hz and higher. Incorporation data are expressed as oscillatory/static (*n* = 12–72). **(C)** Dynamic stiffness amplitude was measured during oscillatory compression experiments. (Reproduced from Sah et al., ref. 182, with permission.)

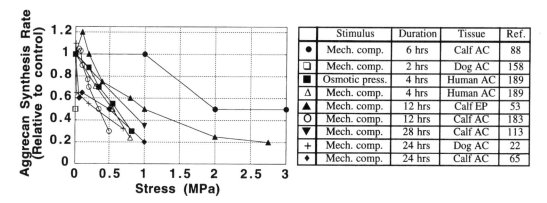

FIG. 3. Summary of the effects of different magnitudes of static physical stimuli (mechanical and osmotic) on aggrecan synthesis rates as measured by the rate of ^{35}S-sulfate incorporation. Data are expressed relative to control studies. Nearly all studies show a trend of decreasing synthesis rates with increasing stress. AC, articular cartilage; EP, epiphyseal plate cartilage. Adapted from Gray et al. (54).

ated with an increase in the density of matrix-associated negative charges, or fixed charged density, which produce an altered osmotic and ionic environment within the extracellular matrix and surrounding the cell (53,107,132, 215). Although transient changes in hydrostatic pressure may occur shortly after loading, the pressure will equilibrate with the external environment for long times after loading, so that the effects of osmotic pressure changes are presumed to dominate over hydrostatic pressure changes. Because a similar inhibition has been observed during mechanical compression of cartilage explants or incubation of cartilage explants in medium containing osmotically active solutes such as polyethylene glycol (189,214,215), the inhibition of biosynthesis by static compression is predominantly associated with tissue consolidation and the associated osmotic effects.[1]

The contributory role of the cartilage extracellular matrix in chondrocyte signaling has been elucidated by studies of cartilage chondrocytes in three-dimensional agarose matrices. In these studies, static compression resulted in an inhibition of biosynthesis similar to that observed in cartilage explants, but only after prolonged culture in which a proteoglycan-rich extracellular matrix had formed (23). At earlier times of culture, static compression did not alter biosynthesis, providing further support for the notion that the biosynthesis changes that occur with static compression are secondary to the associated tissue consolidation.

In studies of cartilage under compression, the regulatory roles of a number of physical factors have been examined, such as matrix stresses or strains, altered electrostatic effects, and decreased hydration or increased solid volume fraction (i.e., associated with a decrease in apparent porosity). One factor that has been discounted as a major regulatory factor in short-term, in vitro experiments is the hindered transport of nutrients or regulatory molecules to the chondrocytes during compression. Evidence for this stems from the findings that the dose-dependent inhibition of aggrecan biosynthesis is not sensitive to sample dimensions and, therefore, to the available pathway for diffusion of regulatory molecules. This finding applies to compression of cartilage test samples of various dimensions, ranging from thin slices of cartilage (200 to 400 μm) to large cartilage explants (5 mm diameter) to full-thickness cartilage from the human femoral head (54,88,97,189).

---

[1]It should be noted, however, that mechanical loading in general does not produce the same internal fluid pressure as osmotic loading (109). It is therefore difficult to make direct comparisons between the results of these biosynthesis studies.

Compression and Release

The biosynthetic responses of cartilage to an applied compression are different after application and removal of the static load (i.e., during the loading and unloading stage). The inhibitory effect of compression occurs within several hours of mechanical equilibration (54,183). However, the release of an applied static compression has more variable effects on subsequent proteoglycan synthesis (22,54, 65,88,97,158,183). The release of a relatively low level of compressive load may result in the return of suppressed proteoglycan synthetic rates to uncompressed control levels (53,65, 113). However, the release of a somewhat higher level of compressive load can lead to a stimulation of proteoglycan biosynthesis to levels higher than that of unloaded control samples (22,65,183). Finally, the application and then release of extremely high levels of compression (50% or 1 MPa) may require a prolonged duration for proteoglycan synthesis rates to return to unloaded control levels or, alternatively, may result in cell death (22,65).

Osmotic Pressure

Proteoglycan synthesis rates have been shown to be maximal when the osmolality of the extracellular media matches the *in situ* osmolality of cartilage (350 to 450 mOsm), suggesting that the normal interstitial environment is optimal for maintaining chondrocyte activity (214,215). These findings are consistent with earlier studies that have shown that the composition of the matrix (e.g., proteoglycan concentration) exerts a strong influence on chondrocyte biosynthetic activity (71, 73,147,187).

In studies of static compression, the regulatory roles of physicochemical factors, such as pH, fixed charge density, and osmotic pressure, appear to predominate over the transient mechanical or electrokinetic factors such as hydrostatic pressure, interstitial fluid flow, or streaming potential. The role of the extracellular ionic environment has been examined by comparing the biosynthetic response of explants subjected to compression with the response to alterations in the extracellular ion composition or osmotic pressure in the absence of mechanical loading (53,189,213, 214). Cartilage explants that were placed under osmotic pressure using various concentrations of polyethylene glycol showed similar decreases in aggrecan synthesis rates to those placed under static compression (189). Although the two loading conditions are not identical (109), both osmotic and mechanical stress also resulted in a similar decrease in tissue water content, suggesting that factors related to hydration were responsible for the observed effects.

In other studies, biosynthesis has been found to be inhibited by increasing the hydrogen ion concentration (decreasing the pH) and reducing the concentration of bicarbonate (53,227), suggesting a pH-mediated inhibition of biosynthesis. More recent data indicate different dynamics of pH-induced and mechanically induced changes in biosynthesis, suggesting that pH is not the persisting mechanism in this process (18,19). It is possible that local changes in fixed charge density are sufficient to cause these changes in pH, despite the relatively high intracellular buffering capacity of chondrocytes (226). Biosynthesis may also be inhibited by deviations in the extracellular osmotic pressure from the normal value of the cartilage matrix. The osmotic pressure in cartilage has been altered by incubation of explants in dilute or concentrated medium (213) or by the addition of sodium chloride (212). Direct osmotic compression of the chondrocytes within cartilage by the addition of sucrose to the bathing medium has been shown to modulate chondrocyte biosynthesis as well (214).

Hydrostatic Pressure

The role of hydrostatic pressure as a physical factor in modulating cartilage biosynthesis can be isolated for study because physiological levels of hydrostatic pressure can be applied without inducing confounding physical factors such as fluid flow, electrokinetic effects, or cyclic cell deformation. High pressures, up to those estimated to occur *in vivo*, have been shown to modulate proteoglycan biosynthesis depending on the amplitude, frequency, and duration of pressurization. Continuous pressures of <3 MPa do not generally affect aggrecan biosynthesis (70,98), although other studies show variable effects in this pressure range (120). During the application of higher pressures for 2 hr (70), aggrecan biosynthesis depended on the amplitude of pressure. In these studies, pressures of 5 to 10 MPa were found to stimulate synthesis relative to nonpressure control samples, although higher pressures of 30 to 50 MPa were found to inhibit biosynthesis. The application of a single pulse of pressure of 10 to 20 MPa for only 20 sec stimulated aggrecan biosynthesis in the subsequent 2 hr but did not markedly alter synthesis at lower pressures or at 50 MPa of pressure. The frequency of applied load appears important because pressure of 5 MPa applied at 0.5 Hz has been found to stimulate biosynthesis, whereas lower frequencies of pressurization (0.017 to 0.25 Hz) did not affect biosynthesis (162). In early studies of embryonic epiphyseal chick cartilage, intermittent pressures of 0.01 to 0.02 MPa applied for an extended period were shown to stimulate chondrocyte growth and proteoglycan biosynthesis (103,218). In these studies, hydrostatic pressurization was achieved through a pressurized gas phase, which also resulted in preferential stimulation of cartilage explants from osteoarthritic tissue but not normal articular cartilage (106). However, because these hydrostatic pressures were applied via a gas phase, it may be that changes in the concentration of dissolved gas, rather than pressure itself, were the stimulatory signal.

Cyclic and Intermittent Compression

Cyclic and intermittent compression of cartilage explants and chondrocyte-seeded three-dimensional agarose matrices can produce a range of effects depending on the characteristics of the loading conditions, such as the loading amplitude and frequency (22,23,97, 104,113,156,158,162,183,217) (Fig. 4). In contrast to static compression, physical factors that may regulate the biosynthetic response to cyclic compression are related to time-varying behaviors, including fluid flow, electric fields, matrix stresses and strains, hydrostatic pressure, and cellular deformations (23,97,183).

Theoretical analyses of cylindrical cartilage explants in the unconfined compression configuration have been performed for the condition of a time-varying compressive load applied to the faces of the explant through two impermeable platens, as is frequently the case in *in vitro* culture systems. For these precise loading conditions, the magnitude of the physical phenomenon is predicted to vary with position within the disk and also with the frequency of applied compression (3,69,94). At very low frequencies, the extracellular matrix may be axially compressed in a radially uniform manner with minimal fluid pressurization. With increasing compression frequency, the magnitudes of the fluid velocity and streaming potential increase at the disk periphery (near the tissue-bath–solution interface) while the hydrostatic pressure increases near the center of the disk. In addition, at the higher frequencies, cyclic changes in cell shape and volume may vary with radial position. In some cases, it may be difficult to distinguish between the effects of signals associated with cyclic compression and time-averaged signals associated with a time-averaged compression, particularly in studies in which frequency and amplitude of the load are varied without controlling the time-averaged load (e.g., 113,158). Nevertheless, a number of studies using a variety of cyclic compression conditions have suggested a potential regulatory role for dynamic physical stimuli.

Cyclic compression protocols in the unconfined compression configuration have been used to study specific physical factors such as fluid flow, streaming potentials, and cell deformation and their role in modulating aggrecan biosynthesis. In protocols with low-magnitude

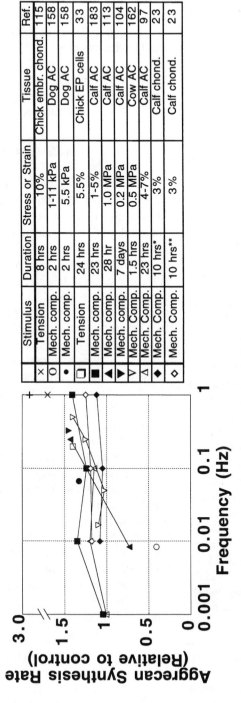

	Stimulus	Duration	Stress or Strain	Tissue	Ref.
×	Tension	8 hrs	10%	Chick embr. chond.	115
○	Mech. comp.	2 hrs	1-11 kPa	Dog AC	158
•	Mech. comp.	2 hrs	5.5 kPa	Dog AC	158
▢	Tension	24 hrs	5.5%	Chick EP cells	33
■	Mech. comp.	23 hrs	1-5%	Calf AC	183
▲	Mech. comp.	28 hr	1.0 MPa	Calf AC	113
▶	Mech. comp.	7 days	0.2 MPa	Calf AC	104
▽	Mech. Comp.	1.5 hrs	0.5 MPa	Cow AC	162
△	Mech. Comp.	23 hrs	4-7%	Calf AC	97
◆	Mech. Comp.	10 hrs*	3%	Calf chond.	23
◇	Mech. Comp.	10 hrs**	3%	Calf chond.	23

FIG. 4. Summary of the effects of different frequencies of cyclic (dynamic) mechanical stimuli on aggrecan synthesis rates as measured by the rate of ^{35}S-sulfate incorporation. Nearly all studies show a trend of increasing synthesis rates with increasing loading frequency. AC, articular cartilage; EP, epiphyseal plate cartilage; *tests were performed 2 days following seeding of chondrocytes in agarose gel; **tests were performed 41 days following seeding of chondrocytes in agarose gel. Adapted from Gray et al. (54).

amplitudes of applied compression, matrix deformation is relatively small, so that biosynthetic stimulation is not likely to occur through mechanisms related to changes in solid volume fraction, such as osmotic effects associated with increased fixed charge density. In the radially unconfined compression configuration of cylindrical test samples, compression frequencies of 0.01 to 1 Hz and amplitudes of 1% to 5% stimulated aggrecan biosynthesis above control levels, whereas lower compression frequencies or amplitudes appear not to elicit a biosynthetic response (23,97,179,181) (Fig. 2). Because the biosynthetic stimulation is highest in the circumferential areas of the cyclically compressed samples, and the peak stress in the experiments was <1 MPa, physical factors such as fluid flow, streaming potentials, and cell deformation, rather than hydrostatic pressure, appear to be responsible for the stimulation of biosynthesis.

In a different test configuration, the central regions of cartilage disks were loaded with a nonporous plane-ended indenter, and a variety of compressive stress amplitudes and frequencies were examined (162). This geometry and test condition do not correspond to that described mathematically by the unconfined compression solution (3), although similar types of physical signals may be expected to occur. Aggrecan synthesis was stimulated beneath and near the loaded site relative to regions away from the loaded site. In another configuration, osteochondral bovine sesamoid samples were cultured and subjected to load against a nylon surface, resulting in contact of a portion of the articular cartilage surface (104). Here, cyclic compression at 0.33 Hz stimulated aggrecan synthesis, especially in the superficial layers of the articular cartilage. In yet another configuration, cartilage disks were compressed between a porous platen and the nonporous base of a culture dish (113). Here, cyclic loads of 1 MPa at a frequency of 0.25 Hz stimulated aggrecan synthesis, whereas a frequency of 0.008 Hz slightly inhibited aggrecan synthesis, emphasizing the sensitivity of the cellular environment to frequency of loading. The generation of physical signals in these experimental geometries, however, has not been well characterized, and it is difficult to assess the role of potential physical regulators of cartilage metabolism. For example, under the same magnitude of applied stress, different loading frequencies will result in different magnitudes of tissue strain. In this sense, cyclic loading experiments that are "load controlled" must be interpreted separately from those that are "deformation controlled."

Tensile Stretch

The response of chondrocytes to tensile stretch has also been examined in two-dimensional cell culture systems (33,115,210). In one model of cyclic tensile stretch, the collagen matrix generated by epiphyseal chondrocytes in high-density culture was stretched at strains of 5.5% at 0.2 Hz, and significant increases were observed in aggrecan synthesis rates following 24 hr of applied strains (33). In other studies, tensile strains of 10% applied to a supportive elastin membrane at 1 Hz resulted in a two- to threefold increase in the rates of aggrecan synthesis in chick sternal chondrocytes (115). Further, agitation of the substrate had similar effects on cellular activity such as stretching of the substrate, implying that fluid motion may have contributed to the observed effects (115). More recent studies have also observed a significant increase in aggrecan synthesis by chondrocytes isolated from rat ribs as induced by tensile deformation of an underlying substrate, although the magnitude of applied strain was not reported (210). It is important to note, however, that even if the strain in the substrate is precisely characterized in studies such as these, the relationship between substrate strain and cellular strain may be complex.

Electric Fields

The role of electric fields on chondrocyte activity has also been studied in culture conditions (1,83,115,124) and has led investigators to hypothesize that mechanically induced electric fields may serve as a mechanism for the regulation of aggrecan biosynthesis. Studies of chick sternal chondrocytes in culture showed that extremely low-level electric currents induced qualitatively similar changes in aggrecan synthesis rates as those induced by cyclic stretching of the substrate, suggesting that similar mechanisms were involved in transducing tension or externally applied electric fields (115). To determine if electric fields modulate cartilage metabolism, it is important to distinguish thermal effects related to the method of electric field application from the effects of the electric fields themselves, because the induction of currents using pulsed electromagnetic fields may be associated with heating (83). In calf cartilage explants, current densities up to 1 mA/cm^2 at frequencies of 1 to 10 Hz did not affect aggrecan biosynthesis (180), whereas higher amplitude current densities of 10 to 30 mA/cm^2 at a frequency of 10 to 1000 Hz stimulated aggrecan biosynthesis (124). These effects were not related to heating because the temperature of the medium was not detectably altered, and there was no evidence for the production of characteristic heat-shock proteins. Pulsed electromagnetic fields, as used to stimulate fracture healing, also appear to stimulate aggrecan biosynthesis in cartilage explants (1). Because of the nature of the electromagnetic stimulus, such protocols would be predicted to induce electric currents of a variety of amplitudes and frequencies within cartilage.

In summary, the results of numerous *in vitro* culture studies have provided significant evidence that changes in the physical environment can modulate the metabolic response of the chondrocyte, whether the cell is within the native tissue or an artificial three-dimensional construct. The application of static changes in the physical environment decreases synthesis rates in a dose-dependent manner (Fig. 3), whereas cyclic and dynamic stimuli increases synthesis rates at higher frequencies (Fig. 4). Although this chapter has focused on aggrecan biosynthesis as a marker of chondrocyte metabolism, there are data available on the biosynthesis of a number of metabolic prod-

ucts, including collagen, noncollagenous proteins, and metalloproteinases. It should be emphasized that biosynthetic regulation of these other matrix molecules by physical factors may not be similar to that of aggrecan (22,54,70,95, 96,104,110,113,183,223). Studies of aggrecan metabolism provide a model system for understanding the involvement of the variety of physical signals associated with static and cyclic compression; a full understanding awaits a more thorough investigation of the long-term influences on aggrecan metabolism as well as the physical influences on other matrix macromolecules.

MECHANICALLY INDUCED SIGNALS AT THE CELL AND MOLECULAR LEVEL

From these *in vivo* and *in vitro* studies, it is evident that mechanical loading has a strong influence on the metabolic activity of the chondrocytes. However, the precise sequence of events and the mechanisms involved in regulating the synthesis and breakdown of matrix components are still unclear. One difficulty in isolating the effects of specific biophysical phenomena on chondrocyte activity is the intrinsic coupling of these phenomena in the physiological situation. Furthermore, the physicochemical, electric, and fluid-flow environments of the chondrocytes will be dependent on the specifics of the loading configuration to which the cartilage is exposed (Fig. 5). In the following sections, we present a review of several biophysical factors that are evoked by mechanical loading of articular cartilage and the potential roles that they may play in signaling mechanisms to the chondrocyte.

Physicochemical Effects

The physicochemical environment within articular cartilage is determined by parameters such as matrix hydration, fixed charge density, interstitial ion concentrations, and activity coefficients for specific ions within the cartilage

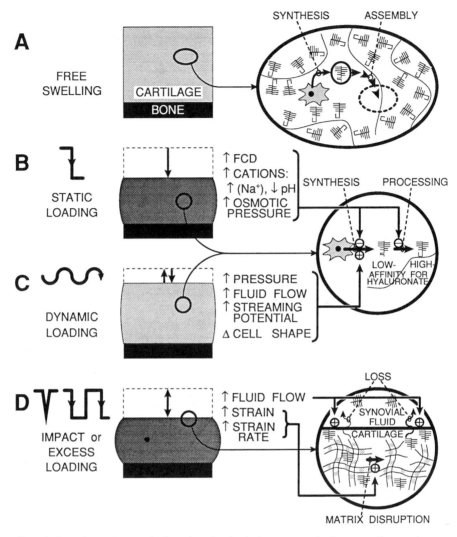

FIG. 5. Regulation of matrix metabolism by physical phenomena in free-swelling and compressed cartilage. **(A)** In free-swelling cartilage, local regions of low proteoglycan content (and low fixed charge density, FCD) attract a relatively low concentration of positive counter-ions (Na^+, H^+, Ca^{2+}) and may thereby stimulate aggrecan synthesis and deposition. **(B)** During static compression, there is an increase in the FCD, the concentration of positive counter-ions, and the osmotic pressure in the tissue, which may inhibit aggrecan synthesis. **(C)** Dynamic loading conditions such as oscillatory or intermittent compression may affect chondrocyte metabolic activity through other biophysical mechanisms such as hydrostatic pressure, fluid flow, streaming potentials, or oscillations in cell shape. **(D)** During excessive compression or impact loading, high levels of strain or strain rate may cause tissue disruption, tissue swelling, increased diffusion, and potentially increased loss of matrix macromolecules through fluid convection. (Reproduced from Sah et al., ref. 182, with permission.)

extracellular matrix (128,129,130,132). The negatively charged groups on the glycosaminoglycans in cartilage influence the electrolyte composition of the interstitial fluid such that the anions are dilute and the cations are con- centrated relative to the external compartments (e.g., synovial capsule). This physicochemical state, which can be described theoretically using Donnan or Boltzmann approaches, confers the tissue with a propensity to swell and is responsible for electrokinetic effects including electroosmosis, streaming potentials, and streaming currents (47,55,59,60,107,128). The swelling pressure in cartilage is directly coupled to the state of stress and strain in the matrix, because the density of negative charges explicitly depends on the water volume fraction and, therefore, on the dilatation of the cartilage matrix (107). As an example, when a cylindrical cartilage explant is deformed in compression by 20%, the negative fixed charge density may increase from 15% to 20% (107), depending on material parameters of the solid matrix such as the Poisson's ratio.

In general, such changes in both the mechanical environment and fixed charge density would be expected to vary spatially through the explant. The associated changes in local ionic environment with compression will give rise to increases in osmotic and swelling pressures and decreases in intratissue pH. These changes in the local physicochemical environment may modify the mechanical behaviors of the tissue, because physicochemical factors have been strongly linked to material parameters such as hydraulic permeability and compressive modulus (4,55,59,60,107,128,132,146). Chondrocyte biosynthetic activity is very sensitive to extracellular osmolarity, suggesting that coupling of the mechanical and physicochemical environments may be important as a process for transducing signals associated with applied loads.

Cell Deformation

One mechanism by which mammalian cells may perceive alterations in their physical environment is through cellular deformation (i.e., changes in shape and volume) (12,86, 178,225). Under physiological levels of matrix deformation, chondrocyte volume *in situ* can be altered by as much as 20% (18,51,62, 68) (Fig. 6). Theoretical predictions and experimental measurements of cellular deformation in response to applied loading also indicate that the magnitude and distribution of cell deformations will vary with depth in the cartilage layer (9,66,68,190). The mechanism

for chondrocyte volumetric decrease may be related to mechanical and osmotic effects associated with matrix compression (62) or may be an active cellular response to loading (51).

Volumetric cell changes in other mammalian cells have been associated with mechanical transduction and signaling through the transport of ions and organic compounds (28,178,188,225). In the chondrocyte, volume also seems to exert a strong influence on biosynthetic activity (215). Cell volume increases significantly by 30% to 40% when chondrocytes are removed from the extracellular matrix (215), and chondrocytes *in situ* will shrink or swell in proportion to changes in the ionic composition of the extracellular matrix. Further, chondrocytes exhibit active volume recovery mechanisms in response to osmotic shock, i.e., a rapid change in the osmotic environment of the extracellular fluid (34). It may be difficult, however, to uncouple direct cellular deformation from ion-specific osmotic activity changes in these studies of volumetric changes induced by osmotic shock, because physicochemical factors are known to be important in regulating chondrocyte activity (see above). Further, rapid changes in the ion concentrations around a chondrocyte are unlikely. Intracellular signaling in response to cell volume changes may be occurring through changes in cell shape and the accompanying deformation of the cell membrane and cytoplasm. It is known that chondrocyte shape influences phenotypic expression (81,151) through what is apparently a secondary response to changes in cytoskeletal architecture (125). Further, stretching of an underlying substrate, which presumably causes changes in the shape of chondrocytes grown on the substrate, has been shown to modify chondrocyte metabolism, proliferation, and second messenger activity (115,210) (see section on Tensile Stretch).

Hydrostatic Pressure

Because of the incompressible nature of the fluid-filled solid matrix at physiological pressures, hydrostatic fluid pressurization of carti-

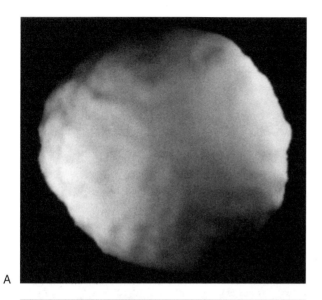

A

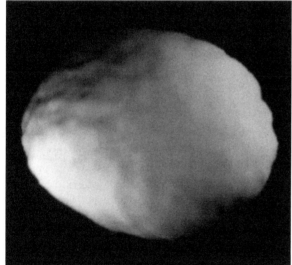

B

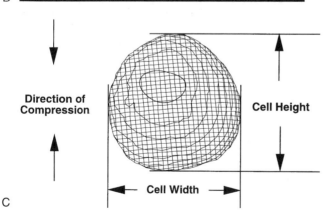

C

FIG. 6. Three-dimensional confocal microscopy images of viable chondrocytes *in situ* from the middle zone of articular cartilage of the canine patellofemoral groove before **(A)** and after **(B)** compression of the extracellular matrix. Chondrocytes were imaged by introducing fluorescein dextran (10,000 Da) into the extracellular medium. This fluorescent indicator diffuses rapidly within the extracellular matrix but is excluded from an intact cell membrane of viable chondrocytes. A series of 32 confocal images spaced at 0.5-μm intervals was recorded of a chondrocyte in the undeformed tissue. The tissue was then compressed in a direction perpendicular to the cartilage surface (as shown in **C**), and the same chondrocyte was imaged again. Three-dimensional reconstructions of the images were used to determine cell height, width, surface area, and volume (62,68). A 15% surface-to-surface compression of the tissue resulted in significant decreases in cell height of 26%, 19%, and 20% and in cell volume of 22%, 16%, and 17% in the surface, middle and deep zones, respectively. Removal of compression resulted in a complete recovery of cell shape and volume. (Reproduced from Guilak, ref. 62, with permission.)

lage will not cause appreciable deformation of the extracellular matrix or chondrocytes (8). Unlike the deforming loads of normal joint loading, hydrostatic pressures will not induce interstitial fluid flow or osmotic changes because no dilatation of the extracellular matrix occurs (64). These points would suggest that the chondrocyte itself is sensitive to the effects of static and intermittent hydrostatic pressures.

Hydrostatic pressure appears to modulate aggrecan biosynthesis through membrane-mediated pathways such as the transport of cations, amino acids, and macromolecules (215). Relatively low hydrostatic pressures (0.006 MPa) have been shown to inhibit the accumulation of cyclic adenosine 3′,5′-monophosphate (cAMP) in isolated chick epiphyseal chondrocytes through a mechanism involving the uptake of calcium ion (Ca^{2+}) (16), and it was hypothesized that these effects were regulated through pressure-induced changes in the structure of various membrane components. It has also been suggested that hydrostatic pressure may alter the action of the membrane Na^+/K^+ pump, thus altering intracellular K^+ concentrations (215). This hypothesis is supported by the finding that hydrostatic pressure has a direct effect on the transmembrane potential of chondrocytes (229). Continuous and low-frequency (<0.08 Hz) pressures of 120 mm Hg (0.016 MPa) caused membrane depolarization in chondrocytes, whereas higher frequency compression (0.33 Hz) significantly increased membrane resting potentials. Both Ca^{2+}-dependent K^+ channels and Na^+ channels were involved in these responses.

In addition to these membrane-related effects, there is evidence for involvement of the cytoskeleton in chondrocyte response to hydrostatic pressure (163,229), although separation of membrane and cytoskeletal effects is difficult because of the interactions between these components. Treatment with cytochalasin B, which disrupts actin microfilaments, abolished pressure-induced hyperpolarization of the chondrocyte membrane, suggesting that the actin cytoskeleton is involved in this

phenomenon (229). Continuous pressures of up to 30 MPa alter the organization of stress fibers, microtubules, and the Golgi apparatus in isolated chondrocytes. Treatment with nocodazole, which inhibits microtubule assembly, has been shown to block pressure-induced alterations of the Golgi apparatus (164). Considering that the extracellular matrix may influence cytoskeletal function (196), differences in chondrocyte shape and cytoskeletal structure may explain the differential response of isolated chondrocytes and explants to hydrostatic pressure (161,215).

Fluid Transport

One mechanism by which joint loading may regulate chondrocyte metabolism is through the induction of interstitial fluid flow. Cyclic and intermittent loading of articular cartilage produce spatial gradients in the hydrostatic fluid pressure within the cartilage matrix, resulting in convective transport and redistribution of the interstitial fluid phase. In explant models, physiological frequencies of compression can generate interstitial fluid flow velocities that are predicted to be in excess of 1 μm/sec (69,94,199). These velocities may be one to two orders of magnitude higher during joint contact and sliding (7) or in degenerative cartilage (191), although little is known regarding actual interstitial flow velocities *in vivo*.

Fluid flow within cartilage may modulate chondrocyte activity by accelerating the transport of solutes and macromolecules that regulate cartilage metabolism. Although the nutrition to the chondrocytes is achieved primarily through diffusion mechanisms, many essential macromolecules exhibit a very low diffusivity within cartilage relative to that in free solution (128,129,153). In addition, macromolecules more massive than several kilodaltons are largely excluded from partitioning into cartilage because of the small "effective pore size" of the extracellular matrix (131, 132). This apparent pore size may be decreased even further in response to matrix deformations that increase the solid volume fraction (e.g., compression) (144–146). In addition, changes in fixed charge density with matrix deformation may affect the diffusion properties, partition coefficients, or matrix permeabilities for select solutes (59,60,107, 108,128,132). Macromolecules that may be affected through such mechanisms and that are important to chondrocyte metabolism include a number of polypeptide growth factors such as insulin-like growth factor I (135,140).

There is little evidence that these factors play a role in transport of small solutes and nutrient molecules, as they diffuse rapidly through the cartilage matrix and are unaffected by matrix loading (128–130,132,189, 209). For these reasons, convective transport associated with time-varying or cyclic loading of articular cartilage may affect chondrocyte metabolism by enhancing the transport of larger molecules (e.g., growth factors, cytokines, or enzymes), as has been demonstrated experimentally (30,153).

In addition, fluid flow may alter chondrocyte metabolism by directly exerting shear stresses on the chondrocyte membrane. This mechanism of cellular signal transduction has been studied extensively in other cells (32,46,149), but there are few studies that report direct evidence of shear stress effects on chondrocytes. In recent studies, shear stresses of 1.6 Pa applied to human chondrocytes in monolayer with a cone-on-plate viscometer caused cellular alignment with the direction of flow and induced a significant elevation of mRNA levels of tissue inhibitor of metalloproteinase (197). Fluid-induced shear also stimulated aggrecan synthesis twofold and increased the length of newly synthesized chains. These findings imply that fluid flow, in and of itself, can modulate chondrocyte activity. An important question that remains is the process by which shear stresses interact at the cellular and intracellular levels to invoke these observed changes.

Electromechanical Transduction

Another physical mechanism by which loading may regulate chondrocyte activity is through mechanical-to-electric transduction phenomena that occur naturally within cartilage. As a result of the negatively charged nature of the cartilage solid matrix, nonuniform deformations in response to applied loads will give rise to gradients in both fluid pressure and ionic composition. Interstitial fluid and ion fluxes will result, with associated electrokinetic phenomena such as streaming potentials and streaming currents (10,48,56,59,122,128, 132). These effects arise from the flow of mobile cations and anions relative to the negative charge groups on the glycosaminoglycans in cartilage, which are restrained from flow by their large size and physical and chemical interactions with the solid matrix. Other examples of electrokinetic phenomena that occur in articular cartilage are mechanical stresses in response to an applied current density (i.e., current-generated stress) and electroosmosis (48). Theoretical models have been developed to describe these phenomena in a variety of experimental geometries and to relate the measured potentials to the charged proteoglycan components of the tissue (41,47,49,59, 60,114,128). The streaming potential of cartilage tissue may be modulated by alterations in the proteoglycan content that result, for example, from enzymatic digestion, modulation of chondrocyte metabolism, or cartilage compression (15,27,50,59; see also Chapter 4).

Although the magnitude and frequency of the electric fields within articular cartilage have not been directly measured *in vivo*, estimates of these field quantities have been made. Peak streaming potentials of 15 mV have been predicted based on estimates of applied loading encountered during normal walking (79,80,132). The spatial gradient in electric potential and the corresponding magnitude of local electric fields are more difficult to estimate, as they would depend on the geometry of the cartilage layer and boundary conditions during joint loading *in vivo* (27, 49,59). However, electric field strengths of up to 1500 V/m and current densities of 100 mA/cm^2 have been estimated to occur in cartilage during loading (47,76,128). Based on more conservative estimates of fluid flow *in vivo*, current densities of 0.1 to 1 mA/cm^2 have also been predicted (180). Estimates of the magnitude and frequency of electric fields that occur naturally within articular cartilage provide a framework for examining the role of electric fields in modulating cartilage metabolism. Because these phenomena are directly related to the magnitude of the interstitial fluid velocity (49,58,60,107), there is some indirect evidence supporting their involvement in elevating biosynthetic activity during cyclic loading (97,115). In addition to flow-mediated electrokinetic effects, several studies have provided evidence that low-level electric fields can directly influence chondrocyte activity (1,21,115,124,152,174). Possible mechanisms through which these fields interact with chondrocytes include gating of voltage-dependent ion channels, hyper- or hypopopolarization of the membrane, or, in some cases, thermal effects.

INTRACELLULAR SIGNALING PATHWAYS

To affect chondrocyte activity and gene expression, all potential physical signals described above must be transduced across the cell membrane to an intracellular biochemical signal. The chondrocyte plasma membrane is the host of numerous receptors, adhesion molecules, and ion channels and thus serves as a critical component of cellular function (121, 184,200,211,224). Hence, it is not surprising that the chondrocyte membrane is apparently involved in multiple physical signaling pathways, including osmotic and ionic changes, cell deformation, and hydrostatic pressure. In this section, we describe a variety of signaling pathways that have been studied in chondrocytes and are potentially involved in the process of transducing physical signals (Fig. 7).

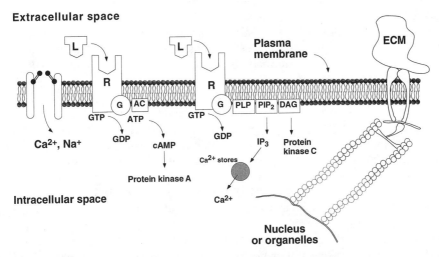

FIG. 7. Potential signaling pathways by which physical factors may be transduced into an intracellular signal. Intracellular signaling may be occurring through one or more of the traditional second messenger systems such as the adenylate cyclase/cAMP system, the IP$_3$ system, or the Ca^{2+} system. The concentrations of these intracellular messengers may be modulated by gating of membrane ion channels (e.g., voltage-activated or stretch-activated channels) or by a G-protein pathway that leads to increased levels of cytosolic cAMP or IP$_3$. Alternatively, transmembrane signaling may be occuring through a direct link between extracellular matrix molecules and intracellular organelles through membrane-spanning molecules (i.e., integrins). R, receptor; G, G protein; AC, adenylate cyclase; GDP, GTP, guanosine 5′-di- or triphosphate; ATP, adenosine triphosphate; cAMP, cyclic adenosine 3′,5′-monophosphate; IP$_3$, inositol triphosphate; DAG, diacylglycerol; PIP$_2$, phosphoinositol phosphate; PLP, phospholipase C.

The plasma membrane in all cells seems to be critical to the transduction of cell deformation and volume change, possibly through mechanosensitive or "stretch-activated" ion channels (141,178). These channels are defined as ion transport pathways whose gating characteristics are dependent on stretch of the plasma membrane (61). By activating or inactivating these channels, cellular deformation or volume change could directly regulate specific ion transport pathways, which could conceivably affect second messenger activity or membrane potential (12,28,178,188,225). Recent studies provide indirect evidence that chondrocytes possess stretch-activated ion channels (228). Furthermore, direct perturbation of the chondrocyte membrane has been shown to cause a rapid increase in the concentration of cytosolic calcium ion ($[Ca^{2+}]_i$) (63), an intracellular second messenger. Stretch-activated ion-channel blockers such as gadolinium or amiloride significantly attenuated the peak increase of fluorescence in deformed cells, suggesting that this calcium signaling was regulated through stretch of the chondrocyte membrane. These findings provide support for the hypothesis that chondrocytes have the ability to transduce isolated deformations in the absence of other matrix-related effects.

Alternatively, chondrocytes may be responding to extracellular matrix deformation by sensing apparent changes in local tissue composition through plasma membrane binding proteins (receptors) for specific macromolecules, such as hyaluronic acid (hyaluronan), aggrecan, collagen, or fibronectin (121, 184,211,224). Changes in the local concentrations or conformations of these molecules through consolidation of the extracellular matrix could significantly affect the kinetics of ligand–receptor binding and ultimately influence cell activity through intracellular second messengers.

These membrane-related phenomena support the involvement of the traditional second messenger pathways and transmembrane enzymatic mechanisms such as the adenylate cyclase system, the inositol triphosphate system, and cytosolic calcium (Fig. 7; see 201 for a review). The transport of even a relatively small number of ions may have a substantial biological effect through second messengers such as cAMP or Ca^{2+}. These messengers could affect levels of protein kinase A or phospholipase C and, subsequently, inositol phosphate metabolism. This would result in the mobilization of Ca^{2+} from intracellular stores and the activation of protein kinase C, affecting phosphorylation of cytosolic proteins.

These pathways appear to be involved in the chondrocyte mechanical signal transduction cascade (201). Calcium is a nearly ubiquitous regulator of cell metabolism and is involved in the control of a large number of cellular functions (24,172). In chondrocytes, it has been suggested that an increase in $[Ca^{2+}]_i$ may initiate matrix vesicle biogenesis (84,175), alter type I and type II collagen ratios (35), and affect proteoglycan synthesis rates (29,39,40,150).

Cyclic AMP, which has been identified as an important mediator of proteoglycan synthesis and cartilage growth (37,139), also seems to play a direct role in the mechanical stimulation of matrix biosynthesis. Constant hydrostatic pressures that inhibit proteoglycan synthesis also inhibit cAMP accumulation through a calcium-mediated process (16,152). Conversely, mechanical factors that increase cAMP levels also seem to increase proteoglycan synthesis rates. For example, intermittent hydrostatic pressures in chondrocyte cell culture systems result in concurrent increases in both cAMP and proteoglycan synthesis rates (219), and continuous tension of chondrocytes causes a rapid increase of cAMP levels (210).

It is important to note that the ultimate second messenger response to mechanical stimuli may be a result of the interaction of multiple signal transduction pathways. For example, cAMP accumulation can be decreased by increased $[Ca^{2+}]_i$ (17), and IP₃ is an important mediator of cytosolic Ca^{2+} release from intracellular stores (138,169). Such signal "cross talk" may include interaction of the adenylate cyclase/cAMP and Ca^{2+} or IP₃ and Ca^{2+} pathways (85,230).

Alternatively, mechanical and physical signaling may be occurring through a transmembrane pathway that bypasses the traditional second messenger cascades. One hypothesis proposes that normal cellular activity and mechanical signal transduction are regulated by a physical connection from intracellular organelles to the extracellular matrix via the cytoskeleton and the proteins of the adhesion plaque (e.g., α-actinin, vinculin, talin) (12,86, 165). The connection between the extracellular matrix and the cytoskeleton is believed to occur through the integrins, a family of membrane-spanning heterodimeric glycoproteins (82). Chondrocytes show strong expression of the β1 and α5 integrin subunits, which mediate cellular attachment to extracellular collagen and fibronectin (121,184). This molecular link provides a physical pathway through which changes in the extracellular mechanical environment could directly alter the shape or structure of the cell nucleus or other organelles (86,166). The direct influence of mechanical forces on nuclear function is not known, although hypothetically, mechanical

signals from the extracellular matrix could modulate nuclear function (e.g., gene expression, mitosis) in a manner that bypasses or complements traditional second messenger systems. For example, direct deformation of the nucleus may be responsible for distortion of nuclear pores and therefore alter the transport of molecules responsible for cell cycling (72). This hypothesis is supported indirectly by the finding that the chondrocyte nucleus is deformed within the cartilage extracellular matrix (62) (Fig. 8).

SUMMARY AND CONCLUSIONS

It is evident that the process of mechanical signal transduction in cartilage involves a complex sequence of mechanical and biochemical processes. Many other detailed studies must be performed before we fully understand the process of mechanical signal transduction in cartilage. In regard to the effects of physical factors on chondrocyte activity, consistent findings among different stud-

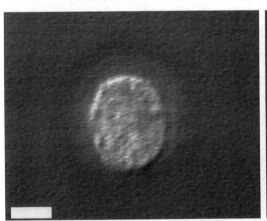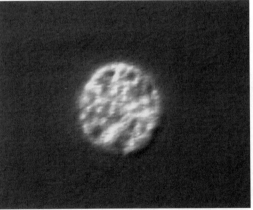

FIG. 8. Digitally enhanced confocal microscopy section through the center of a chondrocyte nucleus *in situ* before **(left)** and after **(right)** 15% compression of the extracellular matrix. Chondrocyte nuclei were stained with acridine orange, and a three-dimensional volume image of the cells and nuclei was recorded before and after application of compression. A 15% surface-to-surface tissue compression resulted in nuclear height and volume decreases of 9% and 10%, respectively, as well as significant changes in nuclear shape. Pretreatment of the tissue with cytochalasin D to disrupt actin microfilament altered the relationship between matrix compression and nuclear height and shape changes but not volume changes, suggesting that osmotic effects may play a role in the observed cell and nuclear volume changes. Scale bar, 3 μm.

ies and model systems suggest the following conclusions:

- The mechanical environment of the chondrocyte plays an important role in the health and function of the diarthrodial joint *in vivo*. Significant deviations from the normal pattern of joint loading result in deleterious and often irreversible changes in the articular cartilage and surrounding tissues.
- Under normal physiological conditions, the chondrocyte population is exposed to changes in the mechanical, physicochemical, and electric environment of the extracellular matrix, resulting in spatial and temporal variations in stress, strain, fluid flow, fluid pressure, osmotic pressure, fixed charge density, pH, and electric field effects within the cartilage extracellular matrix. These physical phenomena have the potential to activate multiple cellular signaling pathways.
- Static compression of articular cartilage results in a suppression of biosynthesis. This effect is presumed to be related to the changes in the physicochemical environment of the chondrocytes in response to matrix deformation, such as osmotic pressure and intratissue pH and/or changes in cell shape. Cyclic or intermittent compression of articular cartilage or chondrocytes *in vitro* significantly increases biosynthetic activity. Indirect evidence suggests that this stimulatory effect is related to factors involving interstitial fluid and ion flows in response to gradients in the mechanical stress–strain field. These factors include enhanced nutrient transport, flow-induced shear stresses, and electrokinetic signals such as streaming potentials.
- Static and intermittent hydrostatic pressure can affect chondrocyte activity in a manner that is dependent on several factors such as the duration, magnitude, and frequency of loading.
- Externally applied electric fields can affect chondrocyte activity, supporting the notion that mechanically induced electric fields *in vivo* may play a role in the process of mechanical signal transduction.
- Cellular shape and volume change in response to extracellular matrix deformation or volumetric changes may affect biosynthesis. Deformations may be transduced to the cell through several different signaling mechanisms, including stretch-activated ion channels on the cell membrane or through a physical link between the extracellular matrix and the cytoskeleton. The plasma membrane is also likely to be involved in the transduction of hydrostatic pressure, osmotic and ionic changes, and extracellular matrix composition. Intracellular signaling in these cases seems to be occurring through transmembrane enzymatic and second messenger pathways (i.e., Ca^{2+}, IP_3, cAMP).

Acknowledgments

The authors would like to acknowledge the support of The Arthritis Foundation (R.L. Sah), The Lord Foundation (L.A. Setton), the Musculoskeletal Transplant Foundation (F. Guilak), The National Institutes of Health (R.L. Sah), The National Science Foundation (R.L. Sah, L.A. Setton), The Whitaker Foundation (F. Guilak, L.A. Setton, R.L. Sah), and the Miami Department of Veteran's Affairs (L.A. Setton). The authors would like to thank Dr. Martha L. Gray for her insightful comments and critical reading of the manuscript.

REFERENCES

1. Aaron, R. K., and Ciombor, D. M. (1993): Enhancement of extracellular matrix synthesis in cartilage explant cultures by exposure to an electric field. *Trans. Orthop. Res. Soc.,* 18:630.
2. Altman, R. D., Tenenbaum, J., Latta, L., Riskin, W., Blanco, L. N., and Howell, D. S. (1984): Biomechanical and biochemical properties of dog cartilage in experimentally induced osteoarthritis. *Ann. Rheum. Dis.,* 43:83–90.
3. Armstrong, C. G., Lai, W. M., and Mow, V. C. (1984): An analysis of the unconfined compression of articular cartilage. *J. Biomech. Eng.,* 106:165–173.
4. Armstrong, C. G., and Mow, V. C. (1982): Variations in the intrinsic mechanical properties of human articular

cartilage with age, degeneration, and water content. *J. Bone Joint Surg. Am.,* 64:88–94.

5. Armstrong, C. G., Mow, V. C., and Wirth, C. R. (1985): Biomechanics of impact-induced microdamage to articular cartilage: A possible genesis for chondromalacia patella. In: *AAOS Symposium on Sports Medicine: The Knee,* edited by G. Finerman, pp. 70–84. W.B. Saunders, St. Louis.

6. Arnoczky, S. P., Warren, R. F., and Kaplan, N. (1985): Meniscal remodeling following partial meniscectomy—an experimental study in the dog. *Arthroscopy,* 1:247–252.

7. Ateshian, G. A., Lai, W. M., Zhu, W. B., and Mow, V. C. (1994): An asymptotic solution for the contact of two biphasic cartilage layers. *J. Biomech.,* 27:1347–1360.

8. Bachrach, N. M., Mow, V. C., and Guilak, F. (1997): The response of articular cartilage to hydrostatic pressure. *J. Biomech.* (in press).

9. Bachrach, N. M., Valhmu, W. B., Stazzone, E., Ratcliffe, A., Lai, W. M., and Mow, V. C. (1995): Changes in proteoglycan synthesis of chondrocytes in articular cartilage are associated with the time-dependent changes in their mechanical environment. *J. Biomech.,* 28:1561–1570.

10. Bassett, C. A., and Pawluk, R. J. (1972): Electrical behavior of cartilage during loading. *Science,* 178:982–983.

11. Behrens, F., Kraft, E., and Oegema, T. (1989): Biochemical changes in articular cartilage after joint immobilization by casting and external fixation. *J. Orthop. Res.,* 7:335–343.

12. Ben-Ze'ev, A. (1991): Animal cell shape changes and gene expression. *Bioessays,* 13:207–212.

13. Benya, P. D., and Shaffer, J. D. (1982): Dedifferentiated chondrocytes reexpress the differentiated collagen phenotype when cultured in agarose gels. *Cell,* 30:215–224.

14. Berjon, J. J., Munera, L., and Calvo, M. (1991): Degenerative lesions in articular cartilage after meniscectomy. *J. Traumatol.,* 31:342–350.

15. Bonassar, L. J., Frank, E. H., Murray, J. C., Paguio, C. G., Moore, V. L., Lark, M. W., Sandy, J. D., Wu, J. J., Eyre, D. R., and Grodzinsky, A. J. (1995): Changes in cartilage composition and physical properties due to stromelysin degradation. *Arthritis Rheum.,* 38:173–183.

16. Bourret, L. A., and Rodan, G. A. (1976): Inhibition of cAMP accumulation in epiphyseal cartilage cells exposed to physiological pressure. *Calcif. Tissue Res.,* 21:431–436.

17. Bourret, L. A., and Rodan, G. A. (1976): The role of calcium in the inhibition of cAMP accumulation in epiphyseal cartilage cells exposed to physiological pressure. *J. Cell. Physiol.,* 88:353–361.

18. Boustany, N. N., Gray, M. L., Black, A. C., and Hunziker, E. B. (1995): Correlation between synthetic activity and glycosaminoglycan concentration in epiphyseal cartilage raises questions about the regulatory role of interstitial pH. *J. Orthop. Res.,* 13:733–739.

19. Boustany, N. N., Gray, M. L., Black, A. C., and Hunziker, E. B. (1995): Time-dependent changes in the response of cartilage to static compression suggest interstitial pH is not the only signaling mechanism. *J. Orthop. Res.,* 13:740–750.

20. Brandt, K. D., Myers, S. L., Burr, D., and Albrecht, M. (1991): Osteoarthritic changes in canine articular cartilage, subchondral bone, and synovium fifty-four months after transection of the anterior cruciate ligament. *Arthritis Rheum.,* 34:1560–1570.

21. Brighton, C. T., Unger, A. S., and Stambough, J. L. (1984): *In vitro* growth of bovine articular cartilage chondrocytes in various capacitively coupled electrical fields. *J. Orthop. Res.,* 2:15–22.

22. Burton-Wurster, N., Vernier-Singer, M., Farquhar, T., and Lust, G. (1993): Effect of compressive loading and unloading on the synthesis of total protein, proteoglycan, and fibronectin by canine cartilage explants. *J. Orthop. Res.,* 11:717–729.

23. Buschmann, M. D., Gluzband, Y. A., Grodzinsky, A. J., and Hunziker, E. B. (1995): Mechanical compression modulates matrix biosynthesis in chondrocyte/agarose culture. *J. Cell Sci.,* 108:1497–1508.

24. Carafoli, E. (1987): Intracellular calcium homeostasis. *Annu. Rev. Biochem.,* 56:395–433.

25. Carney, S. L., Billingham, M. E., Muir, H., and Sandy, J. D. (1984): Demonstration of increased proteoglycan turnover in cartilage explants from dogs with experimental osteoarthritis. *J. Orthop. Res.,* 2:201–206.

26. Caterson, B., and Lowther, D. A. (1978): Changes in the metabolism of the proteoglycans from sheep articular cartilage in response to mechanical stress. *Biochim. Biophys. Acta,* 540:412–422.

27. Chen, A., Nguyen, T., and Sah, R. (1995): Streaming potentials in normal and degraded articular cartilage. *Trans. Orthop. Res. Soc.,* 20:336.

28. Christensen, O. (1987): Mediation of cell volume by Ca^{2+} influx through stretch–activated channels. *Nature,* 330:66–68.

29. Clark, C. C., Iannotti, J. P., Misra, S., and Richards, C. F. (1994): Effects of thapsigargin, an intracellular calcium-mobilizing agent, on synthesis and secretion of cartilage collagen and proteoglycan. *J. Orthop. Res.,* 12:601–611.

30. Cohen, S., Snir, E., Schneiderman, R., and Maroudas, A. (1993): Solute transport in cartilage: Effect of static compression. *Trans. Orthop. Res. Soc.,* 18:622.

31. Cruveilhier, J. (1824): Observations sur les cartilages diarthrodiaux et les maladies des articulations diarthrodiales. *Arch. Gen. Med. (Paris),* 4:161–198.

32. Davies, P. F., and Tripathi, S. C. (1993): Mechanical stress mechanisms and the cell. An endothelial paradigm. *Circ. Res.,* 72:239–245.

33. De Witt, M. T., Handley, C. J., Oakes, B. W., and Lowther, D. A. (1984): *In vitro* response of chondrocytes to mechanical loading. The effect of short term mechanical tension. *Connect. Tissue Res.,* 12:97–109.

34. Deshayes, C. M. P., Hall, A. C., and Urban, J. P. G. (1993): Effects of extracellular osmolality on porcine articular chondrocyte volume. *J. Physiol. (Lond.),* 467:214P.

35. Deshmukh, K., Kline, W. G., and Sawyer, B. D. (1976): Role of calcium in the phenotypic expression of rabbit articular chondrocytes in culture. *FEBS Lett.,* 67:48–51.

36. Donohue, J. M., Buss, D., Oegema, T. R., Jr., and Thompson, R. C., Jr. (1983): The effects of indirect blunt trauma on adult canine articular cartilage. *J. Bone Joint Surg. Am.,* 65:948–957.

37. Drezner, M. K., Neelon, F. A., and Lebovitz, H. E. (1976): Stimulation of cartilage macromolecule synthesis by adenosine 3′,5′-monophosphate. *Biochim. Biophys. Acta,* 425:521–531.

38. Dunham, J., Shackleton, D., Nahir, A., Billingham, M., Bitensky, L., Chayen, J., and Muir, H. (1985): Altered orientation of glycosamnoglycans and cellular changes in the tibial cartilage in the first two weeks of experimental osteoarthritis. *J. Orthop. Res.,* 3:258–268.
39. Eilam, Y., Beit-Or, A., and Nevo, Z. (1985): Decrease in cytosolic free Ca²⁺ and enhanced proteoglycan synthesis induced by cartilage derived growth factors in cultured chondrocytes. *Biochem. Biophys. Res. Commun.,* 132:770–779.
40. Eilam, Y., Beit-Or, A., and Nevo, Z. (1987): Cytosolic free Ca++ as a signal for proteoglycan synthesis and cell proliferation in cultured chondrocytes. In: *Current Advances in Skeletogenesis,* edited by S. Horowitz and I. Sela, pp. 127–139. Heiliger, Jerusalem.
41. Eisenberg, S., and Grodzinsky, A. (1988): Electrokinetic micromodel of extracellular matrix and other polyelectrolyte networks. *Physicochem. Hydrodynam.,* 10:517–530.
42. Elliott, D. M., Setton, L. A., Shah, M. P., Vail, T. P., and Guilak, F. (1996): Effects of meniscectomy on the tensile properties of articular cartilage. *ASME Adv. Bioeng.,* BED-33:247–248.
43. Eyre, D., McDevitt, C., Billingham, M., and Muir, H. (1980): Biosynthesis of collagen and other matrix proteins by articular cartilage in experimental osteoarthrosis. *Biochem. J.,* 188:823–837.
44. Fairbank, T. J. (1948): Knee joint changes after meniscectomy. *J. Bone Joint Surg.,* 30B:664–670.
45. Floman, Y., Eyre, D. R., and Glimcher, M. J. (1980): Induction of osteoarthrosis in the rabbit knee joint: biochemical studies on the articular cartilage. *Clin. Orthop.,* 143:278–286.
46. Frangos, J. A., Eskin, S. G., McIntire, L. V., and Ives, C. L. (1985): Flow effects on prostacyclin production by cultured human endothelial cells. *Science,* 227: 1477–1479.
47. Frank, E., Grodzinsky, A., Phillips, S., and Grimshaw, P. (1990): Physicochemical and bioelectrical determinants of cartilage material properties. In: *Biomechanics of Diarthrodial Joints,* edited by V. C. Mow, A. Ratcliffe, and S. L. Y. Woo, pp. 261–282. Springer Verlag, New York.
48. Frank, E. H., and Grodzinsky, A. J. (1987): Cartilage electromechanics—I. Electrokinetic transduction and the effects of electrolyte pH and ionic strength. *J. Biomech.,* 20:615–627.
49. Frank, E. H., and Grodzinsky, A. J. (1987): Cartilage electromechanics—II. A continuum model of cartilage electrokinetics and correlation with experiments. *J. Biomech.,* 20:629–639.
50. Frank, E. H., Grodzinsky, A. J., Koob, T. J., and Eyre, D. R. (1987): Streaming potentials: a sensitive index of enzymatic degradation in articular cartilage. *J. Orthop. Res.,* 5:497–508.
51. Freeman, P. M., Natarjan, R. N., Kimura, J. H., and Andriacchi, T. P. (1994): Chondrocyte cells respond mechanically to compressive loads. *J. Orthop. Res.,* 12:311–320.
52. Gilbertson, E. M. M. (1975): Development of periarticular osteophytes in experimentally induced osteoarthrosis in the dog. *Ann. Rheum. Dis.,* 34:12–25.
53. Gray, M. L., Pizzanelli, A. M., Grodzinsky, A. J., and Lee, R. C. (1988): Mechanical and physiochemical determinants of the chondrocyte biosynthetic response. *J. Orthop. Res.,* 6:777–792.
54. Gray, M. L., Pizzanelli, A. M., Lee, R. C., Grodzinsky, A. J., and Swann, D. A. (1989): Kinetics of the chondrocyte biosynthetic response to compressive load and release. *Biochim. Biophys. Acta,* 991:415–425.
55. Grodzinsky, A. J. (1983): Electromechanical and physicochemical properties of connective tissue. *Crit. Rev. Biomed. Eng.,* 9:133–199.
56. Grodzinsky, A. J., Lipshitz, H., and Glimcher, M. J. (1978): Electromechanical properties of articular cartilage during compression and stress relaxation. *Nature,* 275:448–450.
57. Grumbles, R. M., Howell, D. S., Howard, G. A., Roos, B. A., Setton, L. A., Mow, V. C., Ratcliffe, A., Müller, F. J., and Altman, R. D. (1995): Cartilage metalloproteases in disuse atrophy. *J. Rheumatol. [Suppl.],* 43:146–148.
58. Gu, W., Lai, W. M., and Mow, V. C. (1993): Theoretical basis for measurements of cartilage fixed-charge density using streaming current and electro-osmosis effects. *ASME Adv. Bioeng.,* 26:55–58.
59. Gu, W. Y., Lai, W. M., and Mow, V. C. (1993): Transport of fluid and ions through a porous-permeable charged-hydrated tissue, and streaming potential data on normal bovine articular cartilage. *J. Biomech.,* 26: 709–723.
60. Gu, W. Y., Rabin, J., Lai, W. M., and Mow, V. C. (1995): Measurement of streaming potential of bovine articular and nasal cartilage in 1-D permeation experiments. *ASME Adv. Bioeng.,* BED31:49–50.
61. Guharay, F., and Sachs, F. (1984): Stretch-activated single ion channel currents in tissue-cultured embryonic chick skeletal muscle. *J. Physiol. (Lond.),* 352:685–701.
62. Guilak, F. (1995): Compression-induced changes in the shape and volume of the chondrocyte nucleus. *J. Biomech.,* 28:1529–1542.
63. Guilak, F., Donahue, H. J., Zell, R., Grande, D. A., McLeod, K. J., and Rubin, C. T. (1994): Deformation-induced calcium signaling in articular chondrocytes. In: *Cell Mechanics and Cellular Engineering,* edited by V. C. Mow, F. Guilak, R. Tran-Son-Tay, and R. M. Hochmuth, pp. 380–397. Springer Verlag, New York.
64. Guilak, F., Hou, J. S., Ratcliffe, A., and Mow, V. C. (1988): Articular cartilage under hydrostatic loading. *ASME Adv. Bioeng.,* BED-8:183–186.
65. Guilak, F., Meyer, B. C., Ratcliffe, A., and Mow, V. C. (1994): The effects of matrix compression on proteoglycan metabolism in articular cartilage explants. *Osteoarthritis Cartilage,* 2:91–101.
66. Guilak, F., and Mow, V. C. (1992): Determination of chondrocyte mechanical environment using finite element modeling and confocal microscopy. *ASME Adv. Bioeng.,* BED-20:21–23.
67. Guilak, F., Ratcliffe, A., Lane, N., Rosenwasser, M. P., and Mow, V. C. (1994): Mechanical and biochemical changes in the superficial zone of articular cartilage in canine experimental osteoarthritis. *J. Orthop. Res.,* 12: 474–484.
68. Guilak, F., Ratcliffe, A., and Mow, V. C. (1995): Chondrocyte deformation and local tissue strain in articular cartilage: a confocal microscopy study. *J. Orthop. Res.,* 13:410–421.
69. Guilak, F., Spilker, R. L., Suh, J. K., and Mow, V. C. (1997): A biphasic finite element model of the mechanical response of articular cartilage to cyclic compression. *J. Biomech. Eng.* (in press).

70. Hall, A. C., Urban, J. P., and Gehl, K. A. (1991): The effects of hydrostatic pressure on matrix synthesis in articular cartilage. *J. Orthop. Res.,* 9:1–10.
71. Handley, C. J., and Lowther, D. A. (1977): Extracellular metabolism by chondrocytes. III. Modulation of proteoglycan synthesis by extracellular levels of proteoglycan in cartilage cells in culture. *Biochim. Biophys. Acta,* 500:132–139.
72. Hansen, L. K., and Ingber, D. E. (1992): Regulation of nucleocytoplasmic transport by mechanical forces transmitted through the cytoskeleton. In: *Nuclear Trafficking,* edited by C. Feldher, pp. 71–86. Academic Press, San Diego.
73. Hardingham, T. E., Fitton-Jackson, S., and Muir, H. (1972): Replacement of proteoglycans in embryonic chicken cartilage in organ culture after treatment with testicular hyaluronidase. *Biochem. J.,* 129:101–112.
74. Hardingham, T. E., Fosang, A. J., and Dudhia, J. (1992): Aggrecan: the chondroitin sulfate/keratan sulfate proteoglycan from cartilage. In: *Articular Cartilage and Osteoarthritis,* edited by K. E. Kuettner, R. Schleyerbach, J. G. Peyron, and V. C. Hascall, pp. 5–20. Raven Press, New York.
75. Hascall, V., Handley, C., McQuillan, D., Hascall, G., Robinson, H., and Lowther, D. (1983): The effect of serum on biosynthesis of proteoglycans by bovine articular cartilage in culture. *Arch. Biochem. Biophys.,* 224:206–223.
76. Hasegawa, I., Kuriki, S., Matsuno, S., and Matsumoto, G. (1983): Dependence of electrical conductivity on fixed charge density in articular cartilage. *Clin. Orthop.,* 177:283–288.
77. Helminen, H. J., Jurvelin, J., Kiviranta, I., Paukkonen, K., Saamanen, A. M., and Tammi, M. (1987): Joint loading effects on articular cartilage: A historical review. In: *Joint Loading: Biology and Health of Articular Structures,* edited by H. J. Helminen, I. Kiviranta, M. Tammi, A. M. K. P. Saamanen, and J. Jurvelin, pp. 1–46. Wright and Sons, Bristol.
78. Hoch, D. H., Grodzinsky, A. J., Koob, T. J., Albert, M. L., and Eyre, D. R. (1983): Early changes in material properties of rabbit articular cartilage after meniscectomy. *J. Orthop. Res.,* 1:4–12.
79. Hodge, W., Fijan, R., Carlson, K., Burgess, R., Harris, W., and Mann, R. (1986): Contact pressures in the human hip joint measured *in vivo. Proc. Natl. Acad. Sci. USA,* 83:2879–2883.
80. Hodge, W. A., Carlson, K. L., Fijan, R. S., Burgess, R. G., Riley, P. O., Harris, W. H., and R.W. M. (1989): Contact pressures from an instrumented hip endoprosthesis. *J. Bone Joint Surg.,* 71A:1378–1386.
81. Holzer, H., Abbot, J., Lash, J., and Holzer, A. (1960): The loss of phenotypic traits by differentiated cells *in vitro.* I. Dedifferentiation of cartilage cells. *Proc. Natl. Acad. Sci. USA,* 46:1533–1542.
82. Hynes, R. O. (1987): Integrins, a family of cell surface receptors. *Cell,* 48:549–554.
83. Iannacone, W. M., Pienkowski, D., Pollack, S. R., and Brighton, C. T. (1988): Pulsing electromagnetic field stimulation of the *in vitro* growth plate. *J. Orthop. Res.,* 6:239–247.
84. Iannotti, J. P., Naidu, S., Noguchi, Y., Hunt, R. M., and Brighton, C. T. (1994): Growth plate matrix vesicle biogenesis. The role of intracellular calcium. *Clin. Orthop.,* 306:222–229.
85. Iino, M., and Endo, M. (1992): Calcium-dependent immediate feedback control of inositol 1,4,5-triphosphate-induced Ca^{2+} release. *Nature,* 360:76–78.
86. Ingber, D. (1991): Integrins as mechanochemical transducers. *Curr. Opin. Cell Biol.,* 3:841–848.
87. Jackson, D. W., McDevitt, C. A., Simon T. M., Arnoczky S.P., Atwell, E.A., and Silvino, N.J. (1992): Meniscal transplantation using fresh and cryopreserved allografts. An experimental study in goats. *Am. J. Sports Med.,* 20:644–656.
88. Jones, I. L., Klamfeldt, A., and Sanstrom , T. (1982): The effect of continuous mechanical pressure upon the turnover of articular cartilage proteoglycans *in vitro. Clin. Orthop.,* 165:283–289.
89. Jurvelin, J., Helminen, H. J., Lauritsalo, S., Kiviranta, I., Saamanen, A. M., Paukkonen, K., and Tammi, M. (1985): Influences of joint immobilization and running exercise on articular cartilage surfaces of young rabbits. A semiquantitative stereomicroscopic and scanning electron microscopic study. *Acta Anat.,* 122: 62–68.
90. Jurvelin, J., Kiviranta, I., Saamanen, A. M., Tammi, M., and Helminen, H. J. (1989): Partial restoration of immobilization-induced softening of canine articular cartilage after remobilization of the knee (stifle) joint. *J. Orthop. Res.,* 7:352–358.
91. Jurvelin, J., Kiviranta, I., Saamanen, A. M., Tammi, M., and Helminen, H. J. (1990): Indentation stiffness of young canine knee articular cartilage—influence of strenuous joint loading. *J. Biomech.,* 23:1239–1246.
92. Jurvelin, J., Kiviranta, I., Tammi, M., and Helminen, H. J. (1986): Effect of physical exercise on indentation stiffness of articular cartilage in the canine knee. *Int. J. Sports Med.,* 7:106–110.
93. Kempson, G. E., Muir, H., Pollard, C., and Tuke, M. (1973): The tensile properties of the cartilage of human femoral condyles related to the content of collagen and glycosaminoglycans. *Biochim. Biophys. Acta,* 297:456–472.
94. Kim, Y. J., Bonassar, L. J., and Grodzinsky, A. J. (1995): The role of cartilage streaming potential, fluid flow and pressure in the stimulation of chondrocyte biosynthesis during dynamic compression. *J. Biomech.,* 28: 1055–1066.
95. Kim, Y. J., Grodzinsky, A. J., Plaas, A. H. K., and Sandy, J. D. (1992): The differential effects of static compression on synthesis of specific cartilage matrix components. *Trans. Orthop. Res. Soc.,* 17:108.
96. Kim, Y. J., Kung, S., Grodzinsky, A. J., Sandy, J. D., and Plaas, A. H. K. (1993): Effects of compression on cartilage link synthesis, aggrecan structure, and core-protein processing: cellular mechanisms. *Trans. Orthop. Res. Soc.,* 9:365.
97. Kim, Y. J., Sah, R. L., Grodzinsky, A. J., Plaas, A. H., and Sandy, J. D. (1994): Mechanical regulation of cartilage biosynthetic behavior: physical stimuli. *Arch. Biochem. Biophys.,* 311:1–12.
98. Kimura, J., Schipplein, O., Kuettner, K., and Andriacchi, T. (1985): Effects of hydrostatic loading on extracellular matrix formation. *Trans. Orthop. Res. Soc.,* 9:365.
99. King, D. (1936): The healing of semilunar cartilages. *J. Bone Joint Surg.,* 54A:349.
100. Kiviranta, I., Tammi, M., Jurvelin, J., Arokoski, J., Saamanen, A. M., and Helminen, H. J. (1992): Articular cartilage thickness and glycosaminoglycan distribution

in the canine knee joint after strenuous running exercise. *Clin. Orthop.,* :302–308.

101. Kiviranta, I., Tammi, M., Jurvelin, J., Arokoski, J., Saamanen, A. M., and Helminen, H. J. (1994): Articular cartilage thickness and glycosaminoglycan distribution in the young canine knee joint after remobilization of the immobilized limb. *J. Orthop. Res.,* 12:161–167.

102. Kiviranta, I., Tammi, M., Jurvelin, J., Saamanen, A. M., and Helminen, H. J. (1988): Moderate running exercise augments glycosaminoglycans and thickness of articular cartilage in the knee joint of young beagle dogs. *J. Orthop. Res.,* 6:188–195.

103. Klein-Nulend, J., Veldhuijzen, J. P., van de Stadt, R. J., van Kampen, G. P., Kuijer, R., and Burger, E. H. (1987): Influence of intermittent compressive force on proteoglycan content in calcifying growth plate cartilage *in vitro. J. Biol. Chem.,* 262:15490–15495.

104. Korver, T. H., van de Stadt, R. J., Kiljan, E., van Kampen, G. P., and van der Korst, J. K. (1992): Effects of loading on the synthesis of proteoglycans in different layers of anatomically intact articular cartilage *in vitro. J. Rheumatol.,* 19:905–912.

105. Kurosawa, H., Fukubayashi, T., and Nakajuma, H. (1980): Load-bearing mode of the knee joint: physical behavior of the knee joint with or without menisci. *Clin. Orthop.,* 149:283–290.

106. Lafeber, F., Veldhuijzen, J. P., Vanroy, J. L., Huber-Bruning, O., and Bijlsma, J. W. (1992): Intermittent hydrostatic compressive force stimulates exclusively the proteoglycan synthesis of osteoarthritic human cartilage. *Br. J. Rheumatol.,* 31:437–442.

107. Lai, W. M., Hou, J. S., and Mow, V. C. (1991): A triphasic theory for the swelling and deformation behaviors of articular cartilage. *J. Biomech. Eng.,* 113:245–258.

108. Lai, W. M., and Mow, V. C. (1980): Drag-induced compression of articular cartilage during a permeation experiment. *Biorheology,* 17:111–123.

109. Lai, W. M., Setton, L. A., and Mow, V. C. (1991): Conditional equivalence of chemical and mechanical loading on articular cartilage. *ASME Adv. Bioeng.,* BED18:481–484.

110. Lammi, M., Inkinen, R., Parkkinen, J., Hakkinen, T., Jortikka, M., Nelimarkka, L., Jarvelainen, H., and Tammi, M. (1994): Expression of reduced amounts of structurally altered aggrecan in articular cartilage chondrocytes exposed to high hydrostatic pressure. *Biochem. J.,* 304:723–730.

111. Lammi, M. J., Hakkinen, T. P., Parkkinen, J. J., Hyttinen, M. M., Jortikka, M., Helminen, H. J., and Tammi, M. I. (1993): Adaptation of canine femoral head articular cartilage to long distance running exercise in young beagles. *Ann. Rheum. Dis.,* 52:369–377.

112. Lane, J. M., Chisena, E., and Black, J. (1979): Experimental knee instability: Early mechanical property changes in articular cartilage in a rabbit model. *Clin. Orthop.,* 140:262–265.

113. Larsson, T., Aspden, R. M., and Heinegard, D. (1991): Effects of mechanical load on cartilage matrix biosynthesis *in vitro. Matrix,* 11:388–394.

114. Lee, R. C., Frank, E. H., Grodzinsky, A. J., and Roylance, D. K. (1981): Oscillatory compressional behavior of articular cartilage and its associated electromechanical properties. *J. Biomech. Eng.,* 103:280–292.

115. Lee, R. C., Rich, J. B., Kelley, K. M., Weiman, D. S., and Mathews, M. B. (1982): A comparison of *in vitro*

cellular responses to mechanical and electrical stimulation. *Am. Surg.,* 48:567–574.

116. Lefkoe, T. P., Trafton, P. G., Ehrlich, M. G., Walsh, W. R., Dennehy, D. T., Barrach, H. J., and Akelman, E. (1993): An experimental model of femoral condylar defect leading to osteoarthrosis. *J. Orthop. Trauma,* 7:458–467.

117. Lefkoe, T. P., Walsh, W. R., Anastasatos, J., Ehrlich, M. G., and Barrach, H. J. (1995): Remodeling of articular step-offs. Is osteoarthrosis dependent on defect size? *Clin. Orthop.,* 314:253–265.

118. Levy, I. M., Torzilli, P. A., and Fisch, I. D. (1992): The contribution of the menisci to the stability of the knee. In: *Knee Meniscus: Basic and Clinical Foundations,* edited by V. C. Mow, D. W. Jackson, and S. P. Arnoczky, pp. 107–115. Raven Press, New York.

119. Linn, F. C., and Sokoloff, L. (1965): Movement and composition of interstitial fluid of cartilage. *Arthritis Rheum.,* 8:481–494.

120. Lippiello, L., Kaye, C., Neumata, T., and Mankin, H. (1985): *In vitro* metabolic response of articular cartilage segments to low levels of hydrostatic pressure. *Connect. Tissue Res.,* 13:99–107.

121. Loeser, R. F. (1993): Integrin-mediated attachment of articular chondrocytes to extracellular matrix proteins. *Arthritis Rheum.,* 36:1103–1110.

122. Lotke, P., Black, J., and Richardson, S. (1974): Electromechanical properties in human articular cartilage. *J. Bone Joint Surg.,* 56A:1040–1046.

123. Lufti, A. M. (1975): Morphological changes in the articular cartilage after meniscectomy: An experimental study in the monkey. *J. Bone Joint Surg.,* 57B:525–528.

124. MacGinitie, L. A., Gluzband, Y. A., and Grodzinsky, A. J. (1994): Electric field stimulation can increase protein synthesis in articular cartilage explants. *J. Orthop. Res.,* 12:151–160.

125. Mallein-Gerin, F., Garrone, R., and van der Rest, M. (1991): Proteoglycan and collagen synthesis are correlated with actin organization in dedifferentiating chondrocytes. *Eur. J. Cell Biol.,* 56:364–373.

126. Manicourt, D. H., Thonar, E. J.-M., Pita, J. C., and Howell, D. S. (1989): Changes in the sedimentation profile of proteoglycan aggregates in early experimental canine osteoarthritis. *Connect. Tissue Res.,* 23:33–50.

127. Mankin, H. J., and Brandt, K. D. (1992): Biochemistry and metabolism of articular cartilage in osteoarthritis. In: *Osteoarthritis: Diagnosis and Medical/Surgical Management,* edited by R. W. Moskowitz, D. S. Howell, V. M. Goldberg, and H. J. Mankin, pp. 109–154. W.B. Saunders, Philadelphia.

128. Maroudas, A. (1968): Physicochemical properties of cartilage in the light of ion exchange theory. *Biophys. J.,* 8:575–595.

129. Maroudas, A. (1970): Distribution and diffusion of solutes in articular cartilage. *Biophys. J.,* 10:365–379.

130. Maroudas, A. (1972): Physical chemistry and the structure of cartilage. *J. Physiol. (Lond.),* 223:21P–22P.

131. Maroudas, A. (1973): Mechanisms of fluid transport in cartilaginous tissues. In: *Adult Articular Cartilage,* edited by M. Freeman, pp. 47–72. Pitman Medical, Tunbridge Wells.

132. Maroudas, A. (1979): Physicochemical properties of articular cartilage. In: *Adult Articular Cartilage,* edited by M. Freeman, pp. 215–290. Pitman Medical, Tunbridge Wells.

133. Maroudas, A. (1990): Determination of the rate of glycosaminoglycan synthesis *in vivo* using radioactive sulfate as tracer: comparison with *in vitro* results. In: *Methods in Cartilage Research,* edited by A. Maroudas and K. E. Kuettner, pp. 143–148. Academic Press, New York.

134. Maroudas, A., Palla, G., and Gilav, E. (1992): Racemization of aspartic acid in human articular cartilage. *Connect. Tissue Res.,* 28:161–169.

135. Maroudas, A., Popper, O., and Grushko, G. (1991): Partition coefficients of IGF-I between cartilage and external medium in the presence and absence of FCS. *Trans. Orthop. Res. Soc.,* 16:398.

136. McDevitt, C., Gilbertson, E., and Muir, H. (1977): An experimental model of osteoarthritis; early morphological and biochemical changes. *J. Bone Joint Surg.,* 59B:24–35.

137. McDevitt, C. A., and Muir, H. (1976): Biochemical changes in the cartilage of the knee in experimental and natural osteoarthritis in the dog. *J. Bone Joint Surg.,* 58B:94–101.

138. Meyer, T., Holowka, D., and Stryer, L. (1988): Highly cooperative opening of calcium channels by inositol 1,4,5-trisphosphate. *Science,* 240:653–656.

139. Miller, R. P., Husain, M., and Lohin, S. (1979): Long acting cAMP analogues enhance sulfate incorporation into matrix proteoglycans and suppress cell division of fetal rat chondrocytes in monolayer culture. *J. Cell. Physiol.,* 100:63–76.

140. Morales, T., and Hascall, V. (1989): Factors involved in the regulation of proteoglycan metabolism in articular cartilage. *Arthritis Rheum.,* 32:1197–1201.

141. Morris, C. E. (1990): Mechanosensitive ion channels. *J. Membr. Biol.,* 113:93–107.

142. Moskowitz, R. W. (1992): Experimental models of osteoarthritis. In: *Osteoarthritis: Diagnosis and Medical/Surgical Management,* edited by R. W. Moskowitz, D. S. Howell, V. M. Goldberg, and H. J. Mankin, pp. 213–232. W.B. Saunders, Philadelphia.

143. Moskowitz, R. W., Davis, W., and Sammarco, J. (1973): Experimentally induced degenerative joint lesions following partial meniscectomy in the rabbit. *Arthritis Rheum.,* 16:397–405.

144. Mow, V. C., Holmes, M. H., and Lai, W. M. (1984): Fluid transport and mechanical properties of articular cartilage: a review. *J. Biomech.,* 17:377–394.

145. Mow, V. C., Kuei, S. C., Lai, W. M., and Armstrong, C. G. (1980): Biphasic creep and stress relaxation of articular cartilage in compression: Theory and experiments. *J. Biomech. Eng.,* 102:73–84.

146. Mow, V. C., Ratcliffe, A., and Poole, A. R. (1992): Cartilage and diarthrodial joints as paradigms for hierarchical materials and structures. *Biomaterials,* 13:67–97.

147. Muir, H. (1983):Proteoglycans as organizers of the intercellular matrix. *Biochem. Soc. Trans.,* 11(6):613–622..

148. Müller, F. J., Setton, L. A., Manicourt, D. H., Mow, V. C., Howell, D. S., and Pita, J. C. (1994): Centrifugal and biochemical comparison of proteoglycan aggregates from articular cartilage in experimental joint disuse and joint instability. *J. Orthop. Res.,* 12:498–508.

149. Nerem, R. M., Harrison, D. G., Taylor, W. R., and Alexander, R. W. (1993): Hemodynamics and vascular endothelial biology. *J. Cardiovasc. Pharmacol.,* 21: S6–S10.

150. Nevo, Z., Beit-Or, A., and Eilam, Y. (1988): Slowing down aging of cultured embryonal chick chondrocytes by maintenance under lowered oxygen tension. *Mech. Ageing Dev.,* 45:157–165.

151. Newman, P., and Watt, F. M. (1988): Influence of cytochalasin D-induced changes in cell shape on proteoglycan synthesis by cultured articular chondrocytes. *Exp. Cell Res.,* 178:199–210.

152. Norton, L. A., Rodan, G. A., and Bourret, L. A. (1977): Epiphyseal cartilage cAMP changes produced by electrical and mechanical perturbations. *Clin. Orthop.,* :59–68.

153. O'Hara, B. P., Urban, J. P., and Maroudas, A. (1990): Influence of cyclic loading on the nutrition of articular cartilage. *Ann. Rheum. Dis.,* 49:536–539.

154. Oegema, T. R., Jr., Lewis, J. L., and Thompson, R. C., Jr. (1993): Role of acute trauma in development of osteoarthritis. *Agents Actions,* 40:220–223.

155. Orford, C. R., Gardner, D. L., and O'Connor, P. (1983): Ultrastructural changes in dog femoral condylar cartilage following anterior cruciate ligament section. *J. Anat.,* 137:653–663.

156. Ostendorf, R. H., van de Stadt, R. J., and van Kampen, G. P. (1994): Intermittent loading induces the expression of 3-B-3(-) epitope in cultured bovine articular cartilage. *J. Rheumatol.,* 21:287–292.

157. Palmoski, M. J., and Brandt, K. D. (1981): Running inhibits the reversal of atrophic changes in canine knee cartilage after removal of a leg cast. *Arthritis Rheum.,* 24:1329–1337.

158. Palmoski, M. J., and Brandt, K. D. (1984): Effects of static and cyclic compressive loading on articular cartilage plugs *in vitro. Arthritis Rheum.,* 27:675–681.

159. Palmoski, M. J., Colyer, R. A., and Brandt, K. D. (1980): Joint motion in the absence of normal loading does not maintain normal articular cartilage. *Arthritis Rheum.,* 23:325–334.

160. Palmoski, M. J., Perricone, E., and Brandt, K. D. (1979): Development and reversal of a proteoglycan aggregation defect in normal canine knee cartilage after immobilization. *Arthritis Rheum.,* 22:508–517.

161. Parkkinen, J. J., Ikonen, J., Lammi, M. J., Laakkonen, J., Tammi, M., and Helminen, H. J. (1993): Effects of cyclic hydrostatic pressure on proteoglycan synthesis in cultured chondrocytes and articular cartilage explants. *Arch. Biochem. Biophys.,* 300:458–465.

162. Parkkinen, J. J., Lammi, M. J., Helminen, H. J., and Tammi, M. (1992): Local stimulation of proteoglycan synthesis in articular cartilage explants by dynamic compression *in vitro. J. Orthop. Res.,* 10:610–620.

163. Parkkinen, J. J., Lammi, M. J., Inkinen, R., Jortikka, M., Tammi, M., Virtanen, I., and Helminen, H. J. (1995): Influence of short-term hydrostatic pressure on organization of stress fibers in cultured chondrocytes. *J. Orthop. Res.,* 13:495–502.

164. Parkkinen, J. J., Lammi, M. J., Pelttari, A., Helminen, H. J., Tammi, M., and Virtanen, I. (1993): Altered Golgi apparatus in hydrostatically loaded articular cartilage chondrocytes. *Ann. Rheum. Dis.,* 52:192–198.

165. Pavalko, F. M., Otey, C. A., Simon, K. O., and Burridge, K. (1991): Alpha-actinin: a direct link between actin and integrins. *Biochem. Soc. Trans.,* 19:1065–1069.

166. Pienta, K. J., and Coffey, D. S. (1992): Nuclear-cytoskeletal interactions: evidence for physical connections between the nucleus and cell periphery and their alteration by transformation. *J. Cell. Biochem.,* 49:357–365.

167. Pond, M. J., and Nuki, G. (1973): Experimentally induced osteoarthritis in the dog. *Ann. Rheum. Dis.,* 32: 387–388.

168. Pritzker, K. P. H. (1994): Animal models for osteoarthritis: processes, problems and prospects. *Ann. Rheum. Dis.,* 53:406–420.

169. Putney, J., Takemura, H., Hughes, A., Horstman, D., and Thastrup, O. (1989): How do inositol phosphates regulate calcium signaling? *FASEB J.,* 3:1899–1905.

170. Radin, E. L., Parker, G. H., Pugh, J. W., Steinberg, R. S., Paul, I. L., and Rose, R. M. (1973): Response of joints to impact loading. III. Relationship between trabecular microfractures and cartilage degeneration. *J. Biomech.,* 6:51–57.

171. Radin, E. L., and Paul, I. L. (1971): Response of joints to impact loading. I: *In vitro* wear. *Arthritis Rheum.,* 14:356–362.

172. Rasmussen, H. (1986): The calcium messenger system. *N. Engl. J. Med.,* 17:1094–1170.

173. Ratcliffe, A., Billingham, M. E., Saed-Nejad, F., Muir, H., and Hardingham, T. E. (1992): Increased release of matrix components from articular cartilage in experimental canine osteoarthritis. *J. Orthop. Res.,* 10:350–358.

174. Rodan, G. A., Bourret, L. A., and Norton, L. A. (1978): DNA synthesis in cartilage cells is stimulated by oscillating electric fields. *Science,* 199:690–692.

175. Rosier, R. N. (1984): The role of intracellular calcium in matrix vesicle biogenesis. *Orthop. Trans.,* 8:238.

176. Saamanen, A. M., Tammi, M., Jurvelin, J., Kiviranta, I., and Helminen, H. J. (1990): Proteoglycan alterations following immobilization and remobilization in the articular cartilage of young canine knee (stifle) joint. *J. Orthop. Res.,* 8:863–873.

177. Saamanen, A. M., Tammi, M., Kiviranta, I., Jurvelin, J., and Helminen, H. J. (1987): Maturation of proteoglycan matrix in articular cartilage under increased and decreased joint loading. A study in young rabbits. *Connect. Tissue Res.,* 16:163–175.

178. Sachs, F. (1991): Mechanical transduction by membrane ion channels: a mini review. *Mol. Cell. Biochem.,* 104:57–60.

179. Sah, R. L., Doong, J. H., Kim, Y. J., Grodzinsky, A. J., Plaas, A. H. K., and Sandy, J. D. (1988): Biosynthetic response of cartilage explants to mechanical and physicochemical stimuli. *Trans. Orthop. Res. Soc.,* 13:70.

180. Sah, R. L., and Grodzinsky, A. J. (1989): Biosynthetic response to mechanical and electrical forces: calf articular cartilage in organ culture. In: *Biology of Tooth Movement,* edited by L. A. Norton and C. J. Burston, pp. 335–347. CRC Press, Boca Raton, FL.

181. Sah, R. L., Grodzinsky, A. J., Plaas, A. H., and Sandy, J. D. (1990): Effects of tissue compression on the hyaluronate-binding properties of newly synthesized proteoglycans in cartilage explants. *Biochem. J.,* 267: 803–808.

182. Sah, R. L., Grodzinsky, A. J., Plaas, A. H. K., and Sandy, J. D. (1992): Effects of static and dynamic compression on matrix metabolism in cartilage explants. In: *Articular Cartilage and Osteoarthritis,* edited by K. E. Kuettner, R. Schleyerbach, J. G. Peyron, and V. C. Hascall, pp. 373–392. Raven Press, New York.

183. Sah, R. L., Kim, Y. J., Doong, J. Y., Grodzinsky, A. J., Plaas, A. H., and Sandy, J. D. (1989): Biosynthetic re-

sponse of cartilage explants to dynamic compression. *J. Orthop. Res.,* 7:619–636.

184. Salter, D. M., Hughes, D. E., Simpson, R., and Gardner, D. L. (1992): Integrin expression by human articular chondrocytes. *Br. J. Pharmacol.,* 31:231–234.

185. Salter, R. B., and Field, P. (1960): The effects of continuous compression on living articular cartilage. *J. Bone Joint Surg.,* 42A:31–76.

186. Sandy, J. D., Adams, M. E., Billingham, M. E., Plaas, A., and Muir, H. (1984): *In vivo* and *in vitro* stimulation of chondrocyte biosynthetic activity in early experimental osteoarthritis. *Arthritis Rheum.,* 27:388–397.

187. Sandy, J. D., Brown, H. L. G., and Lowther, D. A. (1980): Control of proteoglycan synthesis. Studies on the activation of synthesis observed during culture of articular cartilages. *Biochem. J.,* 188:119–130.

188. Sarkadi, B., and Parker, J. C. (1991): Activation of ion transport pathways by changes in cell volume. *Biochim. Biophys. Acta,* 1071:407–427.

189. Schneiderman, R., Keret, D., and Maroudas, A. (1986): Effects of mechanical and osmotic pressure on the rate of glycosaminoglycan synthesis in the human adult femoral head cartilage: an *in vitro* study. *J. Orthop. Res.,* 4:393–408.

190. Setton, L. A., Lai, W. M., and Mow, V. C. (1994): Swelling-induced residual stresses in articular cartilage: A potential role for chondrocyte morphology. In: *Biomedical Engineering: Recent Developments,* edited by J. Vossoughi, pp. 1207–1210. University of the District of Columbia Press, Washington, DC.

191. Setton, L. A., and Mow, V. C. (1995): Contributions of flow-dependent and flow-independent viscoelasticity to the behavior of articular cartilage in oscillatory compression. *Bioeng. Conf.,* BED-29:307–308.

192. Setton, L. A., Mow, V. C., and Howell, D. S. (1995): Mechanical behavior of articular cartilage in shear is altered by transection of the anterior cruciate ligament. *J. Orthop. Res.,* 13:473–482.

193. Setton, L. A., Mow, V. C., Müller, F. J., Pita, J. C., and Howell, D. S. (1994): Mechanical properties of canine articular cartilage are significantly altered following transection of the anterior cruciate ligament. *J. Orthop. Res.,* 12:451–463.

194. Setton, L. A., Mow, V. C., Müller, F. J., Pita, J. C., and Howell, D. S. (1997): Altered material properties of articular cartilage after periods of joint disuse and joint disuse followed by remobilization. *Osteoarthritis Cartilage,* 5:1–16.

195. Shapiro, F., and Glimcher, M. J. (1980): Induction of osteoarthrosis in the rabbit knee joint. Histologic changes following meniscectomy and meniscal lesions. *Clin. Orthop.,* 147:287–295.

196. Sims, J. R., Karp, S., and Ingber, D. E. (1992): Altering the cellular mechanical force balance results in integrated changes in cell, cytoskeletal and nuclear shape. *J. Cell Sci.,* 103:1215–1222.

197. Smith, R. L., Donlon, B. S., Gupta, M. K., Mohtai, M., Das, P., Carter, D. R., Cooke, J., Gibbons, G., Hutchinson, N., and Schurman, D. J. (1995): Effects of fluid-induced shear on articular chondrocyte morphology and metabolism *in vitro. J. Orthop. Res.,* 13:824–831.

198. Sokoloff, L. (1980): *In vitro* culture of joints and articular tissues. In: *The Joints and Synovial Fluid,* edited by L. Sokoloff, pp. 1–27. Academic Press, New York.

199. Spilker, R. L., Suh, J. K., and Mow, V. C. (1990): Ef-

fects of friction on the unconfined compressive response of articular cartilage: a finite element analysis. *J. Biomech. Eng.,* 112:138–146.

200. Stockwell, R. A. (1979). *Biology of Cartilage Cells.* Cambridge University Press, Cambridge.

201. Stockwell, R. A. (1987): Structure and function of the chondrocyte under mechanical stress. In: *Joint Loading: Biology and Health of Articular Structures,* edited by H. J. Helminen, I. Kiviranta, M. Tammi, A. M. K. P. Saamanen, and J. Jurvelin, pp. 126–148. Wright and Sons, Bristol.

202. Stockwell, R. A., Billingham, M. E. J., and Muir, H. (1983): Ultrastructural changes in articular cartilage after experimental section of the anterior cruciate ligament of the dog knee. *J. Anat.,* 136:425–439.

203. Stockwell, R. A., and Meachim, G. (1973): The chondrocytes. In: *Adult Articular Cartilage,* edited by M. A. R. Freeman, pp. 51–99. London: Pitman Medical.

204. Sun, D., Aydelotte, M. B., Maldonado, B., Kuettner, K. E., and Kimura, J. H. (1986): Clonal analysis of the population of chondrocytes from the Swarm rat chondrosarcoma in agarose culture. *J. Orthop. Res.,* 4:427–436.

205. Tammi, M., Kiviranta, I., Peltonen, L., Jurvelin, J., and Helminen, H. J. (1988): Effects of joint loading on articular cartilage collagen metabolism: assay of procollagen prolyl 4-hydroxylase and galactosylhydroxylysyl glucosyltransferase. *Connect. Tissue Res.,* 17:199–206.

206. Tammi, M., Saamanen, A. M., Jauhiainen, A., Malminen, O., Kiviranta, I., and Helminen, H. J. (1983): Proteoglycan alterations in rabbit knee articular cartilage following physical exercise and immobilization. *Connect. Tissue Res.,* 11:44–55.

207. Thaxter, T. H., Mann, R. A., and Anderson, C. E. (1965): Degeneration of the immobilized knee joint in rats. *J. Bone Joint Surg.,* 47A:567–585.

208. Thompson, R. C., Jr., Oegema, T. R., Jr., Lewis, J. L., and Wallace, L. (1991): Osteoarthrotic changes after acute transarticular load. An animal model. *J. Bone Joint Surg. Am.,* 73:990–1001.

209. Torzilli, P. A. (1993): Effects of temperature, concentration and articular surface removal on transient solute diffusion in articular cartilage. *Med. Biol. Eng. Comput.,* 31:S93–S98.

210. Uchida, A., Yamashita, K., Hashimoto, K., and Shimomura, Y. (1988): The effect of mechanical stress on cultured growth cartilage cells. *Connect. Tissue Res.,* 17:305–311.

211. Underhill, C. B. (1989): The interaction of hyaluronate with the cell surface, the hyaluronate receptor and the core protein. In: *The Biology of Hyaluronan,* edited by D. Evered and J. Whelan, pp. 138–149. John Wiley & Sons, Chichester.

212. Urban, J., and Hall, A. (1993): Adaptive responses of chondrocytes to changes in their physical environment. *Trans. Orthop. Res. Soc.,* 18:260.

213. Urban, J. P., and Bayliss, M. T. (1989): Regulation of proteoglycan synthesis rate in cartilage *in vitro:* influence of extracellular ionic composition. *Biochim. Biophys. Acta,* 992:59–65.

214. Urban, J. P., Hall, A. C., and Gehl, K. A. (1993): Regulation of matrix synthesis rates by the ionic and osmotic environment of articular chondrocytes. *J. Cell. Physiol.,* 154:262–270.

215. Urban, J. P. G., and Hall, A. C. (1994): The effects of hydrostatic and osmotic pressures on chondrocyte metabo-

lism. In: *Cell Mechanics and Cellular Engineering,* edited by V. C. Mow, F. Guilak, R. Tran-Son-tay, and R. M. Hochmuth, pp. 398–419. Springer Verlag, New York.

216. van Kampen, G. P. J., and van de Stadt, R. J. (1987): Cartilage and chondrocytes responses to mechanical loading *in vitro.* In: *Joint Loading: Biology and Health of Articular Structures,* edited by H. J. Helminen, I. Kiviranta, M. Tammi, A. M. K. P. Saamanen, and J. Jurvelin, pp. 112–125. Wright and Sons, Bristol.

217. van Kampen, G. P., Korver, G. H., and van de Stadt, R. J. (1994): Modulation of proteoglycan composition in cultured anatomically intact joint cartilage by cyclic loads of various magnitudes. *Int. J. Tissue React.,* 16:171–179.

218. van Kampen, G. P., Veldhuijzen, J. P., Kuijer, R., van de Stadt, R. J., and Schipper, C. A. (1985): Cartilage response to mechanical force in high-density chondrocyte cultures. *Arthritis Rheum.,* 28:419–424.

219. Veldhuijzen, J. P., Bourret, L. A., and Rodan, G. A. (1979): *In vitro* studies of the effect of intermittent compressive forces on cartilage cell proliferation. *J. Cell. Physiol.,* 98:299–306.

220. Velpeau, A. A. L. M. (1837): *Manuel d'anatomie chirurgicale, générale et topographique.* Méquignon-Marvis, Paris.

221. Vener, M. J., Thompson, R. C., Jr., Lewis, J. L., and Oegema, T. R., Jr. (1992): Subchondral damage after acute transarticular loading: an *in vitro* model of joint injury. *J. Orthop. Res.,* 10:759–765.

222. Videman, T., Michelsson, J., Rauhamaki, R., and Langenskiold, A. (1976): Changes in the ^{35}S-sulphate uptake in different tissues in the knee and hip regions of rabbits during immobilization, remobilization and the development of osteoarthritis. *Acta. Orthop. Scand.,* 47:290–298.

223. Visser, N., van Kampen, G., Dekoning, M., and van der Korst, J. (1994): The effects of loading on the synthesis of biglycan and decorin in intact mature articular cartilage *in vitro. Connect. Tissue Res.,* 30:241–250.

224. von der Mark, K., Mollenhauer, J., Mueller, P. K., and Pfaefflea, M. (1985): Anchorin CII, a collagen-binding glycoprotein from chondrocyte membranes. *Ann. N.Y. Acad. Sci.,* 460:214–223.

225. Watson, P. A. (1991): Function follows form: generation of intracellular signals by cell deformation. *FASEB J.,* 5:2013–2019.

226. Wilkins, R., and Hall, A. (1992): Measurement of intracellular pH in isolated bovine articular chondrocytes. *Exp. Physiol.,* 77:521–524.

227. Wilkins, R. J., Hall, A. C., and Urban, J. P. G. (1992): The correlation between changes in intracellular pH and changes in matrix synthesis rates in chondrocytes. *Trans. Orthop. Res. Soc.,* 17:182.

228. Wright, M., Jobanputra, P., Bavington, C., Salter, D., and Nuki, G. (1994): Evidence for stretch-activated ion channels in human chondrocytes. *Bone Miner.,* S1:S37.

229. Wright, M. O., Stockwell, R. A., and Nuki, G. (1992): Response of plasma membrane to applied hydrostatic pressure in chondrocytes and fibroblasts. *Connect. Tissue Res.,* 28:49–70.

230. Yoshimasa, T., Sibley, D. R., Bouvier, M., Lefkowitz, R. J., and Caron, M. G. (1987): Cross-talk between cellular signalling pathways suggested by phorbol ester-induced adenylate cyclase phosphorylation. *Nature,* 327:67–70.

Basic Orthopaedic Biomechanics, 2nd ed.,
edited by Van C. Mow and Wilson C. Hayes.
Lippincott–Raven Publishers, Philadelphia © 1997.

6

Structure and Function of Tendons and Ligaments

Savio L-Y. Woo, Glen A. Livesay, Thomas J. Runco, and Edmund P. Young

Musculoskeletal Research Center, Department of Orthopaedic Surgery, University of Pittsburgh, Pittsburgh, Pennsylvania 15213

Tendons and ligaments are soft connective tissues composed of closely packed, parallel collagen fiber bundles oriented to provide for the motion and stability of the musculoskeletal system. Ligaments connect bone to bone, whereas tendons connect bone to muscle. The myotendinous junction and the bony attachments are complex and vary considerably. Tendons generally have large parallel fibers that insert uniformly into bone. Ligaments have smaller-diameter fibers that can be either parallel, as in the collateral ligaments of the knee, or branching and interwoven, as in the knee cruciate ligaments.

Under microscopic examination, ground substance and fibroblasts are observed in the interfibrillar spaces. Ultrastructural methods further demonstrate detailed hierarchies of fibrillar arrangement down to microfibril size in tendons (10,63) (Fig. 1). A similar arrangement is thought to exist for ligaments. Although it is agreed that ligaments consist of closely packed collagen fiber bundles that are arranged in a more or less parallel fashion along the longitudinal axis of the ligament, concepts concerning the fibrillar and fiber arrangements of ligamentous tissue differ among investigators (9,21,24,27,63).

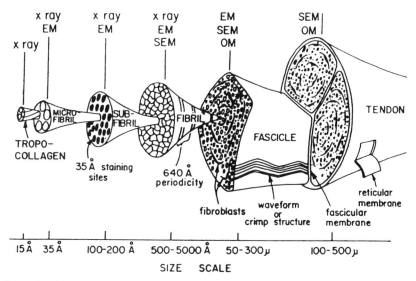

FIG. 1. Schematic of detailed hierarchies of fibrillar arrangements down to the microfibril size. (From Kastelic et al., ref. 63, with permission.)

There are two types of tendon– and ligament–bone insertions: direct and indirect. In the more common direct type of insertion, the tendon or ligament crosses the mineralization front and progresses from fibril through fibrocartilage (usually less than 0.6 mm) to mineralized fibrocartilage (less than 0.4 mm) and finally to bone (Fig. 2A) (24,33). In the second, less common indirect type, the tendon or ligament inserts into bone through the periosteum (Fig. 2B), with short fibers that are obliquely anchored to the bone (24,67,86). Stress and joint motion are important in maintaining the functional integrity of these insertion sites (87,114,118). The details of these interactions are described in a later section.

Tendons and ligaments consist of interdependent aggregations of collagen, elastin,

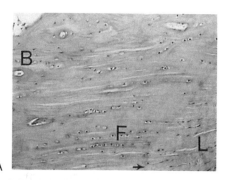
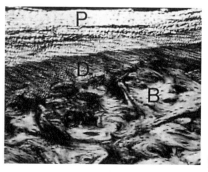

FIG. 2. (A) Photomicrograph of the femoral insertion of rabbit medial collateral ligament (MCL) demonstrating direct insertion. The ligament (L) passes acutely into bone (B) through a well-defined zone of fibrocartilage (F). The line of calcification is indicated by the *arrow*. (Hematoxylin and eosin, ×50) **(B)** The tibial insertion of rabbit MCL demonstrating indirect insertion. The superficial fibrils of the ligament (P) course parallel with the bone (B) and insert in the periosteum. The deeper fibrils (D) course obliquely and insert in the underlying bone. (Hematoxylin and eosin, ×50) (From Woo et al., ref. 148, with permission.)

proteoglycans (PGs), glycolipids, water, and cells. Roughly 70% to 80% of the dry weight of normal tendon or ligament is composed of type I collagen, also found in skin and bone. This collagen is thought to remain relatively inert metabolically, with a half-life of 300 to 500 days (81). Certain components of the collagen molecule may turn over faster than others and may thus be of greater functional importance in adaptations to environmental, traumatic, or pathologic processes (45). Collagen also has the ability to form covalent intramolecular (aldol) and intermolecular (Schiff base) cross-links, which are the keys to its tensile strength characteristics and resistance to chemical or enzymatic breakdown (11,77,112).

The ground substance constituents of tendons or ligaments make up only a small percentage of the total dry tissue weight but are nevertheless quite significant because of their association with water, which represents 60% to 80% of the total wet weight. The water and PGs provide lubrication and spacing crucial to the gliding function at intercept points where fibers cross in the tissue matrix. The role of movement of water in the system is limited by the large PG molecules. These PG molecules are highly negatively charged and possess a large number of hydroxyl groups, which attract water through hydrogen bonding. They contribute important features to the collagen fiber–ground substance interaction (see Chapter 4).

The chemical structure and intermolecular cross-linking of the collagen, its interaction with the ground substance, and the hydrophilic nature of the PGs and collagen fibers are all mechanically significant characteristics. Collectively, they serve to maintain fiber orientation and distance in an organized meshwork for optimal load distribution and response. Tendon and ligament insertions to bone are functionally adapted to distribute and dissipate the forces they carry by passing through fibrocartilage to bone. They are less susceptible to disruption in the transition area than extremes on either side (i.e., bone or periinsertional tissue substance).

Under polarized light microscopy, anterior cruciate ligament (ACL) fibrils, like fibrils comprising other ligaments and tendons, appear in microstructural form in a sinusoidal wave pattern referred to as crimp. Crimping is thought to have significant influence on the biomechanical behavior of ligaments. Yahia and Drouin recently compared the fascicle morphology of canine ACLs and patellar tendons (PTs), using light and scanning electron microscopy (150). They found crimping in both the ACL and PT and presented two models for this pattern, the planar and helical wave structures, representing constituent collagen fibrils either parallel or twisted with respect to the fascicle axis, respectively. The helical waveform was found in both the ACL and PT, whereas the planar waveform was found only in centrally located ACL fascicles. In either form, this pattern has specific biomechanical implications, which are discussed in a later section.

Tendons and ligaments are well suited to the physiological functions they perform. Multiple tendons and ligaments serve a single joint, providing a mechanism for both locomotion and the maintenance of static and dynamic protection of the joint through a wide range of movement. By adding dynamic muscular control, neural feedback mechanisms protect the static stabilizers from displacements beyond their mechanical limits. The parallel fiber arrangement of tendons and ligaments allows early tensile resistance once the "crimp pattern" is straightened.

Like other soft connective tissues, ligaments and tendons are further characterized by a nonlinear mechanical behavior. Their load–deformation or stress–strain behaviors are anisotropic, oriented primarily for the resistance of tensile loads. One simple description of their nonlinear properties employs a model composed of individual linearly elastic components to represent the fibrillar components of the tissue, primarily collagen (Fig. 3A) (119). The collagen fibrils are arranged in varying degrees of crimp so that increasing tensile deformation results in recruitment of additional load-bearing fibrils to resist tensile

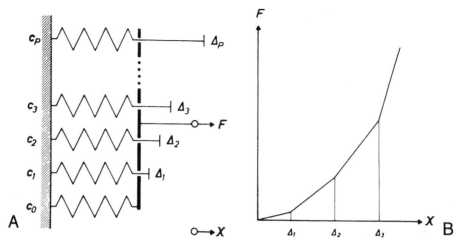

FIG. 3. (A) Model of nonlinear elasticity demonstrating progressive recruitment of individual linear components. **(B)** Resultant nonlinear load–deformation curve. (From Frisen et al., ref. 36, with permission.)

stress. A nonlinear response results as increasing numbers of these components become active with deformation (Fig. 3B).

As with all physiological systems, there are functional adaptations to age, temperature, gender, levels of stress and motion, and any number of other unknown parameters. The mechanism of adaptation may involve changes in content and organization of tendon or ligament substance. Within this chapter the effects of experimental factors, biological factors, and external factors on the apparent biomechanical properties of tendons and ligaments are reviewed and discussed. The flexor tendons and the human ACL will be used as primary examples, as they are among the most widely studied. There is a significant body of literature on other structures, ranging from PT to spinal ligaments.

DETERMINATION OF BIOMECHANICAL PROPERTIES

Because the main function of tendons and ligaments is to transmit tensile loading, experimental studies of the biomechanical properties of these tissues are generally performed in tension. The goal of these tests is to acquire the stress–strain curves of the tendon or ligament substance (from which the mechanical properties are determined) and the load–elongation response for the bone–ligament–bone complex (from which structural properties are obtained). Before discussing these properties and the distinctions that exist between them, it is necessary to present some background information.

Because many factors affect these tensile properties, experimental protocols are devised to minimize the uncertainty introduced by uncontrolled factors (i.e., experimental artifacts). Typically, tensile tests involve gripping the ligament specimen, either directly using clamps or indirectly by gripping the bones to which the ligament is attached, and pulling it in a precise and well-controlled fashion until rupture of the ligament occurs. During the test, the force and elongation applied to the specimen are recorded. Although in most cases the measurement of applied force involves straightforward use of a load cell, other measurements, in particular strain and ligament cross-sectional area, present a number of technical challenges. Some of the techniques and devices created to meet these challenges are introduced in the following sections.

Structural Properties and Mechanical Properties

Clamping of isolated ligament tissue for tensile testing is an inherently difficult task for several reasons. The specimen is often quite short, making it necessary to use a relatively large percentage of the tissue for clamping, leaving little substance for testing. Slipping of the ligament from the clamp is also a problem commonly encountered. Investigators go to great efforts to prevent grip–specimen slipping, such as using specially designed freezing, hydraulic, and pneumatic clamps with roughened gripping surfaces. However, even when slipping is prevented, stress concentrations may develop in the region of the clamp, resulting in premature failure of the specimen. These difficulties may be avoided by rigidly securing attached segments of periinsertional bone, with ligament insertion sites left anatomically intact. Biomechanical testing is then performed on the entire bone–ligament–bone complex.

In discussing the tensile properties of tendons and ligaments (tissue), it is important to distinguish between the structural properties of the tissue–bone complex and the mechanical properties of the tissue. The structural properties (e.g., load, deformation, stiffness, energy absorbed, ultimate load, and ultimate elongation) are measurements of the tensile behavior of the tendon or ligament as a functional organ, a composite bone–tissue complex. Direct experimental measurement of load (using a load cell) and deformation (based on test machine crosshead or clamp-to-clamp displacement) is relatively straightforward. Results of such tensile testing are frequently reported as load–elongation data. These structural properties are, however, dependent on a number of parameters, including (a) the mechanical properties of the tissue substance, (b) the geometry of the tissue (cross-sectional area, length, and shape), and (c) the properties of the bone–tissue and muscle–tissue junctions.

Mechanical properties, on the other hand, are determined from the stress–strain relationship of the ligament substance itself. They are often reported as material coefficients, representing a stress–strain law. These properties reflect collagen fiber organization and orientation, as well as the microstructure of the tissue. The experimental design must ensure that only tissue strain is measured and, when ultimate properties are determined, that failure occurs in the substance (because insertion-site failures measure the ultimate properties of the insertion-site regions and not the ligament substance *per se*). Mechanical properties of the ligament substance are represented by parameters such as the modulus, ultimate strain, and strain energy density.

Tensile failure of a bone–ligament–bone complex occurs within the weakest link of the complex. Thus, failure can occur through any of several mechanisms: fracture through a bone; avulsion, wherein the ligament pulls a small piece of bone free, leaving the insertion sites intact; insertion site failure in which no bone is displaced; and midsubstance rupture of the ligament. Ultimate load and elongation values are meaningful whether failure occurs at the insertion site or within the ligament substance. In contrast, mechanical properties such as ultimate tensile stress and ultimate strain can be determined only if failure occurs within the gauge marks placed midsubstance along the tissue. It is, therefore, important to report failure modes.

Cross-Sectional Area Measurements

Data on mechanical properties of tendons and ligaments have also been compromised by the lack of an ideal method for measuring the cross-sectional area. The irregular, complex shape and geometry of these tissues make direct measurement difficult, and measurement errors can be large.

Several image reconstruction techniques have been described to measure cross-sectional area before tensile testing (30,47,56,85,129), and these can be separated into either contact or noncontact approaches. Contact methods include the use of digital vernier calipers, pressure area micrometers, thickness calipers, and the molding method (96,97). Digital vernier calipers have been used to measure the width and thickness of the ligaments; then the area is calculated on the basis of an assumed ligament shape, usually either a rectangle or an ellipse. This method works well for some ligaments, such as the medial collateral ligament (MCL), that have relatively regular shapes but introduces large errors if used to measure irregular and geometrically complex ligaments such as the ACL (131). The pressure area micrometer method compresses the ligament into a rectangular slot of known width (usually under 0.12 MPa pressure) while the specimen thickness is measured. The cross-sectional area obtained is highly dependent on the amount of pressure applied to the tissue (2,15,31,121). In the thickness caliper method, the tips of a pair of calipers are traversed along the width of both faces of the ligament simultaneously, yielding a thickness profile (104).

To minimize distortion of tissue shape (and therefore the cross-sectional area), many investigators have advocated the use of noncontact methods to determine ligament cross-sectional area. These techniques include the shadow amplitude method (30), the profile method (47,85), and the use of light rays (56). In our laboratory, the laser micrometer system has been used as a method to measure both cross-sectional area and shape of specimens (69,131). The specimen is placed perpendicular to a collimated laser beam, a microprocessor system obtains profile widths as the specimen is incrementally rotated through 180°, and the shape of the ligament is then reconstructed and the cross-sectional area determined. For determination of both the cross-sectional shape and area of the midsubstance region of ACLs, the laser micrometer method has been shown to be highly accurate and reproducible with precision, and the reconstructed shapes match histologic sections very well.

In the attempt to further measure the surface concavities present in many ligaments, particularly near their insertions, a laser-reflectance method was recently introduced to measure the cross-sectional shape and area (18). The laser reflectance transducer (Model LB-70, Keyence Corporation of America, Fair Lawn, NJ) has a measurement range of 60 to 140 mm from the sensor and a resolution of 0.01 mm. The transducer generates a 1-mm-wide beam that strikes the specimen, and its receiver collects the reflected laser radiation. It is mounted on a bearing and rotated 360° around a stationary specimen to collect data for the entire perimeter of the specimen (Fig. 4). A rotary potentiometer continually measures the angular position, while the laser transducer measures the distance to the surface of the specimen. All data are collected and displayed in real time, and the resulting cross-sectional shape is integrated to obtain the area. The accuracy and repeatability of this system were found to be within 2.5% and 1.3%, respectively, on standardized shapes of known cross-sectional area (i.e., circle, circle with square keyway, and circle with triangle keyway).

Because it utilizes reflected laser radiation for specimen measurement and not just a profile, the laser reflectance system is able to detect concavities within the cross-sectional shape of complex ligamentous tissue. The reconstructed cross-sectional shapes of a typical porcine ACL (near the femoral insertion) obtained using the new laser reflectance system and the laser micrometer system are shown overlaid in Fig. 5. When normalized, the laser micrometer cross-sectional area measurements were approximately 110% of the laser reflectance system ($p < 0.05$) and overestimated the area of the ACL because it cannot detect the concavities on the surface. Because the new system is able to detect concavities on the surface of the specimen in a noncontact manner, it provides a more realistic reconstruction of the actual cross-sectional shape.

Strain Monitoring

Accurate experimental measurement of tissue elongation of ligaments and tendons poses a number of hurdles including method of fixation, measurement of dimensions, and isolation of the properties of the tissue from its connecting structures. To avoid introducing possible errors during measurement, optical techniques

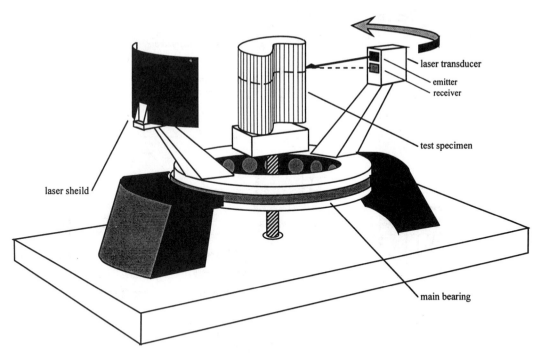

FIG. 4. Schematic diagram of the laser reflectance measurement system, showing the main bearing, the laser transducer, and a sample test specimen. (From Chan et al., ref. 18, with permission.)

to measure tissue strain, such as the video-dimension analyzer (VDA), that require no direct contact with the specimen have been developed (Fig. 6). Before testing, two or more reference lines (gauge lengths) are drawn on the tendon or ligament with Verhoeff's stain perpendicular to the loading axis (143). Testing is then performed, and the data are recorded by video camera and videotape. The taped image is then played back through the VDA system, which superimposes two electronic "windows" over the reference lines. These windows automatically track the movement of the reference lines throughout the test and convert the horizontal scan time between lines into an output voltage. The voltage change expressed as a

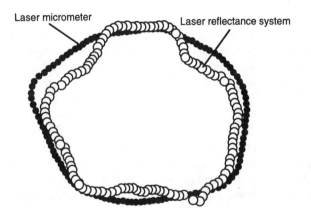

FIG. 5. Reconstructed cross-sectional shapes of a porcine ACL obtained with the laser reflectance system and the laser micrometer system.

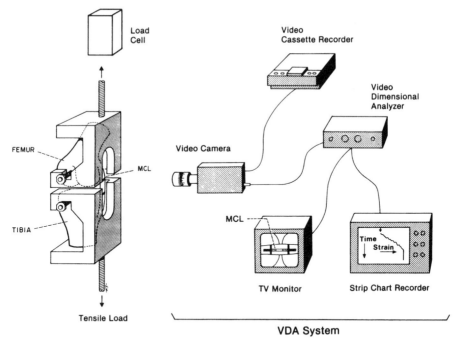

FIG. 6. Experimental apparatus used to measure the tensile strain in the MCL. The VDA system recorded the strain history from the two ligament stain lines (gauge lengths) by means of the video camera, videocassette recorder, dimension analyzer, and strip chart recorder. (From Woo et al., ref. 135, with permission.)

function of the initial voltage can then be calibrated to correspond to percentage strain of the tissue. The frequency response of the VDA system is 120 Hz, and errors in linearity and accuracy are less than 0.5% (136).

More recently, the tracking of small elastin stain markers on the ligament surface has been reported (48,68). Although originally developed primarily for gait analysis, these systems show promise for determining additional components of surface strains during tensile testing. These approaches also possess the advantages of noncontact methods such as the VDA system to measure strains of ligaments and tendons: (a) there is no physical contact with the midsubstance of the specimen during testing; (b) it can measure strains in midsubstance independent of the insertion sites; (c) strain values can be obtained from different regions of the same specimen; (d) video recording of testing permits the data to be analyzed after the test and provides a per-

manent record of the test; and (e) with the advent of high-speed video recorders, high-strain-rate testing can also be videotaped, with strain analysis done at slower playback speeds (92).

CONTRIBUTION OF EXPERIMENTAL FACTORS

The functional support to the joint is provided by a tendon at the muscle–tendon–bone complex and by a ligament at the bone–ligament–bone unit. Clinically, failure in adult tissue–bone complexes is more common by substance tear rather than by avulsion, yet many investigators using cadavers and experimental animals have commented on the difficulty of producing substance injuries and have traditionally stated that the bone is the weakest component of the system (54,78,119,139,151). Some potential factors for such discrepancies arise from experimental procedure and are described below.

Specimen Orientation

The structural properties of the bone–ligament complex are significantly dependent on loading axis. The angle of knee flexion also contributes to the differences in these properties. Figgie et al. (33) compared the structural properties of canine femur–ACL–tibia complex (FATC) tested at 0°, 45°, and 90° of flexion with loading directed along the tibial axis. The ACL was approximately parallel to the loading axis in the 0° case, perpendicular at 90°, and in an intermediate orientation at 45°. The ultimate structural properties were the greatest at 0° of flexion with no observed midsubstance failure. At 90° of flexion, all failures involved some element of substance failure, and the ultimate load values were the lowest. The parallel loading condition was hypothesized to load all fiber bundles simultaneously, resulting in higher ultimate structural properties. The oblique loading condition resulted in progressive fiber failure across the ligament breadth. Similar findings have been demonstrated using the rabbit FATC (139). Loading along the tibial and ACL axes was compared at various knee flexion angles. When the load was directed along the ACL axis, the angle of

knee flexion did not change the ultimate load values, and most failures were by bony avulsion. However, when the load was directed along the longitudinal axis of the tibia, progressive decreases in the structural properties of the bone–ligament–bone complex were found as knee flexion increased (Fig. 7), and failures occurred in the midsubstance. Again, it appears that when the load was applied along the ligament axis, the ligament fibrils were oriented with an even distribution of forces, and maximum strength resulted. Force application along the tibial axis resulted in uneven loading along the ligament, and the fibrils resisting most of the load failed in a progressive fashion.

Specimen orientation is also a significant factor in the structural response of human specimens. Paired younger (22 to 35 years), middle-aged (40 to 50 years), and older (60 to 97 years) donors were tensile tested with the FATC from one knee in the anatomic orientation and the contralateral FATC in the tibial orientation (138). In the anatomic orientation, the natural insertion angles of the ACL were maintained, allowing for a smooth transition of load from bone to ligament as well as a more uniform load distribution within the ligament. The tibial orientation, with insertion angles not maintained, demonstrated more insertion site failures, indicating a nonuniform distribution of tensile load within the ACL. The structural

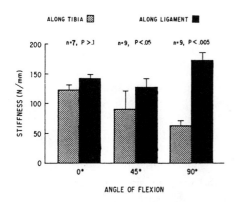
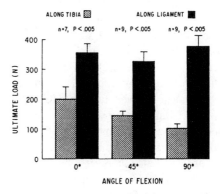

FIG. 7. Variation of structural properties of rabbit FATC obtained at three angles of flexion and two directions of applied loading (tibial axis versus ligament axis). (From Woo et al., ref. 139, with permission.)

properties for the FATCs tested in the anatomic orientation were significantly different from those tested in the tibial orientation, with higher ultimate load, linear stiffness, and energy absorbed at failure. Similar results have also been observed for porcine FATC specimens (72).

Strain Rate

Considerable attention has been given to the effects of the extension rate on the failure mode of a bone–ligament complex. Some investigators feel that the reason others have been unsuccessful in obtaining ligament substance failure is primarily due to the employment of slower strain rates (25,49,86). Others have shown that skeletal maturity can have a significant effect on the failure mode (143). For example, when the rabbit femur-MCL-tibia complex (FMTC) was tested using a relatively low strain rate (0.3%/sec), the animals with open epiphyses all had failures by tibial avulsion. For older animals (12 to 15 months) with closed epiphyses, all failures occurred by substance tear (143). The effect of strain rate on the MCL midsubstance material properties as well as its effect on mode of failure of the FMTC has been investigated using a high-speed video recording system (91,92). The FMTCs from two groups of New Zealand white rabbits—(a) open epiphysis ($3^1/_2$ months old) and (b) closed epiphysis ($8^1/_2$ months old)—were subjected to uniaxial tensile tests at five different extension rates (0.008 to 113 mm/sec), corresponding to strain rates of the ligament substance of 0.01%/ sec to over 200%/sec. For the open epiphysis group, the structural properties of the FMTC were found to be dependent on the extension rate, with the ultimate load and energy absorbed increasing 2.5 and 3.0 times, respectively (Fig. 8). For the closed epiphysis group, the ultimate load and energy absorbed also increased, but to a lesser degree. The mechanical properties of the MCL substance in the prefailure range paralleled the results obtained for the structural properties (Fig. 9). The tensile strength of the MCL in the closed-epiphysis group increased significantly

with strain rate, but by only 60% from the lowest to the highest values. Both the structural and mechanical properties revealed much larger changes as a function of age. Failure modes were significantly affected by skeletal maturity and were independent of strain rate. All failures in animals with open epiphyses occurred by tibial avulsion (therefore, no tensile strength of the MCL substance could be reported), whereas in animals with closed epiphyses, all failures occurred by ligamentous disruption either at midsubstance or near the tibial insertion site. We therefore believe that the age of the animals is a much more important factor in determining failure mode than the strain rate at which the specimen is tested.

Results for the rabbit ACL were similar to those for the MCL. The modulus of the ACL substance measured at 380%/sec was only 31% higher than that measured at 0.02%/sec (26). The PT was found to have a greater sensitivity to strain rate; its modulus increased 94% over the same range of strain rates. Both reports document that failure mode does not change with strain rate. Relative to the large range of strain rates studied, only comparatively small differences in both the mechanical properties of the ligament and tendon substances and structural properties of the bone–ligament–bone complexes were observed. This is in direct contrast to the profound effect that skeletal maturity has on both ligament biomechanical properties and failure modes (91).

Temperature

An important consideration in testing tendons and ligaments is the influence of environmental temperature on their biomechanical behavior. Most tests have been performed with the specimens in air at room temperature. Some investigators immerse the specimen in an aqueous bath, such as an isotonic solution, where pH and temperature can be closely controlled. Rigby et al. (98) suggested that no changes occur in the mechanical properties of ligaments between 0° and 37°C. Apter (8) re-

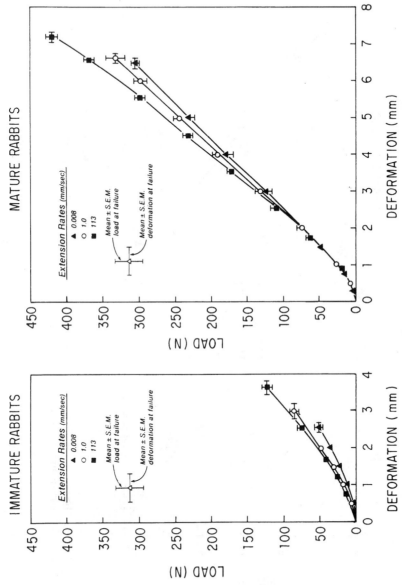

FIG. 8. The structural properties of the FMTC in skeletally immature and mature rabbits as a function of extension rate.

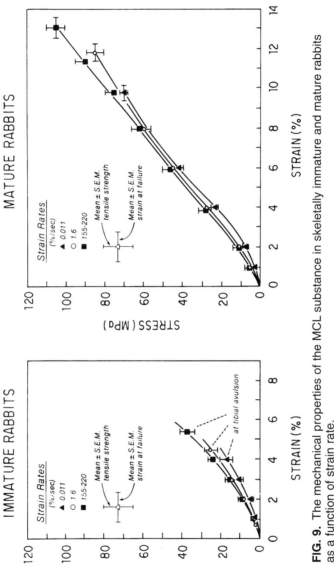

FIG. 9. The mechanical properties of the MCL substance in skeletally immature and mature rabbits as a function of strain rate.

ported that collagen has a negative tempera-ture–elastic modulus relationship from 0° to 70°C. Hunter and Williams (55) found an in-verse relationship between joint stiffness and temperature. We have also observed a similar temperature dependence on ligament proper-ties using the adult canine FMTC (149). The specimen was clamped and submerged in a normal saline bath with a heating and cooling system monitored and controlled by a thermo-stat (accuracy within 0.5°C). Cyclic testing was performed sequentially at temperatures from 2° to 37°C. The results demonstrate that the ligament reflects increasing stiffness in terms of cyclic loading as the temperature de-clines, an effect that can be expressed by a sim-ple linear relationship. For cyclic stress, the re-laxation behavior leveled out to lower values as the testing temperature was increased. It is im-portant to note that between temperature changes, the ligament required between 1 hr and $2^1/_2$ hr to return to its untested, resting characteristics due to the time- and history-de-pendent viscoelastic properties described ear-lier. This may be of particular importance in explaining why our findings differ from those obtained by others. It also demonstrates the ne-cessity of a standardized procedure and that temperature must be reported and controlled, as it can have profound effects on soft tissue behavior.

Hydration

Because ligaments and tendons contain a large amount of water (60% to 80%), their mechanical properties can be expected to vary with hydration. Therefore, their properties are affected by environmental factors such as those commonly used during testing, which include air, a drip environment (air, but with the ligament moistened by saline drip or some other method), and a saline bath (ionic con-centration). For example, rabbit MCLs that contain a greater than normal amount of wa-ter have been shown to experience greater stress relaxation during cyclic loading than those containing less water (19). Ligaments

tested in air are subject to dehydration. Haut and Powlison (50) compared a drip environ-ment with a temperature-controlled saline bath and found that human PTs have a signif-icantly higher strength and modulus when tested in a saline bath than those tested in a drip environment.

CONTRIBUTION OF BIOLOGICAL FACTORS

Tendons and ligaments are subject to a wide variety of stimuli *in vivo*, which are mediated by physiological changes associated with growth and development. A generalized state-ment similar to Wolff's law for bone (127) can also be made regarding the adaptation of ten-dons and ligaments under applied stress and motion. It is therefore reasonable to expect that ligaments and tendons are sensitive to morpho-logic, biomechanical, and biochemical changes in their immediate environment.

Maturation

The effects of skeletal maturity on the prop-erties of tendons, ligaments, and their inser-tions have been demonstrated. Several authors, using rat tail tendons, have shown age-depen-dent increases in collagen fibril size and ulti-mate load (i.e., tensile strength) from puberty to adulthood (49,79,80); afterward, no changes were observed until senescence, where de-creases in these properties may result (88). There exists limited information on changes in human ligament properties as a function of age, however. In one study, four age groups of male New Zealand white rabbits were studied. Animals were aged $1^1/_2$ months (open epiph-ysis by radiologic examination), 4 to 5 months (open epiphysis), 6 to 7 months (closed epiph-ysis), and 12 to 15 months (closed epiphysis). The structural properties of the FMTC were represented by area of hysteresis, load–deformation curves, and ultimate load. The mechanical properties of the MCL substance were expressed by stress–strain curves. The structural properties of the FMTC changed dramatically from 1 to 7 months of age, at which time the magnitude of differences between groups diminished. The mechanical properties of the ligament substance demonstrated relatively early maturation in that by 4 to 5 months of age, the stress–strain curves in the functional range were similar to those of the adults. It was also noted by histologic examination that the tibial insertion site of the MCL is affected by its proximity to the growth plate; rapid remodeling activity in this region weakens the subperiosteal attachment for the younger animals. The failure modes reflect these findings (Fig. 10). All rabbits with open epiphyses failed by tibial avulsion, whereas in animals that had reached skeletal maturity (closed epiphyses), only 15% failed by tibial avulsion.

Aging

In addition to the biomechanical changes observed with skeletal maturation, changes associated with senescence have also been documented. Noyes and Grood (88) found that the structural properties were two to three times greater in young than in old groups of human cadaver FATC preparations. Furthermore, the failure mode of young knees was more commonly by midsubstance failure, whereas older knees failed by bony avulsion. The effects of aging were studied in our laboratory using pairs of human cadaveric knees obtained from young donors (22 to 41 years, mean age 35 years) and older donors (60 to 97 years, mean age 76 years) (138). The FATCs were tested to failure in tension at a knee flexion angle of 30°; one knee of each pair was randomly assigned to be tested alone in the anatomic orientation of ACL with the contralateral knee tested in the tibial orientation. A significant effect of age on linear stiffness was observed, with the linear stiffness of the FATCs tested along the ligament axis being 183 ± 11 N/mm for the younger group and only 158 ± 25 N/mm for the older group. For FATCs tested along the tibial axis, the linear stiffness was 150 ± 19 N/mm for the younger specimens and 127 ± 18 N/mm for the older specimens. Both specimen age and loading axis had a significant effect on ultimate load at failure (Fig. 11). The mean ultimate load of the younger specimens was higher than that of the older specimens, and the mean ultimate

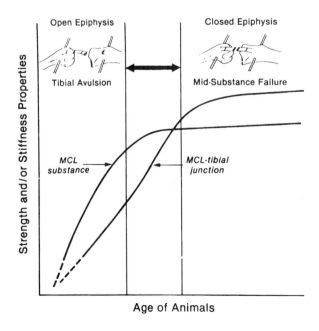

FIG. 10. A schematic diagram depicting the relationship between failure mode and age, hypothesizing the asynchronous rates of maturation between the bone–ligament–bone complex and the ligament substance.

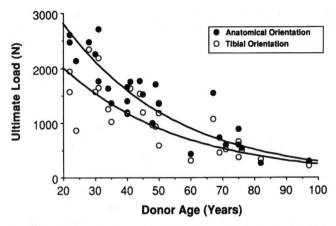

FIG. 11. Ultimate load versus age for human FATC. (From Woo et al., ref. 138, with permission.)

load of the anatomical orientation specimens was higher than that of the tibial orientation specimens. A decrease in ultimate load was seen with increasing age regardless of loading axis, and the difference in ultimate load between the ACL and tibial loading axis decreased with increasing age. The FATC failure mode was affected by both specimen age and loading axis. Older specimens had a higher incidence of midsubstance failure than younger specimens, regardless of loading axis. Specimens tested along the ACL axis had a higher percentage of midsubstance failure than those tested along the tibial axis, regardless of specimen age (57% of the younger age group and 86% of the older age group).

Biomechanical changes in the rabbit FMTC that occur from skeletal maturity to the onset of senescence were further examined in our laboratory (147). Similar to previous findings, significant increases in the stiffness, ultimate load, and energy absorbed to failure of the FMTC were observed during skeletal maturation. However, in contrast to data from the human FATC, the structural properties of the rabbit FMTC showed only a slight decline at the onset of senescence (tested at 48 months of age) as did the modulus of the MCL midsubstance. These changes as a function of age are in direct contrast to the significant decreases in structural properties of the human FATC observed with age.

Immobilization

The effect of stress deprivation on synovial joints can be profound. Intraarticular changes include pannus formation to the point of obliterating the joint space. If the process is allowed to continue, cartilage necrosis is seen in contact areas (101), and cartilage erosion and ulceration occur in noncontact areas (32). Gross inspection of immobilized ligaments and tendons reveals them to be less glistening and more woody in appearance than normal controls. Collagen fiber bundles may be decreased in thickness and number secondary to immobilization. Increased joint stiffness after immobilization is well known clinically and has been demonstrated quantitatively in experimental animals (128). After 9 weeks of immobilization, the amount of torque required to initially extend the rabbit knee and the area of hysteresis were significantly increased (128). Increases in knee joint stiffness have been attributed to adhesions, pannus, and decreased lubrication but probably also include restricted extensibility of loose periarticular weave by fixed contact at strategic sites (1,128). Newly produced collagen fibrils form these interfibrillar contacts and would be expected to restrict normal fiber sliding and motion in extensible structures such as the capsule of the shoulder or posterior aspect of the knee.

In another study, rabbit knees were immobilized and remobilized for varying periods: (a) 9 weeks of immobilization, (b) 12 weeks of immobilization, (c) 9 weeks of immobilization followed by 9 weeks of remobilization, and (d) 12 weeks of immobilization followed by 9 weeks of remobilization (148). Significant changes were found in the structural properties of the FMTC following immobilization. After 9 weeks of immobilization, the ultimate loads and energy- absorbing capabilities of the experimental FMTCs were only 31% and 18%, respectively, of the contralateral controls ($p <$ 0.01). An additional 3 weeks of immobilization further reduced the strength of the FMTC, with the ultimate load reduced to 29% of the control value. After 9 and 12 weeks of immobilization, all the experimental FMTCs failed by tibial avulsion. The ligament substance, itself, is also affected by immobility. Paradoxically, the ligament became less stiff as joint stiffness increased (joint contracture). Stress–strain curves revealed a significant softening of the ligament substance after immobilization (Fig. 12). The mechanical properties of the MCL

substance in the functional range rapidly returned to normal control values as early as 9 weeks following remobilization (Fig. 13). However, the structural properties of the experimental FMT complexes remained inferior to those of controls. Mode of failure for the remobilized limb continued to be disruption at the bony insertion sites, indicating incomplete reorganization at the resorption sites as evidenced by histologic studies of the tibial insertion sites.

Most reports in the literature involving stress and motion deprivation have been concerned with load at failure, with little attention being paid to the mechanical properties of the ligament substance. The rapid recovery of the MCL tissue mechanical properties after remobilization despite the decreased structural properties has important implications not previously revealed. A collagen turnover study further explains the changes seen in the mechanical properties of the ligament tissue (3). Gamble et al. (41) demonstrated the enzymatic adaptation of MCL fibroblasts to a state of catabolism (which may affect all matrix materials) following immobilization. Earlier studies in our laboratory have shown

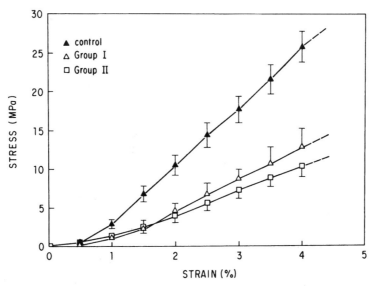

FIG. 12. Mechanical properties of canine MCL from control, 9-week (group 1), and 12-week (group II) immobilization groups. (From Woo et al., ref. 148, with permission).

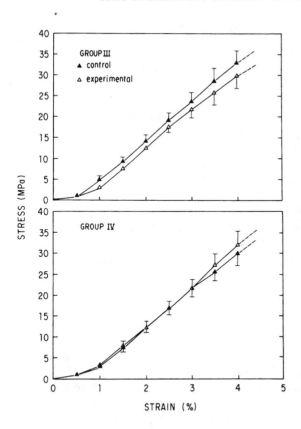

FIG. 13. Mechanical properties of control and experimental (remobilized) MCLs. The experimentals were subjected to 9 weeks of immobilization with 9 weeks remobilization (group III) and 12 weeks of immobilization with 9 weeks remobilization (group IV). (From Woo et al., ref. 148, with permission.)

a large reduction in glycosaminoglycans (GAGs) in the MCLs of immobilized rabbit limbs (1). The significant changes in the mechanical properties of the ligament substance with immobilization may be related to the drastic reduction in GAGs (23). During remobilization, we have observed recovery in the MCL of overall collagen mass and presumably the fiber orientation, and hence, the recovery of the mechanical properties (3). In contrast, the incomplete recovery of the structural properties of the FMTC implies an asynchronous recovery rate at the insertion sites, especially in the subperiosteal region of the tibia.

Recent work has documented significant decreases in the cross-sectional area of rabbit ACL with 9 weeks of immobilization of the knee joint at either 105° or 170° flexion (82). The changes in the tensile properties of the ACL were not as dramatic as with the MCL: there was a slight decrease in the mechanical

properties of the ligament substance for both angles of immobilization, but no statistical significance was demonstrated. On the other hand, the strain at failure was increased 32% to 40% with immobilization. It appears that different soft tissue structures are affected differently by immobilization, and care must therefore be exercised when generalizing specific results to other ligaments or tendons. Obviously, much work remains to be done to increase our understanding of the effects of immobilization and remobilization, in particular, the differences between the overall response of different structures is likely mediated by the cellular response.

Exercise

The effect of exercise on tendons and ligaments has also been investigated, but with often confusing and contradictory results. The cause of discrepancies may include the use of various animal models, inadequate intergroup matching of variables, different experimental procedures, and inconsistent definition of controls and exercised animals. There is a suggestion of decreased water content with a more dull appearance and a slight loss of fiber waviness in ligaments immediately after exercise (117). Increases in cross-sectional area and weight have been reported after certain long-term exercise programs (115). Microscopically, this increase in mass has been proposed to be secondary to fiber bundle hypertrophy (with increased collagen matrix between cell bodies) rather than cellular hyperplasia (113,115). Ligament insertions are particularly sensitive to stress and motion, especially those insertions that insert in concert with the periosteum (5,56). Many of these changes are probably influenced by the specific ligament type, but a spectrum may exist for tissue response to activity level, such that each ligament or tendon has a unique threshold level of activity required to maintain normal homeostatic conditions. Tipton et al. (115) demonstrated definitive improvement in strength of the bone–ligament–bone complex of dogs by keeping animals in open pens. The ultimate loads of these complexes in various models have generally been higher following exercise (17,113,115,151). Similar results were obtained for medial collateral (116, 137,142), lateral collateral (152), and anterior cruciate ligament preparations (86,87).

The effect of short- and long-term exercise on the biomechanical properties of swine digital tendons and the FMTC has been studied (133,145). In the tendon study, swine were randomly divided into two groups that were exercised for 3 months (short-term group) and 12 months (long-term group). The animals were run at speeds of 6 to 8 km/hr over an average distance of 40 km/wk. Nonexercised, age-matched swine were used as sedentary controls. It was found that short-term exercise had little or no effect on the digital extensor tendon properties, whereas the long-term exercise group demonstrated positive changes. There was an increase in cross-sectional area as well as a 22% increase in tensile strength. For the

flexor tendons, the mechanical properties of the tendon substance exhibited no statistical changes, even after 12 months of training. However, the ultimate load of the exercised flexor-tendon complexes increased by 19% secondary to changes at the bony insertion sites. Tipton et al. (113) noted that FMTC of caged, exercised dogs had higher strength/body weight ratios than those from caged, nonexercised controls. In our laboratory, we also examined the effect of long-term (12 months) exercise on the swine FMTC (137,142). Exercise group animals were trained for 1 hr per day at 5 to 6 km/hr plus $^1/_2$ hr at 7 to 8 km/hr every other day. Age-matched nonexercised animals were used as controls. At sacrifice, the FMTC was removed and subjected to tensile testing to failure. Little change was seen in structural properties with exercise, although a small but significant difference was demonstrated when maximum force at failure was normalized for animal body weight (Table 1). No change was found in the concentrations of collagen and elastin in the MCL with exercise.

From these findings we have constructed a hypothesis that schematically describes the homeostatic responses for connective tissues such as tendons and ligaments (Fig. 14). The relationship between the level and duration of stress and motion and the resulting changes in tissue properties and tissue mass can be represented by a series of nonlinear curves. With stress and motion deprivation (immobilization), a rapid reduction in tissue properties and mass may occur. For example, a short period of immobilization of the rabbit knee results in a

TABLE 1. *Comparison of structural properties for control and exercised swine FMTC[a]*

Structural properties	Control ($n = 7$)	Exercised ($n = 10$)
P_{max} (N)	945.0 ± 74.0	1008.2 ± 83.0
Def_{max} (mm)	10.4 ± 0.3	10.0 ± 0.5
A_{max} (N-mm)	4.3 ± 0.4	4.4 ± 0.6
P_{max}/body weight	1.3 ± 0.1	$1.8 \pm 0.2^*$

[a]A significant difference was seen only when ultimate load (P_{max}) was normalized for body weight. Def_{max}, deformation at failure; A_{max}, ultimate energy absorbed. $^*p < 0.05$.

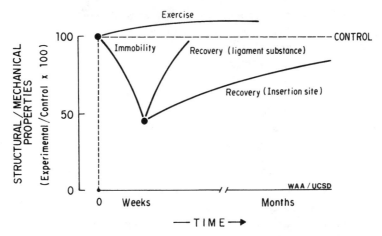

FIG. 14. Schematic curves summarizing the homeostatic responses of the bone–ligament–bone complex when subjected to different levels of physical activity. (From Woo et al., ref. 148, with permission.)

significant alteration in the mechanical properties of the MCL substance and, even more drastically, in the strength of the tibial insertion site. In contrast, the changes resulting from exercise training are not as pronounced. For example, with short-term (3 months) exercise training, the porcine tendon had little change in mass or mechanical properties. Only after long-term (12 months) training were positive responses seen in the strength of the tendon and ligament insertion sites to bone and in the biomechanical properties (and mass) of extensor tendons. In terms of recovery following immobilization, it has been observed that there are differences between the response of the individual tissue constituents and the tissue–bone complex as a whole. The functional integrity of the uninjured, immobilized ligament returns to its normal characteristics quite rapidly following remobilization. However, the recovery of the ligament–bone junction is much slower than that of the ligament substance.

Increased Tension

Altering the stress levels experienced by a ligament can elicit changes in the biomechanical responses of ligamentous tissue (44). In an experimental study, increased tension on the rabbit MCL was accomplished by inserting a stainless steel pin beneath the MCL perpendicular to the long axis of the ligament (44) and developing an increase in *in situ* strain of up to 4%, with a corresponding 2- to 3.5-fold increase of the *in situ* load and stress over those of contralateral controls. However, by 12 weeks, these differences had diminished. In terms of the mechanical properties of the MCL substance, the modulus was lower with increased tension at 6 weeks but became greater than controls at 12 weeks, indicating improved properties of the MCL.

CONTRIBUTION OF EXTERNAL FACTORS

In addition to the factors dicussed above, there exist variables that can further influence the apparent properties obtained from biomechanical testing but that are not always considered. These represent possible alterations introduced during the handling, storage, or preparation of the tissue after harvesting but before experimental testing.

Storage by Freezing

Biomechanical testing of ligaments and tendons has evolved into very complex methodologies. This often requires a considerable period of time for each individual test, and, therefore, storage by specimen freezing becomes a necessity. Consequently, the effects of frozen storage on the mechanical properties of these tissues must be addressed. Furthermore, the results obtained will aid the current clinical interest in using frozen cadaver tendons and ligaments as allografts for transplantation. Several biomechanical studies comparing the properties of fresh soft tissues with those following storage have been conducted, but with conflicting results (76,108,120,125). Most recently, several authors examined the effect of frozen storage for 4 weeks (at $-15°C$) on monkey ACLs. Some authors have found no changes in the structural properties of bone–ligament–bone specimens (88), whereas others reported a slight increase in stiffness (29). A study was designed to evaluate possible changes in the mechanical properties of the rabbit MCL substance and/or of the structural properties of the FMTC following 3 months of limb storage at $-20°C$ (144). Fresh contralateral limbs were dissected immediately at sacrifice and tested as controls.

There were no significant differences between fresh and frozen samples in most of the parameters measured (Table 2), except for the area of hysteresis, where the frozen samples demonstrated significant decreases during the first few cycles of loading and unloading when compared to fresh contralateral controls. These

differences diminished and became insignificant with further cycling. Thus, the area of hysteresis may be a sensitive indicator of minor changes in the properties of bone–ligament complex secondary to storage by freezing. It is conjectured that these changes may result from some insult to cellular integrity or associated ground substance (120) or from changes in fluid flow through the ligament (109). Freezing did not appear to affect the ligament insertion sites, as the mode of failure was not altered between the experimental and the control FMTC. However, it is necessary to reiterate that care must be taken in preparing the tissue sample prior to freezing in order to protect the sample from dehydration. To this end, the ligaments were stored with muscle and other tissue left in place, rather than in the completely dissected state. Each specimen was then double-wrapped in saline-soaked gauze and sealed in airtight plastic bags. Thawing was carried out at refrigerator temperatures ($4°C$) overnight, and specimens were prepared for testing soon after being removed from the refrigerator.

Irradiation

The results of mechanical tests of irradiated PT allografts depend on both the method of graft sterilization and the test environment. Compared with nonirradiated control grafts, modulus and ultimate tensile strength were significantly lower in both freeze-dried irradiated (2 Mrad) grafts and fresh-frozen irradiated (2 Mrad) grafts tested in air (43) or moistened with a saline drip (50). The effects of irradiation on the mechanical properties of the ligaments and tendons are also dose dependent. The ultimate tensile strength, ultimate strain, and strain energy density of goat bone–PT–bone allografts were significantly reduced following 3 Mrad or 4 Mrad, but not 2 Mrad, of irradiation (43,100).

The effect of irradiation on the viscoelastic response of the PT has also been examined. Haut and Powlison (50) compared the amount of stress relaxation in irradiated (2 Mrad) and nonirradiated human PTs and found signifi-

TABLE 2. *Structural properties of the rabbit FMTC (skeletally mature animals) comparing fresh and frozen bone–ligament–bone preparations*

	Fresh ($n = 5$)	Stored 45 days ($n = 5$)
Area of hysteresis		
First cycle (N-mm)	5.86 ± 1.60	2.20 ± 0.54*
Tenth cycle (N-mm)	1.36 ± 0.50	0.58 ± 0.30
Structural properties (at failure)		
P_{max} (N)	368.4 ± 15.0	316.2 ± 22.3
Def_{max} (mm)	6.6 ± 0.5	6.6 ± 0.5
A_{max} (N-mm)	1330.0 ± 200.0	1170.0 ± 200.0

A_{max}, ultimate energy absorbed; Def_{max}, deformation at failure; P_{max} ultimate load (newtons); *$p < 0.05$.

cant differences between the two groups. These radiation-induced changes in ligament and tendon substance are substantiated by biochemical and histologic findings (28). Collagen has been found to be more resistant to extraction after 2 Mrad of irradiation, suggesting that irradiation causes cleavage of polypeptide chains and induces additional cross-linking. However, a 2 Mrad dose of radiation does not cause major disruption of the banding pattern of collagen (28).

NONLINEAR VISCOELASTIC PROPERTIES

Tendons and ligaments display time- and history-dependent viscoelastic properties that reflect the complex interactions of collagen and the surrounding proteins and ground substance. As a result of internal energy dissipation, the loading and unloading curves of these tissues do not follow the same path but instead form a hysteresis loop. Other important viscoelastic characteristics of tendons and ligaments are *creep,* an increase in deformation over time under a constant load, and *stress relaxation,* a decline in stress over time under a constant deformation (Fig. 15). The viscoelastic behavior of tendons and ligaments has important clinical significance. During walking or jogging, the applied strains and strain rates are nearly constant (132,136). Cyclic stress relaxation will effectively soften tissue substance with continuous decreases in peak stress as cycling proceeds. This phenomenon may help to prevent fatigue failure of ligaments and tendons.

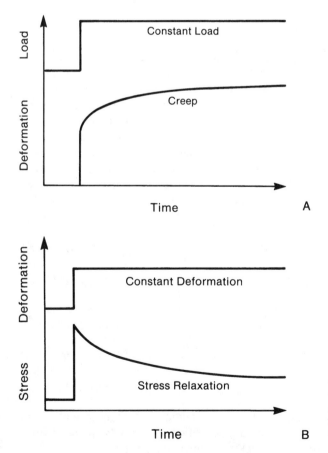

FIG. 15. (A) Schematic representation of creep behavior (increasing deformation over time under a constant load). **(B)** Stress relaxation (decreasing stress over time under a constant deformation).

Similarly, deformation increases slightly during cycles to a constant load, demonstrating creep behavior of tendons and ligaments (124). These changes have been noted clinically with temporary softening of all these tissues and thus increases of test excursion (laxity) in exercised joints. After a short recovery period, there is a return to normal joint stiffness and apparent length.

Quasilinear Viscoelasticity

The quasilinear viscoelastic (QLV) theory developed by Fung has been used successfully in the past to describe these time- and history-dependent viscoelastic properties for many soft tissues (20,40,60,93,107,111,146). This theory has also been used for tendons and ligaments (132,136). Recently, the QLV theory has been further refined to account for a constant strain rate (rather than an infinite strain rate or true step load, which is physically impossible to achieve experimentally) and the subsequent stress relaxation. The QLV theory assumes that the stress relaxation function of the tissue can be expressed in the form

$$\sigma(t) = G(t)\sigma^e(\varepsilon) \qquad (1)$$

where $\sigma^e(\varepsilon)$ is the "elastic response," i.e., the maximum stress in response to an instantaneous step input of strain ε. $G(t)$ is the reduced relaxation function that represents the time-dependent stress response of the tissue normalized by the stress at the time of step input of strain [i.e., $t = 0^+$, such that $G(t) = \sigma(t)/\sigma(0^+)$, and $G(0^+) = 1$].

If the strain history is considered as a series of infinitesimal step strains ($\Delta\varepsilon$), and the superposition principle is accepted as valid, then the overall stress relaxation function will be the sum of all individual relaxations. Thus, for a general strain history, the stress at time t, $\sigma(t)$, is given by the strain history and the convolution integral over time of $G(t)$:

$$\sigma(t) = \int_{-\infty}^{t} G(t-\tau) \frac{\partial\sigma^e(\varepsilon)}{\partial\varepsilon} \frac{\partial\varepsilon}{\partial\tau} d\tau \qquad (2)$$

The lower limit of integration is taken as negative infinity to imply inclusion of all past strain history. In the experimental setting, we can assume that the history begins at $t = 0$. It is evident, then, that once $G(t)$, $\sigma^e(\varepsilon)$, and the strain history are known, the time- and history-dependent stress can be completely described by equation 2. For soft tissues, whose σ–ε relationship and hysteresis are not overly sensitive to strain rates, Fung has proposed the following expression for $G(t)$:

$$G(t) = \frac{1 + C[E_1(t/\tau_2) - E_1(t/\tau_1)]}{1 + Cln(\tau_2/\tau_1)} \qquad (3)$$

where $E_1(y) = \int_y^\infty e^{-z}/z \, dz$ is the exponential integral, and C, τ_1, and τ_2 and are material coefficients. Because tendons and ligaments all possess such properties, this formulation of $G(t)$ has been adopted for some musculoskeletal soft tissues (136).

An exponential approximation has been chosen to describe the elastic stress–strain relationship during a constant strain-rate test:

$$\sigma^e(\varepsilon) = A(e^{B\varepsilon} - 1) \qquad (4)$$

where A and B are material coefficients (136).

As noted previously, it is impossible to experimentally administer an instantaneous strain to the test material, and thus impossible to directly measure $\sigma^e(\varepsilon)$. To better approximate actual experimental conditions, it was necessary to develop a new procedure in which the instantaneous step load is replaced by a ramp load with a constant, finite strain rate γ to a strain level ε at time t_0. The corresponding stress rise during $0 < t < t_0$ can then be written by combining equations 3 and 4 as

$$\sigma(t) = \frac{AB\gamma}{1 + Cln(\tau_2/\tau_1)} \int_0^t \{1 + C[E_1[(t - \tau)/\tau_2] - E_1[(t - \tau)/\tau_1]]\}e^{B\gamma\tau}d\tau \qquad (5)$$

Similarly, the subsequent stress relaxation $\sigma(t)$, from t_0 to $t = \infty$, can be described as

$$\sigma(t) = \frac{AB\gamma}{1 + Cln(\tau_2/\tau_1)} \int_0^{t_0} \{1 + C[E_1[(t - \tau)/\tau_2] - E_1[(t - \tau)/\tau_1]]\}e^{B\gamma\tau}d\tau \qquad (6)$$

These two equations are then normalized by dividing equations 5 and 6 by the peak stress $\sigma(t_0)$ to eliminate constant A.

$$\frac{\sigma(t)}{\sigma(t_0)} = \frac{\int_0^{\min(t,t_0)}\{1 + C[E_1[(t - \tau)/\tau_2] - E_1[(t - \tau)/\tau_1]]\}\varepsilon^{B\gamma\tau}d\tau}{\int_0^{t_0}\{1 + C[E_1[(t_0 - \tau)/\tau_2] - E_1[(t_0 - \tau)/\tau_1]]\}\varepsilon^{B\gamma\tau}d\tau} \tag{7}$$

With data from a stress-relaxation experiment, the material coefficients B, C, τ_1, and τ_2 can be determined by a nonlinear, least-square, curve-fitting procedure (66,70). Constant A can then be computed by using either equation 5 or 6. For a known strain history, these five constants, together with $G(t)$ and $\sigma^e(\varepsilon)$, can then be used to determine the stress at any time t, $\sigma(t)$, by using equation 3. The following example illustrates the method described (66,70). The anteromedial bundles of porcine ACL were stretched to 5% strain at a strain rate of 2.5%/sec and allowed to stress relax up to 2 hr. A typical recording of the stress rise in response to the applied ramp load and the subsequent stress relaxation is shown in Fig. 16. By use of equation 7 and a nonlinear, least-square, curve-fitting procedure, the constants B, C, τ_1, and τ_2 were found to be 0.63 ± 0.002, 0.146 ± 0.07, 0.097 ± 0.01 sec, and 0.808 ± 0.18 ($\times 10^5$ sec), respectively. Constant A was then determined to be 210 ± 36 MPa using equation 5. The time-dependent stress relaxation was then calculated from equation 3 as

$$G(t) = 0.858 - 0.049 \; ln \; t \tag{8}$$

The stress–strain relationship was then obtained using equation 4:

$$\sigma^e(\varepsilon) = 210(e^{0.063\varepsilon} - 1) \tag{9}$$

The theoretical prediction for the reduced relaxation function agrees well with the experimental findings, but these material constants must be verified by a second independent experiment. In this case, a more general cyclic strain history was used. The same anteromedial bundles of the ACL were cycled between 1% and 5% strains at a strain rate of 2.5%/sec for ten cycles. The peak and valley stresses are plotted in Fig. 17 and the QLV theory matches well with the experimental data.

Single Integral Finite Strain Model

Because there are numerous cases in which the deformation of the tissue of interest is finite, a more general continuum model for nonlinear viscoelastic behavior of soft biological tissues is required (61). This model describes finite deformation of a nonlinearly

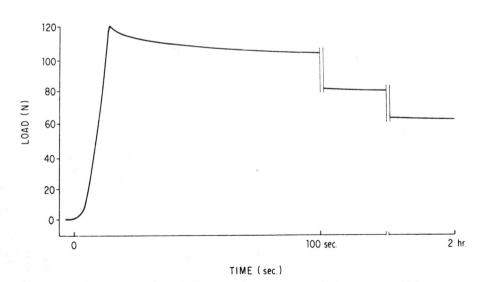

FIG. 16. Typical experimental stress response of porcine anterior cruciate ligament (ACL) anteromedial bundles to applied ramp load and the subsequent stress relaxation.

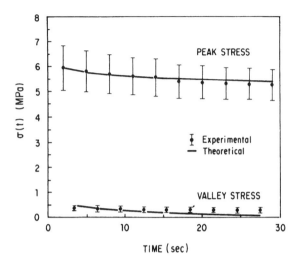

FIG. 17. Theoretical versus experimental peak and valley stress relaxation values for the anteromedial bundle of porcine ACL under cyclic loading. (From Lin et al., ref. 70, with permission.)

viscoelastic material within the context of a three-dimensional model. Called the single integral finite strain (SIFS) viscoelastic model, it is fully nonlinear and reduces to an appropriate finite elasticity model for time zero. Moreover, if linearized, the SIFS model yields the equations for classical linear viscoelasticity. By reducing this model to one dimension and introducing additional assumptions regarding the forms for the relaxation function and stress–strain relationship, QLV can be recovered.

A quite general integral series representation for nonlinear viscoelastic response was proposed by Pipkin and Rogers (94). It is proposed that the same constitutive equation can be applied to the modeling of ligaments and tendons. The development of the current model began with the assumption that the Cauchy stress $\mathbf{T}$ has the form (94)

$$\mathbf{T} = -p\mathbf{I} + \mathbf{F}(t)\left\{\mathbf{R}[\mathbf{C}(t),0]\right.$$
$$\left. + \int_0^t \frac{\partial}{\partial(t-s)}(\mathbf{R}[\mathbf{C}(s),t-s])ds\right\}\mathbf{F}^T(t) \quad (10)$$

where p is the indeterminate part of the stress arising from the constraint of incompressibility, $\mathbf{I}$ is the identity tensor, $\mathbf{F}$ is the deformation gradient tensor, and $\mathbf{C}$ is the Cauchy-Green strain tensor. The symbol $\mathbf{R}$ represents a strain-dependent tensorial relaxation function. The measures of deformation used here

are properly frame indifferent (i.e., independent of the observer). All of the following results are consistent with this requirement, which is sometimes called the principle of objectivity or material frame indifference. The expression given by equation 10 incorporates the assumption that there has been no deformation prior to time $t = 0$. If deformation is allowed for times $-\infty < t < 0$, then the lower limit of integration is changed, and equation 10 becomes

$$\mathbf{T} = -p\mathbf{I} + \mathbf{F}(t)$$
$$\times \left\{\int_{-\infty}^t \frac{\partial}{\partial(t-s)}(\mathbf{R}[\mathbf{C}(s),t-s])ds\right\}\mathbf{F}^T(t) \quad (11)$$

The term $\mathbf{R}[\mathbf{C}(t),0]$ in equation 10 represents an instantaneous deformation occurring at $t = 0$. The strain-dependent tensorial relaxation function in the above equations has the form:

$$\mathbf{R} = \phi_0\mathbf{I} + \phi_1\mathbf{C} + \phi_2\mathbf{C}^2 \quad (12)$$

where ϕ_0, ϕ_1, and ϕ_2 are scalar functions of t and the tensorial invariants of $\mathbf{C}$. If the equations are not linearized, QLV can be obtained by an appropriate selection of ϕ_0, ϕ_1, and ϕ_2. In fact, the formulation of QLV can be obtained as restrictions to one dimension for an infinite number of general models because the choices for ϕ_0, ϕ_1, and ϕ_2 that will yield QLV are not unique.

In general, the ϕ_i should be chosen so that the viscoelastic model will reduce to reasonable limits, such as an accepted model of finite elasticity. Here we are guided, as Fung was previously (39), by the similarities between the elasticity of rubber and of living tissues. The ϕ_i were chosen (126) such that

$$\mathbf{R}[\mathbf{C}(s),\xi] = G(\xi)\{[1 + \mu I(s)]\mathbf{I} - \mu\mathbf{C}(s)\} \quad (13)$$

where

$$I(s) = \mathrm{tr}\mathbf{C}(s) \quad (14)$$

and $G(\xi)$ is a relaxation function. The choice of relaxation function is based on the idea of fading memory; that is, events in the recent past have more influence on the current state of stress than those of the more distant past. Equation 11 can be rewritten by substituting the definitions in equations 13 and 14, as

$$\mathbf{T} = -p\mathbf{I} + C_0\{[1 + \mu I(t)]\mathbf{B}(t) - \mu\mathbf{B}^2(t)\}$$
$$-C_0(1 - \gamma)\int_0^t \dot{G}(t-s)\{[1 + \mu I(s)]\mathbf{B}(t)$$
$$- \mu\mathbf{F}(t)\mathbf{C}(s)\mathbf{F}^T(s)\}ds \quad (15)$$

Here, C_0 is the initial modulus, and $\gamma = C_\infty/C_0$, where C_∞ is the long-time modulus. The relaxation function, $\dot{G}(t-s)$, in the history integral ensures that more recent states of strain have greater weight in determining the stress than earlier states.

Biological tissues such as ligaments and tendons have nonlinear and history-dependent behavior that reflect their complex structure. A typical stress–strain curve has two distinct regions. The initial region, also known as the "toe region," exhibits nonlinearity and low modulus, whereas the second region reflects a greater modulus but a relatively linear stress–strain curve. The term "linear modulus" is sometimes used to refer to the slope of the stress–strain curve in this region. Ligaments and tendons are made up of densely packed collagen fibril bundles that are organized in a parallel fashion along the length of the tissue. Under zero stress, the fibers are crimped. When a ligament is stretched, small initial loads are required to straighten the crimp, and progressively larger loads are required to further elongate the fibers. This phenomenon is called "recruitment."

For uniaxial tension, equation 15 reduces to a single integral equation relating stress to stretch history:

$$\sigma(t) = C_0\left(1 + \mu\frac{1}{\lambda(t)}\right)\left(\lambda^2(t) - \frac{1}{\lambda(t)}\right)$$
$$-C_0(1 - \gamma)\left(\lambda^2(t) - \frac{1}{\lambda(t)}\right)\int_0^t \dot{G}(t-s)\left(1 + \mu\frac{1}{\lambda(t)}\right)ds$$
$$(16)$$

where λ is the stretch ratio at time t. The function $G(t)$ was proposed based on observation in order to capture the physics of the stress-relaxation response exhibited by ligaments and tendons. The relaxation function was selected to be a decreasing function of time

$$G(t) = \frac{\alpha}{(t + \alpha)} \quad (17)$$

Here α is a constant. The shear modulus is assumed to be a function of the invariants of $\mathbf{B}$. For the present case, the following specific form can be used:

$$\mu = \mu_0\left[\left(\lambda^2 - \frac{2}{\lambda}\right)^2 - 9\right] \quad (18)$$

The model was applied to data from uniaxial extension of younger and older human PTs and canine MCLs (61,141). Model parameters were determined from curve-fitting stress–strain and stress–relaxation data and used to predict the time-dependent stress generated by cyclic extensions. Based on the parameters obtained from the stress-relaxation tests, there was very good agreement between model predictions and experimental results for an independent, cyclic stretching test to finite strain.

FUNCTION OF TENDONS AND LIGAMENTS

The kinematics of the musculoskeletal system provide useful insights into the importance of the normal function of ligaments and tendons. In the following section, information obtained for both tendons and ligaments will be reviewed.

Flexor Tendons

The interrelationship of joint rotation and tendon excursion has been studied clinically, experimentally, and analytically. In general, it is well recognized that the greater the distance from the tendon to the joint center or axis of rotation (i.e., the larger the moment arm), the less joint rotation will be generated for a given tendon excursion. The relationship between joint rotation and tendon excursion can be described mathematically (5). From the simple geometric relationship $\Delta\theta = r\Delta s$, the instantaneous moment arm of the tendon in the plane of motion (r) at a specific joint configuration can be obtained from the slope of a plot of tendon excursion (Δs) versus joint rotational displacement ($\Delta\theta$). At the metacarpophalangeal joint, extensor excursion is almost linearly related to the joint angle of rotation. Because the extensor tendon passes the joint by wrapping around the dorsal surface of the metacarpal head, the moment arm is relatively constant throughout the arc of motion. The excursion–rotation relationship for both superficial and deep flexor tendons is relatively linear but becomes slightly curved when the joint is close to full flexion. In other words, the moment arms of these two flexors increase as the joint flexion angle increases. Further, flexor tendon excursion is governed by the constraint of the pulley system (4). Therefore, any alteration in the flexor pulley system will result in a change in the normal relationship.

The normal gliding function of the flexor tendons can be explained in terms of the relative moment arms of the flexor digitorum profundus and superficialis. The moment arms of these tendons are not equal at the proximal interphalangeal (PIP) and metacarpophalangeal (MCP) joints (6,7); thus, for a given degree of flexion, there will be nonequivalent excursions of the two flexors, and any movement of the joints will generate gliding motion be-

tween these tendons. When the distal interphalangeal joint is flexed to 60°, there will be a 4-mm gliding motion between the two tendons in the zone II region (distal palmar crease to the profundus tendon insertion) (Fig. 18). If the proximal interphalangeal joint is flexed to 60°, an additional 1.8 mm of relative gliding motion will be added. Larger motion of the DIP and PIP joints, such as in the "hook" and "fist" positions, will generate the greatest gliding motion between the two flexors (123). The tendon excursion relative to the sheath in zone II has been considered a significant factor in the prevention of adhesion formation following injury.

In our laboratory, the kinematics of the digital flexor tendons in this region was recently studied. Tendon excursion, sheath displacement, and joint rotation were examined in 12 cadaveric human digits using radiopaque markers placed in the flexor digitorum profundus and tendon sheath as well as the metacarpal and three phalangeal bones. Roentgenograms were taken in flexion and extension of the digit, with joint motion allowed first at all joints and then restricted to

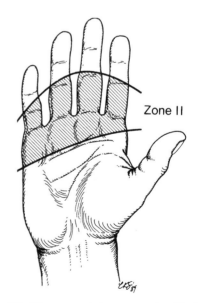

FIG. 18. Diagram of human palm illustrating zone II region–distal palmar crease to the profundus tendon insertion.

only the DIP, PIP, or MCP joint. The changes in the positions of the markers were digitized and stored by computer. The center of rotation, angle of rotation, tendon excursion, and sheath displacement were then calculated. Tendon excursion relative to sheath in zone II was maximized by motion of the PIP joint (1.7 mm/10° of joint flexion) relative to motion at DIP and MCP joints (Fig. 19). Little tendon excursion occurred distal to the joint in motion. In another study using canine digits, tendon excursions at the MCP, PIP, and DIP joints were found to be similar to the results obtained for human specimens, suggesting that the canine may be a suitable model for future studies of tendon kinematics and healing.

Stabilizing Roles of the Ligaments of the Knee

The predominant kinematic characteristics of the knee are determined by the curvatures of the femoral and tibial articulating surfaces as well as by the orientation of the four major ligaments of the knee (62). For example, the important function of the MCL as a stabilizer of valgus knee rotation has previously been reported by several investigators. By applying a predetermined amount of joint rotation and measuring the resultant force or moment, Piziali et al. (95), Seering et al. (103), and Grood et al. (46) compared the changes in the load (or moment) before and after sectioning the knee ligaments and concluded that the MCL was a major restraint to valgus rotation. Other investigators chose to measure joint motion or laxity after applying a specific load or moment and reported conflicting results. Brantigan and Voshell (13) and Nielsen et al. (83,84) found only slight increases in valgus laxity after sectioning the MCL, whereas Kennedy and Fowler (64), Warren et al. (122), Markolf et al. (74), and Mains et al. (73) reported a significant increase in valgus laxity after sectioning of the MCL. Some discrepancies in the data obtained may be attributed to testing devices that overly restrict joint mo-

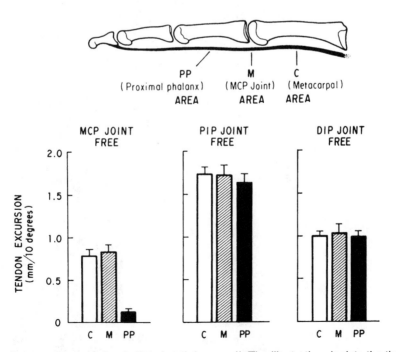

FIG. 19. Tendon excursion relative to the sheath in zone II. The illustration depicts the three regions (PP, M, and C) within zone II for which tendon excursion was determined.

tion. Other reasons may include the different types and methods of force application to the test specimen as well as the species being tested.

To demonstrate this, a study was undertaken to examine the functional roles of the MCL and the ACL and their effects on the kinematics of the canine knee joint after isolated MCL injury (58). Varus-valgus (V-V) joint laxity secondary to the application of a defined bending moment was quantitatively measured in the canine knee joint at 90° flexion using a device that allowed selected degrees of freedom (DOF) of joint motion. When the knee motion was limited to 3 DOF (V-V rotation and proximal-distal and medial-lateral translations), valgus laxity increased significantly (171%) after sectioning the MCL, indicating that the MCL was the primary restraint (Fig. 20). However, when axial tibial rotation and anteroposterior translation were permitted (i.e., increasing the joint motion to 5 DOF), sectioning the MCL resulted in only a 21% increase in valgus laxity, whereas sectioning the ACL resulted in a 123% increase. In this situation, the ACL restrained V-V rotation significantly. This may be due to the fact that internal tibial rotation is coupled with valgus rotation. As a result, in an MCL-deficient

knee, the potential functional deficit in valgus rotation may be compensated for by coupled internal tibial rotation and the remaining structures, especially the ACL. Therefore, the importance of degrees of freedom in the interpretation of test results is evident for complex joints.

Contribution of the ACL to Knee Kinematics

The kinematics of the ACL has received much attention because of its important role in normal knee function as well as in ligament reconstruction. Of particular interest have been the length and loading changes of the ACL during physiological knee motion.

During ACL reconstruction, one of the goals has been to minimize the loads on the graft by seeking an isometric point for graft placement. A number of investigators have examined these isometric or "nearly isometric" positions. Using an electrogoniometer, Hefzy et al. (51) determined the femoral insertion site locations for which the ACL length change was less than 2 mm with knee flexion. These "nearly isometric" insertion sites were contained in a region on the femur, oriented in a proximal–distal direction. The overall shape and orientation were dependent

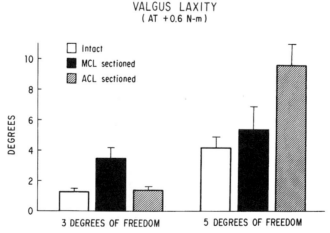

FIG. 20. The increase in valgus laxity after sectioning of MCL versus ACL while permitting 3 DOF versus 5 DOF of the test apparatus. (From Inoue et al., ref. 58, with permission.)

on the tibial insertion site, joint loading, and flexion angle. Sidles et al. (105,106) also examined "nearly isometric" femoral insertion sites and found them to vary with tibial insertion site location.

Variable changes in length among the ACL bundles were examined by Butler et al. (16). These investigators found that such variations depend on the femoral insertion site in flexion and the tibial insertion site during rotation. On the other hand, the importance of isometry during clinical ACL reconstruction has been questioned by other investigators. Sapega et al. (102) challenged the need for truly isometric graft positioning by demonstrating that under motion and loading conditions similar to those in the surgical environment, the ACL exhibits nonisometric characteristics. Using a computer model, Blankevoort and Huiskes et al. (12) found that the actual effects of changing the ACL insertion sites on the loads in the ACL replacement might not be as large as those predicted by models based on the normal knee because alterations in kinematics in the reconstructed knee may compensate for length changes in the ligament.

In our laboratory, we have determined the *in situ* forces without attachment of mechanical devices on, near, or within the ligament. We first began by using a 6-DOF kinematic linkage to measure the *in situ* forces indirectly (53). With this kinematic linkage, the insertions of the ACL were digitized to obtain the lengths of the ACL (or its portions) under anterior–posterior (AP) or V-V loading of the intact knee. These lengths were later correlated to ligament force through tensile testing of ligament portions (52). To avoid alterations in ligament geometry that may have been introduced by the tensile testing of these structures, we then utilized length–force correlations obtained *in situ* to determine ligament forces (110). Because these approaches were both indirect, we then progressed to determining the *in situ* forces in knee ligaments directly and in a noncontact manner. It was further important to develop a methodology in which the *in situ* forces of several soft tissues within the same knee could be determined under complex external loadings

of the joint in order to minimize the effects of inherent interspecimen variability.

Robotic/Universal Force–Motion Sensor System

To accomplish this, we used a robotic manipulator for 6-DOF control of joint motion (38) combined with a universal force–moment sensor (UFS) to determine *in situ* ligament forces (37). Using force–moment control, the robot can learn the exact path of motion of the intact joint under complex loading conditions and then reproduce this motion in a dissected specimen. The UFS, used in conjunction with the robot, can record forces and moments and then yield the magnitude, direction, and the point of application of the *in situ* forces of the ligament. Data obtained under multi-DOF joint loading should help to better characterize the mechanical role of the ligaments during physiological knee motion and will provide data for improved ligament reconstruction and rehabilitation.

Control of 6-DOF joint motion is accomplished using a six-joint serial articulated robotic manipulator (Unimate, PUMA-762). The robot is a position-controlled device, but we can also operate it in a force-controlled mode by using feedback from a UFS (JR3, model 4015) attached to its end-effector. The UFS is a 6-DOF transducer that measures three forces and three moments along and about its Cartesian axes.

During testing, the tibial portion of a knee specimen is rigidly connected to the UFS, which in turn is mounted on the end-effector of the robot. Meanwhile, the femur is fixed relative to the robot base. The robot first "learns" the natural (5-DOF) motion of a test specimen while working in a force-controlled mode. This is accomplished by reacting, iteratively, to forces encountered during a specified test motion (99). The resulting path of motion that is determined is then a series of positions that correspond to the target loading conditions. Thus, during the force-controlled, or learning, phase of the test, the UFS is part of the control system.

After the robot has learned the kinematic motion of the joint, the robot reverts to pure position control. At this point, the UFS is no longer needed for control and is used as a part of the data acquisition system. The robot can exactly repeat a given path of motion, even if the joint has been altered in some way. Reproducing positions before and after cutting a ligament and recording the forces and moments allows determination of the *in situ* force in that structure by the principle of superposition.

We have used this newly developed robotics technology to study the function of the cruciate ligaments. Ten porcine cadaver knee joints were dissected free of musculature, leaving the joint capsule and all ligaments intact. The tibia and femur were cut 20 cm from the joint line and secured within thick-walled aluminum cylinders. The femoral cylinder was then rigidly fixed relative to the robot base, and the tibial cylinder was fixed to the UFS as shown in Fig. 21. Using force–moment control, the robot learned the 6-DOF path of the knee joint between 45° and 90° of knee flexion. In order to minimize the viscoelastic effects, the knee was subject to preconditioning by repeatedly moving it through this range of flexion. With the knee flexed 60°, an A-P load of ±100 N was applied at a rate of 20 mm/min while joint positions were continuously recorded by the manipulator (71). The A-P motion was applied over five cycles, which served to further reduce any viscoelastic effects during this motion. Then

the identical path of 5-DOF motion of the intact knee under A-P loading was reproduced by the robot while the UFS outputs were recorded. Subsequently, the entire ACL was bluntly transected, and the exact path of motion was repeated while the UFS recorded the forces and moments a second time. Using the principle of superposition, the *in situ* forces of the ACL were then determined based on the differences in forces and moments recorded by the UFS before and after the transection.

The use of force–moment control allowed notable tibial rotation under anterior loading. The magnitude and direction of *in situ* forces in the ACL under 100 N of anterior tibial loading was 108 ± 8 N (mean ± SD). This ACL force is lower than that which would be produced if the knee were restricted to single-DOF A-P motion only (71). The direction of *in situ* force for the ACL was also determined. For ease of visualization, this force vector was transformed to spherical coordinates and expressed using two angles, termed elevation (α) and deviation (β); α represents the angle elevated from the tibial plateau, and β represents a medial or lateral deviation from the sagittal plane (Fig. 22). The mean values of these angles were 15° and 6°, respectively, which correspond approximately to the ligament's observed anatomic orientation. The point of application of the *in situ* force in the ACL was centrally located within the ACL insertion site for this unconstrained case.

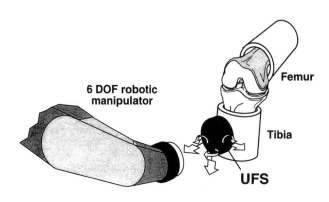

6 DOF robotic manipulator

Femur

Tibia

UFS

FIG. 21. Schematic of the experimental setup showing the robot, the UFS, and the specimen during kinematic testing. (From Livesay et al., ref. 71, with permission.)

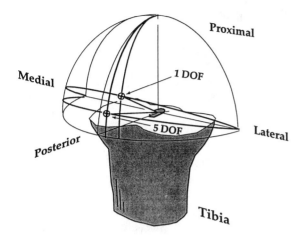

FIG. 22. *In situ* directions for the ACL under 100-N anterior loading, shown from a posterior oblique view of a right knee. Note that the 5-DOF case displays a lower elevation and deviation than the 1-DOF case. (From Livesay et al., ref. 71, with permission.)

Measurement of Ligament Strain During Kinematics

The robotic testing methodology can further be used to examine the *in situ* elongation and strain of the knee ligaments. Because the robotic manipulator can reproduce the complex motion of the knee, we can alter the joint by removing the medial femoral condyle to expose the ACL without affecting the joint kinematics. Video motion analysis equipment can then be used to record and analyze the strains and strain distribution of the ligaments in the dissected knee (e.g., a bone–ligament–bone specimen with the joint capsule and other soft tissues removed). The repeatability of the robot ensures that the joint can be dissected to the point that the ligament becomes visible without altering the path of motion. The use of a noncontact, direct measurement method to obtain these data further enhances their validity.

The video system (VP320/ExpertVision system, Motion Analysis Corporation, Santa Rosa, CA) utilizes multiple cameras to track the positions of optical targets, such as elastin stain markers placed on the ligament surface. In order to find the three-dimensional coordinates of the markers during testing, the system must view each marker in at least two cameras. By using fixed cameras whose positions are precisely known, we can film an object from different directions to determine the coordinates of the object. The motion analysis system can determine the line of sight from any camera to an object in that camera's view. By looking at an object with more than one camera, the system can calculate the intersection of the direction lines to the object, giving its coordinates in three-dimensional space. Thus, it is possible to determine the amount of local elongation that occurs between successive markers on the ligament with a precision of 1% or better.

HEALING OF TENDONS AND LIGAMENTS

The management of damaged ligaments and tendons is one of the most difficult and challenging clinical problems in orthopaedics. Adequate treatment protocols have yet to be determined, and our understanding of the mechanisms of the healing processes remains minimal. The reader is referred to a book for specific reviews of research in this area (130). Descriptions of other types of soft tissue healing have provided a basis for current interests in tendon and ligament healing (14). Two areas of particular clinical interest are (a) the efficacy of repair versus nonrepair, and (b) the effects of motion and activity levels following injury on function.

Flexor Tendons

The digital flexor tendons of the hand are partially surrounded by synovial sheaths that provide lubrication and nutrition for the tendon. Mason and Allen (75) introduced the concept that after tendon injury and repair, the gliding surface between the flexor tendon and its fibrous sheath is compromised as a result of adhesion formation. Three factors are known to contribute to the formation of adhesions: tendon suture, sheath injury, and immobilization. The early stages following repair were characterized by a profound drop in strength, with the lowest values at 4 to 5 days. In contrast, after 13 weeks, the strength of the repair site increased directly in proportion to the stresses applied to it. These findings encouraged clinicians to immobilize tendons for 3 weeks and concentrate on the remodeling stages for stimulation of increased tendon strength and gliding function. The disadvantage of healing precipitated by immobilization is that the remodeling process involves the conflicting needs for both increased strength of the repair and sufficient flexibility of the ingrowing tissue for adequate function. Therefore, it is necessary to explore the fundamental questions regarding the process of tendon healing and the response of the tendon to early mobilization.

In one study (42), the flexor tendons of the second and fourth toes of skeletally mature mongrel dogs were lacerated and repaired using a technique described by Kessler and Missim (65). Animals were divided into three groups to determine the effects of mobilization on repair strength, gliding, and scar remodeling: one group was treated with complete immobilization, a second group with delayed mobilization, and a third group with immediate, controlled, passive mobilization, a protocol similar to the tendon rehabilitation process employed in clinical practice. At sacrifice, the toes of these forepaws were disarticulated at the MCP joints and subjected to biomechanical evaluation. Contralateral control tendons were similarly prepared and tested for comparison. The gliding function of the tendon through the sheath was evaluated using an apparatus designed to measure the angular rotation of the DIP joint when a small load of 1.5 N was applied to the tendon. The tensile properties of the repairs were measured on the basis of the load–deformation relationship of the "tendon–bone composite" (structural properties). The ultimate load and linear slope (stiffness) were determined. The complete immobilization group did not exhibit significant increases in strength of the repaired tendons until 12 weeks postrepair. The delayed, passively mobilized tendons showed increased strength relative to the immobilized tendons at each time interval beyond 3 weeks postrepair. The immediate, controlled, passive mobilization tendons had the best results. Significantly higher values for ultimate load were obtained at each time interval (Fig. 23A). A similar trend was also observed in the stiffness of the load–elongation curves for these tendons. Gliding function (angular rotation per 1.5 N) was greatest in the early mobilization group at both 6 and 12 weeks (Fig. 23B). For the immobilized tendons (group I), the angular rotation 6 weeks after repair was only 21 ± 5% of the intact controls. At 12 weeks, the rotation was further reduced to 19 ± 2%. The delayed mobilization tendons (group II) had better gliding, with angular rotation at 6 and 12 weeks nearly three times that of the immobilized tendons. The angular rotation of the early mobilized repaired tendons (group III) at 6 weeks was 97 ± 16% and at 12 weeks was equal (100%) to that of the controls.

Microangiographic investigation demonstrated that the mobilized groups had vessels that were more normal in density and orientation. Furthermore, scanning electron microscopy showed that the early mobilized tendon and sheath repair sites had a smooth surface and were free of adhesions. Light microscopy also showed that the mobilized tendons had a smooth covering over the repair site by cells from the epitenon at 10 days. This smooth, glistening surface remained unchanged and free of adhesions through 6 weeks. At the ultrastructural level, cells be-

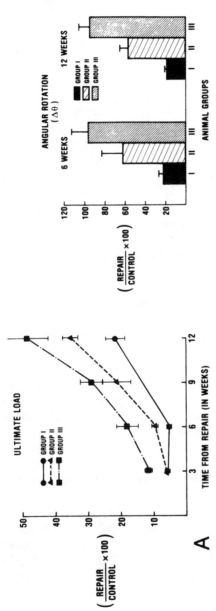

FIG. 23. Comparison of normalized (experimental/control) **(A)** ultimate load and **(B)** angular rotation of repaired canine flexor tendon from immobilization (group I), delayed mobilization (group II), and early mobilization (group III) treatment groups. (From Gelberman et al., ref. 42, with permission.)

tween the tendon ends were active in protein synthesis and collagen production between 3 to 6 weeks. DNA content at the repair site and in the digital sheath was significantly greater in the mobilized groups (42). These studies demonstrated that tensile forces and motion at the repair site provided by controlled passive mobilization appear to accelerate recovery of strength of the repaired tendon. Of equal importance were the improvements in gliding. Prolonged immobilization resulted in decreased range of motion because of scar formation between the repaired tendon and surrounding sheath.

Knee Ligaments

In complete ligament disruptions, free ligament ends usually recoil, with the tortuous, relaxed ligament bodies connected only by hematoma (59). In the first few days following injury, vascular granulation tissue proliferates through hemorrhagic tissues. This is followed by progressive fibrosis for 2 to 3 weeks. At about 1 month, scar formation and maturation begin. Contraction and remodeling of this scar are sufficiently advanced at 6 weeks for some to note "complete healing" (34). However, months or years may be required to approach normality. Tensile tests of healing ligaments suggest that the return to normal strength and elastic stiffness in ligaments is slow (35). The rate of return to normal of structural and mechanical properties in a healing ligament is probably dependent on stress and may therefore be controlled to some extent by levels of physical activity (17,22,118). With repair, there may be alterations in the processes just described. Clayton and Weir (23) and Clayton et al. (22) noted diminution of separation in ligament ends with repair and, therefore, a significant decrease in scar formation. O'Donoghue et al. (90), using a similar model, noted more orderly healing in the early stages as a result of repair. Repaired ligaments appeared "more taut" and had increased collagenization with shorter stages of inflammation and proliferation (90). There is evidence of an early improvement in biomechanical properties of re-

paired ligaments relative to nonrepaired ligaments (23,90). This advantage, however, may not be sustained, as sutured and unsutured ligaments have nearly equal length when measured at rest and comparable failure strength when subjected to exercise (22).

Other biomechanical, biochemical, and histologic aspects of healing of the rabbit MCL have been investigated (35). The study involved complete surgical injuries to the midsubstance of the right rabbit MCLs (experimentals) and only surgical exposure of the contralateral, left MCLs (sham controls). There was no repair or immobilization, and all animals had unrestricted cage activity until sacrificed in groups at 10 days, 3 weeks, 6 weeks, 14 weeks, and 40 weeks after injury. Additional age-, sex-, and activity-matched animals (normal controls) were used at each of these time intervals to provide a baseline of all parameters. Histologic evaluation revealed that healing of the disrupted, nonrepaired ligament is similar to the classic descriptions as detailed earlier. Biochemical results correlated well with the histologic findings (35). Water content was significantly elevated at the injury site but returned to normal after 6 weeks. Glycosaminoglycan (GAG) content was elevated early and remained high at 40 weeks. Collagen content dropped significantly after injury and then steadily recovered but never reached control values. The healing MCLs also contained significant amounts of Type III collagen (scar tissue). The mechanical and structural properties of the healing MCL were persistently different from the sham controls even at 40 weeks postinjury. The healing MCL was larger, weaker, and less stiff in tension than normals.

In a second animal model, three groups of adult mongrel dogs were used to evaluate the effects of both repair versus nonrepair and mobilization versus immobilization on healing of the transected MCL (140). The first group was the early mobilization group in which the MCL of the left knee was transected at the joint line and not repaired. The animals were allowed immediate cage and farm activities for 6, 12, and 48 weeks and were then sacrificed. The second group was the shorter term immobilization group in which the transected MCL was repaired by modified Kessler technique. The knee joint was immobilized for 3 weeks and then remobilized for either 3 or 9 weeks with cage activity. The third group was the longer term immobilization group in which the MCL was transected and repaired as before, but immobilization was extended to 6 weeks. These animals were subsequently remobilized with cage and farm activities for 6 and 42 weeks. The right knees of all animals were sham operated, leaving the MCL intact.

At sacrifice, each knee was then mounted in a device designed to measure V-V laxity at 90° flexion (134). A cyclic torque of ±0.6 N-m was applied to the joint, and the angular deformation θ was recorded. The Δθ value between ± 0.6 N-m was defined as the V-V joint laxity. After laxity testing, all soft tissues except the MCL were removed and the FMTC was subjected to tensile testing to failure (134,135). At 6 weeks postoperatively, all experimental knees had significantly higher V-V laxities (Fig. 24A). At 12 and 48 weeks, the experimental knees from the early mobiliza-

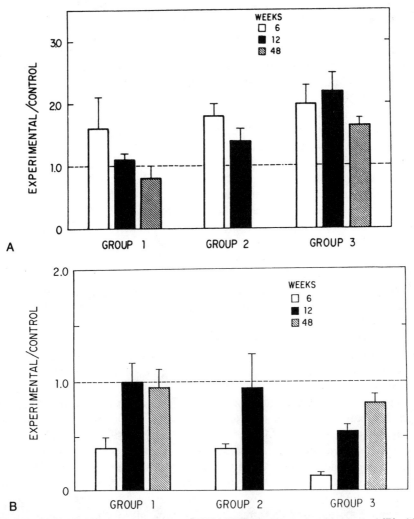

FIG. 24. The normalized (experimental/control) **(A)** V-V laxity for canine knees and **(B)** ultimate load of FMTC during tensile testing as a function of time postoperatively (6, 12, and 48 weeks). Group 1 is the early mobilization group (without repair); group 2 is the short-term immobilization group (with repair); and group 3 is the longer term immobilization group (with repair).

tion group (group 1) achieved the best results, with values similar to those of the controls, whereas the longer term immobilization group continued to exhibit higher V-V laxity (174% of the controls at 48 weeks). An identical trend was observed for the ultimate load (structural properties) of the FMTC (Fig. 24B). In the early mobilization group (group l), the ultimate load of the FMT complex recovered to the level of the control by 12 weeks (98%) and remained at that level up to 48 weeks (105%). The mechanical properties (stress–strain curves) of the healing MCL are detailed in Fig. 25.

At 48 weeks, the tensile strengths of healing MCL for early mobilization and long-term immobilization groups were only 59% and 46% of controls, respectively. There were differences among the three groups with respect to changes in collagen content, collagen types, and reducible cross-links. At 6 weeks, collagen content of experimental MCLs was significantly lower than that of controls, but at 48 weeks, the amount of collagen in the early mobilization group of MCLs was comparable to that in controls. The amount of Type III collagen in the healing area was significantly increased at 6 and 12 weeks. At 48 weeks, the proportion of Type I versus Type III collagen returned to a level comparable to that of the controls. Reducible collagen cross-links in the healing area increased significantly at 6 weeks and increased more at 12 weeks. At 48 weeks, the amount of reducible cross-links in the healing tissue had returned to the level of controls. Both short- and long-term results indicated that surgical repair with subsequent immobilization did not enhance the strength of healing MCL or reduce the V-V laxity. These findings confirmed the clinical practice that primary surgical repair may not be necessary for isolated tears of the MCL (57). These findings further demonstrate that the recovery of the mechanical properties of the healing MCL is slower than that of the structural properties of the FMTC.

Also, the animal species used (dog, rabbit) and postoperative activities (cage versus farm) may have significant effects on the end points of the remodeling process for the healing MCL. It is important to note that ligament healing is very dependent on ligament type. For example, the ACL is not known to heal except in some cases when approximated with sutures. Even then, healing is often incomplete, leading some surgeons to challenge the use of primary repair of the cruciate ligaments (57,89). This experience has led to recent increased interest in the use of autograft, allograft, and xenograft as well as synthetic graft materials to replace the torn ACL in young and active patients. The important question is whether there is a mechanical difference between repaired and nonrepaired ligaments that heal. More studies in this area are needed as well as studies on the healing ligament blood supply, hormones, and other mediators of stress effects. It is hoped that additional investigation will result in a complete understanding of ACL function and nutritional source, so that the success of clinical treatment of ACL injury is not compromised.

SUMMARY AND CONCLUSIONS

Much of our current understanding of the biomechanical properties of ligaments and tendons has come from the development and application of new technologies such as the accurate determination of stress and strain of the ligament substance. These new technical developments have afforded us the ability to examine old ideas more thoroughly and accurately. Even more important is the stimulation that these examinations have provided for exploring new areas. A quasilinear viscoelastic theory for soft tissues has been successfully modified and validated to allow descriptions of tendon and ligament behavior in tension at more realistic strain rates. Through utilization of the laser micrometer system, normal and high-speed video recording, the video dimension analyzer system, and many other bioengineering advances, new insights into the behavior of the biomechanics of ligaments and tendons are presented. The tensile stiffness of ligaments (and probably most muscu-

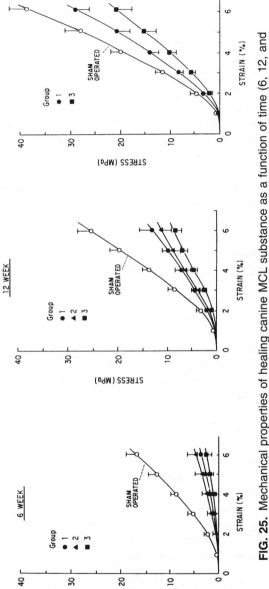

FIG. 25. Mechanical properties of healing canine MCL substance as a function of time (6, 12, and 48 weeks) postoperatively. (Refer to Fig. 24 for group description.)

loskeletal soft tissue) varies in an inverse manner with temperature. This reinforces the need for a standardized testing procedure, as any change in environmental temperature may influence the results.

Other studies described in this chapter include the identification of the differences between the ligament substance and its insertion sites in the presence of various testing conditions and biological factors. The investigations concerning the strain-rate sensitivity of ligaments have reinforced the concept that tensile properties of the ligaments, like those of most other soft tissues, are relatively insensitive to extension rate but are more dependent on the age of the animal. Over four decades of strain rates, all FMTCs from animals with open epiphyses failed by tibial avulsion, whereas those that had reached skeletal maturity failed by tearing of the MCL substance. The mechanical properties of the MCL substance were not as affected by age as the structural properties of the FMTC. Thus, their rates of maturation are asynchronous. Results concerning the homeostatic adaptation of ligaments and tendons to varying activity levels have revealed that each component of the bone–ligament–bone complex has different time-dependent responses to stress. Properties of the ligament substance can completely recover following short-term remobilization, but full recovery of the ligament–bone junction is incomplete after a few weeks and may require many months or years. The response of tendons and ligaments to exercise seems to be type-specific. The mechanical properties of the flexor tendons show no significant changes following prolonged exercise relative to nonexercised controls. However, the extensor tendons demonstrated significant increases as well as tendon hypertrophy. Ligament substance also reveals some changes in the mechanical properties as well as increases in the strength of the bone–ligament junction following exercise.

Kinematic studies demonstrate the importance of normal tendon and ligament integrity to the normal function of joints. The contribution of the MCL as a restraint to valgus rotation in the canine knee joint was seen to be dependent on the degrees of freedom allowed during testing. Under more restricted 3-DOF testing, the MCL provided the primary restraint to an applied valgus moment, whereas under 5-DOF testing, the role of the ACL became more important. With kinematic studies, the role of insertion site location and joint kinematics on the length patterns of the ACL have been clarified. Also, coupled with load–length data, kinematic measurements showed the anteromedial bundle of ACL to be a primary load-bearing structure during anterior loading. The relationships among moment arms, excursions, and gliding functions have been described for the digital flexor tendons. A study of tendon kinematics in zone 2 demonstrated that flexor tendon excursion relative to the sheath was maximized by PIP joint motion and may provide a basis for a more complete understanding of tendon healing and treatment modalities. Indeed, studies concerning tendon and ligament healing continue to generate much new information.

An important observation has been that for an isolated MCL tear, primary surgical repair seems to offer no lasting benefit in terms of V-V laxity or mechanical properties at the healing site. In fact, immobilization proves to be detrimental to the healing process as well as to the overall strength of the bone–ligament–bone complex. The MCL is shown to heal spontaneously, even without reapproximation of the cut ends, and valgus stability is maintained by the remaining joint structures, especially by the ACL. An understanding of the biomechanics of normal tendons and ligaments is an important prerequisite for the study of their healing processes. Normal tendons and ligaments are active biological structures; correlations with morphology, biochemistry, and physiology provide an appreciation of their complexity and functional abilities. Although limited by metabolic activity and blood supply, they are nevertheless able to respond to changes in joint loading and movement.

The development of robotics technology has enabled us to better assess the function of the knee ligaments and to evaluate different techniques for their reconstruction. When we apply more complex external loading conditions to the knee, so that the results mimic sports activities and rehabilitation, the data obtained will improve our understanding of the mechanisms of injury and help in developing protocols for restoring ligament function. This robotics methodology can be further adapted for kinematic study of other synovial joints, such as the human shoulder, where motions are much more complex. As we apply this technology to different areas of joint biomechanics, we look forward to the new and exciting directions in which advances in robotic technology will lead.

The biological and biomechanical story of tendons and ligaments is far from complete, and a wide variety of multidisciplinary studies are needed to optimize their clinical repair or replacement. Improvements in methods of assessment can result from a concerted effort among biologists, biochemists, clinicians, and bioengineers to develop *in vitro* models for the study of normal and injured tendon and ligament with regard to both clinical relevance and a fundamental understanding of structure and function. Further investigations of *in vivo* ligament mechanics and kinematics must be performed. More complex but clinically relevant injury models, including associated injuries to surrounding soft and hard tissues, must be developed. Additional studies are needed to better understand the relationship between tissue loading and tissue remodeling, the cellular response to injury and repair, and other factors responsible for cellular activities (such as growth factors) in both healthy and healing tissues. Clearly, a great deal of work remains to be done in this exciting area.

Acknowledgments

The authors gratefully acknowledge the financial support of RR&D grant A188-3RA of the Veterans Administration, National Institutes of Health grants AR 14918, AR 33097, AR 34264, and AR 39683 and the Malcolm and Dorothy Coutts Institute for Joint Reconstruction and Research. Some of the work detailed here was performed in collaboration with the senior author during his tenure at the University of California, San Diego.

REFERENCES

1. Akeson, W. H., Amiel, D., and Woo, S. L-Y. (1980): Immobility effects on synovial joints: The pathomechanics of joint contracture. *Biorheology*, 17:95–110.
2. Allard, P., Thirty, P. S., Bourgault, A., and Drouin, G. (1979): Pressure dependence of the "area micrometer" method in evaluation of cruciate ligament in cross-section. *J. Biomed. Eng.*, 1:265–267.
3. Amiel, D., Akeson, W. H., Harwood, F. L., and Frank, C. B. (1983): Stress deprivation effect on metabolic turnover of the medial collateral ligament collagen. *Clin. Orthop. Rel. Res.*, 172:265–270.
4. An, K. N., Chao, E. Y., Cooney, W. P. III, and Linschied, R. L. (1979): Normative model of human hand for biomechanical analysis. *J. Biomech.*, 12:775–788.
5. An, K. N., Cooney, W. P., Chao, E. Y., and Askew, L. J. (1983): Determination of forces in extensor pollicus longus and flexor pollicus longus of the thumb. *J. Appl. Physiol.*, 54:714–719.
6. An, K. N., Takahashi, K., Harrigan, T. P., and Chao, E. Y. (1984): Determination of muscle orientations and moment arms. *J. Biomech. Eng.*, 106:280–282.
7. An, K. N., Ueba, Y., Chao, E. Y., Cooney, W. P., and Linschied, R. L. (1983): Tendon excursion and moment arm of index finger muscles. *J. Biomech.*, 16:410–425.
8. Apter, J. (1972): Influence of composition on thermal properties of tissues, In: *Biomechanics: Its Foundations and Objectives*, edited by Y. C. Fung, N. Perrone, and M. Anliker, pp. 217–235. Prentice-Hall, Englewood Cliffs, NJ.
9. Arnoczky, S. P. (1983): Anatomy of the anterior cruciate ligament. *Clin. Orthop. Rel. Res.*, 172:19–25.
10. Baer, E. (1978): The multicomposite structure of tendon collagen: Relationships between ultrastructure and mechanical properties. In: *Proceedings of Third International Congress of Biorheology*, p. 43. La Jolla, CA.
11. Bailey, A. J. (1968): *Comprehensive Biochemistry*. Elsevier, Amsterdam.
12. Blankevoort, L., and Huiskes, R. (1987): The effects of ACL substitute location on knee motion and cruciate ligament strains. *Trans. Orthop. Res. Soc.*, 12:268.
13. Brantigan, O. C., and Voshell, A. F. (1941): The mechanics of ligaments and menisci of the joint. *J. Bone Joint Surg.*, 23A:44–66.
14. Brofkis, J. G. (1972): *The Scientific Fundamentals of Surgery*. Appleton Century Crofts, New York.
15. Butler, D. L., Kay, M. D., and Stouffer, D. C. (1986): Comparison of material properties in fascicle–bone units from human patellar tendon and knee ligaments. *J. Biomech.*, 19:425–432.
16. Butler, D. L., Martin, E. T., Kaiser, A. D., Grood, E. S.,

Chun, K. J., and Sodd, A. N. (1988): The effects of flexion and tibial rotation on the 3-D orientations and lengths of human anterior cruciate ligament bundles. *Trans. Orthop. Res. Soc.,* 13:59.

17. Cabaud, H. E. (1980): Exercise effects on the strength of the rat anterior cruciate ligaments. *Am. J. Sports Med.,* 8:79–86.

18. Chan, S. S., Livesay, G. A., Morrow, D. A., and Woo, S. L-Y. (1995): The development of a low-cost laser reflectance system to determine the cross-sectional shape and area of soft tissues. *ASME Adv. Bioeng.,* BED-31:123–124.

19. Chimich, D., Shrive, N., Frank, C., Marchuk, L., and Bray, R. (1995): Water content alters viscoelastic behavior of the normal adolescent rabbit medial collateral ligament. *J. Biomech.,* 25:831–837.

20. Chun, K. J., and Hubbard, R. P. (1986): Development of reduced relaxation function and stress relaxation with paired tendon. *ASME Adv. Bioeng.,* BED-2:162–163.

21. Clark, J. M., and Sidles, J. A. (1990): The interrelation of fiber bundles in the anterior cruciate ligament. *J. Orthop. Res.,* 8:180–188.

22. Clayton, M. L., Miles, J. S., and Abdulla, M. (1968): Experimental investigations of ligamentous healing. *Clin. Orthop. Rel. Res.,* 61:146–153.

23. Clayton, M. L., and Weir, G. J. (1959): Experimental investigations of ligamentous healing. *Am. J. Surg.,* 98:373–378.

24. Cooper, R. R., and Misol, S. (1970): Tendon and ligament insertion: A light and electron microscopic study. *J. Bone Joint Surg.,* 52A:1–19.

25. Crowninshield, R. D., and Pope, M. H. (1976): The strength and failure characteristics of rat medial collateral ligaments. *J. Trauma,* 16:99–105.

26. Danto, M. I., and Woo, S. L-Y. (1993): The mechanical properties of skeletally mature rabbit anterior cruciate ligament and patellar tendon over a range of strain rates. *J. Orthop. Res.,* 11:58–67.

27. Danylchuk, K. D., Finlay, J. B., and Krcek, J. P. (1978): Microstructural organization of human and bovine cruciate ligament. *Clin. Orthop. Rel. Res.,* 131:294–298.

28. De Deyne, P., and Haut, R. C. (1991): Some effects of gamma irradiation on patellar tendon allografts. *Conn. Tiss. Res.,* 27:51–62.

29. Dorlot, J. M., Ait ba Sidi, M., Gremblay, G. M., and Drouin, G. (1980): Load-elongation behavior of the canine anterior cruciate ligament. *J. Biomech. Eng.,* 102:190–193.

30. Ellis, D. G. (1968): A shadow amplitude method for measuring cross sectional area of biological specimens. In: *21st Annual Conference on Engineering in Medicine and Biology,* p. 51.6. Houston.

31. Ellis, D. G. (1969): Cross-sectional area measurements for tendon specimens—a comparison of several methods. *J. Biomech.,* 2:175–186.

32. Evans, E. B., Eggers, G. W. N., Butler, J. K., and Blumel, J. (1960): Experimental immobilization and remobilization of rat knee joints. *J. Bone Joint Surg.,* 42A:737–758.

33. Figgie, H. E., Bahniuk, E. H., Heiple, G. K., and Davy, D. T. (1986): The effects of tibial–femoral angle on the failure mechanics of the canine anterior cruciate ligament. *J. Biomech.,* 19:89–91.

34. Frank, C. B., Schachar, N., and Ditrich, D. (1983): The

natural history of healing in the repaired medial collateral ligament: A morphological assessment in rabbits. *J. Orthop. Res.,* 1:179–188.

35. Frank, C. B., Woo, S. L-Y., Amiel, D., Gomez, M. A., Harwood, K. F. L., and Akeson, W. H. (1983): Medial collateral ligament healing. A multidisciplinary assessment in rabbits. *Am. J. Sports Med.,* 11:379–389.

36. Frisen, M., Maji, M., Sonnerup, L., and Viidik, A. (1969): Rheological analysis of soft collagenous tissues. Part I: Theoretical considerations. *J. Biomech.,* 2:13–20.

37. Fujie, H., Livesay, G. A., Woo, S. L-Y., Kashiwaguchi, S., and Blomstrom, G. (1995): The use of a universal force-moment sensor to determine in situ forces in ligaments: A new methodology. *J. Biomech. Eng.,* 117:1–7.

38. Fujie, H., Mabuchi, K., Woo, S. L-Y., Livesay, G. A., Arai, S., and Tsukamoto, Y. (1993): The use of robotics technology to study human joint kinematics: A new methodology. *J. Biomech. Eng.,* 115:211–217.

39. Fung, Y. C. (1972): Stress–strain–history relations of soft tissues in simple elongation. In: *Biomechanics: Its Foundations and Objectives,* edited by Y. C. Fung, N. Perrone, and M. Anliker, pp. 181–207. Prentice-Hall: Englewood Cliffs, NJ.

40. Fung, Y. C. B. (1973): Biorheology of soft tissues. *Biorheology,* 10:139–155.

41. Gamble, J. G., Edward, C., and Max, S. (1984): Enzymatic adaptation of ligaments during immobilization. *Am. J. Sports Med.,* 12:221–228.

42. Gelberman, R. H., Manske, P. R., Akeson, W. H., Woo, S. L-Y., Lundborg, G., and Amiel, D. (1986): Flexor tendon repair. *J. Orthop. Res.,* 4:119–128.

43. Gibbons, M. J., Butler, D. L., Grood, E. S., Bylski-Austrow, D. I., Levy, M. S., and Noyes, F. R. (1991): Effects of gamma irradiation on the initial mechanical and material properties of goat bone–patellar tendon bone-grafts. *J. Orthop. Res.,* 9:209–218.

44. Gomez, M. A., Woo, S. L-Y., Amiel, D., Harwood, F. L., Kitabayashi, L. R., and Matyas, J. R. (1991): The effects of increased tension on healing medial collateral ligaments. *Am. J. Sports Med.,* 19:347–354.

45. Grant, M. E., and Prockop, D. J. (1972): The biosynthesis of collagen. *N. Engl. J. Med.,* 286:194–199.

46. Grood, E. S., Noyes, F. R., Butler, D. L., and Suntay, W. J. (1981): Ligamentous and capsular restraints preventing straight medial and lateral laxity in intact human cadaver knees. *J. Bone Joint Surg.,* 63A:1257–1269.

47. Gupta, B. N., Subramanian, K. N., Brinker, W. O., and Gupta, A. N. (1971): Tensile strength of canine cranial cruciate ligaments. *Am. J. Vet. Res.,* 32:183–190.

48. Harner, C. D., Xerogeanes, J. W., Livesay, G. A., Carlin, G. J., Smith, B. A., Kusayama, T., Kashiwaguchi, S., and Woo, S. L-Y. (1995): The human posterior cruciate ligament: An interdisciplinary study. *Am. J. Sports Med.,* 23:736–745.

49. Haut, R. C. (1983): Age-dependent influence of strain rate on the tensile failure of rat-tail tendon. *J. Biomech. Eng.,* 105:296–299.

50. Haut, R. C., and Powlison, A. C. (1990): The effects of test environment and cyclic stretching on the failure properties of human patellar tendons. *J. Orthop. Res.,* 8:532–540.

51. Hefzy, M. S., Grood, E. S., and Noyes, F. R. (1989):

Factors affecting the region of most isometric femoral attachments. Part II: The anterior cruciate ligament. *Am. J. Sports Med.,* 17:208–216.

52. Hollis, M. J., Marcin, J. P., Horibe, S., and Woo, S. L-Y. (1988): Load determination in ACL fiber bundles under knee loading. *Trans. Orthop. Res. Soc.,* 13:58.

53. Hollis, M. J., Takai, S., Adams, D. J., Horibe, S., and Woo, S. L-Y. (1991): The effects of knee motion and external loading on the length of the anterior cruciate ligament: A kinematic study. *J. Biomech. Eng.,* 113:208–214.

54. Horwitz, M. T. (1939): Injuries of the ligaments of the knee joint. An experimental study. *Arch. Surg.,* 38:946–954.

55. Hunter, J., and Williams, M. G. (1951): A study of the effect of cold on joint temperature and mobility. *Can. J. Med. Sci.,* 29:255–262.

56. Iaconis, F., Steindler, R., and Marinozzi, G. (1987): Measurements of cross-sectional area of collagen structures (knee ligaments.) by means of an optical method. *J. Biomech.,* 20:1003–1010.

57. Indelicato, P. A. (1983): Non-operative treatment of complete tears of the medial collateral ligament of the knee. *J. Bone Joint Surg.,* 65A:323–329.

58. Inoue, M., McGurk-Burleson, E., Hollis, J. M., and Woo, S. L-Y. (1987): Treatment of the medial collateral ligament injury, I: The importance of the anterior cruciate ligament on the varus–valgus knee laxity. *Am. J. Sports Med.,* 15:15–21.

59. Jack, E. A. (1950): Experimental rupture of the medial collateral ligament of the knee. *J. Bone Joint Surg.,* 32B:396–402.

60. Jenkins, R. B., and Little, R. W. (1974): A constitutive equation for parallel-fibered elastic tissue. *J. Biomech.,* 7:397–402.

61. Johnson, G. A., Livesay, G. A., Woo, S. L-Y., and Rajagopal, K. R. (1996): A single integral finite strain viscoelastic model of ligaments and tendons. *J. Biomech. Eng.,* 118:221–226.

62. Kapandji, I. A. (1970): *The Physiology of the Joints.* Churchill Livingstone, Edinburgh.

63. Kastelic, J., Galeski, A., and Baer, E. (1978): The multicomposite structure of tendon. *Connect. Tissue Res.,* 6:11–23.

64. Kennedy, J. C., and Fowler, P. J. (1971): Medial and anterior instability of the knee: An anatomical and clinical study using stress machines. *J. Bone Joint Surg.,* 53-A:1257–1270.

65. Kessler, I., and Missim, F. (1969): Primary repair without immobilization of flexor tendon division within the digital sheath. *Acta Orthop. Scand.,* 40:587–601.

66. Kwan, M. K., Lin, T. H.-C., and Woo, S. L-Y. (1993): On the viscoelastic properties of the anteromedial bundle of the anterior cruciate ligament. *J. Biomech.,* 26:447–452.

67. Laros, G. S., Tipton, C. M., and Cooper, R. R. (1971): The influence of physical activity on ligament insertions in the knees of dogs. *J. Bone Joint Surg.,* 53A:275–286.

68. Lee, T. Q., and Danto, M. I. (1992): Application of a continuous video digitizing system for tensile testing of bone–soft tissue–bone complex. *ASME Adv. Bioeng.,* BED-22:87–90.

69. Lee, T. Q., and Woo, S. L-Y. (1988): A new method for determining cross-sectional shape and area of soft tissues. *J. Biomech. Eng.,* 110:110–114.

70. Lin, H.-C., Kwan, M. K., and Woo, S. L-Y. (1987): On the stress relaxation properties of anterior cruciate ligament (ACL). *ASME Adv. Bioeng.,* BED-3:5–6.

71. Livesay, G. A., Rudy, T., Xerogeanes, J. W., Ishibashi, Y., Kim, H.-S., Fu, F. H., and Woo, S. L-Y. (1995): The use of robotic technology to examine the *in situ* forces in the ACL. *Trans. Orthop. Res. Soc.,* 20:647.

72. Lyon, R. M., Woo, S. L-Y., Hollis, J. M., Marcin, J. P., and Lee, E. B. (1987): A new device to measure the structural properties of the femur–anterior cruciate ligament–tibia complex. *J. Biomech. Eng.,* 111:350–354.

73. Mains, D. B., Andrews, J. G., and Stonecipher, T. (1977): Medial and anterior–posterior ligament stability of the human knee, measured with a stress apparatus. *Am. J. Sports Med.,* 5:144–153.

74. Markolf, K. L., Mensch, J. S., and Amstutz, H. C. (1976): Stiffness and laxity of the knee—the contributions of the supporting structures. *J. Bone Joint Surg.,* 58A:583–593.

75. Mason, M. L., and Allen, H. S. (1941): The rate of healing of tendons. An experimental study of tensile strength. *Ann. Surg.,* 113:424–459.

76. Matthews, L. S., and Ellis, D. (1968): Viscoelastic properties of cat tendon: Effects of time after death and preservation by freezing. *J. Biomech.,* 1:65–71.

77. Mechanic, G. L. (1974): An automated scintillation counting system with high efficiency for continuous analysis: Cross-links of $(H^3)NaBH_4$ reduced collagen. *Anal. Biochem.,* 61:349–354.

78. Miltner, L. J., Hu, C. H., and Fang, H. C. (1937): Experimental joint sprain. Pathologic study. *Arch. Surg.,* 35:234–240.

79. Morein, G., Goldgefter, L., Kobyliansky, E., Goldschmidt-Nathan, M., and Nathan, H. (1978): Change in mechanical properties of rat tail tendon during postnatal osteogenesis. *Anat. Embryol. Berl.,* 154:121–124.

80. Nathan, H., Goldgefter, L., Kobyliansky, E., Goldschmidt-Nathan, M., and Morein, G. (1978): Energy absorbing capacity of rat tail tendon at various ages. *J. Anat.,* 127:589–593.

81. Neuberger, A., and Slack, H. G. B. (1953): The metabolism of collagen from liver, bones, skin and tendon in the normal rat. *Biochem. J.,* 53:47–52.

82. Newton, P. O., Woo, S. L-Y., MacKenna, D. A., and Akeson, W. H. (1995): Immobilization of the knee joint alters the mechanical and ultrastructural properties of the rabbit anterior cruciate ligament. *J. Orthop. Res.,* 13:191–200.

83. Nielsen, S., Andersen, C. K., Rasmussen, O., and Andersen, K. (1984): Instability of cadaver knees after transection of capsule and ligaments. *Acta Orthop. Scand.,* 55:30–34.

84. Nielsen, S., Rasmussen, O., Ovesen, J., and Andersen, K. (1984): Rotatory instability of cadaver knees after transection of collateral ligaments and capsule. *Arch. Orthop. Trauma Surg.,* 103:165–169.

85. Njus, G. O., and Njus, N. M. (1986): A noncontact method for determining cross-sectional area of soft tissues. *Trans. Orthop. Res. Soc.,* 11:126.

86. Noyes, F. R., DeLucas, J. L., and Torvik, P. J. (1974): Biomechanics of anterior cruciate ligament failure: An analysis of strain rate sensitivity and mechanics of failure in primates. *J. Bone Joint Surg.,* 56A:236–253.

87. Noyes, F. R., DeLucas, J. L., and Torvik, P. J. (1974): Biomechanics of ligament failure, II. An analysis of

immobilization, exercise and reconditioning in primates. *J. Bone Joint Surg.,* 56A:1406–1418.

88. Noyes, F. R., and Grood, E. S. (1976): The strength of the anterior cruciate ligaments in humans and rhesus monkeys: Age–related and species–related changes. *J. Bone Joint Surg.,* 58A:1074–1082.

89. O'Donoghue, D. H., Frank, C. R., Jeter, G. L., Johnson, W., Zeiders, J. W., and Kenyon, R. (1971): Repair and reconstruction of the anterior cruciate ligament in dogs: Factors influencing long–term results. *J. Bone Joint Surg.,* 53A:710–718.

90. O'Donoghue, D. H., Rockwood, C., and Zarecnyj, B. (1961): Repair of knee ligaments in dogs. I. The lateral collateral ligament. *J. Bone Joint Surg.,* 43A:1167–1178.

91. Peterson, R. H., Gomez, M. A., and Woo, S. L-Y. (1987): The effects of strain rate on the biomechanical properties of the medial collateral ligament: A study of immature and mature rabbits. *Trans. Orthop. Res. Soc.,* 12:127.

92. Peterson, R. H., and Woo, S. L-Y. (1986): A new methodology to determine the mechanical properties of ligaments at high strain rates. *J. Biomech. Eng.,* 108:365–367.

93. Pinto, J. G., and Patatucci, P. J. (1980): Viscoelasticity of passive cardiac muscle. *J. Biomech.,* 102: 57–61.

94. Pipkin, A. C., and Rogers, T. C. (1968): A non-linear integral representation for viscoelastic behavior. *J. Mech. Phys. Solids,* 16:59–74.

95. Piziali, R. L., Rastager, J., Nagel, D. A., and Schurman, D. J. (1980): The contribution of the cruciate ligaments to the load-displacement characterisitics of the human knee joint. *J. Biomech. Eng.,* 102:277–283.

96. Race, A., and Amis, A. A. (1994): The mechanical properties of the two bundles of the human posterior cruciate ligament. *J. Biomech.,* 27:13–24.

97. Race, A., and Amis, A. A. (1994): A molding method to find cross-sections of soft tissue bundles with complex shapes. *Trans. Orthop. Res. Soc.,* 19:783.

98. Rigby, B., Hirai, N., Spikes, J., and Eyring, H. (1958): The mechanical properties of rat tail tendon. *J. Gen. Physiol.,* 53:265–283.

99. Rudy, T. W., Livesay, G. A., and Woo, S. L-Y., and Fu, F.H. (1996): A combined robotic/universal force sensor approach to determine the *in situ* forces of knee ligaments. *J. Biomech.* 29:1357–1360.

100. Salehpour, A., Butler, D. L., Proch, F. S., Schwartz, H. E., Feder, S. M., Doxey, C. M., and Ratcliffe, A. (1995): Dose-dependent response of gamma irradiation on mechanical properties and related biochemical composition of goat bone–patellar tendon–bone allografts. *J. Orthop. Res.,* 13:898–906.

101. Salter, R. B., and Field, P. (1960): The effects of continuous compression on living articular cartilage: An experimental investigation. *J. Bone Joint Surg.,* 42A:31–49.

102. Sapega, A. A., Moyer, R. A., Schneck, C., and Komalahiranya, N. (1990): Testing for isometry during reconstruction of the anterior cruciate ligament. *J. Bone Joint Surg.,* 72A:259–267.

103. Seering, W. P., Piziali, R. L., Nagel, D. A., and Schurman, D. J. (1980): The function of the primary ligaments of the knee in varus–valgus and axial rotation. *J. Biomech.,* 13:785–794.

104. Shrive, N. G., Lam, T. C., Damson, E., and Frank, C. B. (1988): A new method for measuring the cross-sectional area of connective tissue structures. *J. Biomech. Eng.,* 110:104–109.

105. Sidles, J. A., Larson, R. V., Garbini, J. L., Downey, D. J., and Matsen, F. A. III (1988): Ligament length relationships in the moving knee. *J. Orthop. Res.,* 6:593–610.

106. Sidles, J. A., Larson, R. V., Garbini, J. L., and Matsen F. A. III (1987): Ligament length relationships in the moving knee. *Trans. Orthop. Res. Soc.,* 12:269.

107. Simon, B. R., Coats, R. S., and Woo, S. L-Y. (1984): Relaxation and creep quasilinear viscoelastic model for normal articular cartilage. *J. Biomech. Eng.,* 106: 159–164.

108. Smith, J. W. (1954): The elastic properties of the anterior cruciate ligament of the rabbit. *J. Anat.,* 88: 369–380.

109. Stouffer, D. C., and Butler, D. L. (1984): Analysis of crimp unfolding, fluid expulsion and fiber failure in collagen fiber bundles. *ASME Adv. Bioeng.,* 46–47.

110. Takai, S., Livesay, G. A., Woo, S. L-Y., Adams, D. J., and Fu, F. H. (1993): Determination of the in situ loads on the human anterior cruciate ligament. *J. Orthop. Res.,* 11:686–695.

111. Tanaka, T. T., and Fung, Y. C. (1974): Elastic and inelastic properties of the canine aorta and their variation along the aortic tree. *J. Biomech.,* 7:357–370.

112. Tanzer, M. L. (1973): Cross-linking of collagen. *Science,* 180:561–566.

113. Tipton, C. M., James, S. L., Mergner, W., and Tcheng, T. K. (1970): Influence of exercise on the strength of the medial collateral ligaments of dogs. *Am. J. Physiol.,* 218:758–761.

114. Tipton, C. M., Matthes, R. D., and Martin, R. R. (1978): The influence of age and sex on the strength of bone–ligament junctions in knee joints of rats. *J. Bone Joint Surg.,* 60A:230–234.

115. Tipton, C. M., Matthes, R. D., Maynard, J. A., and Carey, R. A. (1975): The influence of physical activity on ligaments and tendons. *Med. Sci. Sports Exer.,* 7:165–175.

116. Tipton, C. M., Matthes, R. D., and Sandage, D. S. (1974): *In situ* measurement of junction strength and ligament elongation in rats. *J. Appl. Physiol.,* 37:758–761.

117. Tipton, C. M., Schild, R. J., and Tomanek, R. J. (1967): Influence of physical activity on strength of knee ligaments in rats. *Am. J. Physiol.,* 221:783–787.

118. Vailas, A. C., Tipton, C. M., Matthes, R. D., and Gant, M. (1981): Physical activity and its influence on the repair process of medial collateral ligaments. *Connect. Tissue Res.,* 9:25–31.

119. Viidik, A. (1966): Biomechanics and functional adaptation of tendons and joint ligaments. In: *Studies on the Anatomy and Function of Bone and Joints,* edited by F. G. Evans, pp. 17–39. Springer, Berlin.

120. Viidik, A., Sanquist, L., and Magi, M. (1965): Influence of postmortem storage on tensile strength characteristics and histology of rabbit ligaments. *Acta Orthop. Scand. [Suppl.],* 79:1–38.

121. Walker, L. B., Harris, E. H., and Benedict, J. V. (1964): Stress–strain relationship in human cadaveric plantaris tendon—a preliminary study. *Med. Elect. Biol. Eng.,* 2:31–38.

122. Warren, R. F., Marshall, J. L., and Girgis, F. (1974): The prime static stabilizer of the medial side of the knee. *J. Bone Joint Surg.,* 56A:665–674.

123. Wehbe, M. A., and Hunter, J. M. (1985): Flexor tendon gliding in the hand: Part II. Differential gliding. *J. Hand Surg.,* 10A:575–579.

124. Weisman, G., Pope, M. H., and Johnson, R. J. (1979): The effect of cyclic loading on knee ligaments. *Trans. Orthop. Res. Soc.,* 4:24.

125. Wertheim, M. G. (1847): Memoirs sur l'elasticité et la cohesion des principaux tissu du corps humain. *Ann. Chim. (Phys.),* 21:385–414.

126. Wineman, A. S. (1972): Large axially symmetric stretching of a non-linear viscoelastic membrane. *Int. J. Sols. Structs.,* 8:775–790.

127. Wolff, J. (1882): *Das Gesetz der Transformation der Kochen.* Hirschwald, Berlin.

128. Woo, S. L-Y., Akeson, W. H., Amiel, D., Convery, F. R., and Matthews, J. V. (1975): The connective tissue response to immobility: A correlative study of the biomechanical and biochemical measurements of the normal and immobilized rabbit knee. *Arthritis Rheum.,* 18:257–264.

129. Woo, S. L-Y., Akeson, W. H., and Jemmott, G. F. (1976): The measurement of non-homogeneous, directional mechanical properties of articular cartilage in tension. *J. Biomech.,* 9:785–791.

130. Woo, S. L-Y., and Buckwalter, J. A., eds. (1988): *Injury and Repair of Musculoskeletal Soft Tissues,* p. 548. American Academy of Orthopaedic Surgeons, Park Ridge, IL.

131. Woo, S. L-Y., Danto, M. I., Ohland, K. J., Lee, T. Q., and Newton, P. O. (1990): The use of a laser micrometer system to determine the cross-sectional shape and area of ligaments: A comparative study with two existing methods. *J. Biomech. Eng.,* 112:426–431.

132. Woo, S. L-Y., Gomez, M. A., and Akeson, W. H. (1981): The time and history dependent viscoelastic properties of the canine medial collateral ligament. *J. Biomech. Eng.,* 103:293–298.

133. Woo, S. L-Y., Gomez, M. A., Amiel, D., Ritter, M. A., Gelberman, R. H., and Akeson, W. H. (1981): The effects of exercise on the biomechanical and biochemical properties of swine digital flexor tendons. *J. Biomech. Eng.,* 103:51–56.

134. Woo, S. L-Y., Gomez, M. A., Inoue, M., and Akeson, W. H. (1987): New experimental procedures to evaluate the mechanical properties of healing medial collateral ligament (MCL). *J. Orthop. Res.,* 5:425–432.

135. Woo, S. L-Y., Gomez, M. A., Seguchi, Y., Endo, C., and Akeson, W. H. (1983): Measurement of mechanical properties of ligament substance from a bone–ligament–bone preparation. *J. Orthop. Res.,* 1:22–29.

136. Woo, S. L-Y., Gomez, M. A., Woo, Y.-K., and Akeson, W. H. (1982): Mechanical properties of tendons and ligaments. I. Quasi-static and nonlinear viscoelastic properties. *Biorheology,* 19:385–396.

137. Woo, S. L-Y., Gomez, M. A., Woo, Y.-K., and Akeson, W. H. (1982): Mechanical properties of tendons and ligaments. II. The relationship of immobilization and exercise on tissue remodeling. *Biorheology,* 19:397–408.

138. Woo, S. L-Y., Hollis, J. M., Adams, D. J., Lyon, R. M., and Takai, S. (1991): Tensile properties of the human femur–anterior cruciate ligament–tibia complex: The effect of specimen age and orientation. *Am. J. Sports Med.,* 19:217–225.

139. Woo, S. L-Y., Hollis, J. M., Roux, R. D., Gomez, M. A., Inoue, M., Kleiner, J. B., and Akeson, W. H. (1987): Effects of knee flexion on the structural properties of the rabbit femur–anterior cruciate ligament–tibia complex (FATC). *J. Biomech.,* 20:557–563.

140. Woo, S. L-Y., Inoue, M., McGurk-Burleson, E., and Gomez, M. A. (1987): Treatment of the medial collateral ligament injury. II: Structure and function of canine knees in response to differing treatment regimens. *Am. J. Sports Med.,* 15:22–29.

141. Woo, S. L-Y., Johnson, G. A., and Smith, B. A. (1993): Mathematical modelling of ligaments and tendons. *J. Biomech. Eng.,* 115:468–473.

142. Woo, S. L-Y., Kuei, S. C., Gomez, M. A., Winters, J. M., Amiel, D., and Akeson, W. H. (1979): Effects of immobilization and exercise on the strength characteristics of bone–medial collateral ligament–bone complex. *ASME Biomech. Symp.,* AMD-32:67–70.

143. Woo, S. L-Y., Orlando, C. A., Camp, J. F., and Akeson, W. H. (1986): Effects of postmortem storage by freezing on ligament tensile behavior. *J. Biomech.,* 19:399–404.

144. Woo, S. L-Y., Orlando, C. A., Gomez, M. A., Frank, C. B., and Akeson, W. H. (1986): Tensile properties of medial collateral ligament as a function of age. *J. Orthop. Res.,* 4:133–141.

145. Woo, S. L-Y., Ritter, M. A., Amiel, D., Sanders, T. M., Gomez, M. A., Garfin, S. R., and Akeson, W. H. (1980): The biomechanical and biochemical properties of swine tendons. Long–term effects of exercise on the digital extensors. *Conn. Tiss. Res.,* 7:177–183.

146. Woo, S. L-Y., Simon, B. R., and Kuei, S. C. (1980): Quasilinear viscoelastic properties of normal articular cartilage. *J. Biomech. Eng.,* 102:85–90.

147. Woo, S. L-Y., Weiss, J. A., and Ohland, K. J. (1990): Aging and sex–related changes in the biomechanical properties of the rabbit medial collateral ligament. *Mech. Aging Devel.,* 56:129–142.

148. Woo, S. L-Y., Gomez, M. A., Sites, T. J., Newton, P. O., Orlando, C. A., and Akeson, W. H. (1987): The biomechanical and morphological changes in the medial collateral ligament of the rabbit after immobilization and remobilization. *J. Bone Joint Surg.,* 69A:1200–1211.

149. Woo, S. L-Y., Lee, T. Q., Gomez, M. A., Sato, S., and Field, F. P. (1987): Temperature dependent behavior of the canine medial collateral ligament. *J. Biomech. Eng.,* 109:68–71.

150. Yahia, L. H., and Drouin, G. (1989): Microscopical investigation of canine anterior cruciate ligament and patellar tendon: Collagen fascicle morphology and architecture. *J. Orthop. Res.,* 7:243–251.

151. Zuckerman, J., and Stull, G. A. (1969): Effects of exercise on knee ligament separation force in rats. *J. Appl. Physiol.,* 26:716–719.

152. Zuckerman, J., and Stull, G. A. (1973): Ligamentous separation force in rats as influenced by training, detraining and cage restriction. *Med. Sci. Sports Exer.,* 5:44–49.

Basic Orthopaedic Biomechanics, 2nd ed.,
edited by Van C. Mow and Wilson C. Hayes.
Lippincott–Raven Publishers, Philadelphia © 1997.

7

Quantitative Anatomy of Diarthrodial Joint Articular Layers

Gerard A. Ateshian and Louis J. Soslowsky

*Departments of Mechanical Engineering and Orthopaedic Surgery,
Columbia University, New York, New York 10032; and Departments of Surgery and Mechanical
Engineering and Applied Mechanics, Orthopaedic Research Laboratories,
University of Michigan, Ann Arbor, Michigan 48109*

In recent years, the development of powerful medical imaging tools has brought a new perspective to the study of diarthrodial joint anatomy. Quantitation of topographic features of articular layers has been made possible by a combination of imaging technologies and geometric modeling tools historically developed for the aerospace and automotive industries. The ability to mathematically describe the three-dimensional geometry of articular layers, such as the femoral and patellar surfaces of the knee (Fig. 1), can be valuable in many respects. Such quantitative representations can be used for basic anatomic studies that describe the fundamental features of various diarthrodial joint surfaces. For example, the characterization of ridges and facets of the retropatellar surface can be determined unequivocally by visualizing its surface curvature maps. Furthermore, by quantifying both the articular surface and subchondral bone geometries of a cartilage layer, it is possible to map the cartilage thickness over the entire surface of the joint. By mapping the proximity of two articulating surfaces, it is also possible to infer the location of contact areas in the joint. Three-dimensional models of diarthrodial joint structures can also be used for characterizing joint mechanics and for simulating normal and pathologic conditions or surgical procedures through geometric modeling, finite element modeling, and multibody modeling. The clinical applications of these tools offer tremendous potential in the areas of diagnosis, monitoring of disease progression, or assessment of surgical outcome. In this chapter, an overview of the methods for quantifying the anatomy of diarthrodial joint articular layers is provided, along with recent applications of these methods in the study of various joints.

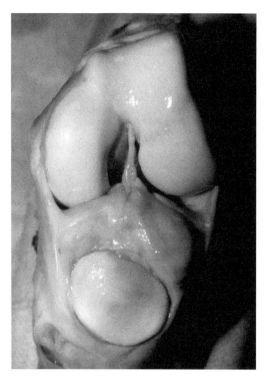

FIG. 1. Typical femoral and patellar articular cartilage layers from a human knee joint. The patella has been reflected down to permit simultaneous visualization of these otherwise contacting surfaces.

TOOLS FOR SURFACE MEASUREMENTS

Many methods have been used to quantify diarthrodial joint surfaces. Mechanical techniques include the production of plastic moldings (82), the production of a silicone rubber mold used to make a plaster casting (79), and the use of a mechanical measuring pin attached to a dial gauge (93). Other methods such as slicing (86) and ultrasound have also been described (78). More recently, such optical techniques as close-range photogrammetry (40) and analytic stereophotogrammetry have been used (5,52). In addition, computed tomography (CT) and magnetic resonance imaging (MRI) technologies have also been used to measure anatomic structures of diarthrodial joints (12,15,29,32,38,71). Similarly, for the determination of articular cartilage thickness,

several methods have been used including measurements obtained from radiographs (3, 44), slicing specimens fixed in formalin (69), successively photographing specimen slices (28,68), and ultrasound (70,78). Two such methods that have shown to be versatile and highly accurate are described in the following sections: stereophotogrammetry and magnetic resonance imaging.

STEREOPHOTOGRAMMETRY

The technique of stereophotogrammetry (SPG) has been in existence almost since the advent of photography. By capturing planar images of a three-dimensional object from two or more directions in space, it is possible to reconstruct the three-dimensional coordinates of that object using only the planar image data. This reconstruction can be achieved using basic principles of projective and perspective geometry. Photogrammetric tools are widely used in constructing three-dimensional geographic maps from aerial or satellite photography. The SPG technique is not limited to the use of the visible light spectrum but can also use radar waves, X-rays, etc. In the medical field, the earliest use of roentgen-photogrammetry (using X-rays) was that by Davidson (24), though its modern application has been pioneered by Selvik (85), who used the method to study the kinematics of the skeletal system. In 1975, Clark et al. (21) employed close-range SPG in the development of prosthetic devices, in particular human aortic valves. Stokes and Greenapple (91) measured three-dimensional soft tissue deformation with SPG, where the noncontacting nature of this method proved to be a distinctive advantage. In gait analysis, photogrammetry has been a standard tool for measuring limb kinematics since the early 1980s.

The first use of SPG for articular surface measurements, however, was by Ghosh (40), who applied standard tools of cartography to reconstructing the three-dimensional topography of the human femoral head and distal femoral surface. In his apparatus, Ghosh projected a fine grid on the articular surfaces, using a slide projector. The grid intersections provided recognizable landmarks on the photographic pair (the stereogram), which were necessary for completing the three-dimensional reconstruction of the articular surface topography. The accuracy reported in these measurements was 0.2 mm. Huiskes et al. (52) and Ateshian et al. (5) developed similar SPG systems for characterizing the topography of knee joint articular surfaces, with accuracies on the order of 0.2 mm and 0.09 mm, respectively, at a 95% confidence level.

The basic apparatus of an SPG system consists of two cameras (or one camera that can be moved to two distinct positions if the measured object is stationary), a calibration frame, a slide projector (or optical spotlight) with a gridded slide (Fig. 2), and a two-dimensional digitizer. The calibration frame, which has a workspace for inserting the object to be measured, is fitted with markers (calibration targets) whose three-dimensional coordinates are known *a priori*. When a stereogram of the object and calibration frame is obtained (Fig. 3), the planar image coordinates of these calibration targets are digitized with the two-dimensional digitizer. From the knowledge of these two-dimensional image coordinates, as well as the corresponding three-dimensional coordinates, the camera parameters can be determined for each camera position. Various procedures exist for performing this camera calibration, based on the collinearity condition (e.g., 39); these procedures can be elaborate, as they aim to compensate for many potential sources of error such as linear and nonlinear lens distortions. Once the camera parameters have been obtained, the digitized stereogram image coordinates of the grid intersections, appearing on the articular surfaces (Fig. 3), can be used to reconstruct their corresponding three-dimensional coordinates. By simply connecting these grid points together, it is possible to visualize the resulting wireframe

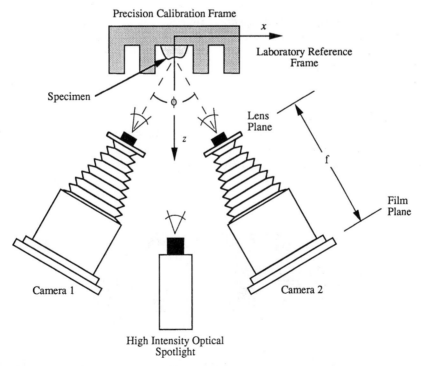

FIG. 2. Schematic of the basic components of a stereophotogrammetry apparatus: cameras, calibration frame, slide projector/optical spotlight, and two-dimensional digitizer (not shown).

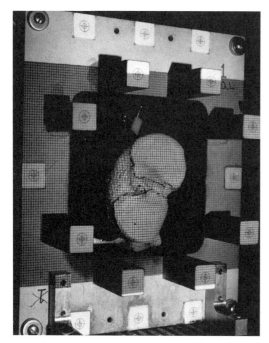
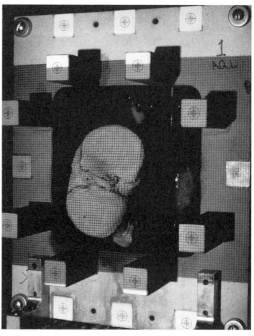

FIG. 3. Typical stereogram of a tibial plateau.

model on a computer graphics workstation (Fig. 4). From these wireframe models, mathematical equations can be generated to represent the articular surfaces, producing geometric models as described below.

ARTICULAR SURFACES FROM MAGNETIC RESONANCE IMAGING

Magnetic resonance imaging (MRI) has been widely used for characterizing the two-dimensional and three-dimensional structure of soft tissues noninvasively. In early orthopaedic applications, emphasis was given to the detection of ligamentous or meniscal injuries; however, the MRI pulse sequences needed to highlight these tissues did not enhance articular cartilage. More recently, there has been a greater emphasis on developing imaging sequences that are more specific to cartilage, providing a good contrast between that tissue and its surroundings

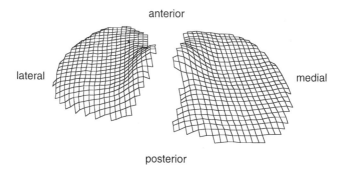

FIG. 4. Wireframe representation of the tibial surface whose stereogram is shown in Fig. 3.

(e.g., 29,75,76,77,95). In particular, fat-suppressed three-dimensional spoiled gradient-recalled echo (GRE) images, or FLASH sequences (depending on the manufacturer's terminology), have been shown to successfully enhance cartilage (Fig. 5). These pulse sequences can be used to generate true proton-density maps that are directly proportional to the water content in the tissue (e.g., 84). These advances have made it possible to generate accurate three-dimensional reconstructions of the articular layers of diarthrodial joints.

One of the challenges of segmenting MR images of cartilage is that water content is not uniform within the tissue; hence, segmentation algorithms that rely on a single gray-scale value for distinguishing surface boundaries (e.g., the popular marching cubes algorithm of Lorensen and Cline [65], which can be used for segmenting bone surfaces on CT images) are not suitable for cartilage.

Hence, fully automated segmentation algorithms for articular cartilage pose a technological challenge that needs to be addressed; to date, the most reliable segmentation tools are still based on manual digitizing. Segmentation of MR images of cartilage, for the purpose of constructing three-dimensional geometric models of the articular surfaces, can be performed in two fundamental ways: (a) from a serial sequence of two-dimensional images or (b) directly from three-dimensional volumetric data. The latter method is more elaborate than the former. Though it can be performed imperfectly by borrowing some of the techniques employed with CT volumetric data for bone, it remains a challenging problem, and much research still needs to be done. Three-dimensional reconstructions from two-dimensional serial sequences may proceed more easily if the sectioning plane is approximately perpendicular to the articular surface, to minimize partial

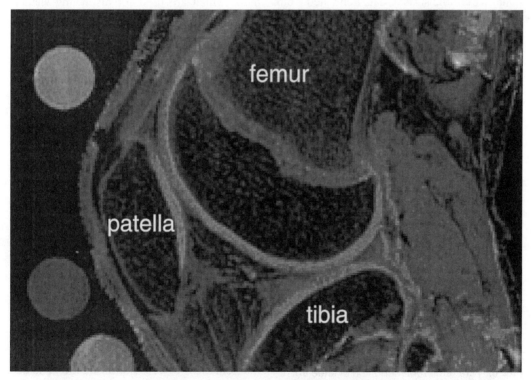

FIG. 5. Typical MR image of a knee joint, with highly contrasting articular cartilage.

volume effects. For example, a retropatellar articular surface is best imaged in the horizontal plane, or even the sagittal plane, but not in the coronal plane. Two-dimensional segmentation tools can be employed to extract the contour of the articular surface as well as that of the subchondral bone in each image slice. The contours from all the images in a serial sequence can subsequently be combined to produce a three-dimensional wireframe representation of the articular layer (Fig. 6). As for the case of surface data generated with SPG, it is possible to derive mathematical representations, or geometric models, of these articular layers from the three-dimensional wireframe data.

GEOMETRIC MODELS OF ARTICULAR LAYERS

The determination of a mathematical representation of the articular layers of a joint is essential in many respects. The three-dimensional wireframe surface data generated from SPG or MRI can be processed to yield much information that can only be extracted from a mathematical representation. These representations are called geometric models, and they can be obtained using various surface-fitting methods. One such method was employed by Scherrer and Hillberry (79), who used the piecewise continuous parametric bicubic patch representation of Coons (23) to interpolate surface data obtained from the canine

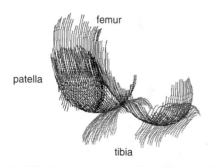

FIG. 6. Wireframe representation of knee articular surfaces obtained from MRI.

glenohumeral joint. The general equation of a bicubic patch is given by:

$$\mathbf{x}(u, v) = \sum_{i=0}^{3} \sum_{j=0}^{3} \mathbf{c}_{ij} \, u^i \, v^j \qquad (1)$$

where $\mathbf{x}$ is the position vector of a point on the bicubic patch at the parametric coordinates (u, v), and $\mathbf{c}_{ij}$ are vector coefficients. For articular surfaces, a large number of patches are used to represent the entire surface, and certain continuity requirements are enforced at the boundaries of adjoining patches. In the piecewise continuous implementation of Coons patches employed by these authors, continuity of the surface tangents was enforced (C^1 continuity). This technique, which is well adapted to gridded wireframes in which each grid cell represents a patch (Fig. 4), was later used by Huiskes et al. (52), Ateshian et al. (5), and Hefzy and Yang (47) for fitting knee joint articular surfaces and by Wood et al. (94) for modeling muscle surfaces. One immediate application of the bicubic representation is to evaluate surface normals, which are used for displaying shaded models of the articular surfaces (Fig. 7). The surface normal is obtained from the normalized cross product of the tangents along each of the two parametric coordinates:

$$\mathbf{n} = \frac{\mathbf{x}_u \times \mathbf{x}_v}{|\mathbf{x}_u \times \mathbf{x}_v|} \qquad (2)$$

where $\mathbf{x}_u = \partial\mathbf{x}/\partial u$ and $\mathbf{x}_v = \partial\mathbf{x}/\partial v$ are the surface tangents along the parametric coordinate directions u and v.

Despite their versatility, piecewise continuous bicubic patches have two drawbacks. First, they do not provide continuity of surface curvatures, which are needed in many applications as described below. Second, they are fitted to the experimental data by interpolation; i.e., the mathematical representation passes exactly through every experimental surface data point. This interpolation becomes problematic because of the inevitable presence of measurement errors, which lead to the creation of ripples in the mathematical representation of the articular surfaces.

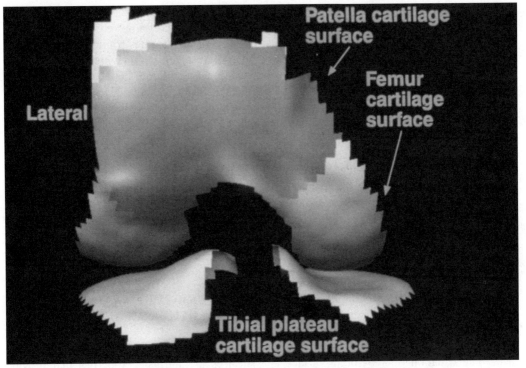

FIG. 7. Shaded models of knee joint articular surfaces.

Though the effect of small ripples may be neglected in some applications, these can be reduced or eliminated by surface approximation. In this approach, the mathematical surface need not pass exactly through every data point but may sufficiently deviate from the data such that it remains smooth. Surface approximation is generally achieved using the method of least squares, in which the root-mean-square (rms) of the residual error between the data points and the mathematical surface is minimized. Rushfeldt et al. (78) used this method to fit the mathematical equation of a sphere,

$$(x - x_o)^2 + (y - y_o)^2 + (z - z_o)^2 = R^2 \quad (3)$$

to articular surface data from the hip joint. In this equation, R is the sphere radius, (x_o, y_o, z_o) are the coordinates of its origin, and (x, y, z) are the coordinates of points on the sphere, relative to some laboratory-fixed coordinate system. Similarly, Soslowsky et al. (88) fitted spherical surfaces to surface data from the

glenohumeral joint; they found that the rms residual error was on the order of 0.2 mm, or less than 1% of the surface radius, and concluded that this joint is well approximated by a spherically shaped geometry. Wismans et al. (93) and Blankevoort et al. (17) used surface approximation to represent the tibial plateau with algebraic surfaces of the form $z = f(x,y)$, where z values measured elevations of surface points relative to the xy plane, and $f(x,y)$ consisted of a bivariate polynomial of degree 6 or 7. These authors reported rms residual errors on the order of 0.3 to 0.5 mm. Although successful in many respects, algebraic representations of this form are not particularly suited for computer implementations because surface slopes parallel to the z-axis have a value of infinity. This difficulty can be avoided with the use of parametric surface representations akin to the bicubic patch of equation 1. For example, Ateshian et al. (6) employed least-squares surface fitting of biquintic parametric patches to represent the articular surfaces of the thumb carpometacarpal joint, with rms residual errors on the order of 0.07 mm (Fig. 8). The equation of a parametric biquintic patch is given by

$$\mathbf{x}(u, v) = \sum_{i=0}^{5} \sum_{j=0}^{5} \mathbf{c}_{ij} \, u^i \, v^j \qquad (4)$$

where, similar to bicubic patches, the c_{ij}'s are vector coefficients. In their study, a single patch was used to represent the entire articular surface, providing continuous higher-order derivatives everywhere within the patch. Although a single biquintic patch could successfully represent the trapezial and metacarpal surfaces with small residual errors, not all articular surfaces of diarthrodial joints could be well approximated by equation 4. In order to combine the usefulness of parametric representations of surfaces with the versatility of piecewise C^2 continous representations, Ateshian (7) used bicubic B-spline surfaces to approximate a wide variety of diarthrodial joint surfaces. The equation of a B-spline surface is given by

$$\mathbf{x}(u, v) = \sum_{i=1}^{n_u} \sum_{j=1}^{n_v} B_i^{k_u}(u) B_j^{k_v}(v) \mathbf{d}_{ij} \quad (5)$$

where d_{ij}'s are B-spline coefficients or control points, n_u and n_v are the numbers of coefficients along each parametric coordinate direction, k_u and k_v are the B-spline orders along those directions ($k_u = k_v = 4$ for bicubic splines), and $B_i^{k_u}(u)$ and $B_j^{k_v}(v)$ are B-spline blending functions. Parametric surfaces, and in particular B-spline surfaces, can be "trimmed" to provide a more realistic smooth boundary, rather than the irregular boundary of a gridded wireframe (e.g., Figs. 4, 7, and 8). Figure 9 illustrates trimmed B-spline surface representations of typical knee articular surfaces. The smooth boundary of a trimmed surface is better suited for finite element modeling of articular layers (90). Figure 10A shows a solid model of the articular layer of a human patella, generated by combining the B-spline representations of its cartilage and subchondral bone surfaces (10), and Fig. 10B shows a finite element mesh of the same layer (33,74). In these figures, a representative contact area contour for a particular joint position is employed as a guide for refining the finite element mesh.

CURVATURE ANALYSIS OF ARTICULAR SURFACES

The curvature characteristics of articular surfaces are intrinsic properties that provide quantitative measures of their shape (30). There are many applications that motivate the calculation of these surface properties. The most straightforward application is the characterization of anatomic features, such as the presence and location of ridges and grooves, as well as sellar (saddle-shaped), ovoid, and flat regions. In their simplest form, these measures provide a snapshot of such features in a joint; for example, they can be used to identify normal features and differentiate dysplastic joint surfaces from a normative data base. Moreover, by use of noninvasive imaging methods

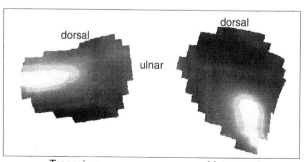

FIG. 8. Shaded models of the thumb carpometacarpal articular surfaces.

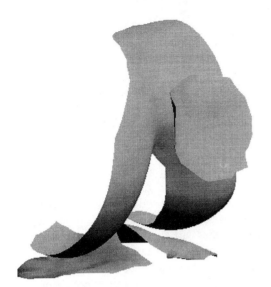

FIG. 9. Shaded models of trimmed *B*-spline surface representations of knee joint surfaces.

such as MRI and CT, changes in these anatomic features can be tracked in patients as a function of time to study joint growth and remodeling. For example, subchondral bone remodeling is known to occur in arthritic joints as well as in congenital dysplasia. Characterizing early changes in the surface curvature of afflicted joints may provide a useful diagnostic tool in a clinical setting; such tools may become more useful as the accuracy of noninvasive imaging modalities increases.

Surface curvatures are also useful in the study of diarthrodial joint congruence and contact mechanics (e.g., 41,53,66). From ba-

sic principles of mechanics, it is recognized that under the same contact load, decreased joint congruence leads to higher cartilage stresses. In canonical contact problems that analyze the contact mechanics of cartilage layers of cylindrical, spherical, or ellipsoidal geometries, the cartilage stresses are directly related to differences in the surface curvatures (i.e., the congruence) of the layers at the point of initial contact (e.g., 4,8,25,26,27,57). Furthermore, in a recent study, it has been shown that cartilage interstitial fluid pressurization, which shields the collagen–proteoglycan matrix from excessive stresses, is promoted by higher congruence of the contacting surfaces (11). Hence, an analysis of the curvature characteristics of diarthrodial joint surfaces can lead to a better understanding of the contact mechanics in joints.

The curvature characteristics at each point of a surface consist of the principal curvatures, κ_{min} and κ_{max}, and their corresponding, mutually orthogonal, principal directions of curvature (30). The inverses of the curvatures are the radii of curvature. A surface that is locally flat has zero curvature along both principal directions ($\kappa_{min} = 0$, $\kappa_{max} = 0$, at any point on a plane); a convex ovoid surface has positive principal curvatures ($\kappa_{min} > 0$, $\kappa_{max} > 0$, as on the outer surface of an egg); a concave ovoid surface has negative principal curvatures ($\kappa_{min} < 0$, $\kappa_{max} < 0$; e.g., on the inner surface of a bowl); a sellar surface has curvatures of opposite signs ($\kappa_{min} < 0$, $\kappa_{max} > 0$; e.g., on a saddle). A sphere has uniform curvatures ($\kappa_{min} = \kappa_{max}$

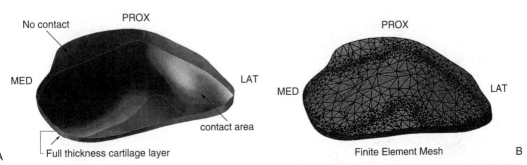

FIG. 10. (A) Solid model of a patellar articular layer with contact area imprint superimposed. **(B)** Finite element mesh of the articular layer with mesh adaptation around the contact area periphery.

= 1/*radius*), and at each surface point every direction is a principal direction. A ridge is characterized by a band of locally high maximum curvatures that follows directions of minimum curvature; similarly, a groove is characterized by a band of locally large negative minimum curvatures that follows directions of maximum curvature. These bands can be seen on maps of the minimum or maximum curvature. Similarly, by starting at arbitrary points on a surface and tracing lines that follow the principal minimum or maximum directions of curvature everywhere, one can produce a map of the lines of curvature, which can facilitate the identification of ridges and grooves. At any surface point of parametric coordinates (u,v), the principal curvatures are the roots of the quadratic equation

$$(EG - F^2)\kappa^2 - (EN + GL - 2FM)\kappa + (LN - M^2) = 0 \quad (6)$$

where $E = x_u \cdot x_u$, $F = x_u \cdot x_v$, $G = x_v \cdot x_v$, $L = x_{uu} \cdot n$, $M = x_{uv} \cdot n$, $N = x_{vv} \cdot \mathbf{n}$, and $x_{uu} = \partial^2 \mathbf{x}/\partial u^2$, etc. Similarly, the principal directions at that point are the roots of

$$(FN - GM)h^2 + (EN - GL)h + (EM - FL) = 0 \quad (7)$$

where $h = dv/du$. These equations can easily be solved, given a parametric representation of the articular surface such as those in equations 1, 4, or 5 (6,14).

Historically, MacConaill (67) was one of the earliest investigators to employ curvature theory for understanding the kinematics of diarthrodial joints from the topography of their articular surfaces. He investigated the conjunct rotation of the bones of a joint during diadochal displacements and noted the opposite conjunct rotations occurring in ovoid versus sellar joints. More recently, Ateshian et al. (6) used curvature analysis to describe the anatomy and congruence of the thumb carpometacarpal (CMC) joint. These authors described the common features that characterize the predominantly saddle-shaped trapezium and metacarpal surfaces; in particular, they observed that lines of curvature were consistently aligned with the dorsovolar and radial–ulnar directions of the joint (Fig. 11), i.e., along the primary motions of flexion–extension and abduction–adduction. Perhaps more significantly, differences were found in the shape of the trapezial articular surface between men and women, with a subset of female joints exhibiting convex ovoid regions on the trapezium rather than the more common sellar topography (Fig. 12). It was also determined that female joints were less congruent than male joints, using a curvature-based global congruence index. These results led to the hypothesis that female CMC joints experience higher cartilage stresses than male joints during light to moderate activities of daily living that involve similar loads for men and women. Such higher stresses may help explain the greater prevalence of osteoarthritis in the female population above the age of 45 (59,64).

The curvature characteristics of the patellofemoral joint articular surfaces have also been determined in recent studies (22,61). Patellar maps of the maximum principal curvatures and the lines of minimum curvature have provided an unequivocal determination of the

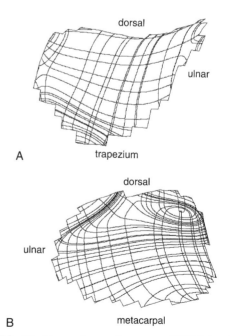

FIG. 11. Lines of curvature on a CMC joint. **(A)** Trapezium. **(B)** Metacarpal.

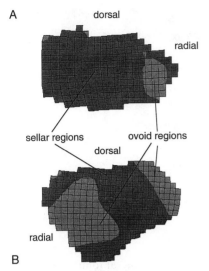

FIG. 12. Gaussian curvature maps of female trapezial surfaces. The Gaussian curvature K is the product of the principal curvatures; i.e., $K = \kappa_{min}\kappa_{max}$. When K is negative, the surface is locally sellar; when it is positive, the surface is ovoid, and its concavity or convexity can be determined from the sign of κ_{min} or κ_{max}. **(A)** Typical sellar trapezial surface. **(B)** Trapezial surface with large convex ovoid region.

existence and location of patellar ridges (Fig. 13). These include a proximal median ridge that extends distally in some specimens, a lateral transverse ridge that extends medially in some specimens, and a secondary ridge that appears in most specimens. No more than one transverse ridge was observed in these studies, which included 31 patellas from 22 cadavers. Paired specimens exhibited remarkable symmetry, as shown in Fig. 14. On the opposing femoral surface, curvature maps confirmed that the trochlea is predominantly sellar within a band centered on the midsagittal plane, with ridges flanking it along its medial and lateral sides (Fig. 15). In all 12 femoral specimens, grooves were observed where the trochlea merges with the condyles, which were more pronounced on the lateral side. It has been suggested that the knee menisci rest against these grooves at full extension (37,72).

CONTACT AREA DETERMINATION FROM PROXIMITY MAPS

Determination of contact areas in diarthrodial joints is a crucial step toward understanding the stress–strain environment and the effects of joint loading on articular cartilage. Although the goal of many rehabilitation and surgical procedures is restoration of normal articular mechanics, little is known regarding the normal or abnormal contact mechanics of many joints. Historically, a variety of techniques have been utilized to measure diarthrodial joint contact areas, including dye staining (42), rubber casting (60,83), piezoresistive transducers (19,20), and Fuji Pressensor Film (e.g., 36,51,87).

Another method, based on evaluating the proximity of articular surfaces to estimate contact areas using experimentally derived geometric models of the joint, has been developed (79,80). In this approach, kinematic data representing relative motion of opposing

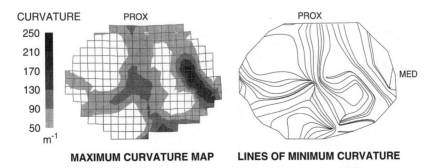

FIG. 13. Maximum curvature map and lines of minimum curvature of a patellar cartilage surface, indicating the presence and location of ridges.

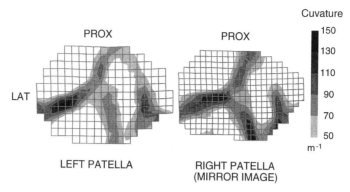

FIG. 14. Maximum curvature maps of matched left and right patellae, demonstrating symmetry of curvature characteristics.

articular surfaces during a specific motion, or with the joint in a series of specified positions, are obtained. Subsequently, articular surfaces are exposed, and their geometry is quantified to create models of the joints. Next, spatial transformations that realign the articular surfaces into the relative positions that they assumed during the motion in question are performed. Finally, by calculating the points of closest proximity between opposing surfaces in this realigned position, contact areas can be estimated. This last step can be accomplished only with the availability of geometric models of the articular surfaces.

Recently, a comparison of contact methods was performed that included dye staining, silicone rubber casting, Fuji film, and an SPG method that utilizes a proximity criterion similar to that described above (9). In this comparison study, both congruent joints (modeled

by bovine glenohumeral joints) and incongruent joints (modeled by bovine lateral tibiofemoral articulations without the menisci) were investigated. All methods provided consistent contact results for the incongruent articulation. However, for the congruent joint, the SPG and Fuji film methods yielded similar results, but the other two methods yielded significantly different contact regions. Some advantages of the SPG method are that it can be used in intact joints and that it can be used repeatedly and quickly through a range of motions. This contact method has been used to quantify contact in joints such as the thumb carpometacarpal, the shoulder glenohumeral, and the knee tibiofemoral and patellofemoral joints. Some results obtained with this method are described below.

For the thumb carpometacarpal joint, contact was determined in the position of lateral

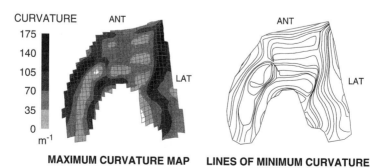

MAXIMUM CURVATURE MAP   **LINES OF MINIMUM CURVATURE**

FIG. 15. Maximum curvature map and lines of minimum curvature of the trochlea.

pinch as well as through a wide range of motion (13). The lateral pinch position produced contact areas predominantly on the central, volar, and volar–ulnar regions of the trapezium and metacarpal. Interestingly, these positions corresponded with positions of SPG-measured cartilage thinning, providing support for the hypothesis that increased contact stresses in these regions may be related to osteoarthritic changes. In the glenohumeral joint, contact was determined through a range of elevation positions (89). Results demonstrated increased contact area through 120° of elevation. In addition, with elevation, humeral head contact was shown to migrate from an inferior region to a superocentral–posterior region while glenoid contact shifts somewhat posteriorly. These results provide the baseline data against which the effect of surgical procedures designed to restore "normal articular mechanics" can be compared. Also in the shoulder, subacromial contact was measured as the relationship between the undersurface of the acromion and the superior surface of the rotator cuff tendons (35). In this study, contact was obtained at the anterolateral edge of the acromion with the arm at the side, which shifted medially with arm elevation. On the supraspinatus tendon, contact was shown to shift from proximal to distal toward the insertion and "critical zone" with arm elevation. This study has significant implications regarding the pathogenesis of rotator cuff damage and the role of extrinsic factors. The SPG proximity-based contact method has also been employed recently for measuring contact in the knee at flexion angles of 0° to 120° degrees, in the open-chain configuration (2); the objective of this study was to investigate the role of the iliotibial band (ITB) on patellar mechanics. It was found that pulling on the ITB generated statistically significant, but quantitatively small, lateral translations of 0.35 mm in the patella; however, the centroid of the contact area was found to shift laterally by approximately 1.47 mm, indicating a disproportionate effect of translation on contact areas and suggesting that kinematic measurements alone cannot be used to assess changes in patellofemoral joint mechanics.

Although the SPG method has some significant advantages, one primary disadvantage is that it is applicable only in the *in vitro* state. Current studies are beginning to apply the concepts developed through the SPG method for use with MRI, whereby proximity of MRI-generated articular surfaces can be used to assess contact areas *in situ* and *in vivo* (12,49). An illustration of this approach is shown in Fig. 16, which displays the proximity-based contact area map for the MRI-generated patellofemoral joint of Figs. 5 and 6.

CARTILAGE THICKNESS MAPS

Cartilage thickness can be readily visualized *in vitro* by sectioning a bone along an appropriate plane and examining the resulting cross sections; thickness maps can be reconstructed from these sections to provide a surface-wide representation of the results, as performed by McLeod et al. (68) on the human tibial plateau and by Eckstein et al. (28) on the human patella. However, this method is prone to errors because results are dependent on the orientation of the sectioning plane. The needle-probe method (50,73), in which the probe is aligned perpendicularly to the surface, is more precise in this respect. In this approach, a load cell connected to a probe records a spike as the needle pierces the cartilage surface and another spike when the needle touches the subchondral bone; the thickness is derived from recordings of the needle displacement between the spikes. This method is practical only when a few measurements are needed. Optical methods have been used to measure the thickness of small plugs of articular cartilage using a microscope; typically, several measurements are made around the plug periphery and averaged to produce a final result (54,70). Ultrasound can also measure the thickness of cartilage by recording the time required for an ultrasound wave to travel between the cartilage and subchondral bone surfaces; the cartilage thickness is derived from the knowledge of the speed of sound in cartilage (70,78). In a recent study,

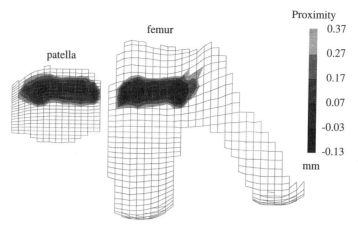

FIG. 16. Proximity-based contact area map for the MRI-generated knee joint articular surfaces of Fig. 6.

Jurvelin et al. (55) compared the needle-probe, optical, and ultrasound methods for measuring cartilage thickness; they found a good correlation between optical and needle-probe methods, though they observed greater scatter with the ultrasound.

Ateshian et al. (5) demonstrated the use of stereophotogrammetry to calculate cartilage thickness maps *in vitro,* in the human knee. In their approach, the cartilage surface was first quantified with SPG, then the cartilage layer was dissolved using a mild solution of sodium hypochloride to expose the underlying subchondral bone. After quantifying the bone surface with SPG, geometric models of the two surfaces were obtained and realigned in a common coordinate system using data from optical targets rigidly fixed to the bone. From these geometric models, they calculated the cartilage layer thickness at various points on the subchondral bone, along directions perpendicular to the bone surface. Using the perpendicular direction to the subchondral bone surface as a geometric reference for measuring cartilage thickness, allows for a more precise method than in-plane thickness measurement methods (e.g., sectioning). Mathematically, this calculation consists of solving the following vector equation:

$$x_{bone} + t\mathbf{n}_{bone} = x(u,v) \qquad (8)$$

where x_{bone} is the position of a point on the subchondral bone surface where the cartilage thickness t is desired, n_{bone} is the unit normal to the bone surface at that point, and $x(u, v)$ is the corresponding point on the cartilage surface. Equation 8 has three scalar component equations which can be solved for the three unknowns u, v, and t. The results of this analysis can be displayed as cartilage thickness maps, as shown in Fig. 17. Similar studies have been conducted on the articular layers of the glenohumeral joint (89) and the thumb CMC joint (13).

More recently, patellar cartilage thickness maps have been obtained noninvasively from MRI by Eckstein et al. (29) who used a three-dimensional fat-supressed FLASH sequence. These authors assessed the accuracy of their MRI thickness measurements against the sectioning method. They found that 81% of their MRI-measured thicknesses over the entire articular surfaces was within 0.5 mm of the sectioning results. Eckstein et al. (29) used in-plane measurements to generate cartilage thickness maps from MRI slices; however, the method used for calculating thickness maps from SPG-generated geometric models as summarized in equation 8 can be used equally well with MRI-generated models of the cartilage and subchondral bone surfaces, as shown in Fig. 18.

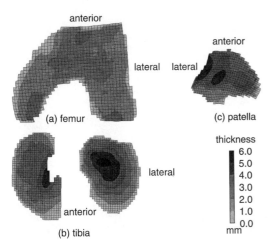

FIG. 17. Thickness maps of the articular layers of a typical knee joint: **(a)** femur, **(b)** tibia, **(c)** patella. Thickness measurements are calculated along a direction perpendicular to the bone surface at every point.

ANATOMICALLY BASED COORDINATE SYSTEMS FOR DIARTHRODIAL JOINTS

The development of quantitative tools for measuring joint kinematics, contact areas, cartilage thickness, and cartilage stresses has brought with it the necessity to describe these measurements in meaningful and reproducible body-fixed coordinate systems. For example, in a patient with patellar malalignment, the success of a corrective surgical procedure can be determined in part by measuring the shift in patellofemoral joint contact areas from pre- and postoperative MRIs. A precise measurement of this spatial shift can be achieved only if a body-fixed coordinate system is defined consistently in both sets of images. Similarly, joint kinematic measurements are best interpreted when they are referred to anatomically based coordinate systems.

Body-fixed coordinate systems can be associated with various bones of a joint by employing topographic measurements of the bone contours as well as the articular surfaces (16,43,62,92). In the case of the knee,

for example, Blankevoort et al. (16) defined coordinate axes for the femur and tibia which are aligned with each other in full extension. The origins of these coordinate systems were determined relative to specific bony landmarks. A similar approach was followed by van Kampen and Huiskes (92) in the case of the patellofemoral joint. However, Blankevoort et al. (16) demonstrated from a parametric analysis that relatively small misalignments in the choice of these coordinate systems may lead to large variations in some of the kinematic measurements. These variations could lead to inconsistent kinematic results among various specimens. Kwak et al. (62) proposed a set of body-fixed coordinate systems for the femur, tibia, and patella, which are derived from three-dimensional geometric data of the bones and their articular surfaces. The articular surface data were derived from SPG, and bone contours were digitized with a coordinate-measurement machine (CMM) (Fig. 19). In this approach, the coordinate axes of the femur, tibia, and patella are no longer necessarily aligned in full extension; thus, for example, the varus–valgus angle of the tibia relative to the femur is derived from the orientation of the femoral and tibial coordinate systems rather than prescribed arbitrarily to be zero when the flexion angle is zero. Blankevoort et al. (18) conducted a kinematic study on seven knee joints, where they compared outcomes using the coordinate systems of Blankevoort et al. (16) and van Kampen and Huiskes (92) against those of Kwak et al. (62). They confirmed that for certain motions, such as mediolateral translation and rotation of the patella as well as internal–external and varus–valgus rotations of the tibia, the differences in the results were very significant (Fig. 20).

COMPUTER SIMULATIONS AND MULTIBODY MODELING OF DIARTHRODIAL JOINTS

Quantitative representations of bones and articular surfaces can be used for mathemat-

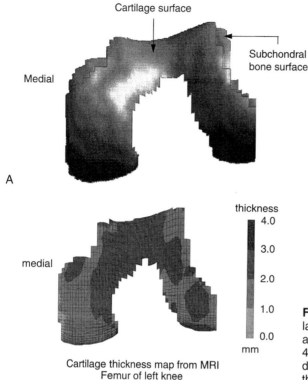

thickness
4.0

3.0

2.0

1.0

0.0

mm

Cartilage thickness map from MRI
Femur of left knee
41 year old female

B

FIG. 18. (A) Geometric models of cartilage and subchondral bone surfaces of a human distal femoral surface from a 41-year-old woman, obtained from MRI data. **(B)** Cartilage thickness map for the same surfaces, calculated from equation 8.

ically modeling diarthrodial joints to predict the normal mechanics and the outcome of simulated injuries, surgical repair procedures, or other pathologic conditions. Generally, these models are created from experimental data and are validated by predicting the outcome of experiments that have actually been performed. If the agreement between the model and experiment is found to be good, it is possible to employ the mathematical model to predict the outcomes of other configurations that have not been tested experimentally. Such computer simulations are becoming more common in orthopaedic research (e.g., 31,34,38,45,46), and some representative examples are described in this section.

As mentioned above, subacromial contact under normal circumstances has been quantified using the SPG method (35). Subsequently, the anterior acromioplasty procedure, which is designed to surgically remove

a portion of the undersurface of the acromion, was simulated on the computer (58). Specifically, various portions of the geometric model of the acromion were removed to simulate the effect of the surgical procedure. Results indicated that "flattening of the anterior ridge" of the acromion was successful in removing subacromial impingement in only three of six specimens, whereas "flattening of the anterior third" was successful in eliminating all impingement. This result indicates that flattening beyond this anterior third is not necessary to achieve relief of acromial impingement. A subsequent study addressed the importance of acromial length on impingement. This study lengthened the geometric model of the acromion by 10 mm and found no change in impingement relative to normal. This result supports the belief that shortening an acromion as part of an acromioplasty procedure is likely unnecessary.

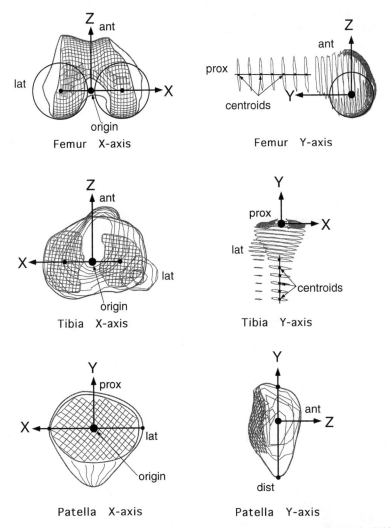

FIG. 19. Body-fixed coordinate systems on the femur, tibia, and patella (62).

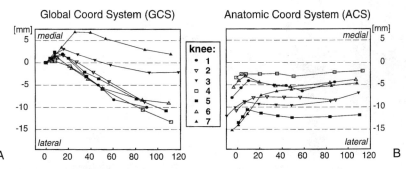

FIG. 20. Mediolateral translation of the patella during flexion from 0° to 120° in six cadaver specimens, using two sets of coordinate systems: **(A)** coordinate axes that are globally aligned with bony landmarks of the knee joint, but which become parallel at full extension; **(B)** body-fixed coordinate systems which are derived from articular and bone surface geometry.

Joint modeling has also been performed using the classical engineering approach of multibody modeling in which bones are assumed to be rigid bodies while cartilage, ligaments, muscles, tendons, and other soft tissue structures are often modeled using springs. For example, models of the knee joint have been described by Wismans et al. (93), Blankevoort et al. (17), Abdel-Rahman and Hefzy (1), Essinger et al. (31), Garg and Walker (38), Hirokawa (48), Heegaard (45), Heegaard and Leyvraz (46), Kwak et al. (63), and others; rigid-body spring models have been described by Schuind et al. (81) for studying force transmission through the wrist. Figure 21 displays a computer rendition of a knee joint model (63) that employs quantitative geometric data for representing bones, cartilage, ligament insertions, and muscle lines of action. By comparing their model predictions with actual experiments simulating open-chain knee exercises in a cadaver knee joint, these authors have shown that predicted displacements and rotations of the patella were within 1 mm and 4°, respectively, of the experimental data over a range of 0° to 90° of knee flexion.

SUMMARY

In this chapter, various applications of quantitative modeling of the anatomy of diarthrodial joints have been reviewed. Because of the rapid and continuing introduction of computer modeling tools from the various fields of engineering into orthopaedic biomechanics, this review does not purport to be exhaustive. Its primary aim is to provide insight into the exciting potential of computer modeling in orthopaedic applications. These exciting advances are occurring simultaneously with advances in noninvasive imaging tools such as CT and MRI, offering the opportunity to employ these techniques *in vivo*. When they fulfill their true potential, these tools can be used in the areas of diagnosis, monitoring of disease progression in conditions such as osteoarthritis, and assessing surgical outcomes.

Acknowledgments

The authors would like to acknowledge the support of the National Science Foundation (ASC-931818). The authors are also grateful to the members of the Knee Group of the Orthopaedic Research Laboratory, Columbia University, for providing many of the data and figures of this chapter; in addition to the lead author, these members include Dr. Christopher Ahmad, Professor Leendert Blankevoort (visiting), Ms. Cerlinde Chahin, Ms. Zohara Cohen, Mr. Thomas R. Gardner, Dr. Ronald P. Grelsamer, Dr. Jack H. Henry, Mr. S. Daniel Kwak, and Professor Van C. Mow. The authors are also indebted to Professor Robert L. Spilker, Professor Mark S. Shephard, and Mr. Bob O'Bara, from the Computational Biomechanics Group at Rensselaer, for their contri-

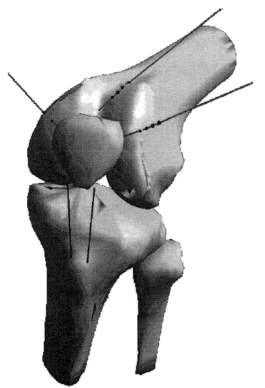

FIG. 21. Multibody model of the knee joint, showing bone and articular surfaces, ligaments, and muscle lines of action.

bution in the area of finite element modeling of diarthrodial joints, and to Dr. Charles M. Peterfy of the University of California, San Francisco, for his contribution in the area of magnetic resonance imaging.

REFERENCES

1. Abdel-Rahman, E., and Hefzy, M. S. (1993): A two-dimensional dynamic anatomical model of the human knee joint. *J. Biomech. Eng.*, 115:357–365.
2. Ahmad, C. S., Kwak, S. D., Grelsamer, R. P., Henry, J., Gardner, T. R., Ateshian, G. A., and Mow, V. C. (1996): The influence of iliotibial band tension on patellar tracking and patellofemoral contact. *Orthop. Trans.*, 20: 119–120.
3. Armstrong, C. G., and Gardner, D. L. (1977): Thickness and distribution of human femoral head articular cartilage. *Ann. Rheum. Dis.*, 36:407–412.
4. Armstrong, C. G. (1986): An analysis of the stresses in a thin layer of articular cartilage in a synovial joint. *Eng. Med.*, 15:55–61.
5. Ateshian, G. A., Soslowsky, L. J., and Mow, V. C. (1991): Quantitation of articular surface topography and cartilage thickness in knee joints using stereophotogrammetry. *J. Biomech.*, 24:761–776.
6. Ateshian, G. A., Rosenwasser, M. P., and Mow, V. C. (1992): Curvature characteristics and congruence of the thumb carpometacarpal joint. *J. Biomech.*, 25: 591–608.
7. Ateshian, G. A. (1993): A least-squares B-spline surface-fitting method for articular surfaces of diarthrodial joints. *J. Biomech. Eng.*, 115:366–373.
8. Ateshian, G. A., Lai, W. M., Zhu, W. B., and Mow, V. C. (1994): An asymptotic solution for the contact of two biphasic cartilage layers. *J. Biomech.*, 27:1347–1360.
9. Ateshian, G. A., Kwak, S. D., Soslowsky, L. J., and Mow, V. C. (1994): A stereophotogrammetric method for determining in situ contact areas in diarthrodial joints, and a comparison with other methods. *J. Biomech.*, 27:111–124.
10. Ateshian, G. A. (1995): Generating trimmed B-spline models of articular cartilage layers from unordered 3D surface data points. 1995 Bioengineering Conference. *ASME*, BED-29:217–218.
11. Ateshian, G. A., and Wang, H. (1995): A theoretical solution for the frictionless rolling contact of cylindrical biphasic articular cartilage layers. *J. Biomech.*, 28: 1341–1355.
12. Ateshian, G. A., Cohen, Z. A., Kwak, S. D., Wang, V. M., Ahmad, C. S., Kelkar, R., Raimondo, R. A., Feldman, F., Miller, T. R., Mun, I. K., Bigliani, L. U., Mow, V. C., and Peterfy, C. G. (1995): Determination of in situ contact areas in diarthrodial joints by MRI. *ASME Adv. Bioeng.* (in press).
13. Ateshian, G. A., Ark, J. W., Rosenwasser, M. P., Pawluk, R. J., and Mow, V. C. (1995): In situ contact areas in the thumb carpometacarpal joint. *J. Orthop. Res.*, 13: 450–458.
14. Beck, J. M., Farouki, R. T., and Hinds, J. K. (1986): Surface analysis methods. *IEEE CG&A*, December:18–36.
15. Belsole, R. J., Hilbelink, D. R., Llewellyn, J. A., Stenzler, S., Green, T. L., and Dale, M. (1988): Mathematical analysis of computed carpal models. *J. Orthop. Res.*, 5:116–122.
16. Blankevoort, L., Huiskes, R., and de Lange, A. (1988): The envelope of passive knee joint motion. *J. Biomech.*, 21:705–720.
17. Blankevoort, L., Kuiper, J. H., Huiskes, R., and Grootenboer, H. J. (1991): Articular contact in a three-dimensional model of the knee. *J. Biomech.*, 24:1019–1031.
18. Blankevoort, L., Kwak, S. D., Ahmad, C. S., Gardner, T. S., Grelsamer, R. P., Henry, J. H., Ateshian, G. A., and Mow, V. C. (1996): Effects of global and anatomic coordinate systems on knee joint kinematics. *Proc. Eur. Soc. Biomech.* 10:260.
19. Brown, T. D., and Shaw, D. T. (1983): In vitro contact stress distributions in the natural human hip. *J. Biomech.*, 16:373–384.
20. Brown, T. D., and Shaw, D. T. (1984): In vitro contact stress distribution on the femoral condyles. *J. Orthop. Res.*, 2:190–199.
21. Clark, R. E., Karara, H. M., Catalogu, A., and Gould, P. L. (1975): Close-range photogrammetry and coupled stress analysis as tools in the development of prosthetic devices. *Trans. Am. Soc. Artif. Int. Organs*, 21:71–78.
22. Colman, W. W., Kwak, S. D., Ateshian, G. A., Grelsamer, R. P., Henry, J. H., and Mow, V. C. (1995): Curvature analysis of the human patellofemoral joint articular surfaces. *Trans. Orthop. Res. Soc.*, 20:694.
23. Coons, S. A. (1967): *Surfaces for Computer-Aided Design and Space Forms*, p. 504. Publication AD-663, Massachusetts Institute of Technology, Cambridge, MA.
24. Davidson, M. (1898): Roentgen rays and localisation. An apparatus for exact measurement and localisation by means of roentgen rays. *Br. Med. J.*, 1898:10–14.
25. Eberhardt, A. W., Keer, L. M., Lewis, J. L., and Vithoontien, V. (1990): An analytical model of joint contact. *ASME J. Biomech. Eng.*, 112:407–413.
26. Eberhardt, A. W., Lewis, J. L., and Keer, L. M. (1991): Contact of layered elastic spheres as a model of joint contact: Effect of tangential load and friction. *ASME J. Biomech. Eng.*, 113:107–108.
27. Eberhardt, A. W., Lewis, J. L., and Keer, L. M. (1991): Normal contact of elastic spheres with two elastic layers as a model of joint articulation. *ASME J. Biomech. Eng.*, 113:410–417.
28. Eckstein, F., Müller-Gerbl, M., and Putz, R. (1992): Distribution of subchondral bone density and cartilage thickness in the human patella. *J. Anat.*, 180:425–433.
29. Eckstein, F., Sittek, H., Gavazzeni, A., Milz, S., Putz, R., and Reiser, M. (1995): Assessment of articular cartilage volume and thickness with magnetic resonance imaging (MRI). *Trans. Orthop. Res. Soc.*, 20:194.
30. Eisenhart, L. P. (1909): *A Treatise on the Differential Geometry of Curves and Surfaces*. Dover, New York.
31. Essinger, J. R., Leyvraz, P. F., Heegard, J. H., and Robertson D. D. (1989): A mathematical model for the evaluations of the behaviour during flexion of condylar-type knee prostheses. *J. Biomech.*, 22:1229–1241.
32. Feldkamp, L. A., Goldstein, S. A., Parfitt, A. M., Jesion, G., and Kleerekoper, M. (1989): The direct examination of three-dimensional bone architecture in vitro by computed tomography. *J. Bone Miner. Res.*, 4:3–11.
33. Flaherty, J. E., Frachioni, M., Huang, L., Ozturan, C., and Shephard, M. S. (1995): Parallel adaptive computa-

tions for soft tissue analysis. 1995 Bioengineering Conference. *ASME Adv. Bioeng.,* BED-29:165–166.

34. Flatow, E. L., Ateshian, G. A., Soslowsky, L. J., Pawluk, R. J., Grelsamer, R. P., Mow, V. C., and Bigliani, L. U. (1994): Computer simulation of glenohumeral and patellofemoral subluxation: Estimating pathological articular contact. *Clin. Orthop.,* 306:28–33.

35. Flatow, E. L., Soslowsky, L. J., Ticker, J. B., Pawluk, R. J., Hepler, M., Ark, J., Mow, V. C., and Bigliani, L. U. (1994): Excursion of the rotator cuff under the acromion. Patterns of subacromial contact. *Am. J. Sports Med.,* 22:779–788.

36. Fukubayashi, T., and Kurosawa, H. (1980): The contact area and pressure distribution pattern of the knee. *Acta Orthop. Scand.,* 51:871–879.

37. Fulkerson, J. P., and Hungerford, D. S. (1990): *Disorders of the Patellofemoral Joint,* pp. 7–12. Williams & Wilkins, Baltimore.

38. Garg, A., and Walker, P. S. (1990): Prediction of knee joint motion using a three-dimensional computer graphics model. *J. Biomech.,* 23:45–58.

39. Ghosh, S. K. (1979): *Analytical Photogrammetry.* New York, Pergamon Press.

40. Ghosh, S. K. (1983): A close-range photogrammetric system for 3-D measurements and perspective diagramming in biomechanics. *J. Biomech.,* 16:667–674.

41. Gladwell, G. M. L. (1980): *Contact Problems in the Classical Theory of Elasticity.* Sijthoff Noorhoff, Germantown, MD.

42. Greenwald, A. S., and O'Connor, J. J. (1971): The transmission of load through the human hip joint. *J. Biomech.,* 4:507–528.

43. Grood, E. S., and Suntay, W. J. (1983): A joint coordinate system for the clinical description of three-dimensional motions: application to the knee. *J. Biomech. Eng.,* 105:136–144.

44. Hall, F. M., and Wyshak, G. (1980): Thickness of articular cartilage in the normal knee. *J. Bone Joint Surg.,* 62A:408–413.

45. Heegaard, J. H. (1993): *Large slip contact in biomechanics: Kinematics and stress analysis of the patellofemoral joint.* Doctoral Thesis, Ecole Polytechnique Federale de Lausanne, Lausanne, Switzerland.

46. Heegaard, J. H., and Leyvraz, P. F. (1995): Computer aided surgery: Application to the Maquet procedure. 1995 Bioengineering Conference. *ASME,* BED-29:221–222.

47. Hefzy, M. S., and Yang, H. (1993): A three-dimensional anatomical model of the human patello-femoral joint, for the determination of patello-femoral motions and contact characteristics. *J. Biomed. Eng.,* 15:289–302.

48. Hirokawa, S. (1991): Three-dimensional mathematical model analysis of the patellofemoral joint. *J. Biomech.,* 24:659–671.

49. Hobatho, M. C., Couteau, B., Darmana, R., Baunin, C., and Cahuzac, J. P. (1994): Contact surfaces of tibiofemoral joints *in vivo.* In *Proceedings of the 2nd World Congress of Biomechanics.* Stichting World Biomechanics, Nijmegen, p. 300.

50. Hoch, D. H., Grodzinsky, A. J., Koob, T. J., Albert, M. L., and Eyre, D. R. (1983): Early changes in the material properties of rabit articular cartilage after meniscectommy. *J. Orthop. Res.,* 1:4–12.

51. Huberti, H. H., and Hayes, W. C. (1984): Patellofemoral contact pressures. *J. Bone Joint Surg.,* 66A:715–724.

52. Huiskes, R., Kremers, J., de Lange, A., Woltring, H. J.,

53. Selvik, G., and van Rens, T. J. G. (1985): Analytical stereophotogrammetric determination of three-dimensional knee-joint geometry. *J. Biomech.,* 18:559–170.

53. Johnson, K. L. (1985): *Contact Mechanics.* Cambridge University Press, Cambridge.

54. Jurvelin, J., Kiviranta, I., Arokoski, J., Tammi, M., and Helminen, H. J. (1987): Indentation study of the biomechanical properties of articular cartilage in the canine knee. *Eng. Med.,* 16:15–22.

55. Jurvelin, J. S., Räsänen, T., Kolmonen, P., and Lyyra, T. (1995): Comparison of optical, needle probe and ultrasonic techniques for the measurement of articular cartilage thickness. *J. Biomech.,* 28:231–235.

56. van Kampen, A., and Huiskes, R. (1990): The three-dimensional tracking pattern of the human patella. *J. Orthop. Res.,* 8:372–382.

57. Kelkar, R., and Ateshian, G. A. (1995): Contact creep response between a rigid impermeable cylinder and a biphasic cartilage layer using integral transforms. 1995 Bioengineering Conference. *ASME,* BED-29:313–314.

58. Kelkar, R., Colman, W. W., Soslowsky, L. J., Pollock, R. G., Flatow, E. L., Bigliani, L. U., and Mow, V. C. (1995): The effect of anterior acromioplasty on rotator cuff contact: An experimental and computer simulation. *Trans. Orthop. Res. Soc.,* 20:22.

59. Kelsey, J. L. (1982): *Epidemiology of Musculoskeletal Disorders.* Oxford University Press, New York.

60. Kurosawa, H., Fukubayashi, T., and Nakajima, H. (1980): Load-bearing mode of the knee joint, physical behavior of the knee joint with or without menisci. *Clin. Orthop.,* 149:283–290.

61. Kwak, S. D., Colman, W. W., Ateshian, G. A., Grelsamer, R. P., and Mow, V. C. (1994): Curvature analysis of the human retropatellar articular cartilage surface. *Adv. Bioeng. ASME,* BED-28:131–132.

62. Kwak, S. D., Blankevoort, L., Ahmad, C. S., Gardner, T. R., Grelsamer, R. P., Henry, J. H., Ateshian, G. A., and Mow, V. C. (1995): An anatomically based 3-D coordinate system for the knee joint. *Adv. Bioeng. ASME,* BED-31:309–310.

63. Kwak, S. D., Ateshian, S. D., Blankevoort, L., Ahmad, C. S., Gardner, T. R., Grelsamer, R. P., and Mow, V. C. (1995): Development of multibody model for diarthrodial joints using accurate 3-D cartilage and bone surfaces. *Ann. Biomed. Eng.,* 23(Suppl. 1):498.

64. Lawrence, J. S., Bremner, J. M., and Bier, F. (1966): Osteoarthrosis: Prevalence in the population and relationship between symptoms and X-ray changes. *Ann. Rheum. Dis.,* 25:1–23.

65. Lorensen, W. E., and Cline, H. E. (1987): Marching cubes: A high resolution 3D surface reconstruction algorithm. *Comput. Graph.,* 21:163–169.

66. Lur'e, A. I. (1964): *Three-Dimensional Problems of the Theory of Elasticity,* edited by J. R. M. Radok. Interscience, New York.

67. MacConaill, M. A. (1946): Studies in the mechanics of synovial joints. *Irish J. Med. Sci.,* 6:223–235.

68. McLeod, W. D., Moschi, A., Andrews, J. R., and Hughston, J. C. (1977): Tibial plateau topography. *Am. J. Sports Med.,* 5:13–18.

69. Meachim, G., Bentley, G., and Baker, R. (1977): Effect of age on thickness of adult patellar articular cartilage. *Ann. Rheum. Dis.,* 36:563–568.

70. Modest, V. E., Murphy, M. C., and Mann, R. W. (1989): Optical verification of a technique for *in situ* ultrasonic

measurement of articular cartilage thickness. *J. Biomech.,* 22:171–176.

71. Moon, K. L., Jr., Genant, H. K., Davis, P. L., Chafetz, N. I., Helms, C. A., Morris, J. M., Rodrigo, J. J., Jergesen, H. E., Brasch, R. C., and Bovill, E. G., Jr. (1983): Nuclear magnetic resonance imaging in orthopaedics: Principles and applications. *J. Orthop. Res.,* 1:101–114.

72. Moore, K. L. (1985): *Clinically Oriented Anatomy,* p. 533. Williams & Wilkins, Baltimore.

73. Mow, V. C., Gibbs, M. C., Lai, W. M., Zhu, W. B., and Athanasiou, K. A. (1989): Biphasic indentation of articular cartilage—II. A numerical algorithm and an experimental study. *J. Biomech.,* 22:853–861.

74. O'Bara, R. M., Shephard, M. S., and Ateshian, G. A. (1995): Geometric model construction and mesh generation for soft tissues in joints. 1995 Bioengineering Conference. *ASME,* BED-29:215–216.

75. Peterfy, C. G., van Dijke, C. F., Janzen, D. L., Gluer, C. C., Namba, R., Majumdar, S., Lang, P., and Genant, H. K. (1994): Quantification of articular cartilage in the knee with pulsed saturation transfer subtraction and fat-suppressed MR imaging: optimization and validation. *Radiology,* 192:485–491.

76. Peterfy, C. G., Majumdar, S., Lang, P., van Dijke, C. F., Sack, K., and Genant, H. K. (1994): MR imaging of the arthritic knee: improved discrimination of cartilage, synovium, and effusion with pulsed saturation transfer and fat-suppressed T_1-weighted sequences. *Radiology,* 191:413–419.

77. Rose, P. M., Demlow, T. A., Szumowski, J., and Quinn, S. F. (1994): Chondromalacia patellae: fat-suppressed MR imaging. *Radiology,* 193:437–440.

78. Rushfeldt, P. D., Mann, R. W., and Harris, W. H. (1981): Improved techniques for measuring *in vitro* the geometry and pressure distribution in the human acetabulum—I. Ultrasonic measurement of acetabular surfaces, sphericity and cartilage thickness. *J. Biomech.,* 14:253–260.

79. Scherrer, P. K., and Hillberry, B. M. (1979): Piecewise mathematical representation of articular surfaces. *J. Biomech.,* 12:301–311.

80. Scherrer, P. K., Hillberry, B. M., and Sickle, D. V. (1979): Determining the *in-vivo* areas of contact in the canine shoulder. *ASME J. Biomech. Eng.,* 101:271–278.

81. Schuind, F., Cooney, W. P., Linscheid, R. L., An, K. N., and Chao, E. Y. (1995): Force and pressure transmission through the normal wrist. A theoretical two-dimensional study in the posteroanterior plane. *J. Biomech.,* 28:587–601.

82. Seedhom, B. B., Longton, E. B., Wright, V., and Dowson, D. (1972): Dimensions of the knee. *Ann. Rheum. Dis.,* 31:54–58.

83. Seedhom, B. B., and Tsubuku, M. (1977): A technique for the study of contact between viscoelastic bodies with special reference to the patello-femoral joint. *J. Biomech.,* 10:253–260.

84. Selby, K., Peterfy, C. G., Cohen, Z. A., Ateshian, G. A., Mow, V. C., Roos, M., Wong, S., Newitt, D. C., van Dijke, C. F., Wendland, M., and Genant, H. K. (1995): *In vivo* MR quantification of articular cartilage water content: a potential early indicator of osteoarthritis. In: *Book of Abstracts: Society of Magnetic Resonance,* Society of Magnetic Resonance, Berkeley, CA, p. 204.

85. Selvik, G. (1974): *A Roentgen stereophotogrammetric method for the study of the kinematics of the skeletal system.* Ph. D. Thesis, University of Lund, Sweden. Reprinted 1989 in *Acta Orthop. Scand.* 60*[Suppl.]:* 232.

86. Shiba, R., Sorbie, C., Siu, D. W., Bryant, J. T., Cooke, D. V., and Wevers, H. W. (1988): Geometry of the humero-ulnar joint. *J. Orthop. Res.,* 6:897–906.

87. Singerman, R. J., Pedersen, D. R., and Brown, T. D. (1987): Quantitation of pressure-sensitive film using digital image scanning. *Exp. Mech.,* March:99–105.

88. Soslowsky, L. J., Flatow, E. L., Bigliani, L. U., and Mow, V. C. (1992): Articular geometry of the glenohumeral joint. *Clin. Orthop.,* 288:181–190.

89. Soslowsky, L. J., Flatow, E. L., Bigliani, L. U., Pawluk, R. J., and Mow, V. C. (1992): Quantitation of *in situ* contact areas at the glenohumeral joint: A biomechanical study. *J. Orthop. Res.,* 10:524–534.

90. Spilker, R. L., Almeida, E. S., Clutz, C., Shephard, M. S., Ateshian, G. A., and Donzelli, P. S. (1993): Three dimensional automated biphasic finite element analysis of soft tissues from stereophotogrammetric data. *ASME Adv. Bioeng.,* BED-26:15–18.

91. Stokes, I., and Greenapple, D. M. (1985): Measurement of surface deformation of soft tissue. *J. Biomech.,* 18:1–7.

92. van Kampen, A., and Huiskes, R. (1990): The three-dimensional tracking pattern of the human patella. *J. Orthop. Res.,* 8:372–382.

93. Wismans, J., Veldpaus, F., and Janssen, J. (1980): A three-dimensional mathematical model of the knee-joint. *J. Biomech.,* 13:677–686.

94. Wood, J. E., Meek, S. G., and Jacobsen, S. C. (1989): Quantitation of human shoulder anatomy for prosthetic arm control—I. Surface modelling. *J. Biomech.,* 22:273–292.

95. Xia, Y., Farquhar, T., Burton-Wurster, N., Ray, E., and Jelinski, L. W. (1994): Diffusion and relaxation mapping of cartilage–bone plugs and excised disks using microscopic magnetic resonance imaging. *Magn. Reson. Med.,* 31:273–282.

Basic Orthopaedic Biomechanics, 2nd ed.,
edited by Van C. Mow and Wilson C. Hayes.
Lippincott–Raven Publishers, Philadelphia © 1997.

8

Lubrication and Wear of Diarthrodial Joints

Van C. Mow and Gerard A. Ateshian

Departments of Mechanical Engineering and Orthopaedic Surgery,
Center for Biomedical Engineering, Columbia University,
New York, New York 10032; and
Departments of Mechanical Engineering and Orthopaedic Surgery,
Columbia University, New York, New York 10032

The three types of joints that exist in the human body are fibrous, cartilaginous, and synovial. Synarthroses, or fibrous joints, are those in which the bony surfaces have very little movement relative to each other. Amphiarthroses, or cartilaginous joints, are those in which the bony surfaces may have some relative movement. Examples of fibrous joints are the junctions of bones in the skull, and examples of cartilaginous joints are those between the two pubic bones of the pelvis, or joints between two vertebral bodies of the spine. Only synovial, or diarthrodial joints, are discussed in this chapter. These joints are different from fibrous or cartilaginous joints in that they allow for a large degree of relative motion between the opposing bones. Some examples of this type of joint are the shoulder, elbow, hip, knee, and ankle.

Diarthrodial joints have some common features. First, they are all enclosed by a strong fibrous capsule (Fig. 1A). Second, the inner surfaces of the joint capsules are lined with a metabolically active tissue, the synovium, which secretes the synovial fluid and the nutrients required by the tissues within the joint. The synovium also absorbs the normal metabolic waste products of cellular activities from these intra-articular tissues. For the human knee shown in Fig. 1, the intra-articular tissues include anterior and posterior cruciate ligaments (not shown), the meniscus, and articular cartilage. The third common feature of diarthrodial joints is that the bone ends are lined with a thin layer of articular cartilage (see Chapter 4 for detailed discussions of articular cartilage). These two linings, i.e., the synovium and the articular cartilage, form the joint cavity that contains the synovial fluid (see refs. 19,101,166 for a detailed description of synovial fluid). The synovial fluid, articular cartilage, and supporting bone form the

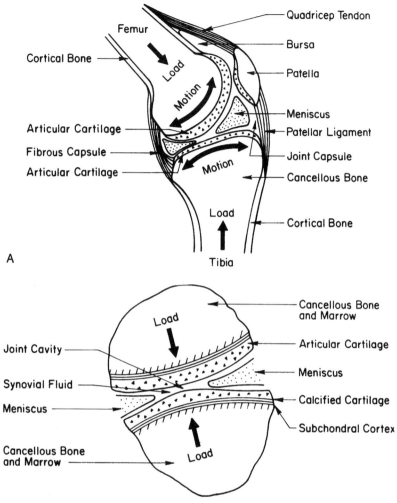

FIG. 1. (A) Schematic representation of the human knee joint showing important anatomic features for mechanical function (142). **(B)** Enlargement of the load-bearing region in the knee, depicting a thin layer of synovial fluid (<50 μm) and two layers of articular cartilage (each <7 mm) (9,142). Each layer of articular cartilage contains approximately 80% fluid.

smooth, nearly frictionless, and wear-resistant bearing system of the body.

Other tissues, such as ligaments and tendons, are also important in providing stability for the joint, maintaining the proper relative positions of the bone ends during motion, and transmitting muscle forces (see Chapters 1 and 2 for a discussion of forces and moments on joints, Chapter 3 for bone, and Chapter 6 for tendons and ligaments).

Although diarthrodial joints are subjected to an enormous range of loading conditions,

the cartilage surfaces undergo little wear and tear under normal circumstances. For example, under high-speed motion, such as during the swing phase of walking or running, the human hip joint sustains loads of slightly more than body weight. However, heel-strike and toe-off may generate forces three to five times body weight across the hip and knee joints (5,43,71,156). In the hip, these forces may yield compressive stresses as high as 18 MPa *in vivo* (84). During prolonged standing, or when a joint is held in a fixed loaded position, moderate fixed loads are also generated (see Chapters 1 and 2).

Human diarthrodial joints must be capable of functioning effectively under these very high loads and stresses (e.g., 1,2,25,43,71, 84) and at generally very low operating speeds (e.g., 5,118,134,156; also see Chapter 2) for seven or eight decades. This demands efficient lubrication processes to minimize friction and to prevent wear of cartilage in the joint. Breakdown of cartilage by either biochemical or biomechanical means may lead to arthritis (see Chapters 4 and 5 for more details).

Tribology is defined as the science that deals with the friction, lubrication, and wear of interacting surfaces in relative motion. Tribology is an interdisciplinary science involving physics and chemistry of the bearing surfaces and fluid and solid mechanics. Biotribology is the branch of tribology that focuses on the understanding of friction, lubrication, and wear phenomena found in diarthrodial joints. Over the past 50 years, many investigators have studied the friction, lubrication, and wear processes in synovial joints (e.g., 13,21,39,45, 48,52,59,79,82,83,101,111–118,129,138,142, 147,149,181,190,196–199,201). Precise and meticulous measurements have been made on the frictional properties of joints (e.g., 34,49, 91,107,110,122,128,193,199,200) and wear properties of cartilage (113,114). Novel lubrication theories have been proposed to describe these extraordinarily efficient frictional and wear properties (14,17,35,44,45, 48,52,59,88,108,111,138,197). Currently, our understanding of the many components of the synovial joint, i.e., articular cartilage, the biochemical and biorheologic properties of synovial fluid, the anatomy of the articulating surfaces of the joint (see Chapter 7 for more details), and the kinematics and load-bearing characteristics of these joints, provides us with the information necessary to understand joint lubrication (see Chapter 2 for more details). This chapter presents our current state of understanding of the friction, lubrication, and wear properties of diarthrodial joints.

MATERIALS OF NATURAL JOINTS

Articular Cartilage

Details of articular cartilage are presented in Chapter 4. For the present purpose, it is sufficient to know that this tissue covers the ends of the articulating bones in the synovial joint. Its thickness varies among species, among joints, and with location within a specific joint (9,10, 29,55,56,152,180,183). Typically, it ranges in thickness from 0.1 to 0.5 mm in rabbit knee joints to 1.0 to 6.0 mm in the human patella or knee trochlea (9,55–57,180). The variation in thickness of this cartilage layer over the joint surface has been quantified using stereophotogrammetry (see Chapter 7). The main functions of this compliant biphasic viscoelastic layer of articular cartilage are to spread the applied load over a large area of the joint (1,2,12, 25,26,28,57,100,172–174) and to minimize the friction and wear of bearing surfaces that result from the continual sliding and rolling movements of the opposing joint surfaces. These functional properties result from the properties of articular cartilage and synovial fluid.

The most important functional aspects of articular cartilage come from its multiphasic nature. The tissue is composed of a porous-permeable solid matrix and an interstitial fluid. The solid phase accounts for 15% to 32% of the wet weight of the tissue, depending on pathology (3,4,6,109,113,120,125,140, 147,148,151,178), and decreases during disease to approximately 10% before total tissue disintegration occurs. The second phase, i.e., water and dissolved ions, comprises approximately 68% to 85% of normal cartilage by wet weight.

The mechanical behavior of articular cartilage has been described by multiphasic theories that take these overall compositional characteristics into consideration. A biphasic model has been developed to describe the deformational behavior of cartilage in terms of two immiscible phases: an elastic, porous-permeable solid matrix phase and an incompressible liquid phase (136,138–141; see Chapter 4 for more details). Interaction between the two phases is modeled by a frictional diffusive drag resulting from the relative velocity between the solid phase and the fluid phase and from the manifested compressive viscoelastic behaviors (e.g., 6,58,85,100,138–150,178,203). A triphasic model has also been developed that describes the interactions between the two immiscible solid–fluid phases as well as with a third miscible ion phase (cations, e.g., Na^+ or Ca^{+2}, and anions, e.g., Cl^-) (67,104; see Chapter 4 for more details). The ions modulate and dictate the swelling behavior of articular cartilage through changes in the Donnan osmotic pressure and charge-to-charge repulsion (104, 125,148). For more details on articular cartilage deformational and swelling behaviors, see Chapter 4.

The solid phase is a porous-permeable, fiber-reinforced composite (Fig. 2). In general, because of the complex organizational arrangement of the collagen network, the inhomogeneous solid phase exhibits anisotropic and nonlinear behaviors in tension, compression, and shear. In confined compression, however, the tissue appears to be isotropic (28,31,92,96,139,147). Although permeability appears to be direction independent, there does exist a variation with depth (125,128). These varying deformational characteristics make cartilage a highly nonlinear

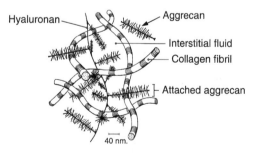

FIG. 2. Schematic representation of the molecular organization of the solid matrix of cartilage. The molecular structural components, collagen, aggrecans, and proteoglycan aggregates, interact to form a porous-permeable fiber-reinforced composite solid matrix. The interstices of this porous solid matrix are filled with water and dissolved ions (139,143).

material and difficult to describe using a theoretical model (147). In compression, articular cartilage obeys the linear isotropic biphasic theory well (18,121,138–140,146). This theory has been used extensively to describe the compressive creep and stress-relaxation behaviors of the tissue and to determine its three material coefficients: permeability, aggregate modulus, and Poisson's ratio. From the predictions of this theory and supportive experimental data, it is known that the compressive viscoelastic creep and stress-relaxation behaviors of normal articular cartilage are primarily governed by interstitial fluid flow and exudation. When a compressive load is applied to the surface of cartilage via a free-draining, porous platen, viscoelastic creep will occur; however, for cartilage, this is caused by the viscous drag associated with interstitial fluid flow (Fig. 3). This fluid transport, as well as pressurization, are essential for normal synovial joint function (see Chapter 4 for more details).

Synovial Fluid

Synovial fluid is a clear, or sometimes slightly yellowish, highly viscous liquid secreted into the joint cavity by the synovium. Small amounts of this fluid are contained in all human and animal synovial joints (20,22,33, 39–41,59,90,97,166). For example, approximately 1 to 5 ml of fluid is contained in a healthy human knee joint. Synovial fluid is a dialysate of blood plasma without clotting factors, erythrocytes, or hemoglobin (40,166) but containing hyaluronate, an extended glycosaminoglycan chain (19,20,74,154,166,168, 185,188), as well as a lubricating glycoprotein (186–190) and wear-retarding phospholipids (79–81,201). Hyaluronan is an unbranched macromolecule whose basic dimer is a disaccharide composed of glucuronic acid linked with N-acetylglucosamine (Fig. 4). A typical hyaluronate chain has a molecular mass from 0.5 to 2 million daltons.

Synovial fluid, like all polymeric fluids, exhibits non-Newtonian flow properties, which

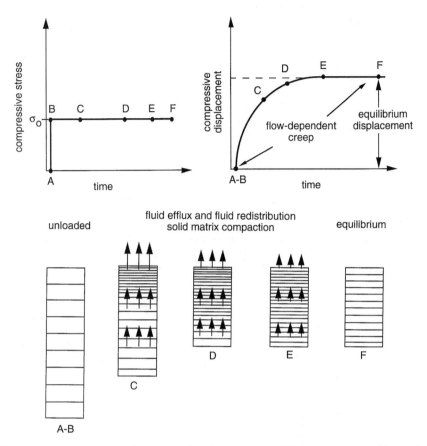

FIG. 3. A constant stress σ_0 (load/area) applied to a sample of the porous-permeable articular cartilage **(top left)**; creep response of the sample under the constant applied stress **(top right)**. The boxes below the loading and creep curves illustrate that creep is accompanied by fluid exudation from the tissue. At equilibrium ($t \to \infty$), fluid flow ceases, and the load is borne entirely by the solid matrix (F).

include an elastic effect, a shear thinning effect, and a normal stress effect (20,22,33,40, 46,60,69,101,153,171,176). These flow properties are similar to those found for other biomacromolecular solutions such as proteoglycans (e.g., 77,145,182,205,206). For example, in bovine knee joints, the apparent viscosity of synovial fluid has been shown to decrease nonlinearly from 10 to 0.02 N-sec/m² as the shear rate increased from 0.1 to 1000 sec⁻¹ (97). Synovial fluids obtained from degenerative joints show reduced apparent viscosity properties compared to those exhibited by normal synovial fluid (19,20,41,60,101,171). Figure 5 demonstrates the variations in appar-

ent viscosity and normal stress with varying shear rates for both normal and pathologic synovial fluids (171). All rheologic coefficients are affected by disease and have been calculated (101,171). These fluid properties play an important role in understanding the lubrication mechanisms in diarthrodial joints (46,51,101,134,136,138,142,153). Synovial fluid not only aids in lubrication but also provides the necessary nutrients for cartilage (105,106,165,166,179). Furthermore, synovial fluid acts as a medium for osmosis between the joint and the blood supply and as protection for cartilage against enzyme activity (39,74,105,106,154).

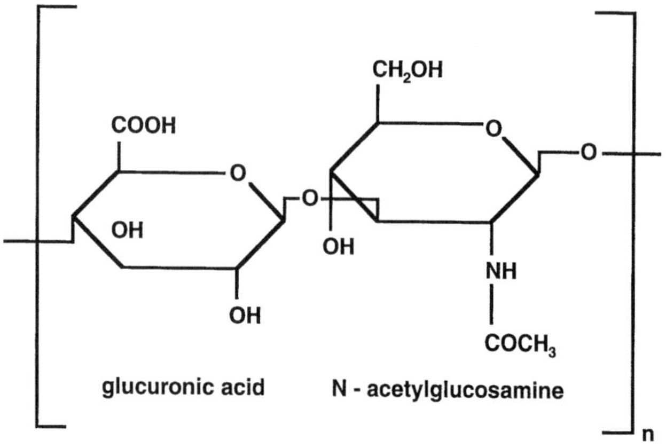

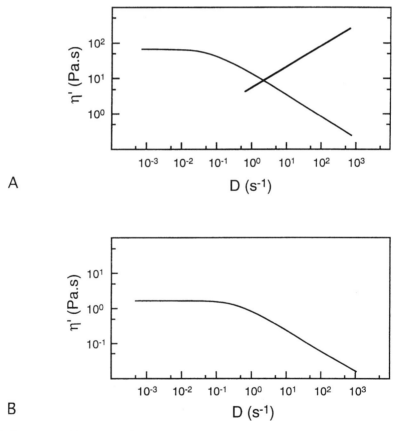

FIG. 4. The repeating disaccharide unit of hyaluronan in synovial fluid. This is a nonsulfated dimer of glucuronic acid with N-acetylglucosamine. Hyaluronan is polymerized into long chains consisting of approximately 2500 of these repeating units with molecular weight ranging from 500,000 to 2,000,000 daltons.

FIG. 5. (A) Shear-rate-dependent viscosity η' and normal stress σ_1 versus shear rate for normal synovial fluid. (Adapted from Schurz and Ribitsch, ref. 171, with permission.) **(B)** Shear-rate-dependent viscosity η' versus shear rate for pathologic synovial fluid. (Adapted from Schurz and Ribitsch, ref. 171, with permission.)

Bone

Bone is a supporting structural element of the body that is more rigid than cartilage and other soft tissues. It consists of an abundant matrix of type I collagen fibers impregnated with minerals, primarily calcium and phosphate compounds. Joints are junctures between the bony segments that permit motion. Detailed descriptions of cortical and cancellous bone are provided in Chapter 3.

Under the uncalcified cartilage layer, there is a very thin layer of calcified cartilage (Fig. 1B). The wavy line in the figure demarcating the uncalcified cartilage from calcified cartilage is the "tidemark" (27,30,162), which provides a gradual transition between the two dissimilar regions of cartilage and appears to have significant biomechanical functions (131,162). It is remodeled during life in response to micro-injuries (30,68,70,160) and advances into the uncalcified cartilage. This remodeling process causes significant thinning of cartilage and alters the state of stress in the tissue (30). The subchondral cortex lies immediately below the thin layer of calcified cartilage. It is a layer of dense, stiff, cortical bone. In the mature animal, it forms a closed cap supporting the cartilage on one side and supported by the cancellous bone on the other. The apparent elastic modulus of the subchondral cortex ranges from 1.0 to 15 GPa (27). For cortical bone, the modulus is approximately 15 GPa. The cancellous bone is softer, less dense, and makes up the bulk of the bone end in the joint capsule. Cancellous bone is highly porous and contains the well-vascularized marrow within its intricate trabecular structure. Its stiffness ranges from 0.1 to 0.5 GPa (27,32,70). One possible mechanism for the initiation of cartilage damage may be the steep stiffness gradient in the subchondral bone caused by healing of trabecular bone fractures (68,94,159,160). According to this hypothesis, large shear stresses are developed at the cartilage–calcified cartilage–subchondral bone junctures, causing deep horizontal splits in the tissue, thus damaging the layer of cartilage. Histo-logic sections of articular cartilage and bone often reveal the existence of blisters in the deep layers of cartilage, presumably caused by the mechanism described above (7,11,30, 150,159,192,195). For a more detailed description of bone, see Chapter 3.

ANATOMIC FORMS OF DIARTHRODIAL JOINTS

A major consideration in determining the frictional characteristics between two surfaces sliding over each other is the topography of the given surfaces. Changes in topographic form affect the way in which loads are transmitted across joints, altering the mode of lubrication in that joint and thus the physiological state of cartilage (28,29).

Macroscopically, approximations are made to ease the mathematical analyses caused by these anatomic effects for studies in lubrication. In two dimensions, articulating surfaces are commonly approximated by a cylindrical surface interacting with a plane. In three dimensions, the simplest approximation used is a sphere in association with a half space (Fig. 6). With the three-dimensional approximation, it has been shown that the radius of an equivalent sphere near a plane can be as high as 1.0 m for hip joints or as low as 0.02 to 0.1 m for the knee joint (48,72,78,134,167). This radius of curvature is important in assessing the feasibility of fluid-film lubrication mechanisms in a given joint.

Microscopically, articular surfaces are relatively rough, as demonstrated from Talysurf tracings and microscopic examinations (37,63, 64,98,99,135,169). These surfaces are much rougher than typical engineering bearings or joint replacement prostheses (50). A quantity called the arithmetic mean deviation, R_a, is used to define surface roughness. It is defined as the average value of the difference of the microscopic surface profile above and below a given reference line (mean line) (Fig. 7). For example, R_a values for articular cartilage range from 1 to 6 μm, while the metal femoral head of a typical artificial hip has a value of approx-

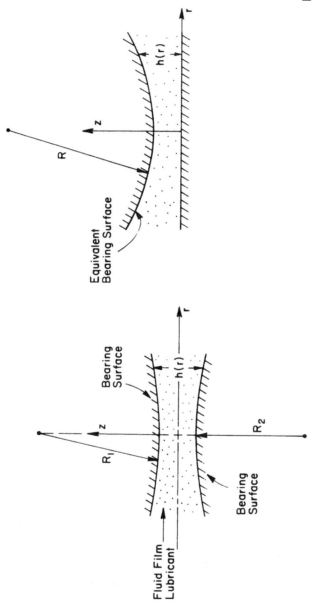

FIG. 6. (A) Two bearing surfaces separated by a thin layer of fluid (usually <20 μm) lubricant in the load-bearing region. The thin film geometry is $h(r)$, and R_1 and R_2 are the radii of curvature of the two bearings. **(B)** Equivalent bearing surface with curved surface of equivalent radius of curvature R and flat surface.

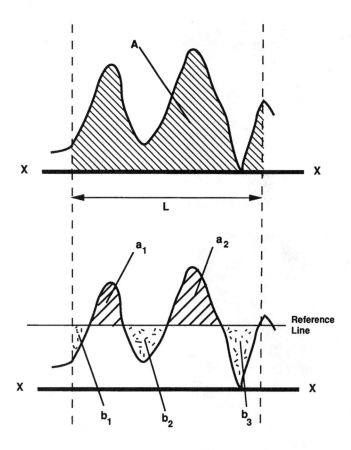

$$R_a = \frac{\text{Sum of areas (a) + Sum of areas (b)}}{L}$$

FIG. 7. Illustration of the concept of the arithmetical mean deviation R_a of a rough surface. (Adapted from Dowson, ref. 50, with permission.)

imately 0.025 μm; i.e., the metal femoral head is much smoother (Table 1). A common terminology is used to describe the levels of topographic roughness of joint surfaces (63,117):

1. Primary anatomic contours.
2. Secondary roughness less than 0.5 mm in diameter and less than 50 μm deep.
3. Tertiary hollows on the order of 20 to 45 μm deep.
4. Quaternary ridges 1 to 4 μm in diameter and 0.1 to 0.3 μm deep.

Topographic features are important in determining the causes of friction associated

TABLE 1. *Typical values of R_a for various surfaces*

Components	R_a (μm)
Plain bearings	
Bearing (bush or pad)	0.25–1.2
Journal or runner	0.12–0.5
Rolling bearings	
Tracks	0.2–0.3
Rolling element	0.05–0.12
Gears	0.25–1.0
Articular cartilage	1.0–6.0
Endoprostheses	
Metal (e.g., femoral head)	0.025
Plastic (e.g., acetabulum)	0.25–2.5

Data from Dowson (50).

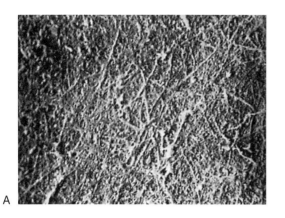

A

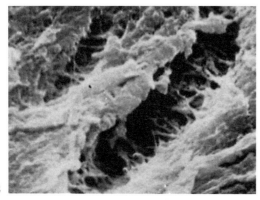

B

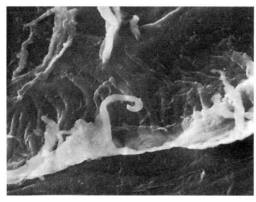

C

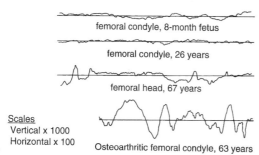

femoral condyle, 8-month fetus

femoral condyle, 26 years

femoral head, 67 years

Scales
Vertical x 1000
Horizontal x 100

D

Osteoarthritic femoral condyle, 63 years

FIG. 8. (A) Scanning electron microscopic view of the texture of normal human articular cartilage surface, showing a dense-pack random arrangement of collagen fibrils at the surface; specimen is a 21-year-old male femoral head retrieved from autopsy and magnified ×3000 (142). **(B)** Typical appearance of articular cartilage surface from an osteoarthritic human specimen showing deep fissures forming, ×3000 (142). **(C)** Scanning electron micrograph of an aging femoral head surface retrieved from the fracture neck of a femur; no OA was detected in this hip joint, ×1000 (142). **(D)** Talysurf tracing of surface roughness for normal young and aging and osteoarthritic cartilage samples (196).

with the articulation, not only when actual contact between two surfaces occurs but also under fluid-film lubrication conditions, where the surface roughness dictates the minimum fluid-film thickness necessary to keep the two moving surfaces completely separated. Scanning electron micrographs of arthritic cartilage depict a large degree of surface irregularity (Fig. 8A–C). Figure 8D shows three Talysurf tracings of surface roughness for fetal, young normal, and aging human femoral and condylar articular surfaces (196). Normal articular surface texture is shown in Fig. 8A, which depicts a tightly woven texture with fine pores. Degenerative tissues often exhibit tears (Fig. 8B) and peelings (Fig. 8C) on their surface. These surface irregularities have profound effects on the lubrication mechanism involved and thus on the friction and the rate of degradation of the articular cartilage.

On the macroscopic level, the types of surface interactions occurring between different joints in the body vary greatly. For example, the hip joint is a deep congruent ball-and-socket joint (84,167); this differs from the glenohumeral joint of the shoulder, which is often described as a shallow ball-and-socket or a minimally constrained articulation (183). Furthermore, these joint shapes differ greatly from that of the distal femur in the knee joint, which is bicondylar in nature, or from the saddle shape of the thumb carpometacarpal or the ankle joints. Furthermore, these anatomic forms can vary with age and disease (29,161,167). The degree of matching between the various bones and articulating cartilage surfaces comprising a joint is a major factor affecting the distribution of stresses in the cartilage and subchondral bone (1,2,10–13,25–29,95). Thus, the precise quantitation of joint anatomy is extremely important. A description of quantitative methods for characterizing the three-dimensional anatomy of articular surfaces is provided in Chapter 7. These methodologies include the calculation of surface radii of curvature and joint congruence, which are useful for tribologic analyses.

MOTION AND FORCES ON DIARTHRODIAL JOINTS

In vivo experimental measurements of the relative motions between articulating surfaces of a joint corresponding to daily activities are limited. Most quantitative information is obtained from gait studies (see Chapter 2 for more detail), which do not provide the detailed information required for lubrication studies (5,38,54,61,156,175,198). Simple calculations show that peak translational speeds between two articulating surfaces can range from approximately 0.06 m/sec between the femoral head surface and the acetabulum surface during normal walking to approximately 0.6 m/sec between the humeral head surface and the glenoid cavity of the shoulder for a baseball pitcher during the throwing motion (134). Assuming, roughly, that synovial fluid film thicknesses are on the order of, or greater than, the surface roughness, e.g., 6 μm, it is estimated that the shear rate found within joints may reach or exceed 10^5 sec^{-1} (45,48, 134,171).

The loads transmitted across a joint may be carried by the opposing joint surfaces via solid-to-solid contact, through a fluid-film layer, or by a mixture of both. As in joint motion, the load on the joint is dependent on the type of activity; i.e., the loading sites change continuously as the articulating surfaces move relative to each other (12,16,25,54,66,127,167, 170,172–174,184). During a normal walking cycle, the human hip, knee, and ankle joints can be subject to loads ranging up to ten times body weight, thus causing very high stresses (1,2,38,84,119,123,132,133). In the lower extremity, the peak loads at the knee and ankle are attained at heel-strike and toe-off and, at the hip, when rising from a seat. The average load on the joint is approximately three times body weight, which lasts maybe as long as 60% of the walking cycle. During the swing phase of walking, only light loads (one to three times body weight) are carried. During this phase, the articular surfaces move rapidly over each other. In addition, extremely high forces occur across the joints in the leg during jumping. Fig-

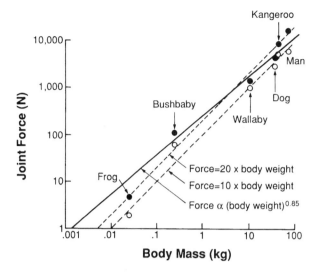

FIG. 9. Maximum joint forces during jumping in the knee *(solid symbols)* and ankle *(open symbols)* of various animals versus body weight. (Adapted from Dowson, ref. 50, with permission.)

ure 9 illustrates the levels of force that can exist in the knees and ankles of different species. For these reasons, the magnitude and duration of the joint loading, as well as the relative motion between the two articulating surfaces, must be considered when lubrication mechanisms are discussed.

FRICTION

Basic Concepts

Friction is defined as the resistance to motion between two bodies in contact. The first type of friction, called surface friction, comes either from adhesion of one surface to another because of roughness of the two surfaces or from the viscosity of the sheared lubricant film between the two surfaces (Fig. 10). In the case of "dry friction," i.e., surface friction without a lubricant, three laws have been postulated by Amonton (1699) and Coulomb (1785):

1. Frictional force *(F)* is directly proportional to the applied load *(W)*.
2. *F* is independent of the apparent area of contact.
3. The kinetic *F* is independent of the sliding speed *(V)*.

These laws help to define a coefficient of friction μ by the simple, well-known equation

$F = \mu W$. The second type of friction, called bulk friction, occurs from the internal energy dissipation mechanisms within the bulk material or within the lubricant. For cartilage, an internal friction is produced by the viscous drag caused when interstitial fluid flows through the porous-permeable solid matrix (100,110,111,139,142,148). Plowing friction is a specific form of internal friction and occurs in diarthrodial joints when a load moves across a joint surface, causing interstitial fluid flow (110,111). Interstitial fluid flow patterns throughout the tissue have been calculated (11,13,137,138). The dissipation related to interstitial fluid flow has been calculated and confirmed experimentally using a material testing protocol for the determination of hysteretic behavior of cartilage in uniaxial compression (141,148).

Measurements of Coefficients of Friction

For friction between articular surfaces, μ has remarkably low values in comparison to other engineering materials (Tables 2 and 3). This friction coefficient μ for articular surfaces of joints has been measured in two ways. First, specially designed "arthrotripsometers" or pendulum devices have been used on intact joints (50,91,110–112,193, 194). The second method involves sliding ex-

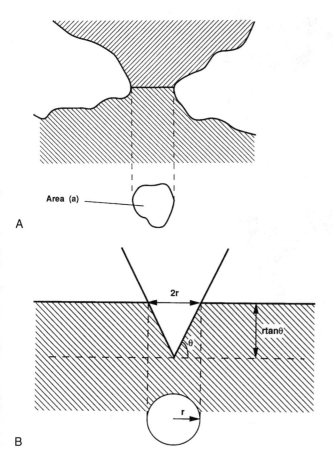

A

B

FIG. 10. (A) Interaction between two asperities of two rough surfaces with similar hardness. For metals, adhesion by welding occurs at these junction sites. Adhesive friction is caused by the energy required to fracture these microwelds. (Adapted from Dowson, ref. 50, with permission.) **(B)** Penetration of a hard conical microasperity on one surface into a softer material of the other surface. A form of plowing friction occurs when the hard asperity is forced to cut through the softer surface. (Adapted from Dowson, ref. 50, with permission.)

cised pieces of cartilage over another surface (122,128,129,186–190,196,197,199,200).

The pendulum-type experimental configuration uses a diarthrodial joint, e.g., the hip, as the fulcrum of a simple pendulum in which one of the joint surfaces rocks freely over the other (Fig. 11A). Such studies have produced coefficients of friction from 0.003 to 0.06 for the combination of both plowing friction and surface friction (e.g., Fig. 11B). Unsworth and co-workers (193,194) demonstrated that when a load is applied to the hip joint suddenly, and synovial fluid is present in the joint cavity, the opposing surfaces approach each other under squeeze-film lubri-

TABLE 2. *Coefficients of friction for typical materials*

Material combination	Coefficient of friction
Gold on gold	2.8
Aluminum on aluminum	1.9
Silver on silver	1.5
Steel on steel	0.6–0.8
Brass on steel	0.35
Glass on glass	0.9
Wood on wood	0.25–0.5
Nylon on nylon	0.2
Graphite on steel	0.1
Ice on ice at 0°C	0.1
UHMWPE on cobalt chrome (artificial joints)	0.01–0.05

Adapted from Dowson (50), with permission.

TABLE 3. *Coefficients of friction for articular cartilage in synovial joints*

Investigator	Coefficient of friction	Joint tested
Charnley (36)	0.005–0.02	Human ankle
McCutchen (128)	0.02–0.35	Porcine shoulder
Linn (110,111)	0.005–0.01	Canine ankle
Unsworth et al. (190)	0.01–0.04	Human hip
Malcom (122)	0.002–0.03	Bovine shoulder

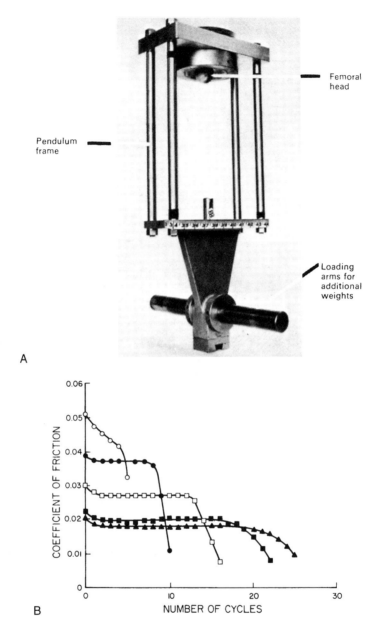

A

B   NUMBER OF CYCLES

FIG. 11. (A) A compound pendulum device with the human hip joint as its fulcrum; this device is used to measure the coefficient of friction between femoral head *(shown)* and the acetabulum *(not shown)* by the decay of the amplitude of the pendulum motion (193). **(B)** A typical set of curves for the coefficient of friction versus the number of cycles from a hip specimen under suddenly loaded, unlubricated conditions (i.e., no synovial fluid). Results show a longer period of swing and a lower coefficient of friction with increasing load (*open circle,* 133.5 N; *solid circle,* 213 N; *open square,* 375 N; *solid square,* 577 N; *solid triangle,* 1020 N) (193). **(C)** Differences of the coefficient of friction between unlubricated and lubricated (with synovial fluid) hip joints at varying applied loads. At a load >90 N, no differences in coefficients of friction were observed (193).

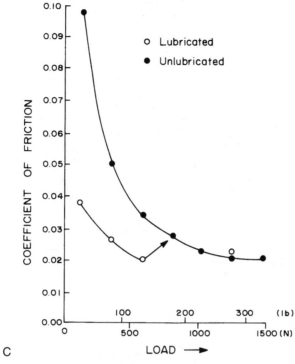

C

FIG. 11. *Continued.*

cation conditions. The evidence presented in support of this mechanism was that frictional resistance increased and then decreased with increasing cycles of oscillation because of the decrease of fluid film thickness with time. They also attempted to prevent squeeze-film action by preloading the joint before the first oscillation, and they observed that the friction coefficient monotonically decreased with increasing oscillations under this configuration; they observed a similar response after wiping away the synovial fluid and applying a sudden load, thus confirming that squeeze-film lubrication occurs only in the presence of an external supply of lubricant (Fig. 11B). The maximum friction coefficients recorded for their tests with and without synovial fluid as a function of joint load are shown in Fig. 11C. These results indicate that the friction coefficient of cartilage decreases with increasing load. Above a threshold of load, synovial fluid causes no difference in the frictional proper-

ties of joints. These authors therefore hypothesized that in the absence of squeeze-film action, lubrication must have been generated from the interstitial fluid in articular cartilage or from boundary lubrication (Fig. 11C).

The second type of experimental configuration involves the sliding of a small piece of cartilage over another surface (e.g., glass, rubber, another piece of cartilage) (122,128, 129,186–190,196,197,199,200). This technique has the advantage that the effects of surface friction can be measured directly, as compared with measuring the combination of surface and plowing friction as was done using the first configuration. When a flat specimen is loaded, no plowing can occur (hypothetically). Malcom (122) tested excised annular plugs from a bovine humeral head against the adjacent glenoid surface under a continuously rotating articulation (Fig. 12A). The coefficient of friction μ from his experiments ranged from 0.002 to 0.03. Fur-

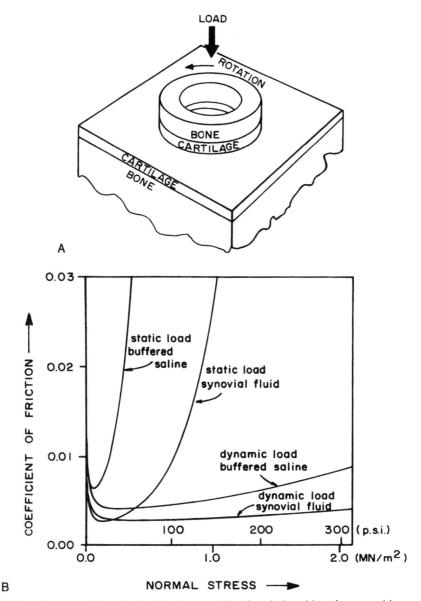

FIG. 12. **(A)** Specimens cut from the bovine humeral head and glenoid surface provide conforming surfaces for studies on interfacial friction. This configuration is effective in preventing plowing friction (122). **(B)** Variation of the coefficient of friction corresponding to the test configuration depicted in Fig. 14A under various lubrication and loading conditions: with and without synovial fluid; static and dynamic (122).

thermore, the interfacial μ had the following characteristics:

1. μ increased with time after application of the load.

2. μ increased with magnitude of the load.

3. μ was lower when synovial fluid was used as the lubricant than with buffer saline.

4. μ was very sensitive to small vertical oscillations of the annular plug of cartilage and actually decreased in magnitude under such motions (Fig. 12B).

This last observation is likely related to pressurization of interstitial fluid caused by the applied dynamic compressive load (122). This topic is addressed further below.

Role of Synovial Fluid

Many experiments have been performed in an attempt to assess the role of synovial fluid or its components in joint lubrication (19,22,33,41,45,46,97,101,176,186–190,196, 197). This role has been difficult to quantify because it differs under varying circumstances and with different material properties of cartilage and synovial fluid.

A series of experiments, in which synovial fluid was passed through filters with various pore sizes and/or treated with various enzymes, were performed. The components separated from filtration were subsequently tested for lubrication efficiency. McCutchen passed synovial fluid through filters with pore sizes of 0.22 μm in an attempt to sieve out the lubricating component of synovial fluid (129). He observed that the residue provided better lubrication than the filtrate. Filters with larger pore sizes of 0.65 μm were also used. In this case, the filtrate was the better lubricant. Thus, he concluded that a macromolecule, presumably a hyaluronate, whose size was between 0.22 μm and 0.65 μm, is a key component responsible for boundary lubrication; nevertheless, this boundary lubricant was observed to be weak and failed to lubricate under high loads. Malcom (122) also noted that above a threshold of applied pressure, frictional properties of cartilage became erratic and nonrepeatable.

Little and co-workers measured an average coefficient of friction of 0.008 in articular cartilage (115). They observed that treating the articular surfaces with a fat solvent increased the coefficient of friction to an average of 0.022. They concluded that boundary lubrication prevailed in joints and was aided by a lipid present in the articular cartilage. Maroudas (124) demonstrated the formation of hyaluronan gels by performing *in vitro* filtration experiments on synovial fluid. Walker and co-workers per-

formed electron micrograph studies of cartilage surfaces where they believed they observed aggregates of hyaluronic acid (197). However, Linn showed that purified hyaluronic acid "lacked lubricating ability" (111).

In several studies throughout the 1970s and 1980s, Radin and co-workers (157) and Swann and co-workers (188–190) analyzed a glycoprotein isolated from bovine and human synovial fluid that they found to provide boundary lubricating ability. They called this synovial fluid constituent LGP-I (lubricating glycoprotein) or lubricin. Using LGP-I at a concentration between 65 μg/ml and 100 μg/ml (190), these investigators observed frictional responses identical to those of normal synovial fluid. More recently, Jay and Hong tested the boundary lubrication ability of a synovial fluid retentate that they believed to be identical to lubricin (90). From latex-on-glass experiments under a 0.03-MPa stress, they observed that the friction coefficient decreased from 0.11 with a 0.9% NaCl solution to a modest 0.07 with lubricin at 260 μg/ml in 0.9% NaCl.

Hills and Butler suggested that phospholipids were the major ingredients responsible for the lubricating ability of synovial fluid, in analogy to their previous findings in pleural movement (79). They indicated that the extraction procedure of Swann and co-workers was unlikely to have excluded phospholipids as contaminants in their lubricin. Hills and Butler demonstrated that these phospholipids were readily adsorbed to hydrophilic solids whose surfaces then became hydrophobic (79). In a subsequent study, Hills showed that dipalmitoyl phosphatidylcholine (DPPC) could rapidly adsorb on glass surfaces, making them hydrophobic (80). The DPPC could not be removed from glass by rinsing with saline but required the use of the same fat solvent as the one employed by Little and co-workers (115), and this was cited as evidence that DPPC is the active boundary lubricant in synovial fluid. Hills also argued that DPPC formed oligolamellar deposits on cartilage rather than monolayers. Williams et al. (201) performed friction tests with and without DPPC using borosilicate surfaces in a reciprocating apparatus. These authors observed that the friction co-efficient in the presence of DPPC was veloc-ity-dependent. Under dry friction, static fric-tion coefficients varied from 0.65 to 0.88, and scratches appeared on the sliding surfaces; with DPPC, average static coefficients of fric-tion were in the range of 0.123 to 0.158, and no scratches were apparent. Hills has also con-firmed the wear-resistant properties of DPPC when used in engineering bearings (81).

These recent developments provide strong evidence that some constituents of synovial fluid act as boundary lubricants. The effec-tiveness of this lubricant appears to be load-dependent as well as velocity-dependent. Un-der the best experimental configurations, however, this boundary lubricant appears to improve the friction coefficient only by a fac-tor of two to six, approximately. These obser-vations are consistent with the previously re-ported differences in friction coefficient when using saline instead of synovial fluid (122,128), which may be attributed to the presence of boundary lubricant in the latter. Hence, it is necessary to further explore the mechanisms that may also contribute to re-ducing the friction coefficient of cartilage in order to explain the wide variations of fric-tional properties reported in the literature (Table 3).

Synovial fluid may also play the role of lu-bricant in fluid-film lubrication, though the vi-ability of this mode of lubrication has not been established unequivocally for diarthrodial joints, as is further discussed below. Several studies (111,112,129,157,187) have shown that hyaluronidase-treated synovial fluid lubricated almost as well as untreated fluid, even though hyaluronidase depolymerizes hyaluronic acid and decreases the viscosity of synovial fluid to that of saline. Such a result suggests that fluid-film lubrication, which is highly dependent on lubricant viscosity, cannot be the primary mechanism responsible for the low frictional coefficient of joints. When trypsin was used to treat synovial fluid (trypsin degrades proteins and glycoproteins but not phospholipids), the coefficient of friction rose significantly while the viscosity remained similar to that of normal synovial fluid (157,187). It remains to be seen whether trypsin could indirectly degrade the ability of DPPC to adsorb to the cartilage sur-face as well. Interestingly, O'Kelly and co-workers (155) obtained results that contra-dicted the previous work; they used a static loading pendulum and a dynamic oscillator designed to reproduce physiological loading patterns and observed that the lubrication properties of synovial fluid treated with hyaluronidase differed significantly from un-treated synovial fluid. Furthermore, they found no evidence that lubrication efficiency was affected if synovial fluid was treated with trypsin to remove glycoproteins. These results suggest that additional mechanisms might be at work that have not yet been de-scribed appropriately.

In summary, very low friction appears to exist within diarthrodial joints even in the ab-sence of synovial fluid or hyaluronate, though synovial fluid contributes to further decreasing the friction coefficient. Further-more, dynamically applied loads, oscilla-tions, or sliding tends to lower the coefficient of friction. However, higher loads may de-crease the friction coefficient (Fig. 11C) or increase it (Fig. 12B).

WEAR

Wear of bearings is a phenomenon of boundary degradation involving progressive loss of bearing substance from the body as a result of mechanical action. The two conven-tional types of wear are fatigue wear and in-terfacial wear. Fatigue wear is independent of the lubrication phenomenon occurring at the surfaces of bearings. It occurs because of the cyclic stresses and strains generated within the cartilage by the application of repetitive loads in joint motion. It is estimated that a typical human joint may experience one million cy-cles of loading in a year. These large cyclical stresses and strains may cause fatigue failure within the bulk material and may grow by an accumulation of microscopic damage within the material. These internal failures within diseased tissues have been observed in the form of collagen fiber buckling and loosening of the normally tight collagen network (23,24). Eventually, the internal failures can extend to the material surface, causing cracks and fissures (23,24,37,147,161). In time, if the rate of damage exceeds that by which the cartilage cells may regenerate the tissue, an accumulation of fatigue microdamage will occur that may lead to bulk tissue failure (147,161). Thus, *in vivo* wear is a balance of mechanical attrition and biological synthesis (89).

Interfacial wear results from solid–solid contact at the surface of bearing materials. There are two basic types of interfacial wear. Adhesive wear is the more common and occurs when a junction is formed between the two opposing surfaces as they come into contact (Fig. 10A). If this junction is stronger than the cohesive strength of the individual materials, fragments of the weaker material may be torn off and may adhere to the stronger material (8,50). Abrasive wear occurs when a soft material comes into contact with a significantly harder material (Fig. 10B). Under these circumstances, the asperities of the harder material surface may cut into the softer counterpart, causing abrasive wear. This harder material may be either the opposing bearing surface or loose particles between the bearing surfaces. When loose particles between the surfaces cause abrasive wear, the process is termed three-body wear.

Wear is measured either as the mass of material removed from interacting surfaces per unit of time or as the volume lost. At present, wear analysis is mostly an empirical science. Therefore, it is difficult to predict either wear rates or their dependence on other physical parameters (8). For biological materials, little quantitative information exists on wear mechanisms or wear rates (114). In general, different types of wear mechanisms produce different wear rates. For example, fatigue wear depends on the frequency and magnitude of the applied loads and on the intrinsic material properties of the bulk material. On the other hand, interfacial wear depends on the roughness of the bearing surfaces, the true size of

the contact area of the two surfaces, and the magnitude of the applied load (8,50). Some general rules on wear have been observed:

1. Wear rates increase with increasing applied normal load.
2. Wear rates increase with increasing sliding contact area between the two opposing bearing surfaces.
3. Wear rate of the softer bearing surface is higher than that of the harder bearing surface.

The function of typical engineering bearings is often impaired if even a relatively small amount of the bearing volume is lost. This is because minute changes of bearing surface geometry affect the hydrodynamics of the thin lubricant film, usually no more than 25 μm thick, in the worn bearing. For hydrated tissues such as cartilage, it is very difficult to quantify either mass loss or volume loss because of the phenomenon of swelling (see Chapter 4). In the 1970s, Lipshitz and co-workers, in a tedious set of experiments, measured wear and wear rates for cartilage using hydroxyproline (collagen) and hexosamine as markers (Fig. 13) (113, 114) and found them to be extremely low. In these *in vitro* experiments, excised cartilage plugs were equilibrated in a buffered saline bath and loaded against a polished stainless steel surface. A steady harmonic sliding motion was imposed for long periods of time (114). Wear was measured by the hydroxyproline and hexosamine contents in the bathing solution, and wear rates were determined. In both the 4.62- and 1.66-MPa cases, the initial wear rate was high, gradually decreasing to a steady state of wear. Removal of load to allow the tissue to recover its interstitial fluid content (located by the arrow in Fig. 13) did not alter the wear rate. This figure also shows that even at high pressures, wear rate was extremely small. This may be because of the large number of redundant, "fail-safe" lubrication mechanisms that exist at the articular surface preventing wear. However, it is likely that once the ultrastructure of the articular surface is damaged and/or proteogly-

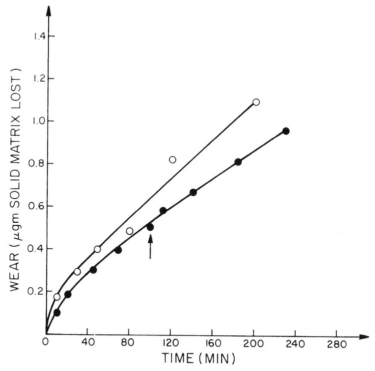

FIG. 13. Variation of wear rate as a function of time (*open circle,* 4.62 MPa; *solid circle,* 1.66 MPa). At the point indicated by the *arrow,* the cartilage plugs were allowed to imbibe fluid overnight. No drop in wear rate was seen, and the wear rate continues without the initial "toe region" (114).

cans are lost, the cartilage becomes softer and more permeable (3,4,6,73,177,178; Fig. 8B,C). Under these conditions, cartilage loses its ability to support load by *hydrostatic* pressure and may not be as efficient in lubrication (138,144). In these cases, fluid-film lubrication is not likely to exist (138), and adhesive and abrasive wear may occur (8,37,161).

Some general conclusions were drawn from the wear studies of cartilage-against-steel plate by Lipshitz and Glimcher (114):

1. Wear rates decrease with time until they reach a constant value; this value is dependent on the applied pressure and the roughness of the opposing stainless steel surface.
2. Wear rates increase with applied normal pressure and with increased relative speed of the opposing surfaces.
3. Wear rates decrease fivefold if the tissue is fixed and stiffened by formaldehyde, which retards abrasive wear.

4. Wear rates decrease tenfold if synovial fluid is used as a lubricant.

Thus, though the role of synovial fluid in fluid-film lubrication may be questionable, its role in reducing the wear rate of articular cartilage against a stainless steel plate is remarkable. This fact may be very important clinically when a femoral head endoprosthesis articulates with the cartilage of the acetabulum. The wear rates determined by Lipshitz and co-workers exhibit large variability and are very sensitive to the laboratory environment, the nature of the test, and the mechanical and chemical nature of the bearing materials. For these reasons, information regarding wear mechanisms is minimal despite the large body of knowledge concerning changes in tissue composition.

Repetitive joint motion and loading could cause cartilage damage and wear (62). Another cause of cartilage damage and wear is high-impact loading (7,47,158,159,163,192,

195). As normal cartilage is compressed, its interstitial fluid pressurizes and contributes to support more than 90% of the applied load (11,13,119,147,148), thus shielding the collagen–proteoglycan matrix from excessive and potentially damaging stresses. However, above a threshold level of stress, the cartilage matrix will fail, creating vertical fissures at the surface as well as horizontal splits at the cartilage–bone interface (7,11,157–160,163,192, 195). For example, a single impact on the patellofemoral joint has been observed to cause cartilage damage at the surface and the tidemark (7) and biological remodeling of cartilage in the region surrounding the tidemark (47). Loss of fluid pressurization near these defects may lead to progressive degeneration of the tissue (150), accelerating the release of wear particles into the joint cavity under *in vivo* conditions. In other experiments, Radin and Paul (158) tested bovine metacarpal–phalangeal joints lubricated with veronate saline in an arthrotripsometer. When a static load of 1000 lb was applied for 5000 hr, no significant wear was evident. However, when a 500-lb static load was combined with a 500-lb periodic impact load, wear was observed in 200 hr. A similar study was repeated and indicated severe cartilage damage because of impact loading (159). Repo and Finlay (163) showed that an impact load larger than a critical value would cause surface fractures on cartilage plugs, and Armstrong and co-workers showed that an impact load greater than 6 kN will cause shear failure at the tidemark of porcine knee joints *in vivo* (7).

HYPOTHESES FOR DIARTHRODIAL JOINT LUBRICATION

Many modes of lubrication have been proposed in attempts to explain the minimal friction and wear characteristics of cartilage found in diarthrodial joints. To be acceptable, each proposed mode of lubrication must be able to account for friction and wear characteristics of these joints under a variety of loading and motion conditions. For fluid-film lubrication, the minimum fluid film thickness predicted by a specific lubrication theory must exceed three times the combined statistical surface roughness of cartilage (e.g., 4 to 25 μm) (76). If the predicted fluid-film gap is too thin to produce fluid-film lubrication under given loading and motion conditions, then boundary lubrication must be present.

Fluid-Film Lubrication

Hydrodynamic Lubrication

In 1932, MacConaill (118) proposed that the two articulating surfaces do not actually come into contact and that the load is transmitted via a thin layer of fluid lubricant, thus explaining the low friction coefficients associated with synovial joints measured later by Jones (91). MacConaill hypothesized that the high viscosity of synovial fluid and the relative motion of the joint surfaces can create the thin wedge-shaped fluid layer required for the hydrodynamic mode of lubrication to operate within the knee. The basic mechanism of hydrodynamic lubrication is shown in Fig. 14A. A high-speed transversely moving surface is required to drag a layer of viscous fluid through a narrowing wedge-shaped gap. This action creates a hydrodynamic pressure in the fluid, generating lift, which forces the two surfaces apart (164). However, this conventional hydrodynamic lubrication theory requires a continuous high-speed relative motion between the two opposing bearing surfaces to provide a substantial load-carrying pressure. Although high-speed motion is occasionally present (e.g., the articulation at the glenohumeral joint of the shoulder of a baseball pitcher), many more activities of daily living involve intermittent and low-speed motions in various joints (34,35). Because of this argument, hydrodynamic lubrication is not likely to be a primary mechanism operating in the joint. Other factors such as deformation of cartilage and interstitial fluid flow may play important roles in determining the modes of joint lubrication.

To quantitatively examine the plausibility of the hydrodynamic mode of lubrication, let us use the mathematical results for the minimum

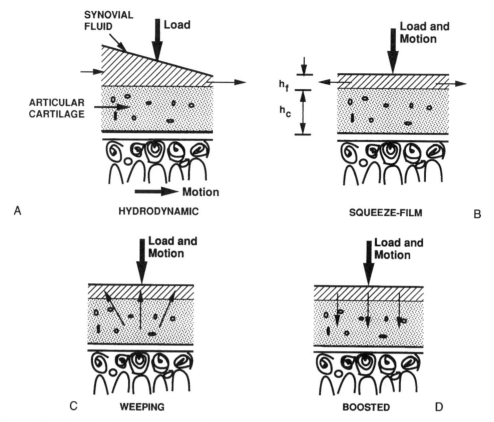

FIG. 14. (A) Schematic representation of hydrodynamic lubrication. Viscous fluid is dragged into a convergent channel, causing a pressure field to be generated in the lubricant. Fluid viscosity, gap geometry, and relative sliding speed determine the load-carrying capacity. **(B)** As the bearing surfaces are squeezed together, the viscous fluid is forced from the gap in the transverse direction. This squeeze action generates a hydrodynamic pressure in the fluid for load support. The load-carrying capacity depends on the size of the surfaces, velocity of approach, and fluid viscosity. **(C)** Weeping lubrication hypothesis for the uniform exudation of interstitial fluid from the cartilage. The driving mechanism is a self-pressurization of the interstitial fluid when the tissue is compressed. **(D)** Direction of fluid flow under squeeze-film lubrication in the boosted mode for joint lubrication.

film thickness and some salient approximations for diarthrodial joint operating conditions. Martin derived the formula for estimating the minimum film thickness for the hydrodynamic lubrication of a long rigid cylinder on a plane (126). His equation for minimum film thickness expression is given by:

$$h/R = 4.9\eta uL/W. \qquad (1)$$

Kapitza derived a similar relationship considering the hydrodynamic lubrication of a sphere on a plane (93). This expression is given by:

$$h/R = 113.7(\eta uR/W)^2. \qquad (2)$$

In both expressions, h is the minimum film thickness, R is the radius of the cylinder or sphere, L is the axial length of the cylinder, η is the viscosity of a Newtonian lubricant, u is the entraining velocity, which is equal to half the sum of the velocities of the interacting surfaces, and W is the load on the bearing (Fig. 15). If the articulating surfaces can be approximated by either a rigid cylinder interacting with a plane or by a rigid sphere on a plane, and if the synovial fluid is considered to be Newtonian with a known constant viscosity, these simplified approximations can be used

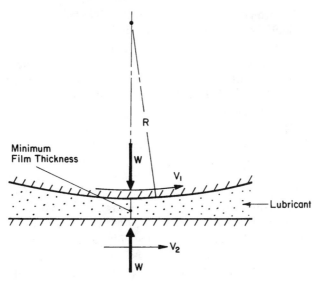

FIG. 15. Cylinder-on-plane bearing configuration: u = entraining velocity = $(V_1 + V_2)/2$; R = effective radius of curvature; W = bearing load supported by the lubricant.

to assess whether hydrodynamic lubrication can work in diarthrodial joints. The calculation of the fluid film thickness under hydrodynamic conditions can be performed with some specific diarthrodial joint examples.

Example 1

For the knee joint during the stance phase of walking, the following values are taken to calculate the minimum fluid-film thickness: R = 0.1 m, L/W = 2 × 10⁻⁵ m/N, u = 0.3 m/sec, and η = 10⁻² N-sec/m².

Using equation 1 and multiplying through by R yields: h = (0.1 m) × (4.9) × (10⁻² N-sec/m²) × (0.3 m/sec) × (2 × 10⁻⁵ m/N); the fluid-film thickness prediction is h = 0.029 μm. This value is too low in comparison with the cartilage surface roughness for an effective fluid lubricant film to be formed between the bearing surfaces.

Example 2

For the hip joint during the swing phase of walking, the following values are taken to calculate the approximate fluid-film thick-

ness: R = 1.0 m, W = 75 kg, u = 0.1 m/sec, η = 10⁻² N-sec/m².

Using equation 2 and multiplying through by R yields:

$$h = (1.0\ \text{m}) \times (113.7) \times [(10^{-2}\ \text{N-sec/m}^2) \\ \times (0.1\ \text{m/sec}) \times (1.0\ \text{m})/(75\ \text{kgf})]^2$$

The fluid-film thickness prediction is h = 0.020 μm. This value for fluid-film thickness is also much smaller than the articular cartilage surface roughness.

It is thus evident that hydrodynamic lubrication cannot operate in these joints under these loading conditions. However, under smaller loads, and during faster motions such as in the swing phase of walking, this mechanism of lubrication may possibly be responsible for lubrication. One should, however, remember that synovial fluid is non-Newtonian and exhibits a shear thinning effect (Fig. 5) (171). Thus, these joint "model" assumptions may be far from reality.

Dintenfass included cartilage deformation in his theory (44,45). This would act to spread the joint load over a larger surface area and would decrease the velocity gradient between the two surfaces. In engineering terminology, this lubrication mode, in which both the viscous resistance of the lubricant as well as the elastic deformation of the bearing surfaces play a prominent role, is called elastohydrodynamic lubrication. For the hip and knee joints, film thicknesses provided by this mechanism have been calculated to be as high as 1.3 and 1.25 μm, respectively (51,75,78).

Although Dintenfass allowed for cartilage deformability, he assumed a simplified deformation field to occur in a homogeneous, linearly elastic half-space. In reality, this deformation occurs in a thin, soft cartilage layer backed by stiff subchondral bone. A layered structure with a rigid backing was studied by Hooke and O'Donoghue (86), who calculated the minimum film thickness for the cylinder and plane approximation using:

$$h/R = [L^{0.2}(\eta u)^{0.6}]/[W^{0.2}(E'R)^{0.4}]. \quad (3)$$

where h, R, L, η, u, and W are as defined previously, and E' is the effective elastic modulus given by:

$$1/E' = (1/2)[(1 - v_1^2)/E_1 + (1 - v_2^2)/E_2]. (4)$$

where E_1, v_1, E_2, and v_2 are the elastic moduli for the two-layer model (86). To see how the deformation of the cartilage might influence the minimum fluid-film predictions, let us use these two equations in an example.

Example 3

For the knee joint during the stance phase of walking, the following values are taken (as in Example 1) to calculate the approximate fluid-film thickness: $R = 0.1$ m, $(L/W) = 2 \times 10^{-5}$ m/N, $u = 0.3$ m/sec, $\eta = 10^{-2}$ N-sec/m^2, and $E' = 10^7$ N/m^2.

Using equation 3 and multiplying through by R gives:

$$h = (0.1 \text{ m}) \times (2 \times 10^{-5} \text{ m/N})^{0.2}$$
$$\times [(10^{-2} \text{ N-sec/m}^2) \times (0.3 \text{ m/sec})]^{0.6}$$
$$/[(10^7 \text{ N/m}^2) \times (0.1 \text{ m})]^{0.4}$$

The fluid-film thickness prediction is: $h = 1.4$ μm.

If cartilage is more compliant, the fluid-film thickness will be greater. Thus, the elas-

tohydrodynamic mode appears more plausible than hydrodynamic lubrication for conditions observed in diarthrodial joints. Nevertheless, the film thicknesses reported for this lubrication mode are still smaller than the combined surface roughness of contacting cartilage layers.

Addressing this issue, Dowson and Jin (52, 53) argued that the surface asperities of articular cartilage would be flattened out under the physiological pressures experienced in joints. They called this mechanism microelastohydrodynamic lubrication (micro-EHL), and they calculated a minimum film thickness on the order of 0.7 μm, but the ratio of this thickness to the flattened composite surface roughness could be as great as 19:1. However, despite providing a possible theoretical mechanism for maintaining full-thickness fluid films between the surfaces, the predictions of the micro-EHL theory yielded smaller friction coefficients than experimental results (53).

Most recently, Kirk and co-workers (98) used environmental scanning electron microscopy (ESEM) to demonstrate that cartilage surfaces are smooth under normal conditions and that the roughness reported in previous EM studies (e.g., 135,161,196,204) resulted from the drying of specimens. Kirk et al. (99) also imaged a groove formed by Talysurf instrumentation on the cartilage surface, suggesting that such measurements (e.g., 191,204) reveal the topography of the collagen ultrastructure underneath the most superficial zone of cartilage. These findings remain to be confirmed; if cartilage is indeed found to be a lot smoother than earlier reported, one of the major obstacles for accepting the viability of EHL will have been overcome. It will then remain to be demonstrated that the frictional properties and their dependence on joint load, congruence, and material properties behave according to EHL theory. For example, to date, EHL theory has not been able to explain the time-dependent variation in the friction coefficient of cartilage in all the configurations tested experimentally (e.g., 116, 122,128,196).

Self-Generating Mechanism

In a study by Mow and Lai, articular cartilage was modeled as a thin-layer biphasic medium supported by a hard bony substrate. In this formulation, normal cartilage was subjected to a constant-width, parabolically distributed normal load sliding over its surface at physiological speeds V (103,138). This load distribution is representative of the hydrodynamic pressure in the synovial fluid film; the authors investigated whether, under this prescribed traction, cartilage could yield its interstitial fluid for use as a fluid-film lubricant. In their original study, these authors employed a parametric analysis in which they varied the load partition factor, which determines the load fractions applied to the solid and fluid phases of the tissue, respectively. Since that study, however, Hou and co-workers (87) demonstrated mathematically that the load is partitioned according to the solid and fluid fractions (or solidity and porosity) of cartilage, assuming an isotropic model of tissue porosity. For this configuration, the formulation of Mow and Lai yielded a "self-generating mechanism" in which fluid was observed

to exude under the leading and trailing edges of the load distribution while it was resorbed into the tissue near the center (Fig. 16A) (138); the exuded fluid at the leading edge would provide a continuous supply of lubricant to maintain a fluid film between the surfaces, thus reducing the friction coefficient.

In this configuration, the effect of cartilage material properties and sliding speed is manifested through the nondimensional parameter $R_h = Vh/H_Ak$, where V is the sliding speed, k is the permeability coefficient of the tissue, H_A is the aggregate modulus of the solid matrix of cartilage, and h is the thickness of the cartilage layer. For normal tissues, R_h ranges from 10^3 to 10^5, and for pathologic tissues (with decreasing H_A and k; see Chapter 4 for more details), R_h decreases. Thus, the amount of fluid expelled into the joint space is a function of the characteristics of the applied load and the properties of the solid matrix of cartilage (Fig. 16B). In this figure, it is assumed that $R_h = 10^4$ for normal cartilage, $R_h = 10^2$ for mildly degenerate cartilage, and $R_h = 1$ for highly degenerate cartilage (138). As degeneration proceeds, a decrease of interstitial fluid flow occurs, thus defeating the self-generating

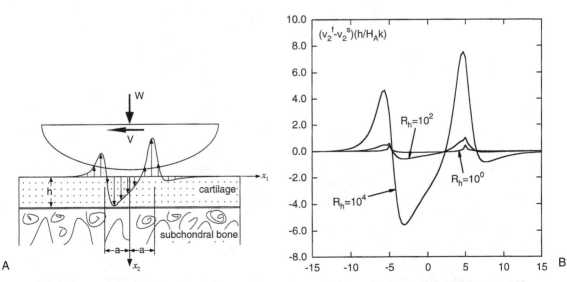

FIG. 16. **(A)** Pattern of predicted fluid exudation and imbibition over the articular surface resulting from a hydrodynamic pressure distribution acting between a biphasic layer of thickness *h(r)* and a moving indenter. Here *V* is the speed of the horizontal translation. **(B)** Fluid efflux from the tissue for various values of the nondimensional parameter $R_h = Vh/H_Ak$.

mechanism. This effect may have significant consequences on the inexorable degeneration process in cartilage during osteoarthritis.

This self-generating mechanism was studied using an optical sliding-contact analytic rheometer, which produced a cinematographic record of the flow pattern (137). In this experiment, strips of cartilage were mounted on a glass slide and loaded normally by a sliding optical glass lens. The flow patterns provided visual evidence for this self-generating lubrication mechanism and supported the theory that articular cartilage can generate a fluid film under slow, moderate loading conditions. This self-generating mechanism may not only contribute significantly to fluid-film lubrication but may also create a mechanically generated circulation system required for the nutrition of chondrocytes in the tissue (105,106,166,179).

Squeeze-Film Lubrication

In squeeze-film lubrication, two bearing surfaces simply approach each other along a normal direction (Fig. 14B). Because a viscous lubricant cannot be instantaneously squeezed out from the gap between the surfaces, a pressure is built up as a result of the viscous resistance offered by the lubricant as it is being squeezed from the gap. The pressure field in the fluid film formed in this manner is capable of supporting large loads. Because the bearing surfaces are deformable layers of articular cartilage, the large pressure generated may cause localized depressions where the lubricant film can be trapped.

In 1967, Fein noted the importance of squeeze-film lubrication and derived expressions for the calculation of film thickness for various parameters using the sphere-on-plane configuration for his mathematical approximation of diarthrodial joints (59). Later, Higginson and Unsworth (78) demonstrated that for two compliant bearing surfaces, squeeze-film lubrication could yield physiologically meaningful squeeze-film times of approximately 60 sec. The squeeze-film time is defined as the theoretical time required to reduce a lubricant film thickness down to a small prescribed minimum film thickness (Fig. 15), usually of the order of the surface roughness. Later, Dowson and co-workers (51) demonstrated that during lightly loaded portions of the swing phase of walking, a film thickness of 2.5 μm would decrease by only 0.06 μm in 0.5 sec after heel strike. Mow (134) addressed the question of the non-Newtonian effects of synovial fluid in squeeze-film lubrication. He demonstrated that these non-Newtonian effects require a larger surface area to support a given load because of the lower peak hydrodynamic pressures that exist during squeeze film for the sphere-on-plane configuration. These non-Newtonian effects act to increase the squeeze-film time.

The viability of squeeze-film lubrication can be assessed from the squeeze-film time, which should be on the order of or greater than physiological loading times, film thickness, as well as film replenishment. In lower extremity joints, where loading is intermittent and inertial effects during the swing phase of a gait cycle may contribute to separating the joint surfaces, squeeze-film action may be viable if it occurs in conjunction with other lubrication modes. In a study of transient EHL using thin layer elastic models for cartilage, Medley et al. (130) and Smith and Medley (181) demonstrated theoretically that a minimum fluid film thickness of 0.7 to 1.0 μm could be maintained during cyclical loading of a joint. This result is significant because it addresses the concern regarding film depletion in fluid-film lubrication, over several cycles of loading, combining both the effects of squeeze-film and EHL actions. Assuming that the concerns about fluid-film thickness in relation to surface roughness can be addressed properly by micro-EHL or another related mechanism, it appears that squeeze-film lubrication does occur in lower-extremity diarthrodial joints under certain load configurations. This theoretical framework provides a cogent interpretation of the experimental results of Unsworth and co-workers (193,194). Further discussion of theoretical squeeze-film analyses is provided below, in the section on boosted lubrication.

Hydrostatic Lubrication

A classical engineering lubrication theory, hydrostatic lubrication, exists in which a pressurized fluid film is maintained between two bearing surfaces via an external pump. McCutchen postulated a similar self-pressurized hydrostatic lubrication or weeping lubrication mechanism for diarthrodial joints (107,108,124) that functions in the absence of an external pump. According to this theory, a lubricant fluid film between the two articulating surfaces is generated by the compression of the articular cartilage layers during joint function. Furthermore, this uniform exudation was assumed to occur over the entire articulating surface under compaction of the tissue (Fig. 14C). In a recent finite element study of a poroelastic spherical cartilage layer against an impermeable steel spherical endoprosthesis, Macirowski and co-workers reported numerical results that purportedly confirm this weeping phenomenon at the contact interface (119).

Boosted Lubrication

Another possible mechanism of lubrication of diarthrodial joints was proposed by Walker and co-workers (197,198) and Maroudas (124). This theory, termed *boosted lubrication,* hypothesizes that as the articulating surfaces approach each other, the solvent component of synovial fluid, i.e., water, passes into the articular cartilage over the entire contact region during squeeze-film conditions, thus leaving a concentrated pool of hyaluronic acid protein complex behind to lubricate the surfaces. It is reasoned that as the size of the gap between articulating surfaces decreases, the resistance of sideways efflux of the lubricant will eventually become greater than the resistance of flow into the articular cartilage (Fig. 14D). Furthermore, because of the small size (20 to 70 Å) of the pores in normal articular cartilage (Fig. 8A), the hyaluronan, with a diameter of its solution domain on the order of 4000 Å, is unable to penetrate the cartilage surface and is left behind in the gap. Thus, with the normal articulating surface acting as an ultrafiltration membrane, only water and small electrolytes are able to pass into the tissue.

Scanning electron microscopic observations indicating the presence of a hyaluronate–protein complex layer under squeeze-film conditions were made by Seller and co-workers (176; Fig. 17). Walker and co-workers noted that this concentrated hyaluronate and protein gel layer might be capable of supporting larger loads for longer periods of time than synovial fluid containing normal hyaluronate and protein concentrations (196). They postulated that this gel could become trapped in the normal roughness present in articular cartilage, forming micro-pockets of concentrated gel on the articulating surfaces that aid in the lubrication process.

Lai and Mow (102) studied this ultrafiltration at the articular surface using a one-dimensional convection–diffusion model for the transport of macromolecules. They obtained quantitative information on the buildup rate of this gel near the articular surface. The rate and the extent of such a buildup depends on the Peclet number ($= VH_o/K$), which characterizes the relative contribution of the diffusion (described by the diffusion coefficient K of hyaluronate in the fluid) versus the convection (with speed V, the rate of descent of the upper surface). Here H_o denotes the original thickness of the fluid. Because the concentration of hyaluronate and large protein molecules can not increase indefinitely in the fluid, at a certain critical concentration, C_{cr}, a three-dimensional molecular network will be formed creating a gel where C_{cr} is a nondimensional concentration given by C/C_o with C_o as the starting concentration in the fluid and C as the dimensional critical concentration. For hyaluronate, the concentration C_o in synovial fluid ranges from 2 to 5 mg/ml, and the critical concentration C may range from 10 to 20 mg/ml, though no firm data exist on this point (138). Thus, estimates of C_{cr} may range from 2 to 10.

Figure 18 shows that during ultrafiltration, as the upper surface descends, a height will be

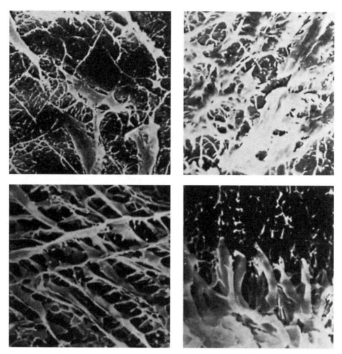

FIG. 17. Scanning electron microscopy showing surface aggregation of dried hyaluronic acid–protein complexes on cartilage surfaces (176).

reached at which the gel begins to form at the lower surface. This gel or molecular network allows the complete passage of the solvent but is impermeable to the macromolecular solutes. Subsequent squeezing results in the growth of the thickness of this gel layer until the remaining gap is filled with the gel at a concentration C_{cr}. Figure 18 demonstrates the growth of the gel layer for various C_{cr} at a Peclet number of 2.5 and with the articular surface being entirely impermeable to large hyaluronate and protein molecules found in the fluid, i.e., N = 1. From Fig. 18, the final thickness h_f of the gel in boosted lubrication may be computed. The final thickness h_f is given by the expression $h_f = H_o\delta(t)$, where $\delta(t)$ is given by the curves for different C_{cr} in Fig. 18. For example, if $H_o = 20$ μm and $C_{cr} = 3.07$, the final thickness of the gel is $h_f = 6.4$ μm.

In 1989, Hou and co-workers formulated the boundary conditions at the cartilage-synovial fluid interface (87). These boundary conditions are required for theoretical

modeling of fluid exchanges between synovial fluid and articular cartilage interstitial fluid, in the cavity of diarthrodial joints. This general formulation considers cartilage to be biphasic (139) and synovial fluid to be viscous non-Newtonian; a "pseudo-no-slip" kinematic boundary condition was proposed based on the principle that the conditions at the interface between a multiphasic mixture and a fluid must reduce to those boundary conditions in single-phase fluid mechanics. These relations have been used to solve the problem of squeeze-film lubrication of a spherical, rigid, impermeable indenter on a cartilage layer supported by a rigid bony substrate (Fig. 19; 88). In this study, Hou and co-workers, assumed that synovial fluid may be modeled as a viscous Newtonian fluid. Their theoretical results demonstrate that fluid-film viscosity is dominant in affecting the fluid flow pattern just after loading when the fluid film is large; when the gap reduces in size, however, the effect of cartilage per-

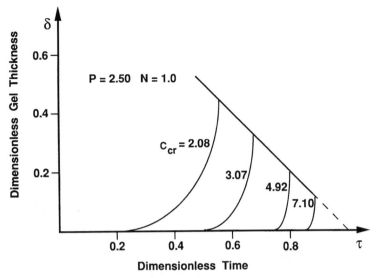

FIG. 18. Predicted rate of growth of the thickness of the hyaluronic acid–protein gel for various critical concentrations (102). The *upper line* represents the instantaneous position of the upper moving surface. Gelling stops when the whole gap is filled with the gel at C_{cr} and $\tau = Vt/H_0$.

meability becomes more significant. Figure 20A shows the location of the indenter surface, pressure distribution, and deformed cartilage surface during squeeze-film. It is seen that the cartilage surface deformation promotes formation of the fluid-film gap. Figure 20B shows the fluid efflux patterns when the minimum film thickness h_{min} is 50 μm and 5 μm. These results indicate that fluid exudation and imbibition occur simultaneously across the cartilage surface, a situation in between the weeping lubrication hypothesis (107,108,128,129) and the boosted lubrication hypothesis (196,197). The fluid lubricant is forced into the cartilage at the high-pressure central region and out of the

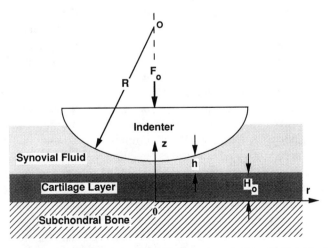

FIG. 19. A model for joint squeeze-film lubrication between a viscous fluid and a thin layer of biphasic material attached to the impervious subchondral bone.

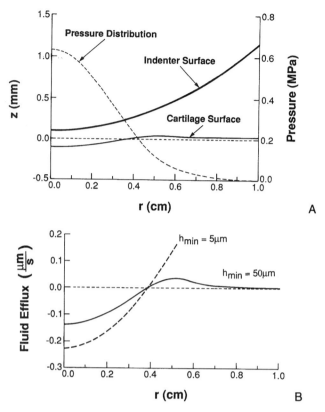

FIG. 20. (A) Theoretical prediction of the squeeze-film problem illustrated in Fig. 19 for pressure distribution, indenter surface, and articular surface deformation. **(B)** Theoretical prediction of fluid efflux pattern at the articular surface for a minimum film thickness of 50 μm and 5 μm.

cartilage in the peripheral region of the squeeze-film gap within the circular load support area. Furthermore, assuming typical values for loads, geometries, and biphasic material properties, calculations show that it takes approximately 2.4 sec to close the gap from 100 μm to 1 μm. If the tissue permeability is increased by one order of magnitude as for diseased cartilage, the squeeze-film time is decreased to 0.9 sec, whereas if the synovial fluid viscosity is increased by two orders of magnitude, the squeeze-film time is increased to 24 sec. Thus, synovial fluid viscosity and cartilage permeability are the two dominant parameters governing the behavior of joints operating under squeeze-film action. Because the synovial fluid was observed to filter into the cartilage layer in the high-pressure central region of the fluid

film, Hou and co-workers conjectured that their mathematical predictions supported the premise of boosted lubrication.

Hlavácek (82,83) elaborated considerably on the biphasic squeeze-film model of Hou and co-workers. He first developed a biphasic model for synovial fluid in which one phase represents the low-molecular-weight substances and is assumed ideal and the other represents the hyaluronic acid protein complex and is assumed viscous and non-Newtonian, obeying a power law. He then employed this theory along with the cartilage biphasic theory of Mow et al. (139) to solve the problem of gel formation during squeeze-film lubrication of cartilage disks. He observed that for normal synovial fluid with a hyaluronic acid concentration of 50 mg/ml, a stable gel layer formed as a result of homogeneous filtration in a model of the hip joint. The typical thickness of this gel layer was found to be 0.1 μm and was observed to be almost independent of the applied load. Models of inflammatory synovial fluid demonstrated significantly smaller gel thicknesses.

From these various studies, the deposition of hyaluronic acid gels on the surface of cartilage appears to be a plausible mechanism in diarthrodial joints. Whether these results validate boosted lubrication remains to be seen, however, in light of the observation by Linn (111) and others that purified hyaluronic acid is not a good lubricant.

Boundary Lubrication

Charnley suggested that a monolayer of lubricant might serve to separate the two articulating surfaces during normal joint function (34–36). Davies and co-workers suggested a variation of this theme in which a thin layer of "structured water" (several water molecules thick) is adsorbed onto the articular surface, thus providing the required boundary lubricant (42). Such mechanisms fall into the category of boundary lubrication (Fig. 21A). In a series of investigations, Swann and Radin (186–190) isolated a single polypeptide chain from synovial fluid that is believed to be the boundary lubricant. This molecule, called lubricin, is a protein–carbohydrate complex comprised of oligosaccharides distributed along the length of a protein core. Its molecular weight is approximately 250,000 daltons (188), and it can be adsorbed to each articulating surface of the cartilage. This monolayer on each surface has a thickness on the order of 10 to 1000 Å and has the ability to carry weight and reduce friction (190). Hills and Butler suggested that the boundary lubricant found in synovial fluid was more likely to be dipalmitoyl phosphatidylcholine (DPPC), a phospholipid (79,80). Whether DPPC was present as a contaminant

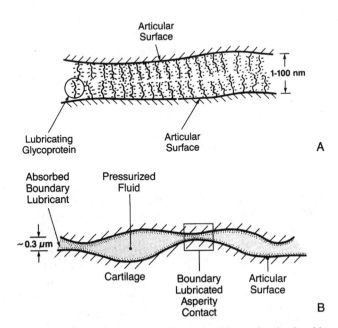

FIG. 21. **(A)** Boundary lubrication of articular cartilage. In this mode, the load is carried by a monolayer of the lubricating glycoprotein, which is adsorbed onto the articular surfaces (142). **(B)** Depiction of mixed lubrication. Boundary lubrication occurs where the thickness of the fluid film is on the same order as the roughness of the bearing surfaces. Fluid-film lubrication takes place in areas with more widely separated surfaces (142).

in lubricin or not, the evidence that these compounds act as effective boundary lubricants is very strong. However, it should be noted that experiments demonstrate that a boundary lubricant can account for a reduction in the friction coefficient by a factor of only two to six (90,115,190,201). Although this is a remarkable effect, it remains that the friction coefficient of cartilage has been shown to vary over a much greater range, e.g., by a factor of 60 (128), within the same cartilage sample as a function of time. Hence, boundary lubrication, which is certain to occur, must be complemented by one or more mechanisms that can explain these observed phenomena. Figure 21B shows a proposed mixed mode of lubrication in which boundary lubrication and fluid lubrication coexist (48). In this mode, with limited solid–solid contact, the frictional coefficient may be minimized, providing an attractive alternative mechanism for joint lubrication.

INTERSTITIAL FLUID PRESSURIZATION AND DIARTHRODIAL JOINT LUBRICATION

Although a considerable amount of research has been done on lubrication mechanisms in diarthrodial joints, there remain many experimental results that have not been successfully predicted within a mathematically tractable theoretical framework. Perhaps the most notable of these is the observed time dependence of the friction coefficient of cartilage during creep or stress-relaxation experiments (122, 128,204). It has been proposed that this time dependence is directly related to the exudation of cartilage interstitial water during tissue creep (122,128). When the tissue has reached its equilibrium creep deformation, i.e., when the interstitial fluid pressure has reduced to zero (139,147,148), the friction coefficient has been shown experimentally to also achieve an equilibrium value (122,204).

Based on these observations, Ateshian (14, 15) proposed a mathematical formulation of a boundary friction model for articular cartilage that uses the theoretical framework of the biphasic theory for articular cartilage (139). The biphasic theory accounts for the fluid stress in the tissue, given by the stress tensor $\sigma^f = -\phi^f p \mathbf{I}$, where p is the interstitial fluid pressure, ϕ^f is the porosity, and $\mathbf{I}$ is the identity tensor; it also accounts for the solid stress $\sigma^s = -\phi^s p \mathbf{I} + \sigma^e$, where $\phi^s = 1 - \phi^f$, and σ^e is the effective (or elastic) stress, which results from the state of strain in the solid collagen–proteoglycan matrix. The total stress in the tissue is given by $\sigma^t = \sigma^s + \sigma^f = -p\mathbf{I} + \sigma^e$; hence, the total stress represents the summation of effect of interstitial fluid pressure and effective stress. At the interfacial contact surface between two biphasic articular layers, the surface traction vector is given by $\sigma^t \mathbf{n}$, where $\mathbf{n}$ is the unit surface normal at the interface. This traction vector can be resolved into a normal traction component, $\mathbf{n} \cdot \sigma^t \mathbf{n}$, and a tangential component, $\tau \cdot \sigma^t \mathbf{n}$, along the direction of relative motion of the surfaces, where τ is a unit vector orthogonal to $\mathbf{n}$. By integrating these traction components over the area A of the contact interface, the normal load W across the articular surfaces and the friction force F tangential to the surfaces, are produced:

$$W = \int \mathbf{n} \cdot \sigma^t \mathbf{n} \, dA \qquad F = \int \tau \cdot \sigma^t \mathbf{n} \, dA. \qquad (5)$$

The effective (i.e., measured) friction coefficient at the surfaces is then given by $\mu_{eff} = F/W$. However, by substituting the expression for σ^t in the above integrals, the normal load W can be separated into a component contributed by interstitial fluid pressure, $W_p = \int -p \, dA$, and another contributed by the effective stress, $W_e = \int \mathbf{n} \cdot \sigma^e \mathbf{n} \, dA$, such that $W = W_p + W_e$; the friction force F is found to depend on the effective stress alone, $F = \int \tau \cdot \sigma^e \mathbf{n} \, dA$. Hence, according to Ateshian (14,15), the friction force may be related to the normal load component W_e through the relationship $F = \mu_{eq} W_e$, where μ_{eq} is the equilibrium friction coefficient in the absence of interstitial fluid pressure. The effective friction coefficient is related to this equilibrium friction coefficient through

$$\mu_{eff} = \mu_{eq} W_e / W = \mu_{eq}(1 - W_p / W). \qquad (6)$$

The simplicity of this expression, which satisfies the interface continuity requirements derived by Hou et al. (87), contrasts with the complexity of calculating the ratio W_p/W for various biphasic contact configurations (14). Furthermore, the value of μ_{eq} need not be constant but may vary with the magnitude of surface roughness or the amount of boundary lubricant present on the articular surfaces; μ_{eq} may even be velocity dependent (122,199–201), load dependent (122), and strain dependent (199).

In the simplest model, where μ_{eq} is assumed to be constant, equation 6 demonstrates that the measured friction coefficient μ_{eff} may be time dependent through the time dependence of the ratio W_p (or W_p/W). For ex-

ample, consider a cylindrical biphasic cartilage plug that is compressed in a confining chamber under a constant applied load W through an impermeable rigid platen rotating with a prescribed angular speed (Fig. 22A). The surface of the plug opposite the platen presses against a rigid porous filter, and interdigitation of the cartilage with the rough surface of the porous filter will prevent it from rotating. A frictional torque will develop at the platen–cartilage interface and can be measured with a torque cell. Under infinitesimal deformation, the frictional torque acting on the specimen produces deformations that are uncoupled from the axial creep deformation of the tissue; hence, an analytic expression for W_p/W can be easily derived for this problem

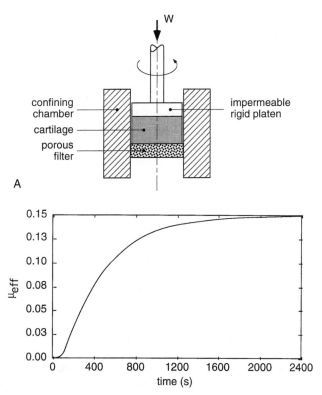

A

B

FIG. 22. **(A)** Confined compression configuration for creep and torsional friction testing. The cartilage plug rests on a rigid porous filter **(bottom)** and is acted on by a rotating smooth-rigid impermeable platen under a constant applied load *W*. The cartilage plug is prevented from rotating at the rough cartilage–porous filter interface. **(B)** The time-dependent effective friction coefficient μ_{eff}, as predicted by the friction model proposed by Ateshian (14–17). In the early time response, when interstitial fluid pressurization is high, the friction coefficient can be very low; however, after the tissue has reached creep equilibrium, the friction coefficient has increased to $\mu_{eq} = 0.15$.

from the governing linear biphasic equations (see Chapter 4). Figure 22B shows the theoretical prediction for the effective friction coefficient μ_{eff} at the cartilage–platen interface using equation 6 and assuming a value of μ_{eq} = 0.15. The results of this simple analysis indicate that the measured friction coefficient may indeed be very low, though it may increase with time to an unremarkable equilibrium value of 0.15. The time constant for this transient response is the same as that of the creep deformation, in agreement with observed experimental results (122,128,204).

Thus, interstitial fluid pressurization can indeed account for producing very low friction coefficients for articular cartilage, even when the equilibrium friction coefficient is not particularly small. Although the theoretical formulation embodied in equation 6 supports part of the premise for weeping lubrication (128), namely, the role of hydrostatic pressurization, it remains that no weeping of interstitial fluid needs to occur toward the contact interface of the sliding surfaces (Fig. 14C) in order to promote low friction coefficients; indeed, in the example analyzed above, fluid efflux occurs in the direction opposite that of the cartilage–platen interface where friction is measured, in contradiction with the mechanism postulated by McCutchen (128). Ateshian (15,17) has also demonstrated the application of equation 6 to problems of rolling contact and contact creep of cylindrical biphasic layers, based on corresponding solutions for W_p/W for these problems (13,95); theoretical predictions from these analyses provide an explanation for the observed decrease of the effective friction coefficient with increasing rolling and sliding joint velocities, as in the experiments of Linn (111), and with increasing joint load, as in the experiments of Linn (111) and Unsworth et al. (193; Fig. 11).

SUMMARY OF DIARTHRODIAL JOINT LUBRICATION

Lubrication acts to keep wear of articular cartilage in diarthrodial joints to a minimum.

Under normal circumstances, with proper lubrication, together with repair by chondrocytes in the tissue, diarthrodial joints can function normally for many decades. However, in pathologic cases, or under conditions of abnormally severe loading, both fatigue and interfacial wear become evident. As the wear process initiates, the tissue becomes more susceptible to both surface and interior damage, thus leading to a progressive degeneration process. Failure of cartilage as a bearing surface results from the loss of balance between the ability of chondrocytes to maintain the tissue (see Chapters 4 and 5) and the wear rate.

A considerable amount of work has been done in the field of diarthrodial joint lubrication, though some of the theories proposed to explain the vast body of experimental data are sometimes contradictory or appear to be limited to particular loading configurations. All of these theories are based on conceptually attractive arguments; however, a critical reading of the literature demonstrates that unequivocal verifications are lacking for many of them. From a theoretical perspective, fluid-film lubrication theories, whether using elastic or biphasic models for cartilage, have been arguably analyzed more thoroughly than any other. This is because of the availability of well-understood equations for fluid-film lubrication for engineering bearings (164). The self-generating mechanism (103,138) may enhance fluid-film lubrication, though theoretical analyses of hydrodynamic lubrication using biphasic articular layers are required to confirm the distinct effectiveness of this proposed mechanism. Boundary lubrication theories are more difficult to formulate, though promising results have been presented recently (14,15,17) in conjunction with the use of the biphasic theory for cartilage (139). The theoretical viability for one of the tenets of boosted lubrication has been demonstrated (82,83,88,102), but the formation of hyaluronan gels on the surface of cartilage has not been shown to explain the low frictional response of joints. Although one finite element study appeared to have confirmed the mechanism of weeping lubrication (119), several others studies have clearly demonstrated that interstitial fluid does not weep out of the cartilage layers into a fluid film under the contact region (11,13,82,83,88).

It is also evident from the literature that several different theories may yield similar predictions of particular experimental results, though few theories can explain the wide variety of observed cartilage frictional properties. Hence, the interpretation of experimental results cannot occur without a proper theoretical formulation of a lubrication theory for cartilage. Any such formulation must be able to predict a variety of experimental outcomes using physically and mathematically consistent equations. This has been, and continues to be, a great challenge in the field of biotribology, and a considerable amount of research is still required to fully understand the physiological lubrication processes *in vivo*.

Acknowledgments

This work was supported in part by grants from the National Science Foundation (EET-8518501, ASC-9318184), the National Institutes of Health (1R29-AR43628-01), and the Whitaker Foundation. Any opinions, findings, and conclusions or recommendations expressed in this publication are those of the authors and do not necessarily reflect the views of the National Science Foundation.

PROBLEMS

1. From Table 3 and Fig. 9, what is the typical range of friction forces acting on a joint surface?

2. From Fig. 13, determine the wear rates of cartilage for the two applied pressures at early times (<40 min) and at late times (>120 min). Explain why it is difficult to measure wear of any bearing surface.

3. What are typical R_a values for articular cartilage versus those for the surfaces of artificial implants? Read the papers by Walker et al. (197) and Sayles et al. (169).

4. Does it seem reasonable that no single lubrication theory can explain the process of lubrication of diarthrodial joints? Why? Provide three important deformational effects each for synovial fluid and articular cartilage that must be considered in understanding joint lubrication.

5. Jones (91) and Charnley (36) used the outcome of pendulum experiments to investigate whether joints were lubricated by a fluid film or by boundary friction. By reading these papers, determine the specific experimental observation these authors used to justify their conclusions. How did Barnett and Cobbold (21) address the contradictory interpretations of these previous authors? What was the corresponding explanation provided by Unsworth et al. (93)?

6. Fluid-film lubrication theories require the knowledge of the lubricant viscosity η in order to calculate the minimum film thickness (e.g., equations 1–3). By estimating the shear rate D of a lubricant film in a joint, can you determine an appropriate value for η from Fig. 5? Are the values used in Examples 1 to 3 appropriate, a little too low, or a little too high?

7. Synovial fluid is non-Newtonian and exhibits a characteristic normal stress σ^1, as shown in Fig. 5. Can this normal stress contribute significantly to load support in a typical joint? (Hint: Use Fig. 9 to estimate loads in human joints, and assume a typical joint contact area of 5 cm^2.)

8. The "flat-on-flat" experimental configuration of the frictional tests by Malcom (122; Fig. 12A) precluded the formation of a wedge-shaped gap necessary for fluid-film lubrication. His results demonstrated that synovial fluid yields a lower friction coefficient than buffered saline (Fig. 12B). What is a likely explanation of that result?

9. McCutchen (128) conducted an experiment in which he observed that the friction coefficient of cartilage against glass increases with time when the surfaces are subjected to a step constant load. He also

demonstrated that separating the contacting surfaces for a few seconds and then loading them again in an identical fashion does not produce identical frictional coefficients. He concluded that squeeze-film lubrication is not responsible for this observed behavior. What explanation can you provide to support this claim?

10. Describe the process of squeeze-film lubrication. How do the permeability and elastic moduli of the solid matrix of cartilage and the viscosity of synovial fluid affect squeeze-film lubrication?

11. Describe the fluid-film lubrication hypotheses proposed by MacConaill and Jones, Dintenfass, McCutchen, and Walker and co-workers.

12. Define elastohydrodynamic lubrication. How does it differ from hydrodynamic lubrication? What is elastorheodynamic lubrication?

13. Describe the "self-lubrication mechanism" for joint lubrication.

14. Other than lubrication, describe the functions for the synovial fluid.

15. What are the main types of wear? Briefly describe how these mechanisms work.

16. In general terms, how do the material properties of articular cartilage change following rupture of the anterior cruciate ligament of the knee (73,178)? How would these material property changes affect cartilage lubrication, wear, and load support?

17. Describe the "stress-shielding effect" in normal articular cartilage.

REFERENCES

1. Ahmed, A. M., and Burke, D. L. (1983): *In-vitro* measurement of static pressure distribution in synovial joints—Part I: Tibial surface of the knee. *J. Biomech. Eng.,* 105:216–225.
2. Ahmed, A. M., and Burke, D. L. (1983): *In-vitro* measurement of static pressure distribution in synovial joints—Part II: Retropatellar surface. *J. Biomech. Eng.,* 105:226–236.
3. Akizuki, S., Mow, V. C., Muller, F., Pita, J. C., Howell, D. S., and Manicourt, D. H. (1986): Tensile properties of knee joint cartilage: I. Influence of ionic condition, weight bearing, and fibrillation on the tensile modulus. *J. Orthop. Res.,* 4:379–392.
4. Akizuki, S., Mow, V. C., Muller, F., Pita, J. C., and

5. Howell, D. S. (1987): The tensile properties of human knee joint cartilage II: The influence of weight bearing, and tissue pathology on the kinetics of swelling. *J. Orthop. Res.,* 5:173–186.
5. Andriacchi, T. P., Ogle, J. A., and Galante, J. O. (1977): Walking speed as a basis for normal and abnormal gait measurements. *J. Biomech.,* 10:261–268.
6. Armstrong, C. G., and Mow, V. C. (1982): Variations in the intrinsic mechanical properties of human articular cartilage with age, degeneration, and water content. *J. Bone Joint Surg.,* 64A:88–94.
7. Armstrong, C. G., Mow, V. C., and Wirth, C. R. (1985): Biomechanics of impact-induced microdamage to articular surface—A possible genesis for chondromalacia patella. In: *AAOS Symposium Sports Medicine: The Knee,* edited by G. A. M. Finerman, pp. 54–69. C. V. Mosby, St. Louis.
8. Archard, J. F. (1980): Wear theory and mechanisms. In: *Wear Control Handbook,* edited by M. B. Peterson and W. O. Winer, pp. 35–80. ASME Publications, New York.
9. Ateshian, G. A., Soslowsky, L. J., and Mow, V. C. (1991): Quantitation of articular surface topography and cartilage thickness in knee joints using stereophotogrammetry. *J. Biomech.,* 24:761–776.
10. Ateshian, G. A., Rosenwasser, M. P., and Mow, V. C. (1992): Curvature characteristics and congruence of the thumb carpometacarpal joint: Differences between male and female joints. *J. Biomech.,* 25:591–607.
11. Ateshian, G. A., Lai, W. M., Zhu, W. B., and Mow, V. C. (1994): An asymptotic solution for the contact of two biphasic cartilage layers. *J. Biomech.,* 27:1347–1360.
12. Ateshian, G. A., Kwak, S. D., Soslowsky, L. J., and Mow, V. C. (1994): A new stereophotogrammetry method for determining *in situ* contact areas in diarthrodial joints: A comparison study. *J. Biomech.,* 27:111–124.
13. Ateshian, G. A., and Wang, H. (1995): A theoretical solution for the frictionless rolling contact of cylindrical biphasic articular cartilage layers. *J. Biomech.,* 28:1341–1355.
14. Ateshian, G. A. (1995): Continuity requirements across a contact interface in the formulation of a boundary friction model for biphasic articular cartilage. *Bioeng. Conf. Trans. ASME,* BED-29:147–148.
15. Ateshian, G. A. (1995): A theoretical model for boundary friction in articular cartilage. In: *Proceedings of the 4th China-Japan-U.S.A.-Singapore Conference on Biomechanics,* edited by G. Yang, K. Hayashi, S. L.-Y. Woo, and J. C. H. Goh, pp. 142–145. International Academic Publishers, Beijing.
16. Ateshian, G. A., Ark, J. W., Rosenwasser, M. P., Pawluk, R. J., Soslowsky, L. J., and Mow, V. C. (1995): Contact areas in the thumb carpometacarpal joint. *J. Orthop. Res.,* 13:450–458.
17. Ateshian, G. A. (1996): A theoretical formulation for boundary friction in articular cartilage. *J. Biomech. Eng.* (in press).
18. Athanasiou, K. A., Rosenwasser, M. P., Buckwalter, J. A., Malinin, T. I., Mow, V. C. (1991): Interspecies comparison of *in situ* intrinsic mechanical properties of distal femoral cartilage. *J. Orthop. Res.,* 9:330–340.
19. Balazs, E. A., Watson, C., Duff, I. F., and Roseman, S. (1967): Hyaluronic acid in synovial fluid: I. Molecular

parameters of hyaluronic acid in normal and arthritic human fluids. *Arthritis Rheum.,* 10:357–376.

20. Balazs, E. A., and Gibbs, D. A. (1970): The rheological properties and biological function of hyaluronic acid. In: *Chemistry and Molecular Biology of the Intercellular Matrix,* Vol. 3, edited by E. A. Balazs, pp. 1241–1253. Academic Press, New York.

21. Barnett, C. H., and Cobbold A. F. (1962): Lubrication within living joints. *J. Bone Joint Surg.,* 44B:662–674.

22. Bloch, B., and Dintenfass, L. (1963): Rheological study of human synovial fluid. *Aust. N.Z. J. Surg.,* 33:108–113.

23. Broom, N. D. (1986): Structural consequences of traumatising articular cartilage. *Ann. Rheum. Dis.,* 45:225–234.

24. Broom, N. D. (1988): The collagen framework of articular cartilage: Its profound influence on normal and abnormal load-bearing function. In: *Collagen: Chemistry, Biology and Biotechnology,* Vol. II, edited by M. E. Nimni, pp. 243–265. CRC Press, Boca Raton, FL.

25. Brown, T. D., and Shaw, D. T. (1983): *In vitro* contact stress distributions in the natural hip. *J. Biomech.,* 16:373–384.

26. Brown, T. D., and Shaw, D. T. (1984): *In vitro* contact stress distribution on the femoral condyles. *J. Orthop. Res.,* 2:190–199.

27. Brown, T. D., and Vrahas, M. S. (1984): The apparent elastic modulus of the juxtarticular subchondral bone of the femoral head. *J. Orthop. Res.,* 2:32–38.

28. Buckwalter, J. A., Rosenberg, L. C., Coutts, R., Hunziker, E. B., Reddi, A. H., and Mow, V. C. (1988): Articular cartilge: Injury and repair. In: *Injury and Repair of the Musculoskeletal Soft Tissues,* edited by S. L.-Y. Woo and J. A. Buckwalter. American Academy of Orthopaedic Surgery Press, Chicago, pp. 456–482.

29. Bullough, P. G. (1981): The geometry of diarthrodial joints, its physiologic maintenance, and the possible significance of age-related changes in geometry-to-load distribution and the development of osteoarthritis. *Clin. Orthop. Rel. Res.,* 156:61–66.

30. Bullough, P., and Jagannath, P. (1983): The morphology of the calcification front in articular cartilage: Its significance in joint function. *J. Bone Joint Surg.,* 65B:72–78.

31. Buschmann, M. D., Jurvelin, J. S., and Hunziker, E. B. (1995): Confined compression of articular cartilage: small-amplitude linear and nonlinear stress responses and the effect of the porous compression platen. *Advances in Bioengineering, Trans. ASME,* BED-31:307–398.

32. Carter, D. R., and Hayes, W. C. (1977): The compressive behavior of bone as a two phase porous structure. *J. Bone Joint Surg.,* 59A:965–967.

33. Caygill, J. C., and West, G. H. (1969): The rheological behavior of synovial fluid and its possible relation to joint lubrication. *Med. Biol. Eng.,* 7:507–516.

34. Charnley, J. (1959): The lubrication of animal joints. In: *Symposium on Biomechanics,* pp. 12–22. Institute of Mechanical Engineers, London.

35. Charnley, J. (1960): How our joints are lubricated. *Triangle,* 4:175.

36. Charnley, J. (1960): The lubrication of animal joints in relation to surgical reconstruction by arthroplasty. *Ann. Rheum. Dis.,* 19:10–19.

37. Clarke, I. C. (1972): The microevaluation of articular surface contours. *Ann. Biomed. Eng.,* 1:31–43.

38. Crowninshield, R. D., Johnston, R. C., Andrews, J. G., and Brand, R. A. (1978): A biomechanical investigation of the human hip. *J. Biomech.,* 11:75–85.

39. Davies, D. V. (1966): Synovial fluid as a lubricant. *Fed. Proc.,* 25:1069–1076.

40. Davies, D. V. (1967): Properties of synovial fluid. *Proc. Inst. Mech. Engrs.,* 181:25.

41. Davies, D. V., and Palfrey, A. J. (1968): Some of the physical properties of normal and pathological synovial fluids. *J. Biomech.,* 1:79–88.

42. Davis, W. H., Jr., Lee, S. L., and Sokoloff, L. (1979): A proposed model of boundary lubrication by synovial fluid: Structuring of boundary water. *J. Biomech. Eng.,* 101:185–192.

43. Dickinson, J. A., Cook, S. D., and Leinhardt, T. M. (1985): The measurement of shock waves following heel strike while running. *J. Biomech.,* 18:415–422.

44. Dintenfass, L. (1963): Lubrication in synovial joints. *Nature,* 197:496–497.

45. Dintenfass, L. (1963): Lubrication in synovial joints: A theoretical analysis, *J. Bone Joint Surg.,* 45A:1241–1256.

46. Dintenfass, L. (1966): Rheology of complex fluids and some observations on joint lubrication. *Fed. Proc.,* 25:1054–1060.

47. Donohue, J. M., Buss, D., Oegema, T. R., Jr., and Thompson, R. C. (1983): The effects of indirect blunt trauma on adult canine articular cartilage. *J. Bone Joint Surg.,* 65A:948–957.

48. Dowson D. (1967): Modes of lubrication in human joints. *Proc. Inst. Mech. Engrs.,* 181:45–54.

49. Dowson, D., Longfield, M. D., Walker, P. S., and Wright, V. (1968): An investigation of the friction and lubrication in human joints. *Proc. Inst. Mech. Engrs.,* 182:68–76.

50. Dowson, D. (1981): Basic tribology. In: *Introduction to the Biomechanics of Joints and Joint Replacement,* edited by D. Dowson and V. Wright, pp. 49–60. Mechanical Engineering Publications, London.

51. Dowson, D., Unsworth, A., Cooke, A. F., and Gvozdanovic, D. (1981): Lubrication of joints. In: *An Introduction to the Biomehanics of Joints and Joint Replacement,* edited by D. Dowson and V. Wright, pp. 120–145. Mechanical Engineering Publications, London.

52. Dowson, D., and Jin, Z.-M. (1986): Micro-elastohydrodynamic lubrication of synovial joints. *Eng. Med.,* 15:63–65.

53. Dowson, D., and Jin, Z. M. (1987): An analysis of micro-elastohydrodynamic lubrication in synovial joints considering cyclic loading and entraining velocities. In: *Proceedings 13th Leeds–Lyon Symposium on Tribology,* pp. 375–386.

54. Eberhart, H. D., Inman, V. T., and Saunders, J. B. de C. (1947): *Fundamental Studies of Human Locomotion and Other Information Relating to Design of Artificial Limbs.* University of California Press, Berkeley.

55. Eckstein, F., Muller-Gerbl, M., and Putz, R. (1992): Distribution of subchondral bone density and cartilage thickness in the human patella. *J. Anat.,* 180:425–433.

56. Eckstein, F., Sittek, H. Milz, E., Schulte, E., Kiefer, B., Reiser, M., and Putz, R. (1995): The potential of magnetic resonance imaging (MRI) for quantifying articu-

lar cartilage thickness—a methodological study. *Clin. Biomech.,* 8:4434–4440.

57. Eckstein, F., Lohe, F., Hillebrand, S., Bergmann, M. Schulte, E., Milz, S., and Putz, R. (1995): Morphomechanics of the humero-ulnar joint: I. Joint space width and contact areas as a function of load and flexion angle. *Anat. Rec.,* 243:318–326.

58. Eisenfeld, J., Mow, V. C., and Lipshitz, H. (1978): The mathematical analysis of stress relaxation in articular cartilage during compression. *Math. Biosci.,* 39: 97–111.

59. Fein, R. S. (1967): Are synovial joints squeeze film lubricated? *Proc. Inst. Mech. Engrs.,* 181:125–128.

60. Ferguson, J., Boyle, J. A., McSween, R. N. M., and Jasani, M. K. (1968): Observations on the flow properties of the synovial fluid from patients with rheumatoid arthritis. *Biorheology,* 5:119–131.

61. Frankel, V. H., and Burstein, A. H. (1971): *Orthopaedic Biomechanics.* Lea & Febiger, Philadelphia.

62. Freeman, M. A. R., and Meachim, G. (1979): Ageing and degeneration. In: *Adult Articular Cartilage,* 2nd ed., edited by M. A. R. Freeman, pp. 487–543. Pitman Medical Publishing, Kent.

63. Gardner, D. L. (1972): The influence of microscopic technology on knowledge of cartilage surface structure. *Ann. Rheum. Dis.,* 31:235–258.

64. Ghadially, F. N., Moshurchak, E. M., and Thomas, I. (1977): Humps on young human and rabbit articular cartilage. *J. Anat.,* 124:425–435.

65. Ghosh, S. K. (1983): A close-range photogrammetric system for 3-D measurements and perspective diagramming in biomechanics. *J. Biomech.,* 16:667–674.

66. Goodfellow, J., Hungerford, D. S., and Zindel, M. (1976).

67. Gu, W. Y., Lai, W. M., and Mow, V. C. (1993): Transport of fluid and ions through a porous-permeable charged-hydrated tissue, and streaming potential data on normal bovine articular cartilage. *J. Biomech.,* 26: 709–723.

68. Guo, X. E., Gibson, L. J., McMahon, T. A., Keaveny, T. M., and Hayes, W. C. (1994): Finite element modeling of damage accumulation in trabecular bone under cyclic loading. *J. Biomech.,* 27:145–155.

69. Gibbs, D. A., Merrill, E. W., and Smith, K. A. (1968): Rheology of hyaluronic acid. *Biopolymers,* 6:777–791.

70. Goldstein, S. A., Wilson, D. L., Sonstegard, D. S., and Mathews, L. S. (1983): The mechanical properties of human tibial trabecular bone as a function of metaphyseal location. *J. Biomech.,* 16:965–969.

71. Greenwald, A. S., and Haynes, D. W. (1972): Weight bearing areas in human hip joint. *J. Bone Joint Surg.,* 54B:157–163.

72. Greenwald, A. S. (1974): Joint congruence—a dynamic concept. In: *The Hip,* edited by W. H. Harris, pp. 3–22. C. V. Mosby, St. Louis.

73. Guilak, F., Ratcliffe, A., Lane, N., Rosenwasser, M. P., and Mow, V. C. (1994): Mechanical and biochemical changes in the superficial zone of articular cartilage in a canine model of osteoarthritis. *J. Orthop. Res.,* 12: 474–484.

74. Hamerman, D., and Schuster, H. (1958): Hyaluronate in normal human synovial fluid. *J. Clin. Invest.,* 37: 57–64.

75. Hamrock, B. J., and Dowson, D. (1978): Elastohydrodynamic lubrication of elliptical contacts for materials of low elastic modulus: I. Fully flooded conjunction. *J. Lubr. Technol.,* 100:236–245.

76. Hamrock B. J. (1994): *Fundamentals of Fluid Film Lubrication.* McGraw-Hill, New York.

77. Hardingham, T. E., Muir, H., Kwan, M. K., Lai, W. M., and Mow, V. C. (1987): Viscoelastic properties of proteoglycan solutions with varying proportions present as aggregates. *J. Orthop. Res.,* 5:36–46.

78. Higginson, G. R., and Unsworth, A. (1981): The lubrication of natural joints. In: *Tribology of Natural and Artificial Joints,* edited by J. H. Dumbleton, pp. 47–73. Elsevier Scientific, Amsterdam.

79. Hills, B. A., and Butler B. D. (1984): Surfactants identified in synovial fluid and their ability to act as boundary lubricants. *Ann. Rheum. Dis.,* 43:641–648.

80. Hills, B. A. (1989): Oligolamellar lubrication of joints by surface active phospholipid. *J. Rheum.,* 16:82–91.

81. Hills, B. A. (1995): Remarkable anti-wear properties of joint surfactant. *Ann. Biomed. Eng.,* 23:112–115.

82. Hlaváček, M. (1993): The role of synovial fluid filtration by cartilage in lubrication of synovial joints. I. Mixture model of synovial fluid. *J. Biomech.,* 26: 1145–1150.

83. Hlaváček, M. (1993): The role of synovial fluid filtration by cartilage in lubrication of synovial joints II. Squeeze-film lubrication: homogeneous filtration. *J. Biomech.,* 26:1151–1160.

84. Hodge, W. A., Fijan, R. S., Carlson, K. L., Burgess, R. G., Harris, W. H., and Mann, R. W. (1986): Contact pressure in the human hip joint measured *in vivo. Proc. Natl. Acad. Sci. USA,* 83:2879–2883.

85. Holmes, M. H., Lai, W. M., and Mow, V. C. (1985): Singular perturbation analysis of the nonlinear, flow-dependent, compressive stress-relaxation behavior of articular cartilage. *J. Biomech. Eng.,* 107:206–218.

86. Hooke, C. J., and O'Donoghue, J. P. (1972): Elasticohydrodynamic lubrication of soft, highly deformed contacts. *J. Mech. Eng. Sci.,* 14:34–48.

87. Hou, J. S., Holmes, M. H., Lai, W. M., and Mow, V. C. (1989): Boundary conditions at the cartilage–synovial fluid interface for joint lubrication and theoretical verifications. *J. Biomech. Eng.,* 111:78–87.

88. Hou, J. S., Mow, V. C., Lai, W. M., and Holmes, M. H. (1992): Squeeze film lubrication for articular cartilage with synovial fluid. *J. Biomech.,* 25:247–259.

89. Howell, D. S., Treadwell, B. V., and Trippel, S. B. (1992): Etiopathogenesis of osteoarthritis. In: *Osteoarthritis: Diagnosis and Medical/Surgical Management,* 2nd ed., edited by R. W. Moskowitz et al., pp. 233–252. W. B. Saunders, Philadelphia.

90. Jay, G. D., and Hong, B.-S. (1992): Characterization of a bovine synovial fluid lubricating factor. *Conn. Tissue Res.,* 28:71–98.

91. Jones, E. S. (1936): Joint lubrication. *Lancet,* 230: 1043–1044.

92. Jurvelin, J. S., Buschmann, M. D., and Hunziker, E. B. (1995): Characterization of the equilibrium response of bovine humeral cartilage in confined and unconfined compression. *Trans. Orthop. Res. Soc.,* 20:512.

93. Kapitza, P. L. (1955): Hydrodynamic theory of lubrication during rolling. *Zh. Tekh. Fiz.,* 25:747–762.

94. Keaveny, T. M., Watchtel, E. F., Guo, X. E., and Hayes, W. C. (1994): The mechanical properties of damaged trabecular bone. *J. Biomech.,* 27:1309–1318.

95. Kelkar, R., and Ateshian, G. A. (1995): Contact creep

response between a rigid impermeable cylinder and a biphasic cartilage layer using integral transforms. *Trans. ASME,* BED-29:313–314.

96. Khalsa, P. S., and Eisenberg, S. R. (1995): Direct measurement of axial and radial confining stresses in articular cartilage during uniaxial confined compression. *Trans. Orthop. Res. Soc.,* 20:519.

97. King, R. G. (1966): A rheological measurement of three synovial fluids. *Rheol. Acta,* 5:41.

98. Kirk, T. B., O'Neill, P. L., and Stachowiak, G. A. (1993): The effects of dehydration on the surface morphology of articular cartilage, *J. Orthop. Rheum.,* 6.2: 75–80.

99. Kirk, T. B., Stachowiak, G. A., and Wilson, A. S. (1994): The morphology of the surface of articular cartilage. In: *Proceedings 2nd World Congress of Biomechanics,* Stichting World Biomechanics, Nijmegen, The Netherlands, I:208a.

100. Kwan, M. K., Lai, W. M., and Mow, V. C. (1984): Fundamentals of fluid transport through cartilage in compression. *Ann. Biomed. Eng.,* 12:537–558.

101. Lai, W. M., Kuei, S. C., and Mow, V. C. (1978): Rheological equations for synovial fluids. *J. Biomech. Eng.,* 100:169–186.

102. Lai, W. M., and Mow, V. C. (1978): Ultrafiltration of synovial fluid by cartilage. *J. Eng. Mech. Div. Trans. ASCE,* 104:79–96.

103. Lai, W. M., and Mow, V. C. (1979): Flow fields in a single layer model of articular cartilage created by a sliding load. *Adv. Bioeng. Trans. ASME,* pp. 101–104.

104. Lai, W. M., Hou, J. S., and Mow, V. C. (1991): A triphasic theory for the swelling and deformation behaviors of articular cartilage. *J. Biomech. Eng.,* 113:245–258.

105. Levick, J. R. (1979): The influence of hydrostatic pressure on trans-synovial fluid movement and on capsular expansion in the rabbit knee. *J. Physiol.,* 331:1–15.

106. Levick, J. R. (1987): Synovial fluid and trans-synovial flow in stationary and moving normal joints. In: *Joint Loading,* edited by H. J. Helminen, et al., pp. 149–186. Wright, Bristol (England).

107. Lewis, P. R., and McCutchen, C. W. (1959): Experimental evidence for weeping lubrication in mammalian joints. *Nature,* 184:1284–1285.

108. Lewis, P. R., and McCutchen, C. W. (1960): Lubrication of mammalian joints. *Nature,* 185:920–921.

109. Linn, F. C., and Sokoloff, L. (1965): Movement and composition of interstitial fluid of cartilage. *Arthritis Rheum.,* 8:481–494.

110. Linn, F. C. (1967): Lubrication of animal joints: I. The arthrotrip-someter. *J. Bone Joint Surg.,* 49A: 1079–1098.

111. Linn, F. C. (1968): Lubrication of animal joints: II. The mechanism. *J. Biomech.,* 1:193–205.

112. Linn, F. C., and Radin, E. L. (1968): Lubrication of animal joints: III. The effect of certain chemical alterations of the cartilage and lubricant. *Arthritis Rheum.,* 11:674–682.

113. Lipshitz, H., Etheredge, R., and Glimcher, M. J. (1975): *In vitro* wear of articular cartilage. I. Hydroxyproline, hexosamine, and amino acid composition of bovine articular cartilage as a function of depth from the surface; hydroxyproline content of the lubricant and the wear debris as a measure of wear. *J. Bone Joint Surg.,* 57A:527–534.

114. Lipshitz, H., and Glimcher, M. J. (1979): *In vitro* stud-

ies of the wear of articular cartilage. II. Characteristics of the wear of articular cartilage when worn against stainless steel plates having characterized surfaces. *Wear,* 52:297–339.

115. Little, T., Freeman, M., and Swanson, S. A. V. (1969): Experiments on friction in the human hip joint. In: *Lubrication and Wear in Joints,* edited by V. Wright, p. 110. Sector, J. B. Lippincott Company, Philadelphia, pp. 110–114.

116. Longfield, M. D., Dowson, D., Walker, P. S., and Wright, V. (1969): "Boosted lubrication" of human joints by fluid enrichment and entrapment. *Biomed. Eng.,* 4:517–522.

117. Longmore, R. B., and Gardner, M. J. (1975): Development with age of human articular cartilage surface structure. *Ann. Rheum. Dis.,* 34:26–37.

118. MacConaill, M. A. (1932): The function of intra-articular fibrocartilages, with special references to the knee and inferior radio-ulnar joints. *J. Anat.,* 66:210–227.

119. Macirowski, T., Tepic, S., and Mann, R. W. (1994): Cartilage stresses in the human hip joint. *J. Biomech. Eng.,* 116:11–18.

120. Mak, A. F. (1986): The apparent viscoelastic behavior of articular cartilage—The contributions from the intrinsic matrix viscoelasticity and interstitial fluid flows. *J. Biomech. Eng.,* 108:123–130.

121. Mak, A. F., Lai, W. M., and Mow, V. C. (1987): Biphasic indentation of articular cartilage: Part I. Theoretical analysis. *J. Biomech.,* 20:703–714.

122. Malcom, L. L. (1976): *An experimental investigation of the frictional and deformational responses of articular cartilage interfaces to static and dynamic loading.* Ph.D. Thesis, University of California, San Diego.

123. Maquet, P. G., van de Berg, A. J., and Simone, J. C. (1975): Femorotibial weight-bearing areas. *J. Bone Joint Surg.,* 57A:766–771.

124. Maroudas, A. (1967): Hyaluronic acid films. *Proc. Inst. Mech. Eng.,* 181:122–124.

125. Maroudas, A. (1979): Physicochemical properties of articular cartilage. In: *Adult Articular Cartilage,* 2nd ed., edited by M. A. R. Freeman, pp. 215–290. Pitman Medical Publishing, Kent.

126. Martin, H. M. (1916): Lubrication of gear teeth. *Engineering,* 102:199.

127. Mattews, L. S., Sonstegard, D. A., and Henke, J. A. (1977): Load bearing characteristics of the patellofemoral joint. *Acta Orthop. Scand.,* 48:511–516.

128. McCutchen, C. W. (1962): The frictional properties of animal joints. *Wear,* 5:1–17.

129. McCutchen, C. W. (1966): Boundary lubrication by synovial fluid: demonstration and possible osmotic explanation. *Fed. Proc.,* 25:1061–1068.

130. Medley, J. B., Dowson, D., and Wright, V. (1984): Transient elasto-hydrodynamic lubrication models for the human ankle joint. *Eng. Med.,* 13:137–151.

131. Mente, P. L., and Lewis, J. L. (1994): Elastic modulus of calcified cartilage is an order of magnitude less than that of subchondral bone. *J. Orthop. Res.,* 12:637–647.

132. Morrison, J. B. (1968): Bioengineering analysis of force actions transmitted by the knee. *Biomed. Eng.,* 3: 154–170.

133. Morrison, J. B. (1970): The mechanics of the knee joint in relation to normal working. *J. Biomech.,* 3:51–61.

134. Mow, V. C. (1969): The role of lubrication in biomechanical joints. *J. Lubr. Technol.,* 91:320–329.

135. Mow, V. C., Lai, W. M., and Redler, I. (1974): Some surface characteristics of articular cartilage, Part I. *J. Biomech.*, 7:449–456.

136. Mow, V. C., and Lai, W. M. (1979): Mechanics of animal joints. *Ann. Rev. Fluid Mech.*, 11:247–288.

137. Mow, V. C., and Lai, W. M. (1979): The optical sliding contact analytical rheometer (OSCAR) for flow visualization at the articular surface. *Adv. Bioeng. Trans. ASME*, pp. 97–99.

138. Mow, V. C., and Lai, W. M. (1980): Recent developments in synovial joint biomechanics. *SIAM Rev.*, 22:275–317.

139. Mow, V. C., Kuei, S. C., Lai, W. M., and Armstrong, C. G. (1980): Biphasic creep and stress relaxation of articular cartilage in compression: Theory and experiments. *J. Biomech. Eng.*, 102:73–84.

140. Mow, V. C., Holmes, M. H., and Lai, W. M. (1984): Fluid transport and mechanical properties of articular cartilage: A review. *J. Biomech.*, 17:377–394.

141. Mow, V. C., Kwan, M. K., Lai, W. M., and Holmes, M. H. (1986): A finite deformation theory for nonlinearly permeable soft hydrated biological tissues. In: *Frontiers in Biomechanics*, edited by G. W. Schmid-Schonbein, S. L.-Y. Woo, and B. W. Zweifach, pp. 153–179. Springer-Verlag, New York.

142. Mow, V. C., and Mak, A. F. (1987): Lubrication of diarthrodial joints. In: *Handbook of Bioengineering*, edited by R. Skalak and S. Chien, pp. 5.1–5.34. McGraw-Hill, New York.

143. Mow, V. C. (1988): Molecular structure and function relationships for articular cartilage. *J. Educ. Inform. Rheum.*, 17:9–13.

144. Mow, V. C., and Rosenwasser, M. P. (1988): Articular cartilage: Biomechanics. In: *Injury and Repair of the Musculoskeletal Soft Tissues*, edited by S. L.-Y. Woo and J. A. Buckwalter, pp. 427–463. American Academy of Orthopaedic Surgery Press, Chicago.

145. Mow, V. C., Zhu, W., Lai, W. M., Hardingham, T. E., Hughes, C., Muir, H. (1989): The influence of link protein stabilization on the viscometric properties of proteoglycan aggregate solutions. *Biochim. Biophys. Acta*, 112:201–208.

146. Mow, V. C., Gibbs, M. C., Lai, W. M., Zhu, W., and Athanasiou, K. A. (1989): Biphasic indentation of articular cartilage—Part II. A numerical algorithm and an experimental study. *J. Biomech.*, 22:853–861.

147. Mow, V. C., Ratcliffe, A., and Poole, A. R. (1992): Cartilage and diarthrodial joints as paradigms for hierarchical materials and structures. *Biomaterials*, 13:67–97.

148. Mow, V. C., Ateshian, G. A., and Ratcliffe, A. (1992): Anatomic form and biomechanical properties of articular cartilage of the knee joint. In: *Biology and Biomechanics of the Traumatized Synovial Joint: The Knee as a Model*, edited by G. A. M. Finerman and F. R. Noyes, pp. 55–81. American Academy of Orthopaedic Surgery, Rosemont, IL.

149. Mow, V. C., Ateshian, G. A., and Spilker, R. L. (1993): Biomechanics of diarthrodial joints: A review of twenty years of progress. *J. Biomech. Eng.*, 115:460–467.

150. Mow, V. C., Bachrach, N. M., and Ateshian, G. A. (1994): The effects of a subchondral bone perforation on the load support mechanism within articular cartilage. *Wear*, 175:167–175.

151. Muir, H. (1983): Proteoglycans as organizers of the intercellular matrix. *Biochem. Soc. Trans.*, 11:613–622.

152. Muller-Gerbl, M. R., Putz, R., Kenn, R., and Kierse, R. (1993): People in different age groups show different hip joint morphology. *Clin. Biomech.*, 8:66–72.

153. Myers, R. R., Negami, S., and White, R. K. (1966): Dynamic mechanical properties of synovial fluid. *Biorheology*, 3:197–209.

154. Ogston, A. G., and Stanier, J. E. (1950): On the state of hyaluronic acid in the synovial fluid. *Biochem. J.*, 46:364–376.

155. O'Kelly, J., Unsworth, A., Dowson, D., Hall, D. A., and Wright, V. (1978): A study of the role of synovial fluid and its constituents in the friction and lubrication of human hip joints. *Eng. Med.*, 7:72–83.

156. Paul, J. P. (1980): Joint kinetics. In: *The Joints and Synovial Fluid*, Vol. II, edited by L. Sokoloff, pp. 139–176. Academic Press, New York.

157. Radin, E. L., Swann, D. A., and Weisser, P. A. (1970): Separation of a hyaluronate-free lubricating fraction from synovial fluid. *Nature*, 228:377–378.

158. Radin, E. L., and Paul, I. L. (1971): Response of joints to impact loading. I: *In vitro* wear. *Arthritis Rheum.*, 14:356–362.

159. Radin, E. L., Martin, R. B., Burr, D. B., Caterson, B. Boyd, R. D., and Goodwin, C. (1984): Effects of mechanical loading on the tissue of rabbit knee. *J. Orthop. Res.*, 2:221–234.

160. Radin, E. L., and Rose, R. M. (1986): Role of subchondral bone in the initiation and progression of cartilage damage. *Clin. Orthop. Rel. Res.*, 213:34–40.

161. Redler, I., and Mow, V. C. (1974): Biomechanical theories of ultrastructural alterations of articular surfaces of the femoral head. In: *The Hip*, edited by W. H. Harris, pp. 23–59. C. V. Mosby, St. Louis.

162. Redler, I., Zimny, M., Mansell, J., and Mow, V. C. (1975): The ultrastructure and biomechanical significance of the tidemark of articular cartilage. *Clin. Orthop. Rel. Res.*, 112:357–362.

163. Repo, R. U., and Finlay, J. B. (1977): Survival of articular cartilage after controlled impact. *J. Bone Joint Surg.*, 59A:1068–1076.

164. Reynolds, O. (1886): On the theory of lubrication and its application to Mr. Beauchamp Tower's experiment, including an experimental determination of the viscosity of olive oil. *Phil. Trans. R. Soc.*, 177:157–234.

165. Rhinelander, F. W., Bennett, G. A., and Bauer, W. (1939): Exchange of substances in aqueous solutions between joints and the vascular system. *J. Clin. Invest.*, 18:1–13.

166. Ropes, M. W., and Bauer, W. (1953): *Synovial Fluid Changes in Joint Disease.* Harvard University Press, Cambridge, MA.

167. Rushfeldt, P. D., Mann, R. W., and Harris, W. H. (1981): Improved techniques for measuring *in vitro* the geometry and pressure distribution in the human acetabulum: I. Ultrasonic measurement of acetabular surfaces, sphericity and cartilage thickness. *J. Biomech.*, 14:253–260.

168. Sandson, J. (1967): Human synovial fluid: Detection of a new component. *Science*, 155:839–841.

169. Sayles, R. S., Thomas, T. R., Anderson, J., Haslock, I., and Unsworth, A. (1979): Measurement of the surface microgeometry of articular cartilage. *J. Biomech.*, 12:257–267.

170. Scherrer, P. K., Hillberry, B. M., and Van Sickle, D. C.

(1979): Determining the *in vivo* areas of contact in the canine shoulder. *J. Biomech. Eng.,* 101:271–278.

171. Schurz, J., and Ribitsch, V. (1987): Rheology of synovial fluid. *Biorheology,* 24:385–399.

172. Seedhom, B. B., and Tsubuku, M. (1977): A technique for the study of contact between visco-elastic bodies with special reference to the patello-femoral joint. *J. Biomech.,* 10:253–260.

173. Seedhom, B. B. (1979): Transmission of the load in the knee joint with special reference to the role of the menisci: I. Anatomy, analysis and apparatus. *Eng. Med.,* 8:207–219.

174. Seedhom, B. B., and Hargreaves, D. J. (1979): Transmission of the load in the knee joint with special reference to the role of the menisci: II. Experimental results, discussion and conclusions. *Eng. Med.,* 8: 220–228.

175. Seireg, A., and Arvikar, R. J. (1975): The prediction of muscular load sharing and joint forces in the lower extremities during walking. *J. Biomech.,* 8:89–102.

176. Seller, P. C., Dowson, D., and Wright, V. (1971): The rheology of synovial fluid. *Rheol. Acta,* 10:2–7.

177. Setton, L. A., Zhu, W. B., and Mow, V. C. (1993): The biphasic poroviscoelastic behavior of articular cartilage in compression: Role of the surface zone. *J. Biomech.,* 26:581–592.

178. Setton, L. A., Mow, V. C., Muller, F. J., Pita, J. C., and Howell, D. S. (1994): Mechanical properties of canine articular cartilage are significantly altered following transection of the anterior cruciate ligament. *J. Orthop. Res.,* 12:451–463.

179. Simkin, P. A., and Nilson, K. L. (1981): Trans-synovial exchange of large and small molecules. *Clin. Rheum. Dis.,* 7:99–129.

180. Simon, W. H. (1970): Scale effects in animal joints. I. Articular cartilage thickness and compressive stress. *Arthritis Rheum.,* 13:244–256.

181. Smith, T. J., and Medley, J. B. (1987): Development of transient elasto-hydrodynamic models for synovial joint lubrication. In: *Proceedings of the 13th Leeds-Lyon Symposium on Tribology,* pp. 369–374.

182. Soby, L., Jamieson, A. M., Blackwell, J., Choi, H. U., and Rosenberg, L. C. (1990): Viscoelastic and rheological properties of concentrated solutions of proteoglycan subunit and proteoglycan aggregates. *Biopolymer,* 29:1587–1592.

183. Soslowsky, L. J., Flatow, E. L., Bigliani, L. U., and Mow, V. C. (1992): Articular geometry of the glenohumeral joint. *Clin. Orthop. Rel. Res.,* 288:181–190.

184. Soslowsky, L. J., Flatow, E. L., Bigliani, L. U., Pawluk, R. J., Ateshian, G. A., and Mow, V. C. (1992): Quantitation of *in situ* contact areas at the glenohumeral joint: A biomechanical study. *J. Orthop. Res.,* 10:524–534.

185. Sundblad. L. (1965): Glycosaminoglycans and glycoproteins in synovial fluid. In: *The Amino Sugars,* Vol. 2A, edited by E. A. Balazs and R. W. Jeanloz, pp. 229–250. Academic Press, New York.

186. Swann, D. A., and Radin, E. L. (1972): The molecular basis of articular lubrication: I. Purification and properties of a lubricating fraction from bovine synovial fluid. *J. Biol. Chem.,* 247:8069–8073.

187. Swann, D. A., Radin, E. L., Nazimiec, M., Weisser, P. A., Curran, N., and Lewinnek, G. (1974): Role of hyaluronic acid in joint lubrication. *Ann. Rheum. Dis.,* 33:318–326.

188. Swann, D. A. (1978): Macromolecules of synovial fluid. In: *The Joints and Synovial Fluid,* Vol. 1, edited by L. Sokoloff, pp. 407–435. Academic Press, New York.

189. Swann, D. A., Radin, E. L., and Hendren, R. B., (1979): The lubrication of articular cartilage by synovial fluid glycoproteins. *Arthritis Rheum.,* 22:665–666.

190. Swann, D. A., Silver, F. H., Slayter, H. S., Stafford, W., and Showe, E. (1985): The molecular structure and lubricating activity of lubricin from bovine and human synovial fluids. *Biochem. J.,* 225:195–201.

191. Thomas, T. R., Sayles, R. S., and Haslock, I. (1980): Human joint performance and the roughness of articular cartilage. *J. Biomech. Eng.,* 102:50–56.

192. Thompson, R. C., Oegema, T. R., Lewis, J. L., and Wallace, L. (1991): Osteoarthritic changes after acute transarticular load. *J. Bone Joint Surg.,* 73A:990–1001.

193. Unsworth, A., Dowson, D., and Wright, V. (1975): The frictional behavior of human synovial joints: I. Natural joints. *J. Lubr. Technol.,* 97:360–376.

194. Unsworth, A., Dowson, D., and Wright, V. (1975): Some new evidence on human joint lubrication. *Ann. Rheum. Dis.,* 34:277.

195. Vener, J. M., Thompson. R. C., Lewis, J. L., and Oegema, T. R. (1992): Subchondral damage after acute transarticular loading: An in vitro model of joint injury. *J. Orthop. Res.,* 10:759–765.

196. Walker, P. S., Dowson, D., Longfield, M. D., and Wright, V. (1968): "Boosted lubrication" in synovial joints by fluid entrapment and enrichment. *Ann. Rheum. Dis.,* 27:512–520.

197. Walker, P. S., Unsworth, A., Dowson, D., Sikorski, J., and Wright, V. (1970): Mode of aggregation of hyaluronic acid protein complex on the surface of articular cartilage. *Ann. Rheum. Dis.,* 29:591–602.

198. Walker, P. S. (1977): *Human Joints and Their Artificial Replacements.* Charles C. Thomas, Springfield, IL.

199. Wang, L. H., Ateshian, G. A. (1995): The velocity and compressive strain dependence of the cartilage equilibrium friction coefficient. *Adv. Bioeng. Trans. ASME,* BED-31:51–52.

200. Wang, H., and Ateshian, G. A. (1996): The normal stress effect of articular cartilage under steady frictional shear persists after removal of the surface zone. *Trans. Orthop. Res. Soc.,* p. 8.

201. Williams, P. F., Powell, G. L., and Laberge, M. (1993): Sliding friction analysis of phosphatidylcholine as a boundary lubricant for articular cartilage. *Proc. Inst. Mech. Engrs.,* 207:59–66.

202. Wismans, J., Veldpaus, F., Janssen, J., Huson, A., and Struben, P. (1980): A three-dimensional mathematical model of the knee-joint. *J. Biomech.,* 13:677–685.

203. Woo, S. L.-Y., Mow, V. C., and Lai, W. M. (1987): Biomechanical properties of articular cartilage. In: *Handbook of Bioengineering,* edited by R. Skalak and S. Chien, pp. 4.1–4.44. McGraw-Hill, New York.

204. Wright, V., and Dowson, D. (1976): Lubrication and cartilage. *J. Anat.,* 121:107–118.

205. Zhu, W., Lai, W. M., and Mow, V. C. (1991): The density and strength of proteoglycan–proteoglycan interaction sites in concentrated solutions. *J. Biomech.,* 24: 1007–1018.

206. Zhu, W., Mow, V. C., Rosenberg, L. C., and Tang, L. H. (1994): Determination of kinetic changes of aggrecan–hyaluronan interactions in solution from its rheological properties. *J. Biomech.,* 27:571–579.

Basic Orthopaedic Biomechanics, 2nd ed.,
edited by Van C. Mow and Wilson C. Hayes.
Lippincott–Raven Publishers, Philadelphia © 1997.

9

Biomechanics of Fracture Fixation

Edmund Y. S. Chao and Hannu T. Aro

*Orthopaedic Biomechanics Laboratory, Johns Hopkins University, Baltimore, Maryland 21205-2196;
and Department of Orthopaedic Surgery, University of Turku, Turku, Finland*

An understanding of basic biomechanical principles is essential throughout the care and management of patients with long-bone fractures. Each of the well-established fixation methods (rigid compression plating; reamed intramedullary nailing, with or without interlocking of the fracture fragments; and external fixation) has advantages and disadvantages as well as special biomechanical characteristics. Vast clinical experience, combined with the data produced from theoretical and experimental studies, has delineated many of the problems related to the biomechanics of these fracture fixation modalities. These findings have, in many cases, resulted in the improved design of the devices, yielding more reliable clinical results. Because of inherent differences, each of these methods seems to be the method of choice in certain fracture cases, and at present there is considerable agreement on the indications and contraindications for each method. Proper surgical technique must be utilized, however, to ensure the desired biomechanical outcome of the fixation and to avoid additional tissue trauma and devascularization at the fracture site.

Currently, satisfactory results have been achieved with long-bone fractures, even for high-grade open fractures. Modern guidelines for the treatment of intraarticular fractures, including anatomic reduction of the fragments and rigid internal fixation, have produced satisfactory results even in difficult situations. Still, in certain types of long-bone fractures, there sometimes are major treatment problems that require special attention, and, of course, operative management of fractures always involves the risk of infection, which can result in the development of chronic osteomyelitis or even in amputation. Undoubtedly, many complications originate from incomplete evaluation of the biomechanical characteristics of the fracture type and the inherent biomechanical limitations and physiological disadvantages of the fixation method selected.

In this chapter, an overview of fracture mechanics of long bones and the healing mechanisms of diaphyseal fractures under stable and unstable mechanical conditions is presented. Special emphasis is placed on the comparison of fracture fixation and bone-healing characteristics related to the use of rigid compres-

sion plates, intramedullary nails, and external fixators.

NORMAL BONE STRUCTURE AND REMODELING

Bone is a living tissue made rigid by the orderly deposition of minerals. It undergoes constant turnover, with simultaneous bone formation and resorption. There are two types of bone: compact (lamellar) bone and cancellous bone (Fig. 1). Lamellar bone exhibits a circular arrangement or "haversian" system. This system results from the formation of a tunnel, generally in a longitudinal direction in long bone, and the filling of the tunnel by layers of collagen that are concentrically organized and are bounded by cement lines. Cancellous bone is made of a network of trabeculae forming large marrow spaces, which contain hematopoietic cells and fat. Such lamellar, nonhaversian bone is made up of alternating bands of collagen oriented at slightly different angles to

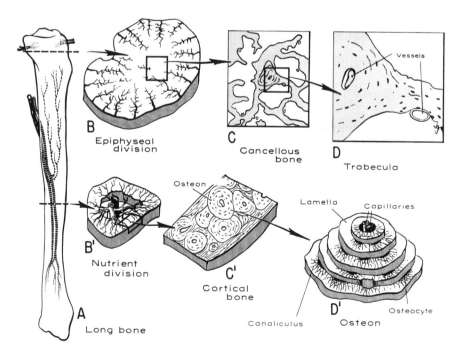

FIG. 1. Schematic diagram of the cancellous and cortical bone structure as related to their vascular network. Cancellous bone contains trabeculae with blood vessels located within and adjacent to the bone tissue. Cortical bone has osteons constructed by concentric lamellae with capillaries located centrally, thus forming the haversian system.

each other. Trabeculae are believed to have an optimal orientation and interconnection to resist compressive load (32).

The cellular components of lamellar and cancellous bone consist of lining cells (inactive osteoblasts), osteoblasts, osteoclasts, and osteocytes. Osteoblasts, derived from mesenchymal precursors, are cuboidal cells with a nucleus that generally lies in the cell opposite to the side of osteoid production. They form a sheet of cells closely packed together, lining the osteoid zone. The osteoid is the unmineralized organic matrix produced by osteoblasts that subsequently undergoes the mineralization process. In mature human lamellar bone, a layer of about 1 mm of osteoid is produced per day (bone appositional rate), and, during the following 10 days, it is subjected to an unknown process of maturation before it calcifies. The mean width of osteoid seams, therefore, is about 10 mm. Mineralization of the osteoid takes place at the mineralization front,

which is a narrow band about 2 to 3 mm in width that separates the osteoid border from the mineralized bone. The collagen fibrils of the osteoid become oriented into the orderly arrangement of lamellar bone except in areas where woven, nonlamellar bone is being laid down. Occasionally, an osteoblast becomes incorporated into the new matrix, connected to the osteoblast layer and more deeply embedded osteocytes by canaliculi. Woven bone, which is generally temporary, is the only type of bone that shows no lamellar pattern if viewed under polarized light microscopy. The collagen layers of woven bone are irregular in arrangement.

Cortical bone remodeling occurs through so-called haversian remodeling (formation of secondary osteons) (Fig. 2). Histologically, it consists of a "cutting cone" formed by a group of osteoclasts functioning in the hemispheric tip of a resorption canal. The close coupling of bone resorption and bone formation is one of the basic phenomena of bone remodeling,

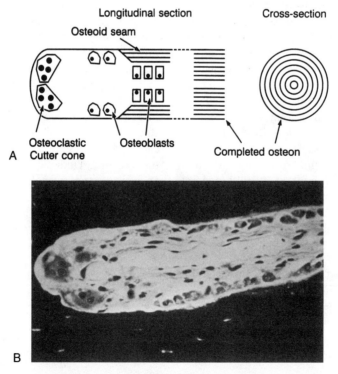

FIG. 2. A schematic diagram **(A)** and histologic section **(B)** illustrating cortical remodeling through the formation of secondary osteons.

which seems to occur not only in lamellar bone but also in cancellous bone. The mechanism of the coupling is poorly understood, but it is generally believed to be mediated through bone cell–derived growth factors.

FRACTURE MECHANISMS OF LONG BONES

Fractures can be classified according to the factors characterizing the force causing the fracture (Tables 1 and 2). Fractures caused by direct forces (Table 1) can be subclassified according to the magnitude and area distribution of the force as well as according to the rate at which the force acts on the bone. Soft tissue injury and fracture comminution are especially related to the loading rate. Trauma energy is dependent on the second power of loading rate, and this energy will be released when a bone fractures. Thus, high-velocity gunshot wounds result in considerably more soft tissue damage and bone comminution than low-velocity gunshot wounds as a result of application of a greater, more rapidly loaded force. The destructive effect of high-velocity bullets is further increased if the impact area (bullet dimension) is decreased.

Fractures caused by indirect forces are produced by a force acting at a distance from the fracture site. When a long bone is loaded, each section of the bone will be subject to both normal and shear stress. When these stresses exceed the limit of the bone, the bone will fracture. Different loads will generate different normal and shear stresses along different orientation planes within the bone. From the morphology of the fracture lines, it is possible to infer the type of indirect injury mechanism (Fig. 3; Table 2).

In general, depending on material strength, the three principal stress planes (maximum tensile stress plane, maximum compressive stress plane, and maximum shear stress plane) dictate the fracture plane and predict when and how the material will fail. Cortical bone as a material is generally weak in tension and shear, particularly along the longitudinal plane. Hence, cortical bone is an anisotropic material because its strength is directionally dependent. This will also influence bone fracture failure under external loads.

The failure patterns of long bones follow basic rules. Under bending, the convex side is under tension, and the concave side under compression. Because bone is more susceptible to failure in tension than in compression, the tension (convex) side fails first. Tension failure then occurs progressively across the bone, creating a transverse fracture without comminution. Occasionally, the cortex under compression breaks as a result of shear stress before the tension failure progresses all the way across the bone; the resulting comminution on the compression side often creates a single "butterfly" fragment or multiple fragments. Under torsion injury, there is always a certain bending moment that prevents the propagation of an endless spiral fracture line. The 45° fracture line (theoretically) is a result of maximum tensile stress acting at a 45° plane. Shear stress may cause small longitudinal cracks on the spiral fracture line. Under experimental conditions, an average fracture angle of a spiral fracture is approximately 30° of the longitudinal axis, and combined axial loading has little effect on the torsional properties of whole bone (48).

TABLE 1. *Classification of fractures of direct injury mechanism*

Type of force	Description of the force	Fracture characteristics
Tapping force	Small force acting on a small area	Nightstick fracture of ulna
Crushing force	High force acting on a large area	Crush fracture with comminution and severe soft tissue injury
Penetrating force	High force acting on a small area	"Open" fracture and minimal to moderate soft tissue disruption
Penetrating-explosive force	High force acting on a small area at a high or extremely high loading rate	"Open" fracture with severe soft tissue disruption and devitalized bone fragments

TABLE 2. *Classification of fractures of indirect injury mechanism*

Fracture type[a]	Example fractures	Injury force
Transverse	Some transverse patella fractures	Tension force
Oblique	Oblique or Y-fractures of the distal femur/humerus	Axial compressive force
Spiral	Spiral fracture of the tibia/humerus with intermittent longitudinal crack lines	Torsional force
Transverse	Transverse shaft fracture of the humerus/tibia, with small butterfly fragment	Bending force
Transverse oblique	Transverse shaft fractures of the tibia with large butterfly fragment	Axial compression and bending

[a]Fracture types are graphically demonstrated in Fig. 3 from right to left.

The susceptibility of a bone to fracture with a single injury is related to its energy-absorbing capacity and modulus of elasticity. The loading rate of bone affects its energy-absorption capacity. Bone undergoing rapid loading will absorb more energy than when loaded at a slower rate (43). However, at very high loading rates there is a decline in energy absorbed (48). The energy absorbed by the bone during loading is released when the bone fractures. This phenomenon helps to explain why injuries with rapid loading involving higher velocities dissipate greater energy and result in greater fracture comminution and displacement. The clinical estimation of fracture energy is of great value. Long-bone shaft fractures resulting from high-energy injuries have a higher rate of bone healing complications than fractures of low-energy injuries. This difference has been explained by the severity of soft tissue injury associated with high-energy injuries. Experimental studies (62) have demonstrated the retarding effect of muscle damage on bone healing.

Clinically, it is well known that spiral and oblique tibial fractures tend to heal faster than some transverse fractures. This difference in the inherent healing rate has commonly been related to the difference in the amount of soft tissue destruction, that is, to the difference of injury mechanism and fracture energy (33). Another variable is the increased surface area of fracture ends in oblique/spiral fractures. *In vitro* experiments have considered the differ-

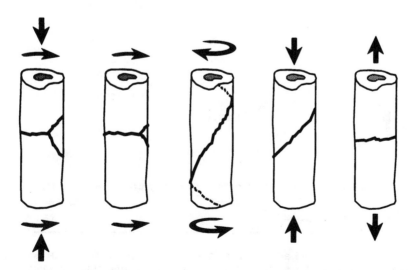

FIG. 3. Typical long-bone fracture morphology corresponding to the type of external load applied to the long bone. The fracture pattern may vary depending upon the magnitude of the composite loading mode involved.

ence in fracture energy under transverse and spiral failure of a loaded bone. Analysis of the load–displacement curves showed no statistically significant difference in the amount of energy absorption at failure (Fig. 4). However, the maximum load to failure was about three times greater on the side of transverse failure. This difference is due to the different stiffness properties of the bone under torsion and bending. Under torsion, the bone exhibited relatively low stiffness and, on average, 23° of deformation before failure. During bending, the bone is relatively stiff and undergoes, on average, only 8° of angulation before failure. Interestingly, the experiment does not suggest any difference in the amount of energy released when a bone develops a transverse or spiral fracture. However, the larger load under bending failure may cause the surrounding soft tissues and periosteum to sustain more damage and thus affect bone fracture healing potential.

The susceptibility of bone to fracture under fluctuating forces (or stresses) is related to its crystal structure and collagen orientation, which reflects the viscoelastic properties of the bone. Cortical bone is vulnerable to both tensile and compressive fluctuating stresses. Under each cycle of loading, a small amount of strain energy may be lost through microcracks along the cement lines. Fatigue load under certain strain rates can cause progressive accumu-

lation of microdamage in cortical bone. When such a process is prolonged, bone may eventually fail through fracture crack propagation. Although bone has rather poor fatigue resistance *in vitro*, it is a living tissue and can undertake a repair process simultaneously. Periosteal callus and new bone formation near the microcracks can arrest crack propagation by reducing the high stresses at the tip of the crack. However, for this repair process to be effective, a relatively low level of stress must be applied and maintained on the bone.

BIOLOGICAL AND BIOMECHANICAL CHARACTERISTICS OF FRACTURE CALLUS

Biological Processes of Fracture Healing

The unique feature of fracture healing is restoration of the original tissue structure with mechanical properties equal to those before fracture. Injured skin, muscle, and tendon are unable to copy such a real regeneration process after injury. Factors that influence fracture healing are both local and systemic (Table 3).

Fracture healing can be considered a series of phases occurring in sequence and also overlapping to a certain extent. The process can be divided into at least three distinct stages: inflammation, reparation, and remod-

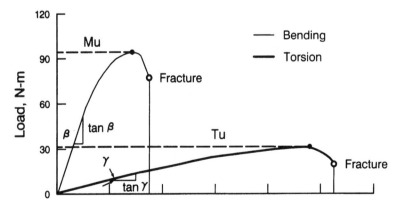

FIG. 4. Comparison of the load and angular deformity curve for canine tibiae under three-point bending and torsional load. Although the total energy to failure under torsion is approximately equal to that produced under bending, the ultimate load to failure for torsion (Tu) was substantially lower than the optimal load to failure through bending (Mu). Such difference in failure load may affect the degree of soft tissue and periosteum damage after bone fracture.

TABLE 3. *Factors influencing fracture healing*

Systemic	Local
Age	Degree of local trauma
Hormones	Vascular injury
Functional activity	Type of bone affected
Nerve functions	Degree of bone loss
Nutrition	Degree of immobilization
	Infection
	Local pathological conditions

eling (21). Fracture healing starts with interfragmentary stabilization by periosteal and endosteal callus formation. The process restores continuity, and bone union occurs by intramembranous and endochondral ossification. Avascular and necrotic areas of fracture ends are replaced by haversian remodeling. The induction and proliferation of undifferentiated periosteal callus tissue is the first critical step in fracture healing by external callus. Formation of such callus will be suppressed by rigid immobilization. Excessive fracture motion will also be equally harmful. Most importantly, the induction and proliferation periods of periosteal callus are finite.

The next critical phase of fracture healing involves the formation of an intact bony bridge between the fragments, and because this involves the joining of hard tissue, it follows that the whole system must become immobile at least momentarily (16). At this stage of healing, inefficient fracture immobilization by flexible stainless steel or plastic intramedullary rods (2,11) or by plates with low axial bending and torsional stiffnesses (67), as well as the presence of excessive fracture gap with no inherent fracture stability (42), may lead to a hypertrophic nonunion. This occurs because of the persistence of fibrous tissue or fibrous transformation of osteogenic callus tissue between the frontiers of bridging external callus. It seems that there is a narrow window for permissible interfragmentary motion, and the use of fixation flexibility as a method of callus stimulation at this stage would be difficult when the fracture-healing pathway has already committed to certain biological and mechanical conditions.

The final phase of fracture healing is governed by Wolff's law where bone is being remodeled back to its original shape and load-carrying strength. Weight bearing is important in order to allow the healing bone to be subject to normal stresses. The remodeling or modeling phase is a slow process, and adequate protection should be recommended to avoid refracture.

Biomechanical Properties of Healing Fractures

During the ossification process of external callus, the total amount of calcium per unit volume of callus shows approximately a fourfold increase, hydroxyproline (an indicator of total collagen content) a twofold increase, and the breaking strength of the callus in a tensile

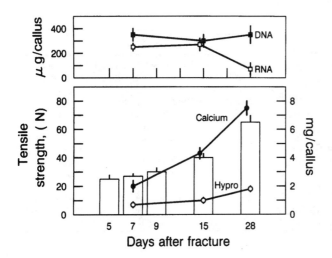

FIG. 5. Time-related change of nucleic acid in terms of DNA and mRNA *(upper diagram)*, calcium, and hydroxyproline contents and the mechanical strength *(lower diagram)* of fracture callus as a function of healing time (rat tibia model, *n* = 6). *Vertical bars* in the lower diagram represent the failure load of the callus in tensile test.

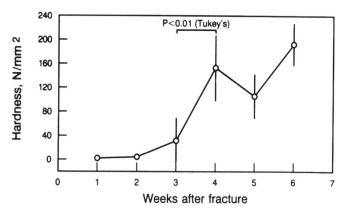

FIG. 6. Time-related change of callus hardness after initial bone fracture (rat tibia model). The increasing hardness with time reflects the differentiation of callus tissue to woven bone (1–4 weeks) and subsequent bone remodeling (4–6 weeks).

test a threefold increase (Fig. 5) (3). However, the chemical parameters of callus production (expressed by DNA and messenger RNA, as shown in Fig. 5) do not correlate with the strength at any time period of healing (45). Radiographic size of the external callus is a poor predictor of fracture strength (44) and does not indicate the quantities of chemical components in the fracture callus at a given healing time (2). The restoration of fracture strength and stiffness seems to be related to the amount of new bone connecting the fracture fragments (measured from the failure plane in the tensile test) rather than to the overall amount of uniting callus (7).

The structural properties of a healing fracture are dependent on the material properties of the uniting callus. To determine the material properties of callus tissue, experiments were performed in which uniform fracture callus specimens were loaded under axial compression using a spherical indenter at a low deformation rate (4,5). The results showed that the staged differentiation and mineralization of fracture callus have a profound influence on its compressive behavior (Fig. 6). Also, there was a high correlation between the hardness of the fracture callus and its mineral content, measured per tissue volume.

Over the whole period of fracture healing, four biomechanical stages can be defined (Table 4). These stages correlate with the pro-

gressive increases in average torque and energy absorption to failure as healing progresses and also with the average healing times (61).

Basic Mechanisms of Bone Fracture Union and Remodeling

In the 1960s, it was discovered that rigid compression plating of an osteotomy inhibits callus formation, and bone ends unite directly by haversian remodeling in contact areas (so-called contact healing) and noncontact areas (so-called gap healing) (52). Subsequently, fracture healing was divided into two patterns: primary bone healing and secondary (spontaneous) fracture healing. Spontaneous fracture

TABLE 4. *The four biomechanical stages of fracture repair*

Stage I	The bone fails through the original fracture site with a low stiffness, rubbery pattern.
Stage II	The bone fails through the original fracture site with a high stiffness, hard tissue pattern.
Stage III	The bone fails partially through the original fracture site and partially through the previously intact bone with a high stiffness, hard tissue pattern
Stage IV	The site of failure is not related to the original fracture site and occurs with a high stiffness pattern.

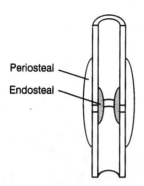

FIG. 7. Schematic diagram illustrating the non-osteonal bone healing mechanism with abundant periosteal callus and a small amount of endosteal callus without osteon formation across the fracture gap. The union of the fracture relies on maturation and remodeling of the periosteal osseous tissue with extensive remodeling processes of the fracture ends.

healing (healing with periosteal and endosteal callus formation) (Fig. 7) was considered "secondary" because, initially, an intermediate fibrous tissue or fibrocartilage is formed between the fracture fragments and only subsequently is replaced by new bone (53).

As a result of bone and soft tissue damage during trauma, the cortical ends at the fracture site are avascular and necrotic during the initial stages of healing. This inevitable vascular compromise does not prevent the avascular fracture ends from playing an important biomechanical role and serving as the mechanical supportive elements for any fixation device. Haversian remodeling has two main functions: (a) the revascularization of necrotic fracture ends and (b) reconstitution of the intercortical union. There are three requirements for the haversian remodeling across the fracture site: (a) exact reduction (axial alignment), (b) stable fixation, and (c) sufficient blood supply. The factors that initiate the dramatic increase of secondary osteons in healing fractures and influence the direction of their growth are not known. Fracture fragments that are deprived of their vascular supply for too long a period of time failed to be remodeled for years (53). This important observation clearly shows that the signal for the growth of secondary osteons after fracture is time limited, corroborating a theory of biochemical induction of haversian remodeling.

The growth of secondary osteons from one fracture fragment to another does not necessarily require intimate contact of fracture fragments. Even after perfect reduction, there are incongruencies at the fracture site that will result in small gaps interspersed with contact areas or even contact points. These gap regions are filled, within weeks after fracture with no lag period, by direct lamellar or woven new bone formation (appositional bone formation) (53). The boundary between the new bone and the original cortex is the weak link of the union process at this stage of healing (4,5). Secondary osteons use the gap tissue as a scaffold to grow from one fragment to another. Although this is the crucial step for the final union, the growth of secondary osteons results, paradoxically, in a transitory compulsory reduction of cortical bone density. The new bone in the gap also shows a similar "porotic change" as a part of the union process with the fragments (Fig. 8) (4,5).

In any form of fracture fixation, bone fragments under load will experience a certain amount of relative motion that, by unknown mechanisms, determines the morphologic features of fracture repair. Perren (46) proposed a hypothesis (so-called interfragmentary strain hypothesis) that refines the notion that the tissue response is affected by the local mechanical environment. This theory is not entirely consistent with the experimental results produced in the validation studies (18). The interfragmentary strain is defined as the ratio of the relative displacement of fracture ends (d, d', and d'') versus the initial gap width (G) (Fig. 9). Interfragmentary strain is believed to govern the type of tissue that forms between the fracture fragments. According to the theory, a balance between the local interfragmentary strain and the mechanical characteristics of the callus tissue is the determining factor in the course of both primary bone healing and spontaneous fracture healing (Fig. 10).

It is important to realize that interfragmentary strain is inversely proportional to the fracture gap size. In the presence of a small

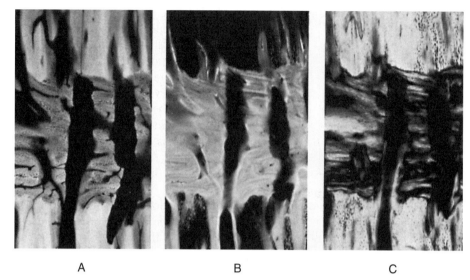

A   B   C

FIG. 8. Histologic appearance of gap healing with osteons crossing the osteotomy gap (canine tibia model). **A:** Microradiograph of gap healing with osteons. **B:** Ultraviolet light microscopy of the same section. **C:** Polarized light microscopy of the same sections. Note transverse orientation of collagen fibers in the gap.

gap, moderate interfragmentary motion can increase the strain to the extent that the progress of tissue differentiation is not possible. To circumvent this situation, small sections of bone near the fracture gap may undergo resorption, thus making the fracture gap larger and reducing the overall strain (Fig. 11). This important biological response is histologically evident in gap-healing areas of fractures treated by rigid external fixation (Fig. 12) (4,5).

The original interfragmentary strain theory considered only longitudinal strains associated with the applied interfragmentary strain. Analytic three-dimensional analyses (22) revealed that interfragmentary motion applied to a plate–bone–gap system resulted in a complex gap deformation and multidirectional principal strains. However, the interface between the fracture fragment ends and the gap tissue represented a critical plane of high distortion containing maximum principal strain magnitudes

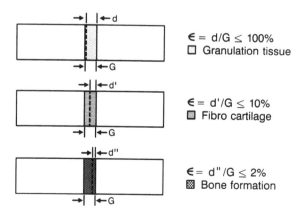

$\epsilon = d/G \leq 100\%$
□ Granulation tissue

$\epsilon = d'/G \leq 10\%$
▨ Fibro cartilage

$\epsilon = d''/G \leq 2\%$
▨ Bone formation

FIG. 9. The concept of interfragmentary strain theory as reflected by the type of tissue formation as a function of the magnitude of the strain occurring in the tissue located in the fracture gap. The strain (ϵ) is defined as the ratio of the fragment relative motion (d, d', d'') and the original gap (G) between the bone fragments. Fracture healing results in a gradual decrease of interfragmentary motion (d, d', d''). Different tissues can sustain different maximum tensile strains before failure.

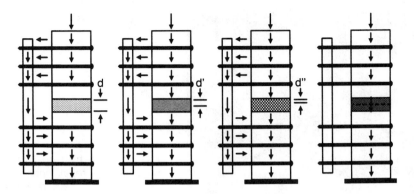

(d>d'>d" Gap motion decreases due to tissue transformation)

FIG. 10. Adaptation of the interfragmentary strain theory to explain fracture healing under external fixation. When the fracture gap tissue has a low modulus, bone stress will pass mainly through the fixation pins and the side bar, bypassing the fracture gap. As the fracture callus begins to mature, more bone stress will pass through the fracture site, thereby releasing the load passing through the external fixation side bars.

and severe endosteal-to-periosteal strain gradients. With bone resorption and callus formation, the largest strain reductions (up to 50%) occurred in these gaps, confirming the original hypothesis.

During the past few years, several experimental studies of external fixation with controlled mechanical conditions of osteotomy healing (1,4,5,30,63) have suggested that there are many combinations of the healing processes. Also, clinical experience has indicated that "callus-free healing" after dynamic compression plating (DCP) is not the rule (54).

Therefore, a modified bone union classification (Table 5) is considered in place of the oversimplified terms "primary bone healing" and "secondary bone healing." The modified classification emphasizes the mechanism of cortical reconstruction (osteonal versus nonosteonal union). In addition, the classification includes contact healing, which can occur with or without external callus, and the gap healing

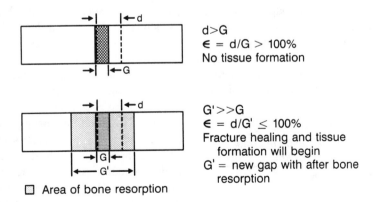

$d>G$
$\epsilon = d/G > 100\%$
No tissue formation

$G'>>G$
$\epsilon = d/G' \leq 100\%$
Fracture healing and tissue
    formation will begin
$G' = $ new gap with after bone
    resorption

☐ Area of bone resorption

FIG. 11. The extension of the interfragmentary strain theory in large fracture gaps. Under such situations, the bone near the fracture gap will undergo a resorption process in order to increase the fracture gap, thus decreasing the overall tissue strain (ϵ). Consequently, the tissue maturation may occur if the interfragmentary motion can be maintained at a low level. d, interfragmentary motion; G, original fracture gap; G', fracture gap after bone end resorption.

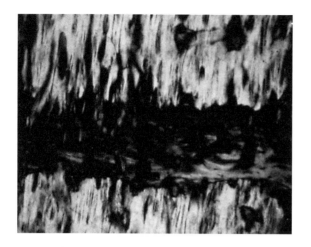

FIG. 12. The histologic appearance of bone fracture repair under rigid external fixation with constant fracture gap. Newly formed woven bone has a transverse orientation. The rough edge at the cortical ends represents bone resorption.

mechanism, which can be achieved when the fracture ends are not in intimate contact (Figs. 13 and 14). The gap healing mechanism also can occur with or without external callus formation (2). The term of primary bone union was originally a radiographic definition, where the lack of external callus formation and the gradual disappearance of the narrow fracture line served as the main criteria (53). This clinically accepted terminology is maintained in the modified classification. Accordingly, secondary bone union means a healing mechanism of substantial radiographic external callus formation. The histologic criteria for the gap healing mechanisms are (a) the formation of lamellar bone in the fracture gap with perpendicular orientation of collagen to the bone axis and (b) the growth of secondary osteons through this lamellar bone from one fragment to another. Nonosteonal bone union includes all the healing patterns that do not exhibit the

TABLE 5. *Classification of bone union mechanisms*

I. Nonosteonal bone union
II. Osteonal bone union
    Primary bone healing
      a. Primary contact healing
      b. Primary gap healing
    Secondary bone healing
      a. Secondary contact healing
      b. Secondary gap healing

direct growth of osteons across the fracture site. The reasons for nonosteonal bone union are (a) axial malalignment, (b) excessive fracture gap, or (c) unstable fixation in the presence of axial alignment. The critical gap size is not completely known but seems to be within the limit of 1 mm as previously suggested (53).

The biomechanical basis for the modified classification is the crucial role of cortical reconstruction to regain the ultimate bone union strength. Cortical reconstruction is the best radiologic indicator of bone union strength (44). The strength of bone union seems to be related to the number of osteons crossing the union site (17). However, it is still unproved whether osteonal fracture healing shortens the time to the return of normal bone strength and stiffness compared with nonosteonal fracture healing. During early stages of fracture healing, the formation of external callus is mechanically sound to cover the lag period before the activation of haversian remodeling during osteonal bone repair, indicating the benefits of secondary, osteonal bone healing. Static compression of bone fragments is not a prerequisite of contact healing. Dynamic compression of bone fragments (obtained by axial dynamization of external fixation without jeopardizing the torsional and bending rigidity of fixation) results in contact healing with periosteal callus formation (5).

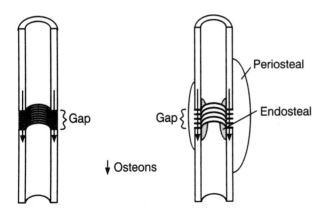

FIG. 13. Schematic diagrams illustrating primary *(left)* and secondary *(right)* gap healing mechanisms under rigid external fixation. The primary healing mechanism does not show substantial radiographic external callus formation. The *arrows* indicate the intracortical secondary osteons' bridging direction across the fracture gap. Formation of periosteal callus under rigid external fixation is related to high axial compression through weight bearing.

The challenge of biomechanical research on fracture healing is to improve the biomechanics of fracture fixation so that, after satisfactory reduction, a fracture can heal through the secondary bone union mechanism. This goal seems to be relevant for the improvement of both plate fixation (67) and external fixation methods (14). This question is less critical in intramedullary nailing. Reamed intra-

medullary nailing results in axial alignment of the bone fragments while permitting axial dynamic compaction, and thus, the nailed fracture heals with external callus followed by osteonal reconstruction of the cortex.

MECHANICAL PROPERTIES OF INTERNAL AND EXTERNAL FIXATION DEVICES

An increasing variety of devices for both internal and external fixation of fractures has made it necessary to quantify the rigidity of the fixation they provide in order to properly evaluate their effects on fracture healing. The structural rigidity (or stiffness) of a fixation device can be determined *in vitro* using a universal mechanical testing machine. The device is applied to an osteotomized cadaver or synthetic bone. The bone ends of the device–bone system are then loaded under axial compression, bending in two planes, and in torsion. During each mode of loading, the load-versus-deformation curve is recorded and subsequently analyzed to define the three basic stiffness parameters: axial, bending (flexural), and torsional stiffness. In each load–deformation curve, the slope of the linear portion of the curve is defined as the fixation rigidity or stiffness (Fig. 15).

By using this type of testing procedure of device–bone systems, it is possible to compare the stiffness of different types of fixa-

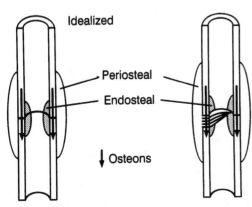

FIG. 14. Schematic diagrams illustrating the secondary contact healing mechanism. This bone-healing pattern is characterized by periosteal callus formation and direct cortical reconstruction by secondary osteons. Even under contact healing, as illustrated on the right diagram, there will be small gaps asymmetrically located around the circumference of the bone cortex. Thus, contact healing does not imply that the entire cortex will undergo the contact healing mechanism. Primary contact healing (not shown) is characterized by equivalent direct cortical reconstruction but without substantial periosteal new bone formation.

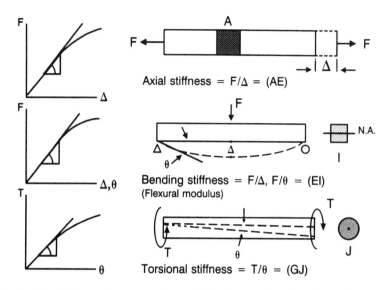

FIG. 15. Using the load deformation curve for each loading mode, the slope of the linear portion of the curve will be used to define the structural rigidity or stiffness property of the intact bone or the bone fragments fixed with either internal or external fixation devices.

tion. In an experimental study (Fig. 16) (64), plate fixation, intramedullary nailing, and external fixation devices of two different configurations were compared. The study utilized osteotomized cadaver canine tibias, and the stiffness of each fixation device was expressed as a percentage of the intact bone stiffness. The stiffness patterns of the different fixation methods were mismatched. The plated bones behaved like intact bones under the different loading conditions. The stiffness properties of the external fixators with full pins or half pins were different in magnitude, but they followed a similar pattern. Osteotomies stabilized by fluted intramedullary rods showed, compared with other devices, low bending and torsional stiffnesses. In this experiment, bone ends were in contact during loading. Therefore, the measured distraction stiffness values in this particular experiment describe the inherent axial stiffness of each method in the absence of fracture contact.

Mechanical Performance of External Fixation

As evident, the axial stiffness of external fixation tends to be low. The axial stiffness of

most frames and pin configurations (using simulated clinical dimensions) varies between 2,000 and 4,000 N/cm (10,15,24,41), which means partial weight bearing (about 20 kilograms) causes 0.5 to 1.0 mm axial cyclic movement of fracture fragments if the fracture ends are not in contact. This biomechanical characteristic of external fixation emphasizes the importance of considering the effects of weight bearing together with the frame and pin configuration used (Fig. 17) and the modes of fracture reduction. Using *in vitro* standard testing conditions, it is possible to determine how the mode of fracture reduction (contact with or without compression versus neutralization) and the type of fracture (stable versus unstable) affects the stability of a fixation method. In the *in vitro* experimental model, paired canine tibias were used. One bone of each pair was osteotomized and fixed with a unilateral external fixator. Osteotomy was performed transversely in five pairs of bones (a model of stable fracture), and an oblique osteotomy (45°) was performed in the other five pairs of bones. The rigidity of fixation provided by the fixator was compared with the contralateral intact bone. The osteotomized bone was loaded in

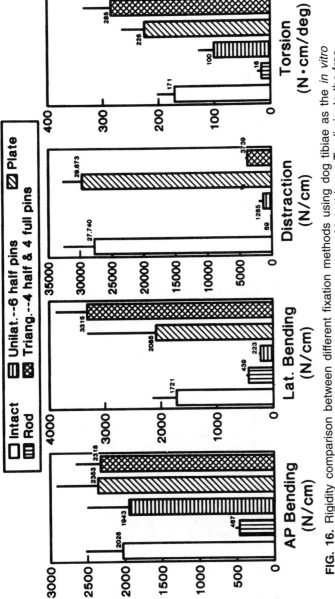

FIG. 16. Rigidity comparison between different fixation methods using dog tibiae as the *in vitro* model. All the fixation stiffness values are compared with that of intact bone. To eliminate the fracture site effect, only distraction was included in the axial loading mode (64).

Legend:
□ Intact 🎜 Unilat.--6 half pins ▨ Plate
▥ Rod ▧ Triang.--4 half & 4 full pins

AP Bending (N/cm)
- Intact: 2028
- Rod: 467
- Unilat.: 1643
- Plate: 2353
- Triang.: 2318

Lat. Bending (N/cm)
- Intact: 1721
- Rod: 439
- Unilat.: 223
- Plate: 2065
- Triang.: 3315

Distraction (N/cm)
- Intact: 27,740
- Rod: 69
- Unilat.: 1285
- Plate: 26,673
- Triang.: 3739

Torsion (N·cm/deg)
- Intact: 171
- Rod: 16
- Unilat.: 100
- Plate: 226
- Triang.: 285

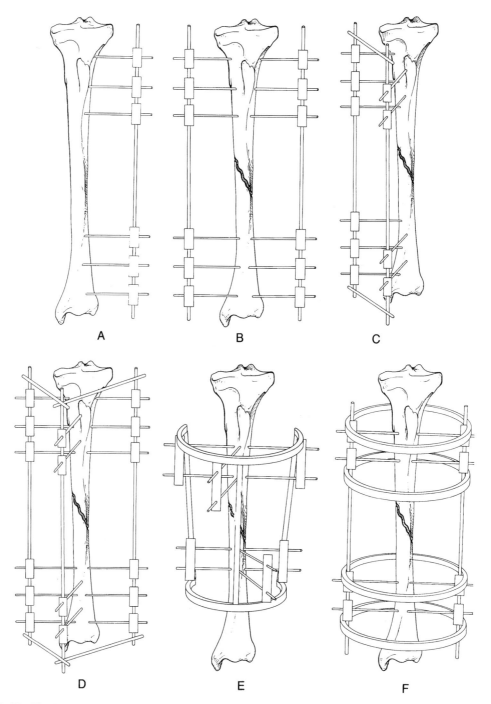

FIG. 17. The basic frame configurations and pin arrangements in external fixation. **A:** Unilateral half-pin device. **B:** Bilateral or quadrilateral full-pin device. **C:** Triangular half-pin device. **D:** Triangular full-pin plus half-pin device. **E:** Semicircular full-pin and half-pin device. **F:** Circular full-pin and half-pin device. The full pins in configurations **E** and **F** can be replaced by K-wire under high tension.

contact mode of fixation (osteotomy ends in contact) as well as in the presence of fracture gap. The results showed that simulated stable fractures (transverse osteotomies) fixed in the contact bone behaved like contralateral intact bones in all loading modes except in anteroposterior bending. On the other hand, axial stability was much greater in contact healing and in the stable fracture configurations. These findings emphasize that the axial rigidity of the bone–fixator system is crucially dependent on the type of fracture and the modes of reduction.

During the past few years, there has been an increasing interest in circular external fixation configurations (Fig. 17E and F), especially for certain reconstructive procedures. These devices generally use four pairs of crossed Kirschner wires (diameter approximately 2 mm or less) that are held under high tension by screws on circular or semicircular frames. The wires can be oriented at different angles across the bone, and tension in the pins provides fixation rigidity. Mechanical performance of the Volkov–Oganesian fixator using pretensioned K-wires (41) showed low overall fixation stiffness, especially in the axial direction, relative to the standard Hoffman–Vidal quadrilateral frame (Fig. 18). As expected, the bending stiffness of the frame was

independent of the loading direction. Consequently, the device showed a high anteroposterior bending stiffness, which is usually low in unilateral and bilateral noncircular configurations. The rigidity of the circular frame device with K-wires is dependent on wire tension, wire group separation on either side of the fracture, and ring diameter. This type of fixator also exhibited a nonlinear stiffness behavior mainly due to the large deflection of the thin wires (28). A disadvantage of this type of fixation, aside from the complexity of the frame and its application, is the possible sliding action of the bone fragment over the wires during functional loading. The use of threaded wires can eliminate such motion, but the threads may significantly weaken the strength of the wire as it must sustain extremely high tension due to pre-tension plus loading.

The stiffness of an internal fixation system can be achieved in a bone-external fixator system if adequate reduction (contact of fracture surfaces) can be achieved. Table 6 includes the major factors in determination of external fixation rigidity. These variables have different effects on the axial, bending, and torsional stiffness, and varying these key parameters to achieve a desired fracture stability is possible. In general, bilateral configurations (using full

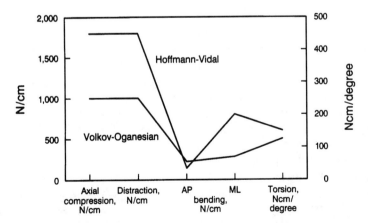

FIG. 18. Comparison of fixation stiffness between the Hoffmann–Vidal quadrilateral fixator and the Volkov–Oganesian semicurcular fixator with cross K-wires. Aside from the slight increase in AP bending, the K-wire device showed significant reduction in medial lateral bending and axial loading. The small axial stiffness is the basic characteristic of an external fixation utilizing cross K-wires.

TABLE 6. *Key factors in increasing the rigidity of external fixation*

Increased pin diameter
  Increased pin number
  Decreased side-bar separation
  Decreased pin separation
  Increased pin group separation

pins) show 50% higher overall rigidity than unilateral configurations (using half pins). However, unilateral external fixators with increased pin diameter (15) or with one-plane or two-plane frame geometries (6) can provide stiffness characteristics comparable to bilateral configurations. Knowledge of the mechanical performance of external fixators is essential if one considers adjusting (decreasing or increasing) the stiffness of external fixation as a means to manipulate bone healing progress.

In the clinical situation, the overall rigidity of a fixation system is dependent on both the frame used and on the pin configuration (Fig. 17). A theoretical model can be used to predict the mechanical performance of standard unilateral or bilateral fixators under any combination of pin and frame parameters (13,35). Many aspects of the fracture-fixation construct bear on the amount of interfragmentary motion. This, in turn, influences the mode of fracture healing. Equally important factors are the type of fracture, the accuracy of reduction, the amount of physiological loading, and the performance of the pin–bone interface. These facts are true regardless of the fixation employed.

Clinical experience (23,29) as well as both two-dimensional and three-dimensional finite element analyses (13,34,35) have clearly identified the biomechanical and other factors that are involved in the pathogenesis of pin loosening and subsequent infection. The results of recent animal experimental studies (4,5,49) have corroborated and also expanded the theoretical predictions. This knowledge has aided efforts to improve the design of fixators and fixation pins, and clinically it gives measures to prevent pin tract complications.

Biomechanically, there are four distinct factors to improve the performance of the pin–bone interface (Table 7) There seems to be a race between the gradually increasing load-carrying capacity of a healing bone and failure of the pin–bone interface. Under various loading modes, pins are primarily subjected to bending. In unstable fractures, the bone stress at the pin tract can approach a very high level, which may create localized yielding failure. Such stresses can be reduced by increasing the bending rigidity of the pin (high-modulus pin material, large pin diameter), reducing the side-bar separation, and applying a full-pin configuration. Half-pins generate high stress primarily at the entry cortex. Stress-related pin–bone failures of half-pins occur mainly at the entry cortex. According to analytic studies, the location of maximum stress within a pin group varies according to the loading mode. To avoid high pin–bone interface stresses, weight bearing should be avoided in fractures without cortical contact. Axial dynamization of an external fixator, on the other hand, restores the cortical contact in stable fractures and thus decreases the pin–bone stresses. Undoubtedly, the surgical pin insertion technique must also play a very important role for the uneventful performance of the pin–bone interface. If the pin insertion technique is inadequate (such as eccentric location of the pins or thermal necrosis of the bone tissue from the use of a power drill), the loosening and failure at the pin–bone interface can be predicted. The measurement of pin insertion torque, at least with the use of tapered fixation pins, seems to be a good indicator if the applied pin is eccentrically (through one cortex) in the bone.

TABLE 7. *Biomechanical factors in prevention of pin-tract problems*

Pin geometry and thread design
  Bone thread preparation
  Pin insertion technique
  Pin-bone stress

Mechanical Performance
of Compression Plate Fixation

The importance of accurate reduction of fracture fragments and the secure permanent contact of fracture fragments is a general principle in fracture management. The goal of bringing the entire fracture surfaces into contact and compressing the fracture surfaces by a fixation device is the widely known principle of rigid compression plating (Table 8). This principle was developed to improve the rigidity of plate fixation, i.e., to prevent the micromotion of fracture fragments that results in fracture end resorption (46). Fracture end resorption jeopardizes the rigidity of plate fixation by reducing contact between the fragments. Rigidly plated bones cannot shorten and establish contact; thus a gap is left, which may result in delayed union.

Interfragmentary compression means any type of constant, static compression exerted across the surfaces of fracture fragments. Two basic principles of action of interfragmentary compression are preload and friction between the plate and the bone cortex and between the bone fragment surfaces. Preloading means

creating compression that will prevent any separation of the fracture surfaces as long as the amount of preload is greater than the functional load (bending or distraction) that tends to separate the fragments. Friction prevents axial sliding under distraction and tangential displacement under shear or torsion. Table 8 summarizes the important principles of compression plate application.

An undesirable consequence of the use of rigid compression plates is postunion osteopenia, which means porotic transformation of the cortex beneath the plate with a net decrease of bone mass and with impaired mechanical properties of the healed bone. This phenomenon has been described in great detail in experimental studies (8,56,59,60,67). It has been related to the occurrence of refractures after plate removal. Most investigators believe that the structural change is secondary to the overprotection of the underlying bone from normal stresses ("stress protection"). Experimental studies have offered three potential solutions, reviewed by Woo and coworkers (67), to overcome these disadvantages: (a) continue to use rigid plates but modify the timing of plate removal, (b) use biologically degradable materials for internal fixation plates, and (c) use a fracture fixation system of reduced rigidity. The main problem of nonrigid systems is that such fixation may fail to ensure the main goal of treatment, i.e., union of the fracture.

The prevalence of postunion osteopenia in plated human fractures is unknown. There is also some controversy about the mechanism causing postunion osteopenia. In animal studies, comparatively large plates are often applied to small bones, and the amount of stress protection has been out of proportion (19,20). The concept that cortical transformation under the plate is related to the "stress protection" includes an assumption that the applied rigid plate is still firmly attached to the underlying bone months or even years after surgery. Recently, Cordey and Perren (19,20) suggested that the limit of frictional transmission between a plate and bone may be reached under certain loading conditions, resulting in

TABLE 8. *Biomechanical principles of rigid compression plating*

Plate positioning: Plate should be applied such that acting forces tend to close the fracture site (applying the plate to the convex or tensile surface of the bone).
Interfragmentary compression: Fixation should produce a sufficiently high amount of compression to increase rigidity and to counteract tension and shear forces under functional load.
Prebending of plate: Use of prebent plates results in more uniform compressive contact stresses across the fracture site, initially to prevent opposite cortex opening.
Plate screws: To allow screws engaging the full cortex. It is important to use screws close to the fracture site to reduce unsupported length.
Lag screw compression fixation: A screw may also be used to compress fracture surfaces as a "lag screw." Lag screw compression fixation, protected by a neutralization plate, reduces fracture gap displacement and thus promotes primary or osteonal bone fracture healing.

Adapted from refs. 31 and 47.

plate loosening, followed by bone resorption and cortical thinning under the plate. At present, there are no data to show how rigidly a plate is fixed to a human bone, for example, 2 years after plating. Experimental studies (36) have shown low removal torques of screws in plated bones at 16 to 32 weeks, suggesting that plates are not firmly pressed on bones after a certain time period. Using quantitative bone densitometry, Schwyzer et al. (54) performed computed tomography of human tibias after fracture plate removal (about 18 months after plating of a fracture). The bone density at the fracture site was reduced by an average of 8%, which was not considered to increase the risk of refracture. The average bone loss was offset by an increase in the total area of the bone.

Mechanical and Biological Characteristics of Intramedullary Nails

In 1940, Kuntscher introduced the closed intramedullary nailing technique of the femur and, in 1950, added reaming of the medullary canal to improve the contact between the nail and the cortical wall for better stability of the fixation (39). Reaming allows the placement of a large nail that resists bending, thus allowing early mobilization of the limb without plaster support. At present, there is an increasing agreement that Kuntscher's method, supplemented with interlocking design, is the treatment of choice for essentially all closed fractures of the femur located between the lesser trochanter and femoral condyles, regardless of the fracture pattern or degree of comminution (66).

Intramedullary nailing has some favorable biomechanical features. A proper nailing technique, including the correct point of pin insertion and prevention of eccentric reaming of the medullary cavity (65), places the neutral axis of the nail–bone structure at the center of the bone itself. Axial alignment, a natural consequence of the introduction of a fitted medullary nail after reaming, restores the load-bearing capacity of a bone with a frac-

ture in the isthmus region of the shaft, allowing protected early weight bearing. Plate fixation, after perfect reduction, also restores such an anatomic condition but does not allow weight bearing until partial bone union has occurred because the neutral axis of the plate–bone system is along the plate, and dynamic forces may result in fatigue breakage of the plate or the screws under bending or torsion.

The intramedullary fixation is mainly based on elastic three-point contact in a longitudinal direction, and reaming prepares a cylindrical channel of uniform diameter for a firm fit of the nail. Outside the isthmus region, the medullary cavity is large, and conventional Kuntscher nailing does not generally provide sufficient rotational stability in proximal and distal fractures. In addition, in comminuted fractures, a regular nail does not prevent axial telescoping and hence may cause fracture collapse and loss of reduction. To overcome these biomechanical difficulties, the interlocking intramedullary nail concept was introduced (Fig. 19). The biomechanical characteristics of interlocking nails are different from those of conventional closed Kuntscher nails (37,38), and functional rehabilitation must be adjusted to complement the unique biomechanical characteristics of the nailing technique. Following insertion of threaded bolts on both sides of the fracture (so-called static interlocking nailing), forces are transmitted from the intact bone tube proximally via the bolt through the nail which span the fracture site and back to the intact cortical bone anchored distally by the transverse locking bolts. This type of fixation, without cortical contact, does not allow immediate weight bearing (37) because of the risk of nail fatigue failure. Interlocking nails can also be used to stabilize transverse and short oblique fractures above and below the isthmus using the bolts to lock the smaller fracture fragment (so-called dynamic interlocking nailing).

Fractures of the subtrochanteric region of the femur represent a difficult biomechanical problem in trauma surgery. The subtrochanteric region is an area of high stresses caused

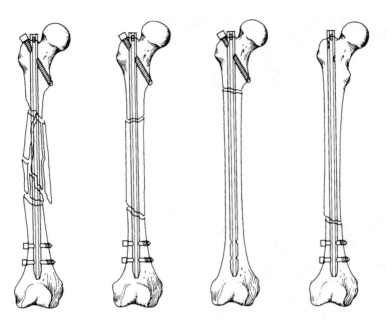

FIG. 19. Common fracture types amenable by interlocking intramedullary nailing using either proximal or distal, or both, interlocking features.

by bending moments and compressive forces. Fixation systems for fractures in this region are exposed to high stresses, even without ambulation. Flexion and extension of the hip, even while in bed, can produce forces at the femoral head as large as 2.5 to 3 times body weight, whereas slow walking can result in hip forces of up to 4.9 times body weight (51). Comminution of subtrochanteric fractures can further increase the stress applied to the implant because a comminuted bone cannot act as a load-sharing part of the fixation system. Tencer et al. (58) made a comparative study to evaluate the stabilization of simulated subtrochanteric fractures by different intramedullary and plate fixation implants (Fig. 20). They measured the torsional and bending stiffnesses of the implant-bone systems and compared these stiffness values with intact bone values. They also determined the maximum load-carrying capacity (failure load) of each device in combined bending and compression, a simulation of the action of weight bearing. All the intramedullary devices (including two types of interlocking nail and multiple Enders pins) showed low torsional

stiffness (maximum of 5% control of intact femur), whereas the plate–bone systems (blade plate or compression hip screw) had higher torsional stiffness (about 50% that of intact bone). In bending, all devices except Enders pins were about 80% as stiff as intact femora. As shown in Fig. 21, an interlocking nail system provided the highest failure loads under simulated weight bearing (between 300% and 400% of body weight). It should be emphasized that this study did not include fatigue testing of the bone–device system, which usually is the clinical cause of implant failure in subtrochanteric fractures.

Clinical experience (9,27,55) has indicated a high success rate in the treatment of subtrochanteric features of the femur by the use of interlocking nails. These results indicate that although the interlocking designs prevent relative rotation between the nail and the cortex, they do not change the inherent low torsional stiffness of the nail itself. This feature, in the case of intramedullary fixation, does not seem to be detrimental to bone-healing results. However, changes in nail designs (elimination of posterior slot) have been made to

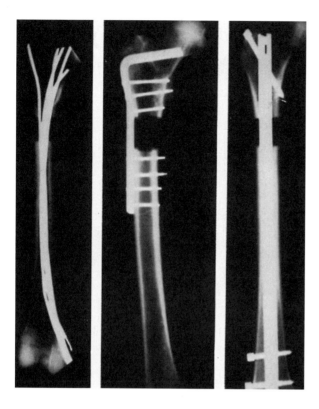

FIG. 20. Rigidity comparison for subtrochanteric fracture using Enders nails *(left)*, blade plate *(middle)*, and the Grosse-Kempf interlocking nail *(right)*.

improve torsional rigidity of the device (37,57). Such change may be efficacious because the slotted section provides the essential flexibility needed for the nail to follow the medullary cavity, whereas the combination of the slot and the cover-leaf profile (of the original Kuntscher nail) aids in fixation between the implant and bone. It should be emphasized that a low torsional stiffness of a device is not synonymous with torsional instability of the fixation system, which reflects uncontrolled motion between the nail and bone.

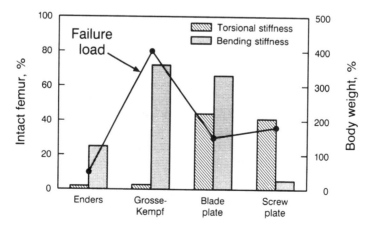

FIG. 21. Comparison of intramedullary and plate fixation devices in fixation of unstable subtrochanteric fractures of the femur. The bending stiffness (indicated by *bars* and expressed in percent of intact femur) and the failure load (indicated by *dots* connected by *lines* and expressed in percent of intact femur and percent of body weight) were highest for the Grosse-Kempf interlocking nail.

CHARACTERISTICS OF FRACTURE HEALING UNDER INTERNAL AND EXTERNAL FIXATION

The following series of animal experimental studies were done to evaluate the biomechanical and morphologic characteristics of fracture healing and remodeling under plate fixation, intramedullary nailing, and external fixation. Each experiment involved a paired comparison of fixation devices with different stiffness properties or a paired comparison of the different fixation modes of the same external fixator. The experiments were carried out using the same fracture model (canine tibial shaft osteotomy) to eliminate other variables (such as the extent of soft tissue injury, the variation of fracture surface, the accuracy of reduction, and the type of fracture configuration) influencing bone healing.

The purpose of these experiments was not to show the superiority of any particular device or fixation mode over another. Instead, the experiments were designed to demonstrate the model of healing expected by each type of fixation rigidity under standardized, uncompromised healing conditions. Under clinical fracture-healing conditions, the fixation rigidity and the type of fixation are major variables influencing the outcome of the treatment. The use of intraanimal comparison in statistical analysis also minimizes the many interanimal variables, such as individual differences in functional activity and loading magnitude. It must also be emphasized that the studies of external fixation do not represent only the healing modes provided by external fixators. External fixation, allowing a controlled adjustment of fixation rigidity, is an important experimental tool to study the mechanical factors influencing fracture healing, and the data can be used to improve the designs of other fixation devices.

Plate Fixation Versus Intramedullary Fixation

Rand et al. (50) compared the effects of compression plating (eight-hole DCP) and intramedullary nailing after reaming (fluted Sampson rod) on the vascular supply of the canine tibial osteotomy site and on the rate and quality of osteotomal union. Rod-fixed osteotomies healed by periosteal callus, whereas plate-fixed osteotomies showed predominantly endosteal callus formation (Fig. 22). There were no significant differences in bone porosity between the fixation methods. The plated osteotomies displayed higher torsional stiffness values than rod-fixed osteotomies at 90 days ($p < 0.005$), but this difference was no longer apparent at 120 days. Maximum torque values of the plated osteotomies were significantly higher at 90 days ($p < 0.01$), but this difference also disappeared by 120 days.

This experiment confirmed that bone union occurs through different mechanisms after intramedullary rod fixation and plate fixation. Interestingly, rigid plate fixation improved the recovery of mechanical properties at the early phases of healing, although the rigidity of

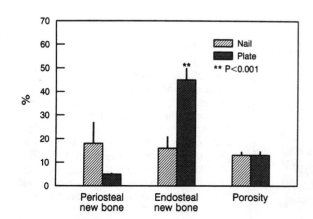

FIG. 22. Comparison of new bone formation and porosity between intramedullary nailing and compression plate fixation (canine tibial osteotomy model). Significantly higher endosteal new bone formation occurred on the plated side. IM nail fixation produced higher periosteal new bone formation.

plate fixation inhibited periosteal callus formation. The time needed for the return of normal strength and stiffness was, however, the same between the two methods, indicating that the end result of the different healing patterns was biomechanically indifferent.

Plate Fixation Versus External Fixation

Lewallen et al. (40) compared compression plating (eight-hole prebent DCP) and unilateral external fixation (Sukhtian–Hughes design). The fixator was applied using six stainless steel Schanz screws, 4 mm in diameter. *In vitro* mechanical testing showed that the plate–bone system was significantly more rigid than the external fixator–bone system in all testing modes except in lateral bending (in the plane of the pins), where the external fixator was more rigid. *In vivo* study showed that the use of both methods led to osteotomy union by 120 days. However, the maximum torque and stiffness of the plated osteotomies were significantly higher than those of the external fixator side ($p < 0.05$ and $p < 0.01$, respectively). Histologically, there was more porosity ($p < 0.05$) on the external fixator side relative to paired osteotomies treated with compression plates (Fig. 23). The external fixator side also had significantly less intracortical new bone ($p < 0.01$). Higher bone turnover on the fixator side was accompanied by higher blood flow ($p < 0.05$, compared with the plated side).

This experiment showed that rigidity is an important factor in early bone healing. Exter-

nal fixation was shown to increase bone resorption and to decrease intracortical bone formation relative to rigid compression plating. This study, as well as the study of Rand et al. (50), did not show porotic transformation of the cortical bone in the canine tibia beneath a rigid plate, suggesting that such a phenomenon must be a late effect and unrelated to changes in blood flow that occur during initial stages of healing.

Unilateral External Fixation with Different Rigidity

The study of Wu et al. (68) compared the healing pattern of osteotomies fixed with more rigid (six half-pins) and less rigid (four half-pins) unilateral external fixator configurations. The Sukhtian–Hughes model fixator was used, and the pins were 4-mm stainless steel Schanz screws. *In vitro* testing showed that the axial, torsional, and lateral bending stiffness of the four-pin configuration was about 70% that of the six-pin configuration. The anteroposterior bending stiffness in the four-pin side was only 50% that of the six-pin side. *In vivo* study showed increased periosteal callus formation in the four-pin side, based on the planimetry of sequential radiographs. At 120 days, the osteotomies treated by the two configurations did not show significant differences in the maximum torque to failure or in stiffness. Histologically, the four-pin side showed increased porosity of the osteotomy area ($p < 0.05$ compared with the six-

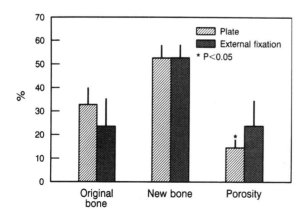

FIG. 23. The relative amounts of original cortical bone, new bone, and porosity between the plated side and the external fixation side in a midtibial canine osteotomy model. The porosity in the external fixation side was higher when compared to the compression plated side. This finding may reflect the higher fracture site movement and nonosteonal bone healing mechanics under the less rigid external fixation.

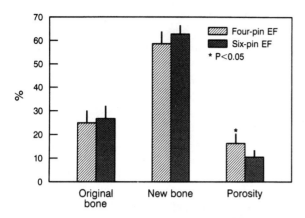

FIG. 24. New bone formation and bone porosity comparison in a four-pin (less rigid) versus six-pin (more rigid) unilateral external fixation configuration (canine tibial osteotomy model). The intracortical porosity was significantly higher in the less stiff four-pin fixator side.

pin side) (Fig. 24). The incidence of pin loosening was significantly higher in the four-pin side than in the six-pin side.

This experiment confirmed that less rigid external fixation results in enhanced periosteal callus formation but, at the same time, increases bone porosity without any beneficial effects on the mechanical recovery. This study also showed that the low initial stiffness of external fixation increases the potential for pin–bone interface problems.

Compression Versus No Compression Under External Fixation

The study by Hart et al. (30) focused on examining the effects of constant compression on osteotomy healing. The static compression of 80 N was applied across the tibial osteotomy site by the Sukhtian–Hughes unilateral external fixator. The contralateral side

was treated with the same fixator, but the osteotomy ends were not in intimate contact (osteotomy gap 20 μm). The fixator was applied using a six-pin configuration (4.5-mm custom-made titanium self-tapping pins). *In vitro* study showed that the static compression of osteotomy ends increased the rigidity of fixation, especially in lateral bending and torsion. All the osteotomies were healed at 90 days. No statistical differences were observed between the paired osteotomies in mechanical testing or in histologic analysis (Fig. 25). The osteotomy-site blood flow did not show any significant differences. On both sides, periosteal new bone formation was less in the mediolateral plane than in the anteroposterior plane, which seemed to correlate inversely with the amount of bending stiffness of the unilateral external fixator. Some of the osteotomies, regardless of the mode of fixation, showed haversian remodeling across the os-

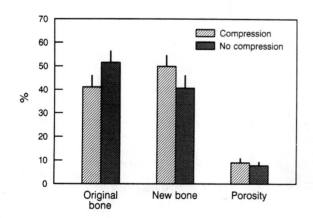

FIG. 25. Static compression did not change new bone formation and porosity at the osteotomy site under external fixation (canine tibial model).

teotomy site through a contact or gap type of healing mechanism.

This study showed that compression, applied through an external fixation system, increases the rigidity of fixation. Relative to the rigidity of the intact tibia, this increase was small, and no significant biological or biomechanical benefits were observed for the bone union process. Therefore, static compression does not seem to enhance healing when adequate rigidity and small fracture gap are maintained by the fixator system.

Unilateral Versus Bilateral, Two-Plane External Fixation

The study of Williams et al. (63) was designed to compare bilateral, two-plane external fixation to unilateral external fixation. The two-plane fixator included two full transfixation pins and two half-pins above and below the site of osteotomy. The unilateral fixator was the Sukhtian–Hughes fixator with six titanium half-pins. *In vitro* testing showed that the bilateral, two-plane configuration significantly improves the torsional stiffness as well as the bending stiffness in the plane perpendicular to the plane of half-pins of the unilateral fixation. In the animal study, the bilateral two-plane configuration induced less periosteal callus formation, and the *in vivo* measurement of osteotomy stiffness showed higher values on this side than on the unilateral fixation side. The ratio of static to dy-

namic bone scan activity, which served as an indicator of bone turnover, was increased at the early stages of osteotomy healing on the side of unilateral external fixation. Histologically, at 13 weeks, the bilateral two-plane fixation side showed cortical restoration more frequently by haversian remodeling across the osteotomy site. The porosity of the osteotomy site was also lower on the side of bilateral fixation ($p < 0.05$) (Fig. 26). Torsional testing showed that the osteotomies fixed with the more rigid bilateral two-plane fixation were stiffer ($p < 0.025$) than those fixed with unilateral fixation, but no statistical difference was observed in the maximum torque to failure.

This study confirmed higher-rigidity external fixation results in osteotomy healing with less callus formation and stiffer union during the healing process. The results agree with the previous experimental data on internal and external fixation, indicating that the healing pattern of a bone osteotomy can be altered by the rigidity of fixation.

Constant Rigid Versus Dynamic Compression Under External Fixation

Under external fixation, the rigidity of the fixator causes mechanical stimulation at the fracture site through relative displacement of the fracture ends. Such stimulation can be classified into three categories:

1. *Static stimulation:* The compressive load applied to the fracture site on weight

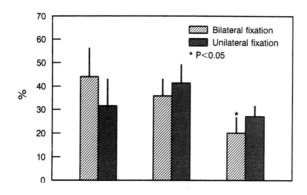

FIG. 26. Comparison of new bone formation and bone porosity between the bilateral full-pin plus half-pin fixation configuration and the unilateral half-pin fixator. Porosity was significantly higher in the less rigid unilateral external fixator.

bearing. When the load is removed, the fracture gap will return to its neutral mode.

2. *Dynamic stimulation:* This is achieved by releasing the axial displacement constraint from the side bar of the fixator, thus allowing uniform axial compression of the fracture ends under loading while the stiffness properties in bending and torsion are maintained. The fracture gap will remain closed even when the load is removed. This is also defined as "dynamization."

3. *Controlled stimulation:* The axial displacement is introduced cyclically by a computer-controlled actuator through either displacement or load control. Such axial dynamization does not require weight bearing.

The study of Aro et al. (5) was designed to examine the effects of dynamic axial compression on bone healing after a short initial period (2 weeks) of a neutralization mode of rigid fixation. *In vitro* studies showed that the introduction of axial dynamization did not alter the fixation rigidity under torsion or bending, while axial compressive load was transmitted through the bone. *In vivo*, dynamization reduced the osteotomy gap and induced contact healing with periosteal callus formation. Nondynamized, rigidly fixed bones healed through a gap healing mechanism with or without external callus, whereas the distribution of external callus was nonuniform around the osteotomy site. The paired comparison of the control and dynamized osteotomies showed no statistical differences in the total quantity of external callus. At 90 days, both sides showed a high rate of cortical reconstruction through haversian remodeling, and no differences were observed in the histologic composition of new bone formation and bone porosity (Fig. 27) as well as in osteotomy-site blood flow and bone scan activity at this postunion stage. Intracortical porosity was low on both sides, with minimal endosteal new bone formation. The torsional strength and stiffness of the healed tibias were not significantly different from those of intact tibias (Fig. 28). The dynamization decreased pin loosening, measured by pin removal torque, among pins closest to the osteotomy site. The overall clinical, radiographic, and biomechanical performance of the tapered pin appeared to be good, with well-formed new bone within the pin thread space. Such pin tract behavior may be related to the thread design in the tapered pin, since no tapping is necessary to create the threads in the bone.

This study showed that the axial readjustment of external fixation rigidity during the bone healing process can facilitate contact osteonal bone healing. The results of the rigidly fixed control side showed that rigid external fixation can completely prevent periosteal callus formation. The fast healing of the bones, compared with the previous studies of external fixation, demonstrated the efficiency of os-

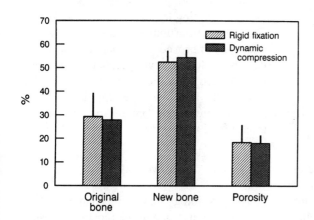

FIG. 27. Comparison of rigid external fixation under neutralization and dynamic compression modes. No significant differences were found in new bone formation and bone porosity.

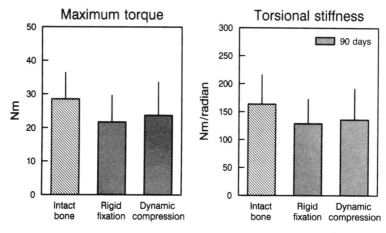

FIG. 28. The maximum torque to failure of the bone union site and torsional stiffness of the healed tibia after 90 days were found to be similar to intact bone strength and stiffness. There was no difference between the rigidly fixed and dynamized sides of the experimental model.

teonal bone healing and the stability of the fixation used in this experiment. Undoubtedly, the tapered pin design with increased shank diameter plays an important part in this achievement. Furthermore, the experiment confirmed the theoretical prediction that rigid external fixation does not cause postunion osteopenia, dissimilar to rigid plate fixation. The dynamization maneuver, relying on the ability of the bone to transmit axial load, appears to reduce pin-bending load and, subsequently, the risk of pin–bone interface failure.

General Comments on the Mechanism of Fracture Healing

The experimental studies reviewed above seem to suggest the following:

1. The rigidity of fixation is an important factor governing not only whether the fracture will heal but also the mechanism through which bone union will take place.

2. The biological and biomechanical pathways to osseous union can be attenuated by changing the rigidity of fixation during the treatment course. However, when and how to alter the rigidity in order to promote more efficient bone remodeling remains to be elucidated. Additional animal experiments performed under different mechanical environments are needed to understand the cellular activities at this early stage of fracture repair.

3. Internal and external fracture fixation devices, as dictated by their biomechanical characteristics, can lead to the same final result of fracture union, but perhaps through slightly different biological processes.

4. Plate fixation favors endosteal healing, whereas intramedullary fixation and less rigid external fixation encourage periosteal healing. Rigid external fixation reduces periosteal callus formation and thus relies on cortical reconstruction with concomitant endosteal healing. Axially dynamized external fixation facilitates secondary contact healing, i.e., direct cortical reconstruction with periosteal new bone formation.

5. Under external fixation, fluctuating stress induced by unstable fixation and the associated fracture gap movement is an important contributing factor in pin-tract loosening. Careful pin insertion technique, increased pin diameter, improved pin geometry and thread design, the load-carrying capacity of the healing fracture, and the magnitude of loading through the bone ends are other key determinants in preventing pin loosening and pin-tract infection.

SUMMARY

The physiology and biomechanics of bone fracture union is one of the most widely studied subjects in orthopaedic surgery. Although much has been written and discussed, many fundamental issues still remain controversial and poorly understood. One of the possible reasons for such deficiency may be related to the inevitable clinical influence on basic research. Frequently, scientific inquiries were stimulated by the introduction of a new treatment modality or device. Very few well-thought-out hypotheses and systematic investigations were conducted to validate the unique characteristics associated with the new device or treatment principles. Furthermore, well-developed techniques or devices for specific applications often tended to overexpand their indications, even at the risk of contradicting the original working principles. These potential pitfalls must be carefully avoided in order to ensure the quality and originality of research in the field of bone fracture repair.

Each bone fracture fixation method, either internal or external, has its specific advantages and disadvantages according to its original development concept and specific indications. No single method or device can be so universal as to be applicable for any fracture type and location. It is therefore logical to select the best treatment modality and fixation device according to the clinical conditions of the patient.

The present chapter has thoroughly documented the fact that bone fracture union can follow several pathways to the final stage. The choice of which healing mechanism will be utilized should be based on many factors. Clinical factors, such as the patient's expectation and his or her compliance with treatment, degree of tolerance, socioeconomic considerations, etc., are likely to play important roles in the selection of fixation method. A biological system appears to have a high level of tolerance and adaptability to even the most adverse conditions. If the fundamental biomechanical and biological principles for any fracture fixation modality are well understood and carefully applied with the "personality of the fracture" in mind, successful bony union is the rule. Table 9 summarizes these considerations.

Compression plate fixation may have potential drawbacks, such as stress shielding bone osteopenia and refracture after plate removal, but its advantages in many special circumstances appear to outweigh these considerations. Redesigning the plate geometry or material composition in order to minimize its axial stiffness would appear contradictory to the underlying principle of compression plate rigid fixation. On the other hand, lack of torsional rigidity in intramedullary nail fixation should not be regarded as an intrinsic deficiency of such a method because the functional principle of intramedullary nailing is to promote axial compaction of the bone ends at the fracture site. Increasing torsional rigidity of the nail (fluted cross section) or fixation (interlocking feature) may reduce the axial stimulation characteristics inherent in such methods of fracture fixation. Therefore, in changing the structural properties of any internal fixation devices, the benefits to be gained may be overshadowed by the loss of certain fundamental working principles on which the original fixation concept was based.

Although some surgeons have had reservations concerning the use of external fixation for fracture treatment, based mainly on the fear of pin tract infection and fracture nonunion, much of the clinical experience and basic

TABLE 9. *Biomechanical considerations in operative treatment of long-bone fractures*

Evaluation of fracture mechanism and trauma energy by studying the injury history and the radiographic appearance of the fracture.

Attention to possible local stress riser that may predispose the bone or the device to fracture.

Recognition of possible systemic factors or underlying diseases that could affect the quality (material properties) of the fractured long bone.

Selection of the fixation method to achieve the preferred fracture stability and the associated bone healing mechanism.

Following the established operative technique according to the biomechanical principles upon which the fixation device was designed.

Staged hardware removal and loading protection in order to allow bone defect repair and remodeling.

science research results have proven that such concern was unfounded. Many of the potential benefits of external fixation, such as dynamization and the change of fixation stiffness, are not yet fully appreciated. Additional research and well-organized clinical trials must be performed. Pin-tract problems can be controlled, but the surgeon utilizing such a device must be familiar with the techniques and clinical care of the patients. On the other hand, external fixation also has its limitations and unavoidable shortcomings from a clinical point of view. It would be a disservice to the external fixation technique to overextend its indications and employ it on certain patients with specific clinical conditions that are more amenable to another form of treatment.

Finally, the importance of balancing between the biomechanical properties and the biological behavior of different fracture fixation methods has been demonstrated. Understanding this knowledge and the application techniques associated with each fixation modality is the prerequisite to selecting the optimal treatment for each patient. This should provide the impetus for surgeons, bioengineers, and medical scientists to continue collaborative basic and applied research. A better understanding of how bone repairs itself under variable conditions and environ-ment can help identify bone union enhancing and inhibiting factors. Ultimately, noninvasive fracture repair-monitoring techniques can be developed to ensure successful treatment outcome and efficient functional recovery.

APPENDIX: BASIC BIOMECHANICAL DEFINITIONS AND TERMINOLOGY

The following list of basic definitions and terminology is useful in the discussion of biomechanics of bone fracture fixation (12,25,26).

Deformation: A change in shape or size of a structure or any part of it.

Normal strain: A measure of localized size change during material deformation. It is expressed by dividing the final length change of a line oriented in a certain direction by its original length at a point in or on a deformable body; hence, it is dimensionless.

Shear strain: A measure of the change of angle of two orthogonal and intersecting lines at a point in or on a deformable body. It is expressed in radians and, therefore, is dimensionless.

Normal stress: The intensity of the internal forces normal to a plane passing through a point in the body, expressed as force per unit area (Fig. 29). Tensile stress is positive,

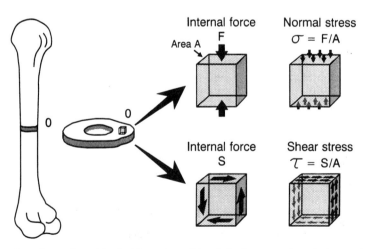

FIG. 29. When long bone is subjected to external load, both normal and shear stresses occur in each location of the bone, and their magnitude is dependent upon the orientation of the material plane on which the stress is to be determined.

and compressive stress is negative. Commonly used units are pounds per square inch (psi) or newtons per square meter (N/m^2 = Pa). 1 MPa = 10^6 Pa = 1 $N/mm^2 \cong$ 145 psi.

Shear stress: The intensity of the internal forces parallel to a plane passing through a point in the body, expressed as force per unit area (Fig. 29), the same as normal stress.

Stress–strain curve: A diagram in which corresponding values of stress and strain (obtained through simple tension, compression, or shear tests) are plotted against each other when a material specimen is tested until failure. Usually, stress is plotted along the ordinate, and strain is plotted along the abscissa (Fig. 30).

Moduli of elasticity: The ratio of stress to corresponding strain below the proportional limit (a point on the stress–strain curve beyond which the stress is no longer proportional to strain). If the test is under tension or compression, the stress–strain ratio is defined as the *Young's modulus.* If the test is in pure shear, it is called the *shear modulus* or *modulus of rigidity.* The units of these moduli are the same as those of stress. For isotropic materials, only two moduli are needed to completely define the material.

Elastic limit: If the stress exceeds a certain value, the test specimen will not completely recover its original size or shape when the applied force is removed. This stress is defined as the *elastic limit* of the material (Fig. 30). The linear portion of the stress–strain curve below this value is defined as the *linear elastic range,* and the nonlinear part is called the *nonlinear elastic range.* The elastic limit is also called the *yield stress.*

Ultimate stress: The maximum attainable stress of a material beyond which an increase in strain occurs without an increase in stress or the material will fail through fracture (Fig. 30). Such stress is also called the strength of the material.

Elastic deformation and plastic deformation: If the applied load is removed from a test specimen, the structural deformation disappears. Such deformation is defined as *elastic.* If, on removal of the load, a permanent deformation occurs in or on the structure, the deformation is called *plastic.* When strain is used to describe material deformation, there will be elastic strain and plastic strain defined in similar fashion.

Ductility: The ability of materials to deform plastically before fracturing.

Brittle material: A material that can sustain only limited strain before fracturing.

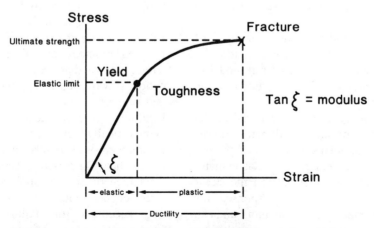

FIG. 30. Typical stress and strain relationship commonly observed in bone or implant materials used in orthopaedic surgery. The slope of the linear portion in the stress–strain curve, expressed as tan ξ, represents the Young's modulus of the material.

Hardness: The resistance of a material surface to deformation under indentation or scratching by an object with specific shape and size.

Strain energy (per unit volume): The area under the stress–strain curve. If the specimen is loaded beyond the elastic limit, upon unloading, the area under the unload curve is defined as the *elastic strain energy density,* and the remaining area under the stress–strain curve during the initial loading process is called the *plastic strain energy density*, which represents the energy dissipated during plastic deformation.

Modulus of resilience: The strain energy at the point of the elastic limit.

Toughness: The strain energy at the point of ultimate stress.

Fatigue: A progressive, localized, permanent microstructural change occurring in a material under repeated load that may culminate in cracks or complete fracture after a sufficient number of fluctuations.

Stress ratio: In a cyclic fatigue test, the ratio of the minimum stress (compressive stress is smaller than tensile stress because of its negative sign) to the maximum stress. A stress ratio of −1 is the worst fatigue loading condition.

Endurance limit: In a fatigue test, the stress level below which no fracture can be obtained, regardless of the number of loading cycles applied.

Creep: Time-dependent increase in strain in a material under constant stress.

Relaxation: Time-dependent reduction of stress in a material under constant strain.

Hookean body (elastic): A material model in which strain is directly proportional to the applied stress.

Newtonian body (viscous): A material model in which rate of strain is directly proportional to the applied stress.

Kelvin body: In modeling a viscoelastic material, the strain is dependent on the stress rate and has a time-delayed response. This type of material has shape memory and can return to its original dimension with time after the stress is removed.

Maxwell body: In modeling a viscoelastic material, the strain is dependent on the stress rate, but the material can have an instantaneous response. The material has no memory and will remain permanently deformed.

Hysteresis loop: When a material is cyclically loaded in the elastic range, a small amount of energy (per unit volume) is dissipated during each loading cycle, which causes the loading and unloading curves to be noncoincident. The loops formed by these lines are called hysteresis loops. The area within the loop represents the energy dissipated per unit volume.

Combined stresses: A structure under the influence of different types of loading simultaneously is often analyzed separately according to the individual load, and the resulting stresses at the same location can be combined to form the state of stress of the structure. Such analysis is defined as linear superposition.

Stress concentration factor: Geometric irregularities such as holes, notches, and sharp corners as well as sudden changes in material properties may produce high localized stresses in structural members under loading. The ratio of the true maximum stress caused by these *stress risers* to the nominal stress calculated at that point by the ordinary formulas of mechanics is called the *stress concentration factor.*

Three-point versus four-point bending: A simply supported beam having only one load applied between the end supports is called *three-point bending.* The maximum bending moment, and thus the bending stress, is located at the point of load application. If two loads are applied between the end supports, the beam is under four-point bending. If the two loads are equal and symmetrically located, the maximum bending moment will be distributed evenly between them. Three-point bending has the advantage of ease in application, but the stress concentration from load application may accentuate the failure mechanism. Four-point bending minimizes the stress effect, but it must have sufficient length to accommodate two loads between the supporting end points.

Axial stiffness (AE): In an axial loading test of a structure with cross-sectional area A and material elastic modulus E, the slope of the linear portion of the load–deformation curve is defined as the axial stiffness of the structure or the resistance of axial deformation on loading.

Bending stiffness or flexural modulus (EI): In a bending test of a specimen with unknown elastic modulus E and cross-sectional area moment of inertia I, the slope of the linear portion of the load–deformation curve provides a measure of bending resistance, and such a parameter is defined as the bending stiffness or flexural modulus of the beam.

Torsional stiffness (GJ): In a torsional test of a specimen with shear modulus G and polar area moment of inertia J, the slope of the linear part of the torque–rotation curve provides a measure of its torsional resistance or the structural parameter, torsional stiffness.

Area moment of inertia (I): The sum of the products obtained by multiplying each element of the infinitesimal subareas (A_i) of the cross-sectional area A and the square of the distance from its centroid to centroidal axes of the entire area A:

$$I_x = \sum_{i=1}^{n} x_i^2 A_i$$

with respect to the y axis through the centroid of A;

$$I_y = \sum_{i=1}^{n} x_i^2 A_i$$

with respect to the x axis through the centroid of A, where x_i and y_i are the distances from the centroid of the subarea A_i to the centroidal reference x,y axes of the entire area A. For these quantities to be accurate, A_i must be very small.

Polar moment of inertia (J): An area moment of inertia where the reference axis is normal to the plane of the area and through its centroid. For an irregular area, J_o (the subscript o designates the centroid location) can be approximated from:

$$J_o = \sum_{i=1}^{n} x_i^2 A_i$$

where r_i is the radial distance between the centroid of the infinitesimal subarea A_i and o, and

$$r_i^2 = x_i^2 + y_i^2$$

$$J_o = I_x + I_y$$

This quantity can be used to describe the resistance to torsion applied to a cylindrical structure.

REFERENCES

1. Aalto, K., Holmstrom, T., Karaharju, E., Joukainen, J., Paavolainen, P., and Slatis, P. (1987): Fracture repair during external fixation. Torsion tests of rabbit osteotomies. *Acta Orthop. Scand.,* 58:66–70.
2. Aro, H., Eerola, E., and Aho, A. J. (1985): Determination of callus quantity in 4-week-old fractures of the rat tibia. *J. Orthop. Res.,* 3:101–108.
3. Aro, H. (1985): *Fracture healing in the rat tibio-fibular bone with special reference to the effects of denervation.* Doctoral Thesis, University of Turku, Turku, Finland, Kirjapaino Pika OY.
4. Aro, H., Wippermann, B., Hodgson, S., Wahner, H., Lewallen, D., and Chao, E. (1989): Prediction of properties of fracture callus by measurement of mineral density using micro-bone densitometry. *J. Bone Joint Surg.,* 71-A:1020–1039.
5. Aro, H., Kelly, P. J., Lewallen, D. G., and Chao, E. Y. S. (1990): The effects of physiologic dynamic compression on bone healing under external fixation. *Clin. Orthop. Rel. Res.,* 256:260–273.
6. Behrens, F., Johnson, W. D., Koch, T. W., and Kovacevic, N. (1983): Bending stiffness of unilateral and bilateral fixator frames. *Clin. Orthop. Rel. Res.,* 178:103–110.
7. Black, J., Perdigon, P., Brown, N., and Pollack, S. R. (1984): Stiffness and strength of fracture callus. Relative rates of mechanical maturation as evaluated by a uniaxial tensile test. *Clin. Orthop. Rel. Res.,* 182:278–288.
8. Bradley, G. W., McKenna, G. B., Dunn, H. K., Daniels, A. U., and Statton, W. O. (1979): Effects of flexural rigidity of plates on bone healing. *J. Bone Joint Surg.,* 61-A:866–872.
9. Brien, W., Wiss, D. A., Peter, K., and Merritt, P. O. (1987): Subtrochanteric fractures of the femur: Treatment with locked medullary nails. In: *Proceedings 54th Annual Meeting American Academy of Orthopaedic Surgery,* p. 121. AAOS, San Francisco.
10. Briggs, B. T., and Chao, E. Y. S. (1982): The mechanical performance of the standard Hoffmann–Vidal external fixation apparatus. *J. Bone Joint Surg.,* 64-A:566–573.
11. Brown, S. A., Gillet, N. A., and Broaddus, T. W. (1984): Biomechanics of fracture fixation by plastic rods with transverse screws. In: *Biomechanics: Current Interdisciplinary Research,* edited by S. M. Perren and E. Schneider, pp. 475–480. Martinus Nijhoff, Dordrecht.
12. Chao, E. Y. S. (1976): *Notes on Principles of Orthopedic Biomechanics.* Biomechanics Laboratory, Department of Orthopedics, Mayo Clinic/Mayo Foundation, Rochester, MN.

13. Chao, E. Y. S., Kasman, R. A., and An, K. N. (1982): Rigidity and stress analyses of external fracture fixation devices—a theoretical approach. *J. Biomech.,* 15(12): 971–983.

14. Chao, E. Y. S. (1983): Fissazione externa e guardigione delle fratture: Proprieta biomeccaniche di strumenti diversi. In: *Attulita in Traumatologia,* edited by L. Ricciardi and A. Gaggi, pp. 191–206. Bologna, Italy.

15. Chao, E. Y. S., and Hein, T. J. (1988): Mechanical performance of standard Orthofix external fixator. *Orthopedics,* 11:1057–1069.

16. Charnley, J. (1970): *The Closed Treatment of Common Fractures.* E & S Livingstone, Edinburgh.

17. Claes, L., Burri, C., Gerngross, H., and Mutschler, W. (1985): Bone healing stimulated by plasma factor XIII. Osteotomy experiments in sheep. *Acta Orthop. Scand.,* 56:57–62.

18. Claes, L., Wilke, J. H., and Kemper, F. (1987): Interfragmentary strain and bone healing: an experimental study. In: *Proceedings International Society of Fracture Repair,* Helsinki and Stockholm, August 31–September 2, pp. 64–65.

19. Cordey, J., and Perren, S. M. (1986): Limits of plate on bone friction in internal fixation of fractures. In: *Proceedings 5th Meeting European Society for Biomechanics,* September, Berlin, p. 102.

20. Cordey, J., Perren, S. M., and Steinemann, S. (1986): Parametric analysis of the strain distribution in bone after plating. In: *Proceedings 5th Meeting European Society for Biomechanics,* September, Berlin, p. 103.

21. Cruess, R. L., and Dumont, J. (1975): Fracture healing. *Can. J. Surg.,* 18(5):403–413.

22. DiGioia, A. M., Cheal, E. J., Hayes, W. C., and Perren, S. M. (1987): Biomechanics of bone resorption, callus formation and medullary pressurization in healing plated fractures. *Trans. Orthop. Res. Soc.* San Francisco, p.100.

23. Edwards, C. C. (1983): Staged reconstruction of complex open tibial fractures using Hoffmann external fixation. *Clin. Orthop. Rel. Res.,* 178:130–161.

24. Finlay, J. B., Moroz, T. K., Rorabeck, C. H., Davey, J. D., and Bourne, R. B. (1987): Stability of ten configurations of the Hoffmann external-fixation frame. *J. Bone Joint Surg.,* 69-A:734–744.

25. Frankel, V. H., and Burstein, A. H. (1970): *Orthopaedic Biomechanics.* Lea & Febiger, Philadelphia.

26. Frankel, V. H., and Nordin, M. (1980): *Basic Biomechanics of the Skeletal System.* Lea & Febiger, Philadelphia.

27. Garbarino, J. L., Brumback, R. J., Poka, A., and Burgess, A. R. (1987): Closed interlocking nailing of subtrochanteric fractures. In: *Proceedings 54th Annual Meeting American Academy of Orthopaedic Surgery,* San Francisco, p. 121.

28. Gasser, B., Wyder, D., and Schneider, E. (1987): The stiffness behaviour of the circular, wire-based frame in contrast to conventional external fixators. *Proceedings International Society for Fracture Repair,* Helsinki and Stockholm, August 31–September 2, pp. 95–96.

29. Green, S. A. (1981): *Complications of External Skeletal Fixation: Causes, Prevention and Treatment.* Charles C. Thomas, Springfield, IL.

30. Hart, M. B., Wu, J-J., Chao, E. Y. S., and Kelly, P. J. (1985): External skeletal fixation of canine tibial osteotomies. Compression compared with no compression. *J. Bone Joint Surg.,* 67-A:598–605.

31. Hayes, W. C. (1980): Basic biomechanics of compression plate fixation. In: *Current Concepts of Internal Fixation of Fractures,* edited by H. K. Uhthoff, pp. 49–62. Springer-Verlag, Berlin.

32. Hayes, W. E., and Snyder, B. D. (1981): Toward a quantitative formulation of Wolff's law in trabecular bone. In: *Mechanical Properties of Bone,* edited by S. C. Cowin, pp. 43–68. ASME, New York.

33. Heppenstall, R. B., Grislis, G., and Hunt, T. K. (1975): Tissue gas tensions and oxygen consumption in healing bone defects. *Clin Orthop. Rel. Res.,* 106:357–365.

34. Huiskes, R., Chao, E. Y. S., and Crippen, T. E. (1985): Parametric analyses of pin–bone stresses in external fracture fixation devices. *J. Orthop. Res.,* 3:341–349.

35. Huiskes, R., and Chao, E. Y. S. (1986): Guidelines for external fixation frame rigidity and stresses. *J. Orthop. Res.,* 4:68–75.

36. Hutzschenreuter, P., and Brummer, H. (1980): Screw design and stability. In: *Current Concepts of Internal Fixation of Fractures,* edited by H. K. Uhthoff, pp. 244–250. Springer-Verlag, Berlin.

37. Kempf, I., Karger, C., Willinger, R., Francois, J. M., Cornet, A., Renault, D., and Bonnel, F. (1984): Locked intramedullary nailing—improvement of mechanical properties. In: *Biomechanics: Current Interdisciplinary Research,* edited by S. M. Perren and E. Schneider, pp. 487–492. Martinus Nijhoff, Dordrecht.

38. Klemm, K. W., and Borner, M. (1986): Interlocking nailing of complex fractures of the femur and tibia. *Clin. Orthop. Rel. Res.,* 212:89–100.

39. Kuntscher, G. (1965): Intramedullary surgical technique and its place in orthopaedic surgery. My present concept. *J. Bone Joint Surg.,* 47-A:809–818.

40. Lewallen, D. G., Chao, E. Y. S., Kasman, R. A., and Kelly, P. J. (1984): Comparison of the effects of compression plates and external fixators on early bone healing. *J. Bone Joint Surg.,* 66-A:1084–1091.

41. McCoy, T. M., Chao, E. Y. S., and Kasman, R. A. (1983): Comparison of mechanical performance in four types of external fixators. *Clin. Orthop. Rel. Res.,* 180:23–33.

42. Muller, J., Schenk, R., and Willenegger, H. (1968): Experimentelle Untersuchungen uber die entstehung reaktiver Pseudarthrosen am Hunderadius. *Helv. Chir. Acta,* 1/2:301–308.

43. Panjabi, M. M., White, A. A., and Southwick, W. O. (1973): Mechanical properties of bone as a function of rate of deformation. *J. Bone Joint Surg.,* 55-A(2): 322–330.

44. Panjabi, M. M., Walter, S. D., Karuda, M., White, A. A., and Lawson, J. P. (1985): Correlations of radiographic analysis of healing fractures with strength: a statistical analysis of experimental osteotomies. *J. Orthop. Res.,* 3:212–218.

45. Penttinen, R. (1972): Biochemical studies on fracture healing in the rat with special reference to the oxygen supply. *Acta Chir. Scand. [Suppl.],* 432.

46. Perren, S. M. (1979): Physical and biological aspects of fracture healing with special reference to internal fixation. *Clin. Orthop. Rel. Res.,* 138:175–196.

47. Perren, S. M., and Cordey, J. (1980): Mechanics of interfragmentary compression by plates and screws. In: *Current Concepts of Internal Fixation of Fractures,* edited by H. K. Uhthoff, pp. 184–191. Springer-Verlag, Berlin.

48. Peterson, D. L., Skraba, J. S., Moran, J. M., and Green-

wald, A. S. (1984): Fracture of long bones: rate effects under singular and combined loading states. *J. Orthop. Res.,* 1:244–250.

49. Pettine, K. A., Kelly, P. J., Chao, E. Y. S., and Huiskes, R. (1986): Histologic and biomechanical analysis of unilateral external fixator pin–bone interface. *Trans. Orthop. Res. Soc.,* 472.

50. Rand, J. A., An, K. N., Chao, E. Y., and Kelly, P. J. (1981): A comparison of the effect of open intramedullary nailing and compression-plate fixation on fracture site blood flow and fracture union. *J. Bone Joint Surg.,* 63-A:427–442.

51. Rydell, N. W. (1966): Forces acting on the femoral head prosthesis: a study on strain gauge supplied prostheses in living persons. *Acta Orthop. Scand. [Suppl.],* 88.

52. Schenk, R., and Willenegger, H. (1963): Zum histologischen Bild der sogenannten Primarheilung der Knochenkompakta nach experimentellen Osteotomien am Hund. *Experientia,* 19:593.

53. Schenk, R. K. (1986): Histophysiology of bone remodeling and bone repair. In: *Perspectives on Biomaterials,* edited by O. C. C. Lin and E. Y. S. Chao, pp. 75–94. Elsevier Science, Amsterdam.

54. Schwyzer, H. K., Cordey, J., Brun, S., Matter, P., and Perren, S. M. (1984): Bone loss after internal fixation using plates, determination in humans using computed tomography. In: *Biomechanics: Current Interdisciplinary Research,* edited by S. M. Perren and E. Schneider, pp. 191–195. Martinus Nijhoff, Dordrecht.

55. Shifflett, M. W., and Bray, T. J. (1987): Subtrochanteric fractures treated by Zickel and Grosse–Kempf nailing. In: *Proceedings 54th Annual Meeting American Academy of Orthopaedic Surgery,* San Francisco, p. 121. AAOS Publishing, Rosemont, IL.

56. Slatis, P., Karaharju, E., Holmstrom, T., Ahonen, J., and Paavolainen, P. (1987): Structural changes in intact tubular bone after application of rigid plates with or without compression. *J. Bone Joint Surg.,* 69-A:516–522.

57. Taylor, J. C., Russell, T. A., LaVelle, D. G., and Calandruccio, R. A. (1987): Clinical results of 100 femoral shaft fractures treated with the Russell–Taylor interlocking nail system. In: *Proceedings 54th Annual Meeting American Academy of Orthopaedic Surgery,* San Francisco, p. 155.

58. Tencer, A. F., Johnson, K. D., Johnston, D. W. C., and Gill, K. (1984): A biomechanical comparison of various methods of stabilization of subtrochanteric fractures of the femur. *J. Orthop. Res.,* 2:297–305.

59. Uhthoff, H. K., and Dubuc, F. L. (1971): Bone structure changes in the dog under rigid internal fixation. *Clin. Orthop. Rel. Res.,* 81:165–170.

60. Uhthoff, H. K., and Finnegan, M. (1983): The effects of metal plates on post-traumatic remodeling and bone mass. *J. Bone Joint Surg.,* 65-B:66–71.

61. White, A. A. III, Panjabi, M. M., and Southwick, W. O. (1977): The four biomechanical stages of fracture repair. *J. Bone Joint Surg.,* 59-A:188–192.

62. Whiteside, L. A., and Lesker, P. A. (1978): The effects of extraperiosteal and subperiosteal dissection. II: On fracture healing. *J. Bone Joint Surg.,* 60-A:26–30.

63. Williams, E. A., Rand, J. A., An, K. N., Chao, E. Y. S., and Kelly, P. J. (1987): The early healing of tibial osteotomies stabilized by one-plane or two-plane external fixation. *J. Bone Joint Surg.,* 69-A:355–365.

64. Williams, E. A., Hein, T. J., and Bronk, J. T. (1988): *Comparison of fixation rigidity in canine tibia using different internal and external devices.* Unpublished data, Department of Orthopedics, Mayo Clinic/Mayo Foundation, Rochester, MN.

65. Winquist, R. A., Hansen, S. T., and Clawson, D. K. (1984): Closed intramedullary nailing of femoral fractures. *J. Bone Joint Surg.,* 66-A:529–539.

66. Wiss, D. A. (1986): Editorial comment. *Clin. Orthop. Rel. Res.,* 212:2–3.

67. Woo, S. L. Y., Lothringer, K. S., Akeson, W. H., Coutts, R. D., Woo, Y. K., Simon, B. R., and Gomez, M. A. (1984): Less rigid internal fixation plates: Historical perspectives and new concepts. *J. Orthop. Res.,* 1:431–449.

68. Wu, J. J., Shyr, H. S., Chao, E. Y. S., and Kelly, P. J. (1984): Comparison of osteotomy healing under external fixation devices with different stiffness characteristics. *J. Bone Joint Surg.,* 66-A:1258–1264.

Basic Orthopaedic Biomechanics, 2nd ed.,
edited by Van C. Mow and Wilson C. Hayes.
Lippincott–Raven Publishers, Philadelphia © 1997.

10

Biomechanics of the Human Spine

James A. Ashton-Miller and Albert B. Schultz

*Biomechanics Research Laboratory, Department of Mechanical Engineering and Applied Mechanics,
University of Michigan, Ann Arbor, Michigan 48109-2125*

Spine disorders are the most prevalent cause of chronic disability in persons less than 45 years of age and are second only to natural childbirth in accounting for hospital stays of patients under age 65 (183,209). In 1983, over 250,000 surgeries were performed on the spine in the United States (218). Although a small proportion of these concern the correction of congenital and idiopathic spine deformities, most relate to low-back and cervical spine disorders. The annual prevalence of low-back disorders in the U.S. population is about 15% to 20%; at any given time, back problems temporarily disable about 1% and chronically disable a further 1% of the population (10). In 1992, the annual costs associated with back pain in the United States ranged from $20 to $50 billion (179). Although the cause of most low-back disorders remains unknown, there is a clear association between strenuous work and lifting and the frequency and severity of spine disorders (9,77,146,171). For example, workers performing frequent heavy lifts from twisted positions have six times the risk of an acute lumbar disk prolapse of those who perform lighter work (128). These statistics and others confirming an association between heavy work and low-back disorders justify studies of the biomechanics of the human spine. However, it should also be noted that a large prospective study demonstrated that nonphysical factors such as job satisfaction and psychological attributes were also found to be important outcome predictors (38,39). A discussion of the range of treatment options that are available (40) is beyond the scope of this chapter.

This chapter reviews present knowledge of the basic biomechanics of the spine, emphasizing experimental measurements and techniques of biomechanical model analysis.

COMPONENTS OF THE TRUNK MUSCULOSKELETAL SYSTEM AND THEIR MECHANICAL PROPERTIES

The trunk musculoskeletal system consists of the spine, rib cage, and pelvis as well as associated fascia and musculature. The spine itself consists of 24 semirigid presacral vertebrae that are separated by relatively flexible intervertebral disks. Together with seven intervertebral ligaments that span each set of adjacent vertebrae, two synovial joints on each vertebra, called the zygapophyseal or facet joints, act to constrain relative motion.

The spine is divided into four regions: cervical, thoracic, lumbar, and sacral (Fig. 1). The thoracic spine serves as an integral part of the rib cage. Twelve pairs of ribs articulate posteri-

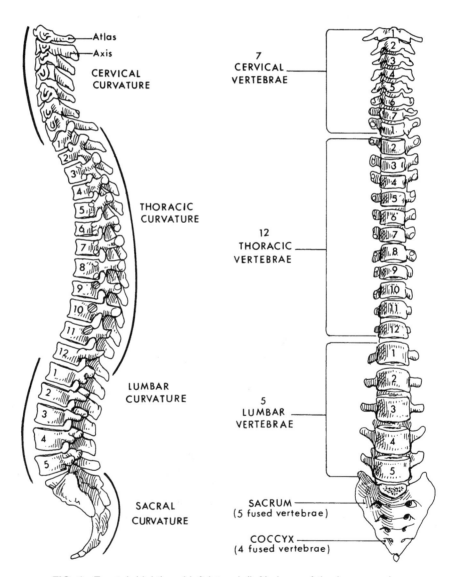

FIG. 1. Frontal *(right)* and left lateral *(left)* views of the human spine.

orly with the spine at the costovertebral joints; the upper ten pairs of ribs also articulate anteriorly with the sternum at the costosternal articulations. Movements of the rib cage relative to the thoracic spine occur during respiration, especially during strenuous activity. The sacral–coccygeal region is formed by nine vertebrae fused into a single bony mass that articulates with the right and left ilia (or innominate bones) to form the pelvis. The ilia articulate with the sacrum at the sacroiliac joints and with each other at the pubic symphysis. Enlargement of the birth canal at childbirth is the only time that appreciable movement of one ilium, relative to the other, normally occurs.

Bones and Joints

Vertebrae

With the exception of the upper cervical vertebrae, C-1 and C-2 (also known as the atlas and axis), each vertebra consists of an anterior structure known as the vertebral centrum and a complex configuration of posterior and lateral structures (note the lumbar vertebrae example, Fig. 2). This configuration is comprised of the structurally significant neural arch, made up of the pedicles and laminae that complete the spinal canal and the spinous and transverse processes, which serve primarily as muscle attachment sites. Each vertebra also has right and left superior and inferior articular processes, which in adjoining pairs constitute the right and left facet joints.

The vertebral centrum consists of trabecular bone surrounded by a thin cortical shell with an average thickness of 0.35 mm (244a). The centrum primarily resists compression and shear loading. Studies have shown that compression is carried mainly by the vertebral trabecular bone (see Vertebral Strengths, below). The superior and inferior margins of the vertebra, called vertebral endplates, average less than 0.5 mm in thickness (244a). In the young adult a thin layer of hyaline cartilage about 1 mm thick covers the central region of the endplate. Neither the vertebra nor the endplate is rigid. Studies have shown that under a 7500-N compressive load (as might occur in heavy lifts), the endplate can deflect up to 0.5 mm, reflecting a strain in the central vertebral trabecular bone of up to 3% (53).

Upper Cervical Vertebrae

The structures of the C-1 and C-2 vertebrae are highly specialized to facilitate a wide

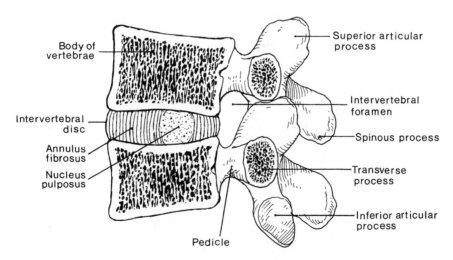

FIG. 2. Lumbar spine motion segment. Medial view of right half when sectioned in the midsagittal plane. Ligaments are omitted for clarity.

range of movements of the head (occiput). For this reason, their forms differ markedly from those of the other vertebrae. The C-1 vertebra, which supports the skull, is a ring-shaped bone with well-developed superior facet joints. The centrum of C-2, the dens, is elongated vertically and forms a longitudinal axis about which C-1 and the occiput rotate. The motion around this axis is constrained by the strong transverse and odontoid ligaments and the Occ–C1 and C1–2 facet joints. The biomechanical role of the alar ligaments has been investigated using both experimental (196) and computer simulation (115) studies. It has recently been shown, for example, that both alar ligaments must be intact to limit axial atlantoaxial joint rotation (71).

Intervertebral Disk

The largest avascular structure in the human body, the intervertebral disk, acts as a flexible spacer between adjacent vertebrae and carries significant compressive loads resulting from gravitational and muscular forces. Contrary to what was thought some years ago, the disk does not behave as a thin-walled cylinder under internal hydraulic pressure. Rather, the normal disk behaves as a thick-walled, deformable annulus, which until degenerate, contains fluid under pressure (117).

The disk consists of two regions, the inner nucleus pulposus and the outer annulus fibrosus (Fig. 3). The nucleus pulposus is formed from a strongly hydrophilic proteoglycan gel that is enmeshed in a random collagen matrix. Marchand and Ahmed showed that the annulus consists of 15 to 26 distinct layers of discontinuous concentric lamellae, the thicknesses of which increase markedly with age; they are arranged so that the orientation of the collagen fibers relative to the longitudinal axis of the spine alternates in successive layers (148). When they viewed the annulus from above, they reported many discontinuities: in any 20° circumferential sector, approximately half the laminae terminate or originate. When the annulus is viewed radially, the collagen is seen to be arranged in 20 to 60 bundles over the height of the disk. From the periphery inward, the proportion of type I collagen decreases, whereas that of type II increases (49,93). The lamellae become progressively less distinct as they merge with the central nucleus pulposus. Systematic radial and circumferential variations in its mechanical properties have been ascribed to variations in regional biochemical composition and structural properties (36,246) as well as to its poroelastic behavior (133).

In adults, the proportion of type I collagen in the posterior annulus progressively increases in the three caudal lumbar levels (48). This has been taken as possible evidence for remodeling of the disk structure in response to stress.

When an axial load is applied to a disk, the external forces are resisted by several mecha-

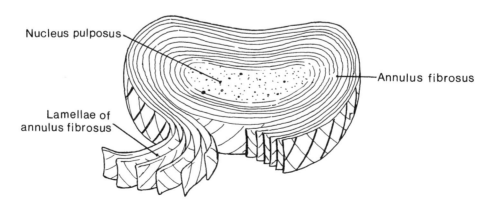

FIG. 3. Intervertebral disk sectioned to expose the annular organization.

nisms, including an elevated nucleus pressure (174). When the disk is in a steady state of hydration, the osmotic swelling pressure developed by the hydrated proteoglycans contained in the nucleus balances the applied stress. If the applied stress increases, water is driven out of the disk until a new steady state is reached. If, on the other hand, the applied stress is reduced, the disk rehydrates accordingly (Fig. 4). Disks taken at surgery have been shown to have a lower fluid content in the nucleus and higher fluid content in the outer annulus than disks removed at autopsy, presumably because of minimal applied compression loading (257). Under compression, the nucleus loses water over time. For example, Adams and Hutton (5) have shown *in*

vitro that in 4 hr the annulus and nucleus can lose up to 15% and 10% of their free water, respectively. Cyclic compression loading can further increase this loss and consequently decrease disk height by a factor of two (293); it is partly responsible for the well-known diurnal changes in standing height (80).

Ecklund and Corlett (87) have shown *in vivo* that the total decrease in disk height that occurs after standing for $1\frac{1}{2}$ hr can be regained in about 15 min by lying supine. These workers found that over the course of a day the total spinal height loss can reach about 1 cm, especially if heavy loads are lifted. The loss in height can be described by a Kelvin spring–dashpot model and is given by $y = A_1 + A_2 e^{-kt}$, where t is time and A_1, A_2, and k are de-

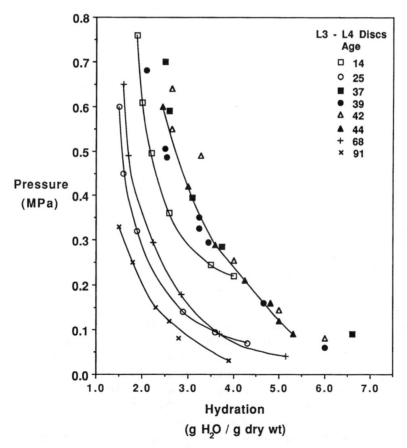

FIG. 4. Human intervertebral disk hydration versus osmotic swelling pressure. (From Urban and Mc-Mullin, ref. 277, with permission.)

termined experimentally. For example, in one subject, A_1, A_2, and k were found to be 1876.5 mm, 14.1 mm, and 0.186 hr^{-1}, respectively.

The maximum cell density in the disk is known to be determined by the nutritional supply (240). Nutrition of the disk is accomplished by diffusion through two main routes: via the blood vessels surrounding the annulus and via the capillary beds adjacent to the cartilaginous endplates. The area of the endplate available for diffusion is approximately 40% of the total vertebral area (72,113,276). Matrix synthesis of ^{3}H-proline and ^{35}S-sulfate in the bovine coccygeal disk has been found to be highest at the inner annulus and lowest in the outer annulus (192); those rates were load sensitive, increasing with increasing load and then decreasing on further load. Further work is needed to understand how changes in disk nutrition associate with degenerative changes commonly found in the annulus and endplates. Sclerotic bone associated with endplate fractures might well be expected to adversely affect the efficacy of the endplate diffusion route, for example.

Facet Joints

The main role of the facet joints is to limit excessive intervertebral shear and torsion motions of the intervertebral segment. Although much low-back pain in the young adult may be discogenic in origin, in the older spine with degenerative changes it is possible that the facet joints, relatively small posterior structures, may also be involved. Investigators have noted the rich afferent innervation of the facet capsules with the associated possibilities for signaling pain (25). Moreover, conditions such as spondylolysis seem to stem from a fatigue fracture of the posterior elements.

There is a gradual and characteristic change in the three-dimensional orientation of the facet joint surfaces from the cervical region through the thoracic region to the lumbar region (199,292). The kinematic constraints provided by the facet joints are particularly pronounced in the cervical spine, where they

cause marked coupling between lateral bending and axial torsion motions. This is the only region where such coupling is significant. The facet joint surfaces themselves are often nonplanar. In the upper lumbar spine, the opposing surfaces of the facet joints are oriented approximately in the sagittal plane, thus limiting axial rotation. More caudally, their orientation is almost in the frontal plane. Computerized tomography (CT) scans can be used to measure the angles subtended by the facet joint surfaces. For example, the average angle between left and right facet surfaces in the transverse plane increases from 74° at L3–4 to 96° at L4–5 and 106° at L5–S1 (278). However, large variability exists at the L5–S1 level: values ranging from about 36° to 180° have been reported (26). In the lumbar spine the area of each facet ranges from 100 to 350 mm^2 and varies with facet orientation (94). The right and left facet joint orientations are not necessarily symmetric about the midline. For example, in 3000 spinal radiographs, 23% of patients exhibited asymmetry at the three lower levels (46). Most patients showed asymmetry of less than 10°, but facet asymmetry, known as facet tropism, can range up to 42° (94). *In vitro* studies show that simultaneous compression and anterior shear cyclic loading can lead a vertebra to rotate to the side of the more oblique facet (75).

The mechanical properties of the lumbar facet joints were studied by Skipor and coworkers (247) in order to estimate the loads carried by the facet joints in different situations. One way of estimating the amount of load sharing between the disk and the facets is by using mathematical models (15,241,242, 297). These models are usually validated by comparing predicted behavior (with and without posterior elements) with experimental measurements (see Motion Segment Stiffnesses, below). These studies show that the facets carry 10% to 20% of the spinal compressive load in an upright standing position and more than 50% of the anterior shear load on the spine in a forward-flexed position. The facets have been shown to resist anterior shear forces up to 2 kN without failure (76).

The contact pressure between facet joint surfaces can be measured *in vitro* by introducing a pressure-sensitive film that registers the average pressure over time or by using a miniature pressure transducer to record the instantaneous fluid pressure under load in this fluid-containing synovial joint (90,142). These techniques have been used to demonstrate that in torsion the facet under compression was loaded most heavily. The relationship between the applied moment and experimentally measured pressure increased linearly and ranged from 4 to 26 Nm/kPa among specimens. The highest facet pressures were recorded under combined torsion, flexion, and compression. Facet joint pressures also increased with a reduction in disk height; the average peak pressure was found to rise 36% for a 1-mm loss in disk height, and 61% for a 4-mm loss in disk height (85).

By categorizing the loads carried by the facets in carefully controlled experimental conditions, studies such as these may help to suggest or clarify the etiology of clinical disorders, and may answer questions such as whether spondylolysis is caused by fatigue fracture of the pars interarticularis (74).

Sacroiliac Joints

Reviews of the literature describing the anatomy and morphology of the sacroiliac joints and their articular surfaces and associated ligaments are given by Ashton-Miller and colleagues (22) and Vleeming and colleagues (282,283).

Vertebral Strengths

Many measurements of vertebral compression strength have been made (291). These studies show an increase in compression strength as one moves caudally, from 1.5 kN at C-3 to 2.0 kN at T-1, 2.5 kN at T-8, 3.7 kN at T-12, and to 5.7 kN at L-5. The ultimate vertebral compressive strength has been shown to increase by 380 N from L-1 to L-4 (109). McBroom and colleagues (152) demonstrated

that most of the vertebral ultimate compressive strength is derived from the strength of the cancellous bone; removing the entire cortex weakened the vertebra by only 10%. Variation in ultimate compressive strength between individuals can be large in adults. For example, Hutton and co-workers (118) found a range greater than one order of magnitude, from 0.8 kN to 15.6 kN. Recently, Brinckmann and co-workers (51) showed a linear correlation between ultimate compressive strength of lumbar vertebrae and a parameter equal to bone density times endplate area, as determined by CT scanning. The ultimate compressive strength has been estimated to within 1-kN accuracy using CT methods (52). Because bone density was found to remain essentially constant throughout the thoracic and lumbar spine, the craniocaudal increase in ultimate compressive strength results from the increase in cross-sectional area of the vertebrae. Brinckmann and colleagues have demonstrated convincingly that the fatigue life of vertebrae, indicated by the initial endplate failure, depends on the compressive load range (Table 1). This has implications for setting guidelines for safe repetitive lifting in the work place. Quantitative computed tomography is a useful technique for estimating the fatigue strength of vertebrae *in vivo* because of the ease with which bone density and endplate area can be estimated. The probability of failure *in vitro* within 5000 cycles, estimated to be equivalent to 2 weeks of athletic training, increases from 36% at a loading range 30% to 40% of ultimate compressive strength (UCS) to 92% at a loading range of 60% to 70%

TABLE 1. *Probability (%) of vertebral fatigue in the lumbar spine*

Load level (%UCS)[a]	Cycles of failure				
	10	100	500	1000	5000
30–40%	0	0	21	21	36
40–50%	0	38	56	56	67
50–60%	0	45	64	82	91
60–70%	8	62	76	84	92

[a]UCS, ultimate compressive strength. Data from Brinckmann et al. (51).

UCS. Vertebral bone mineral density has also been shown to correlate with trunk extensor muscle strength (244). Hence, it is reasonable that competitive weight lifters exhibit significantly increased vertebral bone mineral density (103) due to adaptive remodeling of their vertebrae caused by exposure to large loads.

Motion Segment Stiffnesses

Knowledge of the load-displacement behavior of the spine and its components is required for biomechanical analyses of spine function. For convenience, tests of spine mechanical properties have traditionally used short lengths of spine consisting of two vertebrae and their intervening soft tissues. These are called spine motion segments or spine functional units. In most cases the load-displacement properties are obtained by gripping the lower vertebra securely, applying known test forces or moments or both to a point on the upper vertebra, and measuring the resulting displacements (195). In this way the coefficients of the flexibility matrix can be measured directly. Table 2 gives averaged stiffness values for each spine region. Load-displacement data have also been recorded for whole spine segments, including the complete ligamentous lumbar spine. In the next four sections we consider the load-displacement behavior of each region of the spine.

Cervical Spine

The properties of the occiput–C1–C2 complex were studied for the first time by Goel

and co-workers (100). They found that a test moment of 0.3 Nm produced rotations ranging from only 3° in lateral bending to 14.5° at Cl–2 in axial torsion and 16° at Occ–C1 in extension. Translations occurring in these upper segments under loads up to 1.5 Nm have also been reported. Moroney and colleagues (167,168) found lower cervical spine motion segments to be an order of magnitude stiffer than upper cervical segments. Stiffness was greatest in axial torsion and least in flexion.

Many severe neck injuries are associated with vertebral body fractures as well as intervertebral joint dislocations resulting from a sudden flexion–compression loading of the cervical spine (262,298). The presence of a compression fracture is evidence that the axial compressive load exceeded the ultimate compressive strength of the vertebrae. *In vitro* tests of complete intact cervical spine specimens have shown that commonly observed cervical fractures can be produced under conditions in which the cervical spine lordosis is removed and the spine is rapidly loaded under axial compression (300). Under such conditions the cervical spine can fail by buckling (208): with the head constrained at impact, an anterior, posterior, or lateral "bowing" of the middle cervical region can occur under the compression loading. The direction in which it buckles will be determined principally by how the head is constrained (173) at impact as well as the axis of least cervical bending stiffness (for example, flexion, extension, or one of the two lateral bending directions). Although there is no time for the cervical muscles to respond during most impact loadings of the cervical spine, anticipatory pretensing

TABLE 2. *Average stiffness values (N/mm and Nm/deg) for the adult human spine*

Spine level	Comp	Shear (ant/post)	Lat	Bending (flex/ext)	Lat	Axial torsion	Reference
Occ–C1	—	—	—	0.04/0.02	0.09	0.06	100
C1–2	—	—	—	0.06/0.05	0.09	0.07	100
C2–7	1317	125/55	33	0.4/0.7	0.7	1.2	168
T1–12	1250	86/87	101	2.7/3.3	3.0	2.6	195
L1–5	667	145/143	132	1.4/2.9	1.6	6.9	34, 237
L5–S1	1000	78/72	97	2.1/3.0	3.6	4.6	159

of muscles up to about 50% of their maximum activation can result in a fivefold increase in muscle stiffness (125,245), thereby increasing instantaneous spine-bending resistance. Although this muscle stiffness will increase spine resistance to buckling, it comes at the cost of also increasing spine compression (see section on Biomechanical Model Analyses for mechanism by which spine muscle activity increases spine compression). Experimental and theoretical studies are therefore needed to investigate how the threshold for spine fracture is affected by the level of cervical spine muscle coactivation immediately before and during impact.

Thoracic Spine

The properties of the isolated adult thoracic spine have been reported by Panjabi and colleagues (195) and others. They found average stiffness values ranging from 100 N/mm in lateral shear to 900 N/mm in anterior or posterior shear to 1250 N/mm in compression. Rotational stiffnesses were about 2 to 3 Nm/° in flexion, extension, lateral bending, and axial torsion.

Lumbar Spine

The overall static load-displacement behavior of lumbar spine motion segments has been well documented (34,237). In these studies, the stiffness of intact spine motion segments was in the range of 600 to 700 N/mm in axial compression and 100 to 200 N/mm in anterior, posterior, or lateral shear; however, there was considerable intraindividual variation. Test forces ranged from 86 N in shear to 400 N in compression and were applied at the vertebral body center. Rotational stiffnesses ranged from 1.0 to 2.0 Nm/° in flexion, extension, and lateral bending and 6.8 Nm/° in axial torsion when test moments of 4.7 Nm were used. To simulate the compression loading of the spine *in vivo*, these results were obtained with a 400-N compressive preload. More recently, the lumbosacral (L5–Sl) spine

motion segment has been found to have lower shear stiffnesses (0.5 to 0.75 times), larger bending stiffnesses (1.4 to 3.3 times), and less stiff torsion resistances (1.5 times) than L1–5 lumbar segments (159). We have demonstrated that compressive preloads of the magnitude likely to act *in vivo* can lead to a significant stiffening of the motion segment (123).

The influence of the posterior elements has been investigated by first testing intact motion segments and then excising the pedicles and retesting the motion segment without the posterior elements. Not surprisingly, this always leads to a decrease in stiffness. For example, McGlashen and co-workers (159) found that removal of the posterior elements resulted in 1.7-fold increase in shear translations in response to a given shear force, a 2.1-fold increase in bending rotations in response to a given moment, and a 2.7-fold increase in axial rotation in response to a given axial torsion moment. The behavior of lumbar motion segments under larger shear and with bending and torsion loads of up to 1000 N and 100 Nm have also been examined. Although shear load-displacement behavior remained linear, moment behavior was found to be slightly nonlinear at the higher loads (23).

The mechanical response of the disk to loads has been measured in terms of both internal and external strains. Stokes and Greenapple (258) used a photogrammetric technique to measure surface strains of the annulus fibrosus. Some of the larger strains were measured under torsion, where a 17-Nm load resulted in tensile strains of 9%, well under the 25% ultimate strain of the annulus in tension. Martin and colleagues (149) used an array of 0.5-mm-diameter steel spheres to visualize the movements of the annulus and nucleus under various loads. With a resolution of 0.125 mm, the method showed that the nucleus moves posteriorly in flexion and anteriorly in extension. Disk bulge under load, of course, has clinical relevance for sciatic and stenotic symptoms. *In vitro* (216), the typical increase in disk bulge under load is small: less than 1 mm of bulge under 1000 N compression. Posterior disk bulge is greatest in extension and least in flexion.

Sacroiliac Joints

The mechanical properties of the sacroiliac joints (35,106,249) have received little attention compared to their anatomic, histologic, and clinical characteristics, which were reviewed extensively by Bellamy and co-workers (31). Adult sacroiliac joints were found to exhibit stiffnesses of 100 to 300 N/mm for superior, inferior, anterior, and posterior shear of the sacrum relative to the ilium. Bending stiffness was lowest in axial torsion, 7 Nm/°; higher in extension, 12 Nm/°; and largest in flexion and lateral bending, 16 and 30 Nm/°, respectively (22). Thus, depending on the test direction, these joints have from 0.05 to 7.00 times the stiffness of intact L1–5 lumbar motion segments. No test data are available for the load-displacement behavior of the pubic symphysis. The effects of joint stiffness and pelvic dimensions on mechanical behavior of the intact pelvis have been investigated by Scholten and co-workers using models (221). The recorded motions of these joints *in vivo* is modest: namely, one or two degrees (259). A novel hypothesis, which still requires experimental testing, has been been advanced concerning the stabilization of the sacroiliac joints in physically strenuous upright activities through the coordinated activity of the trunk, pelvic, and hip muscles; these structures are thought to exert a medially directed resultant load on the joints, forcing their articular surface irregularities to "interlock," thus increasing their resistance to the significant cephalocaudad shear loads (282).

Rib Cage Components

The load-displacement properties of adult ribs and costovertebral and costosternal articulations have been measured. In general, for the costosternal articulations, a 7-N test force applied at a point 1 cm lateral to the cartilage gave rise to displacements of about 5 to 20 mm in the superior/inferior or anterior/posterior directions (233). Similarly, for the costovertebral articulations, the same test load applied to the rib about 5 cm from the vertebral body resulted in similar displacements of the loading point in the anterior/posterior and superior/inferior directions but only 1-mm displacement in the lateral direction. Human ribs are themselves flexible. A 7-N test force applied transversely to the end of a rib whose other end is gripped securely causes displacements of about 30 and 60 mm in upper and lower thoracic ribs, respectively (232). These data have been used to validate computer models of the ribcage under various types of loads (see section on Biomechanical Model Analyses).

Ligaments

Spinal ligaments pass between each vertebra along the length of the spine and function to limit excessive joint motion. These ligaments include the anterior and posterior longitudinal ligaments, the ligamentum flavum, the inter- and supraspinous ligaments, and the intertransverse ligaments. The facet joint capsules also act as tension-bearing structures between the articular processes (247). Although most ligaments run the length of the spine, the supraspinous ligament does not extend caudally past L-5 (112).

The tensile properties of isolated spinal ligamentum flavum have been reported by Nachemson and Evans (176); Tkaczuk (269) studied the anterior and posterior longitudinal ligaments, and Waters and Morris (288) have studied the inter- and supraspinous ligaments. Ligamentum flavum demonstrated a pretension in the range of 5 to 18 N, depending on age, and a failure stress in the range of 2 to 10 MPa at strains of 30% to 70%. The longitudinal ligaments failed at about 20 MPa, carrying loads of 180 N (posterior) and 340 N (anterior).

One way to examine the mechanical role of ligaments in spine motion segments is to repeatedly apply a standard load, say a flexion moment, to the motion segment while sequentially sectioning ligaments from posterior to anterior (201). Panjabi and colleagues (197) showed that when lumbar motion segments are loaded in flexion under a moment of 15 Nm, strains in ligaments furthest from the axis of rotation can reach nearly 20%.

Hormonal factors are known to affect collagenous tissue laxity. For example, a relationship has been identified between ligamentous laxity and those women who, later in pregnancy, developed back pain (193).

Muscles

The trunk musculature, though complex, may be divided into the posterior wall musculature (erector spinae or paravertebral muscles), the respiratory or intercostal muscles between adjacent ribs, and abdominal wall muscles comprised (from inside out) of the intertransversus, the interior and exterior obliques, and, anteriorly, the rectus abdominis. The most superficial layer of trunk muscles on the posterior and lateral walls are primarily broad muscles connecting to the shoulder blades, upper extremities, and head: the rhomboids, latissimus dorsi, pectoralis, and trapezius. Finally, some of the lower trunk muscles, such as transversus abdominis, attach to a strong superficial fascial sheet, the lumbodorsal fascia, which may be thought of as a three-layered tensile load-bearing structure that inserts onto the upper pelvic borders. The anatomy of this fascia has been reviewed by Bogduk and Macintosh (42). The diaphragm is a large dome-shaped muscle attached to the lower ribs and to the thoracolumbar spine via the crura and forms the boundary between the lungs and the contents of the abdominal cavity. Its action on the spine has not been included in any model to date. The iliopsoas muscles originate on the anterior aspect of the lumbar spine to pass across the hip joint to the inside of the femur.

The histochemical composition of a muscle can determine its rate of tension development, fatigue characteristics, and power output. Vertebral muscle composition has been reviewed by Bagnall and co-workers (27), who found 50% to 60% type I muscle fibers. Interestingly, 11% more type I fibers were found on the left side of L-5 than on the right in asymptomatic persons. One possible explanation for this may be the dominance of right-handedness, which inevitably increases left-side paravertebral muscle loading.

Striated muscle is almost never injured in isometric or shortening contractions; it can be injured when it is activated and forcibly lengthened (57). Under such conditions, striated muscle can develop at least 50% larger forces than under isometric conditions (154,287), a fact that has not escaped the notice of athletes or anyone using that phenomenon to jerk a heavy load off the ground, hence increasing the potential for injury to the ultrastructure of specific sarcomeres. Depending on the severity of the injury, 1 to 4 weeks is required for the complete recovery of the muscle structure and function (56). That this time span is consistent with the clinical finding that 33% of patients with acute back pain reported pain lasting less than 1 month (81) should not be overlooked. It is therefore instructive to consider situations in which back muscles might be forcibly lengthened and therefore placed at risk for injury.

Problem

Give an example of the conditions under which one might expect the erector spinae to be at greatest risk for injury. For simplicity, consider a sagittally symmetric task.

The erector spinae are most likely to be injured when they are used in a strenuous effort to decelerate the trunk when it is flexing and to accelerate it into extension. Consider what happens, for example, following a trip that leads to a severe stumble or fall. Once the trip is detected the erector spinae become maximally active in an attempt to arrest the forward momentum of the trunk. Let us assume that the level of neural recruitment is maximal. The erector spinae are undergoing a lengthening contraction, and the tension they develop will rise above maximal isometric values in proportion to their initial rate of elongation (65).

Finally, when that force has acted long enough to arrest further trunk flexion, it will lead to trunk extension relative to the pelvis. The greatest risk for muscular injury occurs at the instant of peak erector spinae tension (57), because that is when the internal stress is greatest. The later section on Biomechanical Model Analysis will use mathematical models to explain why this peak tension in turn places the vertebrae under considerable compression loading, so much so that the vertebrae in some individuals can be placed at risk for a fracture.

Mathematical models of the spine often require detailed descriptions of the origin and insertion points of muscles and muscle slips, their anatomic and physiological cross-sectional areas, and even their fiber lengths and fiber types. For example, none of the lumbar back muscles can exert torsional moments greater than 2 Nm about the lumbar spine: it is the oblique abdominal muscles that are the principal axial rotators of the trunk (145). The detailed anatomy of trunk muscles is being updated continually (41,43,44,134,166). Intraindividual differences and changes in muscle lever arms with different body postures may now be taken into account (144,190,273, 275). Magnetic resonance imaging has led to the *in vivo* estimation of muscular lever arms about the cervical and lumbar spine (157,184, 270,273), although the lines of action of muscle fibers in muscles such as the erector spinae remain difficult to visualize because spatial resolution remains limited in whole body images.

Nervous System Tissues

Relatively little attention has been given to the biomechanics of neural tissues associated with the spine. Olmarker and collaborators (192) have studied the effect of pressure on intrathecal spinal nerve root blood flow. Certain movements of spine motion segments are known to affect the foraminal area available for the exiting spinal nerve roots. For example, extension reduces the size of the foramen by at least 20% (202). In some older individuals with spinal stenosis, this can cause nerve root entrapment (220), resulting in sciatic symptoms on standing and in trunk extension (252). This phenomenon is primarily a compression phenomenon and contrasts with a second mechanism that can cause sciatic symptoms in younger and middle-aged adults in relation to tension in the nerve root. To understand this we examined the mechanical factors that determine *in situ* the contact force between a spinal nerve root and a simulated disk protrusion (254,256). Those studies describe the trilamellar arrangement of Hoffmann ligaments that constrain the thecal sac and nerve root above the disk, while the foraminal attachments are known to constrain the extrathecal nerve root distal to the disk. Because the nerve root is thereby constrained above and below the herniated disk, much like a stiff rubber band stretched over the protrusion, the contact force tending to compress the nerve root unilaterally was found to increase with increasing simulated disk protrusion magnitude, even for increases in protrusion of as little as 1 mm. It was also found to increase with increasing disk height and to decrease with decreasing disk height. Because of the known diurnal loss in disk height over the course of the day (see Intervertebral Disk) (212), the latter explains the clinical finding that patients whose sciatica is related to nerve root tension commonly report sciatic symptoms as being worst in the early morning and less severe after an hour of being upright. It also helps to explain why, when chemonucleolysis is effective in alleviating sciatic symptoms, success is almost always correlated with a disk height reduction induced by the chemonucleolysis (253).

MEASUREMENTS OF SYSTEM BEHAVIOR

Spine Configuration

The spine is approximately straight when viewed frontally because each vertebra and disk is approximately symmetric about the sagittal plane. A slight lateral deviation or scoliosis is common because no structure in the body has perfect symmetry. In a lateral view, the spine exhibits four curves (127). In the cervical and lumbar spine, each curve is concave backward-a lordosis. Cervical lordosis ranges from 2° to 24° with an average of 9° (102). In the thoracic and sacral spine, each curve is concave forward kyphosis. The thoracic kyphosis normally averages 39°, with 93% of kyphoses ranging from 22° to 56°. Most of the thoracic kyphosis results from slight wedging of the vertebral bodies; a thoracic disk tends to have endplates that are approximately parallel (284). Wedging over three or more thoracic vertebrae that exceeds 15° is considered abnormal and occurs in conditions such as Scheuermann's kyphosis. Normal lumbar lordosis averages 57°, with 93% ranging from 38° to 75° (284). There are no significant differences in the angle of lordosis between males and females (95).

The lumbosacral angle was defined by Ferguson as the angle that the plane of the upper S-1 endplate makes with the horizontal. In an upright stance, this angle averages 41° in the adult male, with 95% of individuals lying within the range of 26° to 57° (110).

Anthropometry

Anthropometry is the study of human size and form. Mathematical models of the spine often require the linear dimensions and shape of the spine and trunk as input data. These may be obtained from a variety of sources.

Lanier (135) examined the overall geometry of macerated vertebra; Brandner (47) studied disk and vertebral dimensions during growth. On a more global scale, marked variations exist between individuals: Fig. 5 demonstrates the variation in sagittal curvatures of a sample of 18 adolescent girls with a mean age of 12 years. The equation of a fifth-order

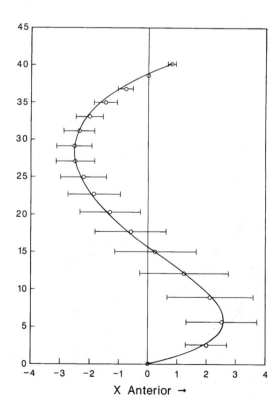

FIG. 5. Normal variation in shape of the adolescent spine. Mean (denoted by *o*) and standard deviation (denoted by *bars*) of vertebral center coordinates (cm) are given. Note that the *y* axis is oriented vertically and the *x* scale is expanded. *Solid line* is fifth-order regression line whose equation is given in section entitled Anthropometry. Data are for 18 adolescents between the ages of 10 and 18 years of age (24).

polynomial regression ($r^2 = 0.80$) fitted to the coordinate values is

$$x = 1.02030y - 0.12767y^2 + 0.00543y^3 - 0.10504 \times 10^{-3}y^4 + 0.83552 \times 10^{-6}y^5$$

where x is the anterior offset in millimeters and y is the distance in millimeters superior from the center of S-1. Table 3 gives the average vertebral center coordinates and angle of disk inclination for these spines.

Linear and cross-sectional dimensions can be measured directly from subjects using calipers (161). These have been used to scale cadaveric segmental mass and inertia data from other sources, such as Clauser and colleagues (64) or McConville and co-workers (153).

Ranges of Motion

Many techniques have been developed to measure spine range of motion *in vivo*. Most are noninvasive and use measurements from surface landmarks (165), pantographs (294), and goniometry (89). Although often quick and convenient, these techniques yield results that are reproducible only to within 7% to 12% (163). They give a reasonable approximation of total spine motions but a poor indication of actual intersegmental spine motions and so are not as reliable for the latter purpose as radiologic techniques (150,211). For this reason we review only radiologic data (Table 4).

Lumbar Spine

Perhaps the most thorough range of motion studies of the lumbar spine region are those of Pearcy and Tibrewal (206) and Pearcy and collaborators (204). These workers carefully standardized test subject postures and used radiographic methods to determine the average maximal intersegmental rotations at L5–S1. In flexion and extension these were found to be 9° and 5°, respectively, whereas in axial rotation and lateral bending, the average was 2° and 3°, respectively.

Thoracic Spine

One of the only studies of thoracic range of motion is that of Bakke (28), who found that total intersegmental flexion–extension movement does not exceed 5°. At each end of the thoracic spine, the motions are similar to those of the cervical and lumbar regions (28). In lateral bending, motions are limited to 4° or less.

TABLE 3. *Mean (SD) coordinates of vertebral body centers in healthy individuals*

Level	x (cm)	y (cm)	θ (°)[a]
T1	0.80 (0.22)	40.13 (0.15)	26.85 (7.75)
T2	0.0	38.47	26.85 (6.12)
T3	−0.77 (0.17)	36.78 (0.11)	24.03 (5.13)
T4	−1.46 (0.33)	35.01 (0.19)	20.03 (4.97)
T5	−2.01 (0.44)	33.11 (0.34)	15.35 (4.33)
T6	−2.36 (0.49)	31.17 (0.33)	9.39 (3.41)
T7	−2.52 (0.59)	29.15 (0.39)	3.82 (3.98)
T8	−2.49 (0.64)	27.07 (0.41)	−2.40 (4.03)
T9	−2.32 (0.75)	24.90 (0.38)	−6.57 (4.54)
T10	1.86 (0.89)	22.64 (0.40)	−8.95 (5.19)
T11	1.31 (1.02)	20.25 (0.37)	−11.22 (5.49)
T12	−0.60 (1.22)	17.72 (0.31)	−12.33 (5.76)
L1	0.24 (1.40)	14.99 (0.35)	−13.40 (4.94)
L2	1.22 (1.50)	12.10 (0.40)	−13.43 (4.65)
L3	2.11 (1.45)	8.96 (0.44)	−8.18 (4.42)
L4	2.51 (1.18)	5.46 (0.47)	2.07 (7.57)
L5	1.99 (0.69)	2.48 (0.40)	19.13 (11.00)
S1	0.0	0.0	42.46 (10.57)

[a]θ is the inclination of the upper endplate with the x axis, which is horizontal; a positive angle denotes an inclination below the horizontal. Data from Ashton-Miller and Skogland (24).

TABLE 4. *Average segmental range of motion (°) at each spine level*[a]

Level	Flexion	Flexion/ Extension	Extension	Lateral bending	Torsion
Occ–C1	13[b]		13[b]	8[b]	0
C1–2	10[b]		9	0[b]	47
C2–3	8		3	10[b]	9
C3–4	7		9	11	11
C4–5	10		8	13	12
C5–6	10		11	15	10
C6–7	13		5	12	9
C7–T1	6		4	14	8
T1–2	5		3	2	9
T2–3		4		3	8
T3–4		5		4	8
T4–5		4		2	8
T5–6		5		2	8
T6–7		5		3	8
T7–8		5		2	8
T8–9		4		2	7
T9–10		3		2	4
T10–11		4		3	2
T11–12		4		3	2
T12–L1		5		3	2
L1–2	8		5	6	1
L2–3	10		3	6	1
L3–4	12		1	6	2
L4–5	13		2	3	2
L5–S1	9		5	1	1

[a]Cervical and thoracic data from ref. 291. Cervical data from ref. 132 unless otherwise specified. Thoracic data from ref. 28. Values are total flexion/extension values. Lumbar data from refs. 204, 206.
[b]Data from ref. 291, p.65.

Torsional data are not available, probably because of difficulties of measuring planar radiographs to a precision of better than 5° (84).

Cervical Spine

Kottke and Mundale (132) studied the range of motion of the lower cervical vertebrae *in vivo* (Table 4). Ranges of motion for the upper cervical spine have not been thoroughly documented (86), but estimates are given by White and Panjabi (291).

Measurements of Intact Trunk Properties *In Vivo*

The bending stiffness of the trunk has been measured *in vivo* in flexion by Scholten and Veldhuizen (222). They applied three-point bending forces to the trunk, which was supported at the pelvis and shoulder region.

Bending stiffness was found to be 0.153×10^8 N/mm^2 or roughly ten times that of the isolated spine. This illustrates how much the rib cage, fascia, and passive muscle tissues serve to stiffen the isolated spine, even in the fully relaxed supine individual.

Trunk Proprioception

Upright posture in humans requires the head to be maintained over the pelvis. The neuromuscular motor control system responsible for this relies on afferent feedback from many sources, including the spine and trunk articular, muscular, and cutaneous sensors as well as the vestibular organs. Trunk proprioception, the ability to sense where the top of the spine is relative to the pelvis, is thus derived from this feedback. Some patients, such as children with certain types of scoliosis, can unknowingly develop a lateral trunk "imbalance" whereby T-1 is offset laterally from S-1 by several centimeters. Why such patients can not sense their asymmetric posture is presently unknown. Indeed, relatively little is known about the accuracy of trunk proprioception, even in the healthy individual. Ashton-Miller and colleagues (17) showed that trunk proprioception improves with age in healthy children so that by adulthood, the top of the spine can be reliably repositioned within 1° of the upright. For a flexible column with some 25 joints, this is impressive accuracy. The threshold for detecting axial torsion is less than 1° (263), whereas proprioceptive accuracy has been found to be slightly worse in the sagittal plane than the frontal plane (158). To examine mechanisms, trunk proprioception acuity has also been compared with the spine in the vertical plane and in the horizontal, gravity-free, plane (122).

Disk Injury

One of the most common causes of back and extremity pain is compression of the dura and/or nerve roots by disk prolapse, particularly in the cervical region and at the lowest lumbar levels. It is not known what causes a disk to prolapse. Disk protrusion and subsequent prolapse may be related to excessive loading that leads to disk degeneration and fatigue failure of the inner posterior annular fibers (4,7,49). Two studies have identified a genetic predisposition to disk herniation in the young (213,279), and a recent study in adults has demonstrated that the odds ratio of a lumbar disk herniation is approximately tenfold higher in relatives of a patient with a proven disk herniation than in matched controls (217). The mechanism of genetic expression is presently unknown. For example, except for a possible association between lifting free weights and cervical prolapse, sports such as recreational baseball, softball, golf, bowling, swimming, diving, jogging, or racquet sports do not seem to be associated with an increased risk for disk herniation (172). Even disk degeneration, as scored by magnetic resonance (MR) imaging, was not sig-

nificantly more extensive in men who exercised more than two times per week for 24 years than in their identical twin who exercised significantly less (280).

A recent review (2) of the quasistatic loading conditions known to cause posterior disk prolapse examined combined axial compression, flexion, and lateral bending. Such loading can cause up to 50% increases in the tensile strain in the posterior annulus (205), significant posterior annulus thinning (6), and increased hydrostatic pressure in cadaver lumbar disks. Cyclic loading of the disk in combined flexion, rotation, and compression at 1.5 Hz has been shown to produce annular protrusion and/or prolapse *in vitro* in an average of only 7 hr (274). Abrupt increases in axial compression combined with hyperflexion have also been shown to cause vertebral failures (160) and failure of the posterior annulus in previously intact lumbar disks (3,4). This is supported by computer simulations that have identified annulus fibers as being particularly susceptible to failure under large lumbar anterolateral bending loads (239). A recent study suggests that disk prolapse may occur relatively late in the degeneration process, after radial fissures have formed in the annulus. These fissures are thought to form conduits along which disk fragments may be expelled with motions involving less than 10° of rotation (55). It is worth noting that these findings generally pertain to lumbar disks from cadavers under 50 years of age; the absence of hydrostatic nuclear pressure in the more degenerate lumbar disks of older cadavers usually precludes this type of discal injury because of the fibrocartilaginous nature of their nucleus. A different mode of failure can, however, occur in older disks involving inward (238), not radial, buckling of the inner annulus under compressive loading (107,261), as a result of the absence of nuclear hydrostatic pressure. In one possible scenario, this could result in a fatigue failure of the inner annulus fibers on repeated loading with damage accumulation because of little or no remodeling potential in that region.

Several studies have attempted to investigate how changes in disk integrity can affect the load-displacement behavior of the disk and spine motion segment (198). Brinckmann and colleagues (51) found that sectioning the posterior inner annulus fibers to within 1 mm of the periphery results in a small localized bulge of only 0.5 mm in that region under compression loading, a clinically irrelevant amount. This evidence supports the argument that the adult annulus acts as a thick-walled rather than a thin-walled cylinder. On overload, they found, the endplate failed before the injured annulus failed. These findings are consistent with endplate failure as a possible precursor to disk degeneration because such a failure may disrupt disk nutritional pathways from the vertebra. However, the links among endplate failure, symptoms, and pain are not well established. Experimental models of disk degeneration have been produced by incising the outer annulus of quadruped disks (8,136,141,162,194, 207): although the site of the original outer annular injury heals with fibrocartilage, the disk degenerates within a few months with lasting structural and compositional changes.

In quadruped animals, the enzymatic removal of the nucleus pulposus by injection has been found to cause a significant loss in disk height and an increase in disk flexibility in bending and torsion (255,285). Moreover, changes in facet joint cartilage have been demonstrated subsequent to enucleation (45). This is one model of disk degeneration that seems useful clinically because disk degeneration usually precedes derangement of the facet joints (58).

Finally, another type of disk injury that can occur is related to failure of the superior or inferior endplate, usually from failure of the underlying cancellous bone. Because the elasticity of the cancellous bone returns the endplate to its original configuration when the injurious load is removed, these failures can be next to impossible to spot visually even in the sectioned specimen, let alone radiographically. Following such an endplate fracture, intraosseous pressure has been shown to increase in the vertebral body (299), a condition that has been shown experimentally to create severe low-back pain (251).

Effects of Age

Growth increases both trunk mass and inertia. Although most data on body segment mass and inertia are for adults, some estimates are available for children (124). With the advent of MR scanners, more data should become available in the future.

Not surprisingly, the immature spine is more flexible than the adult spine; the adolescent spine, for example, is from one to ten times more flexible, depending on the direction of the applied load (24). Growth also affects the angulation of the cervical facets; in the C-2 region the initial angulation of the facets to the sagittal plane increases from about 30° to nearly 80°, whereas in the lower cervical spine the change is from about 60° to 80° (191).

Growth has only a subtle effect on the magnitude of thoracic kyphosis or lumbar lordosis. Thoracic kyphosis decreases by 11% and 13% in boys and girls, respectively, between 8 and 11 years and increases thereafter by 28% and 27%, respectively, by the age of 16 years (295). Lumbar lordosis increases by about 10% from the age of 7 to 17 (284). During this time the spine increases in length by about 26% (248).

In the mature individual, cervical lordosis increases significantly in men between ages 20 and 40 (16° to 22°) and in women between ages 20 and 50 (15° to 27°) (102). In the elderly, increased thoracic kyphosis and decreased lumbar lordosis occur, partially through a decrease in overall disk height (164). This loss in disk height is attributable to two factors—disk degeneration and an increased curvature of the vertebral endplate, often from osteoporotic changes in the vertebral cancellous bone (91). There is also a significant trend toward increasing midbody transverse diameter of the lumbar vertebrae with age, amounting to 14% between the ages of 20 to 80 years in men (91).

In considering other age changes in the mature spine, one should distinguish between the relatively minor changes that represent natural aging, more significant atrophic changes associated with inactivity, and more significant changes associated with disease. In general, when changes in overall mobility are associated with natural aging, they first become evident in the most challenging of physical activities (226). As an example, although 50% of young adult men are willing to lift a 500-N weight, only 15% of men aged between 60 and 65 years may be willing to do so (62).

In regard to age changes at the organ level, it is well known that the strength of bone is proportional to its mineral density. In general, trabecular bone density starts to decrease in the fourth decade, with losses of up to 30% being observed in elderly men and up to 50% in elderly women (151). When a loss in bone density does occur with age, the lumbar vertebrae have been demonstrated to be susceptible to compression failures (37,50). In men, for example, when average vertebral bone density has decreased to 105 mg/ml as measured using quantitative computer tomography, there is a 25% risk of a vertebral fracture, whereas at 45 mg/ml the fracture risk rises to 99% (215). In women, the risk of a vertebral fracture rises 2.2-fold or more for every standard deviation loss in bone mass in postmenopausal women, whether it is measured using dual-photon absorptiometry or quantitative computer tomography (73). Expressed another way, a postmenopausal woman with a bone mineral content that is two standard deviations below the mean value for her age has a 20% risk of spine fracture during the next 3.6 years (73). Osteoporotic fractures lead to an average reduction in anterior and midvertebral height of 25% (99); because the posterior height of the vertebra remains unchanged, this reduction will usually cause a local increase in kyphosis. As far as the functional consequences of osteoporosis are concerned, women with osteoporotic fractures of the spine have been shown to be three times more likely to have difficulty with activities of daily living such as descending stairs, lifting, bending, and walking (104), presumably from activity-related discomfort and/or pain.

Spinal ligaments, as typified by the anterior and posterior longitudinal ligaments, undergo changes of 7%, 28%, and 22%, in elasticity, residual deformation, and energy dissipation, respectively, between the second and seventh decades (269).

It is not uncommon for muscle strength to decrease with advancing age. For example, an approximately 30% loss in isometric strength in the trunk extensors and flexors has been noted between the fourth and eighth decades of life, with the most rapid loss occurring after 50 years of age (60,281). Much of this strength loss can likely be explained by the 30% loss in trunk muscle cross-sectional areas in muscles such as the psoas major and erector spinae over a similar time span (120). We have also found a 30% to 40% loss in the rate of developing isometric strength with age, which appears to be linked to a change in muscle contractility (265). If this finding in the ankle muscles is also found valid in the trunk muscles, it would mean that the rapid deceleration or acceleration of the trunk relative to the pelvis in emergent situations such as a fall would become increasingly challenging with age.

Even in frail elderly, striated muscle retains its ability to gain strength with training, and, depending on the baseline value, strength increases of up to 100% have been recorded in as little as 10 weeks (96). The fact that increases in elderly muscle strength of 20% to 60% were associated with increases in muscle cross-sectional area of approximately 20% (214) suggests that at least some of this increase may be related to improved coordination and/or cognitive factors.

Degeneration

Disk degeneration is usually graded *in vivo* using qualitative radiographic measures of osteophytes and loss of disk height. More recently, magnetic resonance imaging offers a method for quantifying the loss of hydration within the disk (290). Macroscopic disk degeneration *in vitro* is graded by visual inspection and classified according to one of four grades according to Nachemson's scheme (174). Degeneration starts in the second decade of life and continues steadily thereafter (Fig. 6). The gradual yellowing of the disk that occurs with age is apparently contributed by modification of proteins linked to the collagen (115). Loss of nuclear material is characteristic of degeneration. An experimental study has shown that the disk and its intradiscal pressure are sensitive to loss of nuclear material: loss of just 1 g of nuclear tissue results in a disk height loss of about 0.8 mm and an increase in annular bulge of 0.2 mm (54). The risk for disk degeneration has been shown to be increased in the presence of facet tropism (asymmetry) (188).

Does degeneration affect spine mechanical properties? In one study, Nachemson and co-workers (181) found no effect of degeneration on lumbar vertebral behavior. In another, larger study, Koeller and colleagues (131) also found little effect of age on compression stiffness but did find an increase in creep in elderly spines. So, at present, it appears that degeneration in itself does not lead to dramatic changes in disk mechanical properties. Although increased lumbar laxity at low loads, chiefly in the so-called "neutral zone,"

has recently been reported in degenerated disks (200), these results are unlikely to be of much significance because compressive preloads of a magnitude similar to those acting *in vivo* are already known to stiffen such disks (123). With the advent of osteophytes, however, one can expect stiffness to increase by a factor of two (167).

The Relationship of Mechanical Factors to Some Clinical Conditions

Spondylolysis and Spondylolisthesis

Spondylolysis refers to a defect in the pars interarticularis, which may be dysplastic, and results in elongation, thinning, and eventual breakage of this structure. A number of theories have been proposed for the pathogenesis of spondylolysis, including heredity and fatigue failures. Certainly, a higher prevalence of spondylolysis has been demonstrated among relatives of patients with this condition (296). Spondylolysis is rarely observed before the age of 5. Its incidence increases

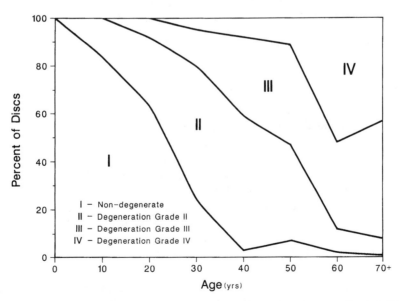

FIG. 6. Percentage of intervertebral disks in each degeneration grade by age. Grade I disks are non-degenerate, whereas grade IV disks are severely degenerate, as defined by Nachemson (174). Data are for 600 disks (19).

from 4.4% in 6-year-old children to 5.8% in adults (98). Certain athletic activities are known to be associated with significant increases in the risk of developing spondylolysis. For example, a fourfold increase in the prevalence of spondylolysis has been observed in female adolescent gymnasts; this rate (i.e., 20.7%) was similar to that found in male high school and university athletes (116,121). Cricket fast bowlers are also at risk for developing spondylolysis: this activity involves repeated near-maximal accelerations and asymmetric motions of the trunk from a position of extension into axial twisting and anterolateral bending on the run (97). The caudal spine level seems to be particularly predisposed to spondylolysis: in one series of 255 patients, 226 (88.6%) had spondylolysis occurring at the L5–S1 level; in the remainder it occurred at the L4–5 level (219).

What mechanical factors are involved? Troup (272) and Cyron and Hutton (75) proposed that repeated extension of the spine, particularly when combined with compression loading, can lead to a fatigue fracture of the pars interarticularis. If the intensity, duration, or rate of the activity increases sufficiently to produce bony microfractures in the pars interarticularis that accumulate faster than can be repaired, a fatigue fracture seems to be a reasonable mode of failure. At present, conclusive proof of this pathogenesis is not available.

Spondylolisthesis is the slippage of one vertebra on another. Usually this results from a defect in the pars interarticularis, a defect in the pedicle, an elongation of the pars and pedicle, or degeneration of the disk. Again, this usually occurs at the L5–S1 level. Degenerative spondylolisthesis at the L4–5 level has been associated with sagittal orientation of the facet joints (105).

Segmental Hypermobility Versus Spine Instability

Much confusion exists in the orthopaedic and spine biomechanics literature concerning the term "spine instability." This is a term that is poorly defined and often misused (21). In mechanical terms, an unstable structure is one in which a small load causes a large (sometimes catastrophic) increase in displacement. Another way of describing this behavior is to say that the structure has experienced a drastic loss of stiffness. A fracture or tumor can cause such behavior. But spines that are classified clinically as having "instability" just because their segmental motions are a few millimeters or degrees more than normal do not exhibit signs of mechanical instability. In regard to these issues, Ashton-Miller and Schultz have argued:

> that the spine is seldom mechanically unstable, rather for many cases that are discussed clinically, it is spine segment hypermobility that is the relevant concept. Decreased spine segment stiffness, evidenced by larger-than-normal vertebral motions on standardized radiographs, should be termed "segmental hypermobility" not "segmental instability" or "spinal instability." Indeed, the measurement of "motion" by itself, without also measuring the associated applied loads (forces and/or moments) that induce the motion, is not fully meaningful, because observed motions always depend on applied loads and loads that produce those motions are seldom quantified, especially *in vivo*. We suggest ways to standardize spine loads when evaluations of segmental hypermobility are to be made. Finally, the definition and measurement of spine segmental hypermobility should be independent of (a) its possible causes (e.g., disk degeneration) and (b) its possible consequences (e.g., neurological deficits) (21).

Thus, loads *and* motions, not just motions, are needed to quantify the stiffness, the flexibility, and, therefore, the instability of the spine. Attempts have been made *in vitro* to quantify hypermobility in the cervical spine in terms of such measurements (201).

In summary, the term "spinal instability" should be reserved for a very specific mechanical behavior, most often associated with trauma, very severe osteoarthrosis, tumor, infection, or iatrogenic causes. It should not be used just to describe segmental motions that are modestly larger than normal, nor should it be used to describe symptomatology. If a spine segment does not display catastrophic displacements, defined in one study as exceeding 12° (185), under known standardized loadings typical of daily activities, then it does not exhibit signs of mechanical instability.

Trunk Muscle Strengths

Maximum isometric voluntary strengths of the lumbar trunk muscles have been reported by several groups (161,234,250). The mean moments that healthy young adult males can develop about low lumbar motion segments in an upright standing position are on the order of 200 Nm in attempted trunk extension, 150 Nm in attempted trunk flexion or lateral bending, and 90 Nm in attempted twisting. The strengths of healthy young adult females are approximately 60% of these values.

The passive moment resistances developed by lumbar motion segments in bending or twisting motions of a few degrees are only a few newton-meters (see Lumbar Spine, above). In upright positions, where motion segments are rotated only a small amount, these passive resistances are negligible compared to the moments that can be actively developed by the trunk muscles. However, when substantially rotated, lumbar motion segments can develop passive moment resistances on the order of 60 Nm (23). In configurations involving substantial bending or twisting of the spine, passive bending resistances are no longer negligible.

While maximum isometric strengths faithfully reflect the strength available to perform tasks slowly, they may not always reflect the strength available during tasks requiring rapid movements because of the well-known Hill hyperbolic relationship describing the reduction of muscle contractile force with increasing muscle fiber shortening velocity. Recognizing this, several investigators have reported lifting strengths and lumbar trunk muscle strengths in tasks in which the trunk is moved at constant angular rates (130,186). Smith and collaborators (250), however, found that when the trunk is moved at rates up to 120°/sec, lumbar trunk strengths are quite similar to strengths measured isometrically. A

review of trunk isokinetic strength test results has appeared (187).

Moroney and co-workers (167) measured the maximum voluntary isometric strength of neck muscles. In healthy, young adult subjects, mean strength was on the order of 26 Nm in attempted neck extension, 10 Nm in attempted flexion, 13 Nm in attempted lateral bending, and 9 Nm in attempted twisting. Thus, neck muscle voluntary strengths are an order of magnitude smaller than lumbar trunk muscle strengths.

As mentioned already, muscle properties are significantly affected by aging. After age 30 years, for example, isometric muscle strength is known to decrease by from 18% to 40% by age 65 years (for example, see review by Chaffin and Ashton-Miller [60]).

Myoelectric Measurements

The loads imposed on spine motion segments and the muscle contraction forces developed in physical task performances cannot be measured directly *in vivo*. However, they can be quantified indirectly by measurements of intradiscal pressures (see Disk Pressures, below) and measurements of myoelectric signals. The latter arise because motor nerves engender muscle contractions through the transmission of electrical signals. Such signals are called myoelectric activities. Semiquantitative measurements of spine myoelectric activities have been reported by many groups, including Walters and Partridge (286) in the anterior abdominal muscles, Carlsöo (59) in an array of trunk muscles, Morris and colleagues (169), Pauly (203), Donisch and Basmajian (83) in the back muscles, and Ashton-Miller and colleagues in studying cervical muscle response to acute pain (16).

Quantitative measurements of trunk muscle activities have been reported by Andersson and colleagues (11), Schultz and colleagues (236), and Pope and colleagues (210). Such measurements have demonstrated that the recruitment patterns of trunk muscles vary in a repeatable manner at a given spine level when the direction of an external moment is changed in a systematic manner (137). Myoelectric signals are noisy, and their absolute values are affected by many variables that cannot easily be controlled. However, when signals are averaged over subject populations and compared on a relative basis from task to task, they can more readily be interpreted quantitatively. The papers last cited used these ideas to interpret the measured activities. A chief use of such measurements is for the validation of biomechanical model analyses (see Rigid-Body Models, below) of muscle contraction forces.

Disk Pressures

Nachemson (174) demonstrated that the pressure developed within the nucleus pulposus of a nondegenerated cadaver lumbar intervertebral disk is nearly proportional to the compressive load on the motion segment containing that disk. This intradiscal pressure is approximately 1.5 times the compression load divided by the transverse cross-sectional area of the disk. Schultz and colleagues (237) showed that other modes of loading seldom modify this proportionality substantially. Thus, measurements of intradiscal pressure provide a means to estimate spine compression loads. Even in cadaveric motion segments, intradiscal pressure has been shown to increase by 100% from the erect posture to the fully forward flexed posture, partly as a result of tension generated in the posterior intervertebral ligaments in such postures (1). Such increases in intradiscal pressure cause the vertebral endplate to deflect into the vertebral body (53) and, when combined with additional compressive loads, can even cause failure of the endplate (114).

Nachemson and Morris (177) used intradiscal pressures to determine *in vivo* compression loads on the lumbar spine resulting from task performances. Subsequent studies have been reported or reviewed by Nachemson and Elfström (175), Andersson and co-workers (12), Nachemson (178), and Schultz and colleagues (230). Pressures within the nucleus of the L-3 disk are typically 300 kPa in

relaxed upright standing configurations, corresponding roughly to a compression equal to the weight of the body segments superior to L-3, and more than four times this value in relatively modest exertions. A chief use of intradiscal pressure measurements has been the validation of biomechanical model predictions (see Rigid-Body Models, below) of spine loads.

Trunk Cavity Pressurization

It was recognized as early as 1900 that trunk cavity pressurization is sometimes used to relieve loads on the spine (9). Davis (78), Bartelink (29), and Morris and collaborators (170) contributed some of the earlier reports of abdominal cavity pressure measurements during physical task performances. Typically, during a heavy exertion, abdominal cavity pressure peaks are on the order of 13.3 kPa (100 mm Hg), and Eie and Wehn (88) found cavity pressures in a weight lifter as high as 26.7 kPa (200 mm Hg). Morris and colleagues (170) reported thoracic cavity pressure measurements as well and analyzed the load-relieving effects of such pressures.

Scaled anatomic cross sections show that the area of the abdominal cavity is on the order of 50% of the product of lumbar trunk width times depth, or approximately 300 cm^2 in an average-size male adult (92). A cavity pressure of 13.3 kPa then yields a resultant force of approximately 400 N. The cavity cross-section centroid lies anterior to the intervertebral disk center at a distance that is approximately 42% of trunk depth, or about 8.4 cm. So, large abdominal cavity pressures can produce flexion-relieving moments about a lumbar intervertebral disk center on the order of 34 Nm. This is particularly true when the transversus abdominis, rather than the rectus abdominis muscle, is the abdominal wall muscle most highly correlated with abdominal cavity pressure (68).

Measurements of abdominal cavity pressures during task performances have been proposed as indicators of spine load (79,147).

However, some evidence indicates that this may not be an accurate measure (230,271), and whether abdominal cavity pressurization actually reduces loads on the spine has been questioned (180). One might speculate that a possible role for the increased abdominal wall muscle activity and simultaneously raised intraabdominal pressure during heavy exertions may be to help stiffen the spine and trunk (267).

BIOMECHANICAL MODEL ANALYSIS

Rigid-Body Models to Determine Trunk Loads

Studies that seek to examine the role of mechanical factors in low-back pain epidemiology or to design industrial work schemes to reduce worker back muscle fatigue, for example, require knowledge of the loads placed on the trunk structures when a physical task is performed. The easiest and safest route to that knowledge is biomechanical model analysis. Tasks that are performed slowly can be modeled effectively using concepts of rigid-body equilibrium, and those performed rapidly are examined more appropriately using concepts of rigid-body dynamics. Morris and co-workers (170) were among the first to attempt a biomechanical analysis of quasistatic trunk loads. King (129) reviewed many of the biomechanical model analyses that have been reported in the literature on the musculoskeletal system. The relevant ideas will be illustrated through calculations of lumbar trunk internal loads, but similar ideas can be used to calculate internal loads on any musculoskeletal system structures. The following section illustrates the use of one modeling approach.

Cross-Section Muscle Models

Animals move and exert forces on their surroundings through the use of their muscles. Cross-sectional muscle models, based on concepts of rigid-body equilibrium, allow analyses to be made of effects produced by muscular contraction. This section illustrates analyses that determine the external loads that can be resisted or developed when lumbar trunk muscles are contracted with known tensions. The following sections illustrate the converse; that is, they show what sets of muscle tensions are required to resist or develop a known external load. The former analyses are relatively simple; the latter are often more complicated.

Figure 7 shows a model of ten single-equivalent muscles through a transverse section of the lumbar trunk at the L-3 level (236). Note that a horizontal plane through L-3 does not intersect bony structures other than those of the spine. This is a convenient reference plane because analysis of load transmission paths through multiple bony structures may be quite complex. Table 5 details representative values of the areas, centroidal locations, and lines of action of those muscles. Similar data have been gathered by others (157,184). Table 6 presents the equations of equilibrium that describe the net force and moment developed by these muscles about the center of the L-3 intervertebral disk. Solutions of these equations serve to predict how a physical task performance will load the structures of the trunk. These equations incorporate the assumption that the lumbar motion segment can resist compression and shear forces but not significant bending moments. This is because, although the passive bending resistance developed by a lumbar motion segment in small rotations is only a few newton-meters per degree, net moments are often on the order of 100 Nm.

Calculation of Net Reactions from Given Contraction Forces: Estimates of Isometric Trunk Strengths

The muscle cross-section model just described, or similar models, can be used to estimate maximum isometric trunk strengths. When muscles are contracted with known forces, the model equations can be used to compute the resulting net reaction force. The

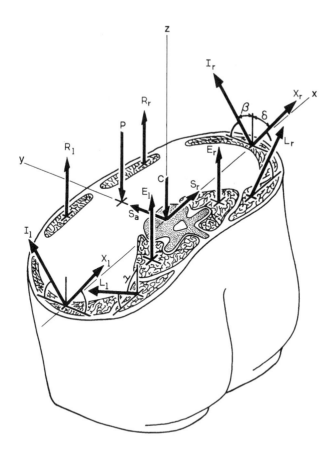

FIG. 7. Schematic representation of a lumbar trunk cross-sectional model with ten single-equivalent muscles. The muscle equivalents represent the rectus abdominis (R), the internal (I) and external (X) oblique abdominal, the erector spinae (E), and the latissimus dorsi (L) muscles. C, S_a, and S_r are the motion segment compression and shear forces resulting from weight and muscle forces. P is the force resulting from intraabdominal pressure within the abdominal cavity.

TABLE 5. *Data incorporated into the ten single equivalent muscle L-3 cross-sectional model*

Muscle	Symbol	Line of action	Area ratio per side[a]	Location of centroid	
				Anteroposterior offset ratio[b]	Lateral offset ratio[c]
Rectus abdominis	R	Longitudinal	0.0060	0.540	0.121
Internal oblique abdominals	I	Inclined 45° to longitudinal, in sagittal plane	0.0168	0.189	0.453
External oblique abdominals	X	Inclined 45° to longitudinal, in sagittal plane	0.0148	0.189	0.453
Erector spinae	E	Longitudinal	0.0389	0.220	0.179
Latissimus dorsi	L	Inclined 45° to longitudinal, in frontal plane	0.0037	0.276	0.211

[a]In ratio to trunk width times trunk depth.
[b]From vertebral body center, in ratio to trunk depth.
[c]From vertebral body center, in ratio to trunk width.
   The vertebral body center lies in the midsagittal plane at 0.66 times the trunk depth from the anterior-most edge of the cross section.

TABLE 6. *The equations of equilibrium that govern the ten-muscle cross-sectional model of Fig. 7[a]*

Equations of force equilibrium:

$$F_x = S_r + (L_r - L_l) \leftrightarrow \sin \gamma$$
$$F_y = S_a = (I_l + I_r) \leftrightarrow \sin \beta - (X_l + X_r) \leftrightarrow \sin \delta$$
$$F_z = (E_l + E_r) + (R_l + R_r) + (L_l + L_r) \leftrightarrow \cos \gamma + (I_l + I_r) \leftrightarrow \cos \beta + (X_l + X_r) \leftrightarrow \cos \delta - C$$

Equations of moment equilibrium:

$$M_x = (R_l + R_r) \leftrightarrow y_r + [(I_l + I_r) \leftrightarrow \cos \beta + (X_l + X_r) \leftrightarrow \cos \delta] \leftrightarrow y_o - (E_l + E_r) \leftrightarrow y_e - (L_l + L_r) \leftrightarrow \cos \gamma \leftrightarrow y_l$$
$$M_y = (R_l - R_r) \leftrightarrow x_r + [(I_l - I_r) \leftrightarrow \cos \beta + (X_l - X_r) \leftrightarrow \cos \delta] \leftrightarrow x_o + (E_l - E_r) \leftrightarrow x_e + (L_l + L_r) \leftrightarrow \cos \gamma \leftrightarrow x_l$$
$$M_z = [(I_r - I_l) \leftrightarrow \sin \beta + (X_l - X_r) \leftrightarrow \sin \delta] \leftrightarrow x_o + (L_r - L_l) \leftrightarrow \sin \gamma \leftrightarrow y_l$$

[a]F_x, F_y, F_z are the net reaction force components.
M_x, M_y, M_z are the net reaction moment components.
C, S_a, S_r are the motion segment compression and shear forces.
E_l, L_l, R_l, I_l, X_l are the forces in the left-side erector spinae, latissimus dorsi, rectus abdominis, and internal and external oblique muscles.
E_r, L_r, R_r, I_r, X_r are the corresponding right-side muscle forces.
β, δ, γ are the angles shown in Fig. 7.
x_e, x_l, x_r, x_o are the positive distances from the y axis for the corresponding muscles.
y_e, y_l, y_r, y_o are the corresponding distances from the x axis.

maximum isometric intensity (in units of stress: force per unit cross-sectional area, also termed "specific tension" by muscle physiologists) that human muscles can develop has been reported by Ikai and Fukunaga (119) to range from 400 to 1000 kPa, and we have used the latter value for illustrative purposes in our own models. In light of recent studies, those values, which are widely used, may be overestimated. For example, it has recently been shown that under volitional recruitment human striated muscle maximally develops up to 279 kPa (kN/m²) in the direction of the muscle fibers (182). As confirmation, this value is consistent with animal muscle, which, under supramaximal electrical stimulation, can develop up to 294 kPa (65), with type I and type II muscle fibers developing similar values (143). Using muscle cross sections from single whole-body MR cross-sectional scans can lead to a 40% underestimate of the physiological cross-sectional area (126) in uni- and bipennate muscles, leading to an inflated estimate of specific tension. Clearly, specific tension values as high as 1000 kPa are overestimates for parallel-fibered muscle. Other errors in estimating specific tension include (a) ignoring load sharing by fascia or tendon inadvertently included in the muscle MR cross section as "muscle," (b) incorrectly calculated muscle physiological cross-sectional area, (c) underestimating the muscle lever arms used to calculate the muscle force from maxi-

mum trunk strength tests, and (d) failing to ensure that the strength tests were truly isometric. In one study, increases in specific tension of 20% were observed in lengthening contractions at joint rotations of 120°/sec, whereas reductions in specific tension approaching 40% were observed in shortening contractions at 30°/sec (126).

In maximum attempted extension, the only muscles included in this model that can contribute force are the latissimus dorsi and the erector spinae. Assume that no other muscles contract in such an attempt. Then, in a person with L-3 level trunk frontal and sagittal diameters of 30 cm and 20 cm, respectively, at a 1000-kPa intensity, the latissimus muscle on each side can develop (Table 5) 222 N and the erector muscles 2334 N.

If these values are substituted into the formulas for force and moment equilibrium in Table 6, it is found that such contractions would develop an extension moment of 223 Nm.

Problem

What extension moment can be developed at a 1000-kPa intensity in the cross-sectional model if only the erector spinae muscles contract? (Answer: 206 Nm)

---

[1]Expositions similar to this are given by Schultz (223, 224) and by Ashton-Miller and Schultz (20).

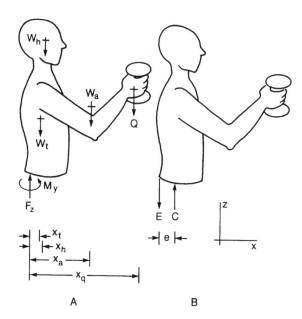

FIG. 8. Free-body diagram for a simple weight-holding task. **(A)** Q is the weight held, W's are the weights of the various body segments, and the x's are their distances anterior to the intervertebral disk center. F_x and M_y are the nonzero components of the net reaction. **(B)** E is the contraction force in the back muscles, and C is the compression on the intervertebral disk. E and C together must provide the required F_z and M_y.

In maximum attempted flexion, the rectus abdominis and the internal and external oblique muscles might be contracted in this model. At a 1000-kPa intensity, these muscles could produce a flexion moment of 180 Nm. These model-predicted maximum strengths in attempted extension and flexion are in good agreement with mean measured values of those strengths (see Trunk Muscle Strengths, above). Now, suppose that in an attempted lateral bend, all muscles on one side contract with an intensity of 1000 kPa. The lateral bending moment component of the net reaction is then 330 Nm. However, in the absence of other external moments, the cross section would not be in equilibrium because six of the ten modeled muscles do not have longitudinal lines of action. When those muscles contract, they produce flexion/extension, lateral bending, and twisting moments simultaneously. In the case of attempted lateral bending, these last two net moment components would be 22 and 20 Nm.

Similarly, if a maximum twisting moment is developed by fully contracting the internal oblique and latissimus muscles on one side and the external obliques on the other, the twisting moment would be 190 Nm under the specified circumstances. However, the twisting moment would be accompanied by a 42 Nm net flexion

and a 21 Nm net lateral bending moment that would need to be equilibrated. In the extension and flexion attempts, lateral bending and twisting moments did not arise because of the bilateral symmetry of the model.

Calculation of Contraction Forces and Internal Loads from Given Net Reactions: Simple Case[1]

An illustration of a simple internal load calculation is afforded by an analysis of a sagittally symmetric weight-holding task. To gauge the muscle contraction forces needed and the loads this task imposes on the lumbar trunk structures, consider the free-body diagram (Fig. 8A) of the body segments above the imaginary transverse plane at the L-3 level. The net reaction across the transverse plane required to keep the upper body segments in equilibrium consists of the force F_z and the moment M_y. The values of these follow from the equations expressing longitudinal force and flexion–extension moment equilibrium:

$$F_z = W_a + W_h + W_t + Q$$
$$-M_y = x_a W_a + x_h W_h + x_t W_t + x_q Q \quad (2)$$

where the Ws represent the weights of the arms, head, and trunk; Q represents the weight held; and the x's represent the moment arms of these forces about the center of the L-3 spine motion segment. Appropriate values of those weights might be 60, 40, 250, and 50 N; and those moment arms 20, 5, 1, and 40 cm, respectively. In that case, $F_z = 400$ N, and $M_y = 36.5$ Nm.

Once the net reaction is known, it is possible to calculate the internal loads required for static equilibrium. Assume that the required net reaction is developed solely by a spine compression force C and an equivalent back muscle tension E acting over moment arm e (Fig. 8b). Balance of force and moment now requires that

$$F_z = C - E$$
$$-M_y = -eE \qquad (3)$$

An appropriate value of e is 6.5 cm. Then, for the data given above, $E = 562$ N, and $C = 962$ N. Note that this spine compression is about 2.4 times the superincumbent body weight. Its value is dictated largely by the need to balance moments.

Calculation of Contraction Forces and Internal Loads from Given Net Reactions: Other Cases

Calculations of net reactions from given contraction forces are called "statically determinate" because the number of unknowns is fewer than the three equations of force and three equations of moment equilibrium available to find them. The major use of trunk cross-section muscle models is for problems that are "statically indeterminate," where the number of unknowns exceeds the total number of equations of equilibrium. In these problems, the net reaction moments are given, and a set of muscle contractions that can produce them, along with the other resulting internal loads, are determined. In the ten-muscle model, for example, there are ten unknown muscle contractions, but only three equations of force equilibrium and three equations of moment equilibrium.

Such statically indeterminate calculations can be made in a number of ways, but only one technique is briefly described here. In this technique, two quantities are optimized in two successive applications of linear programming. In the first linear program, the contraction intensity for which solutions exist is first minimized, subject to the constraints that equilibrium be satisfied and that no contraction force can be negative. In the second linear program, a set of contraction forces that minimize the value of spine compression is calculated, subject to the above two constraints plus the requirement that the maximum contraction intensity used at this stage cannot exceed the value first calculated. Details of these calculations are given by Bean and co-workers (30). Only illustrative results from voluntary strength calculations are presented here.

When estimates of maximum voluntary strengths are made by this double linear programming technique for attempted extension and attempted flexion, results identical to those calculated in the section Calculation of Net Reactions, above, are obtained. This should not be surprising because, in the former calculations, an equilibrium state was achieved.

For attempted lateral bending, the maximum moment that can be developed under the above assumptions is found to be 260 Nm, compared to the 330-Nm value previously obtained. The reason for this is that, along with the contraction of all the model muscles on one side, two muscles on the opposite side are also contracted in order to bring the net flexion–extension and twisting moments to zero. Similarly, in attempted twisting, the maximum moment is found to be 167 Nm, compared to the 190 Nm previously obtained. Note that these model-estimated lateral bending and twisting strengths are well in excess of measured values (see Trunk Muscle Strengths, above), illustrating shortcomings in current models of tasks involving lateral bending and twisting. Current models of this kind also do not predict trunk structure loadings in heavy exertions very well (229). However, for many common physical tasks, biomechanical models do predict trunk structure loadings reasonably well, as confirmed by lumbar intradiscal pressure measurements (230) (see Disk Pres-

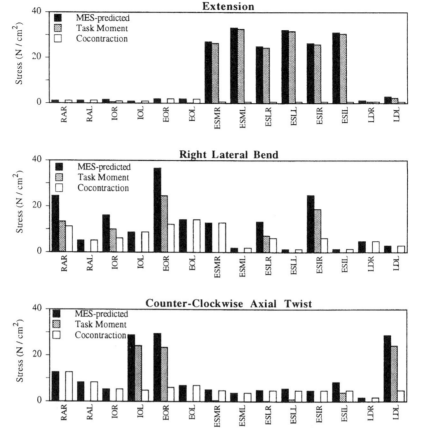

FIG. 9. The pattern of predicted trunk muscle activity *(solid bars)* varies with the direction of the isometric exertion attempted [extension **(top)**, right lateral bend **(middle)**, or axial torsion **(bottom)**]. Results are from a recent EMG-driven, L-3 level, cross-sectional trunk model study (267). The figure also shows how much of each muscle's effort actually contributes to generating useful moment in the intended direction *(gray bar)* and how much contributes to the cocontraction synergy *(open bars)* required to balance moments developed in other directions by the other active muscles. Note the amount of cocontraction, and hence additional spine loading, used in lateral bend or axial twist tasks.

sures, above). The sensitivity of such models to variations in anthropometry and posture has also been explored (61).

Trunk muscle myoelectric signal data have been employed to increase the accuracy of biomechanical models used to predict lumbar spine loads and lumbar trunk muscle contraction forces. These "EMG-driven" models were first developed by McGill and co-workers (155,156). This kind of model has been used in our laboratory to examine the effects of cocontraction of lumbar trunk muscles during physical exertions (225,264,266–268). Thelen and colleagues (267) estimated that cocontractions

contributed 16% to 19% to the sum of the lumbar muscle forces developed during attempted slow and rapid trunk extensions and two to three times that much during attempted trunk lateral bending and axial twisting (Fig. 9).

The use of more complex models to investigate trunk structure loads is justified only in situations where simpler models fail to capture the mechanics essential to the situation. For one example of circumstances under which a simple model predicts trunk loads approximately as well as a complex one, Thelen and colleagues (264), using a 14-muscle biomechanical model of the L3–4 trunk cross section and accounting for inertial effects in the rapid pulling tasks they investigated, predicted that a peak dynamic extension moment of 49 Nm would impose a peak dynamic compression load on the L3–4 motion segment of 1328 N. Using the simple, single equivalent muscle model governed by equations 2 and 3 and assigning to weight Q the perhaps unrealistic value of 164 N, compared to its 50-N value in the example that earlier illustrated the use of this model, would produce a static trunk extension moment $(-M_y)$ also 49 Nm in magnitude. Use of equations 2 and 3 then predicts a net vertical force (F_z) of 514 N, an erector muscle contraction force (E) of 980 N, and a spine compression (C) of 1494 N. This spine compression differs by approximately 11% from the value obtained from the much more sophisticated model of Thelen and colleagues. Moreover, to better reflect the conditions in the experiments of Thelen and colleagues, if one subtracts the 164-N spine compression attributable to weight Q, then the two predictions of spine compression are almost identical. However, the mechanics of generating extension moments are mechanically simple, so this agreement is not surprising. On the other hand, the simple model, in contrast to the sophisticated one, is incapable of investigating lateral bending and twisting.

All models have their limitations, and these single lumbar level models are no exception. One limitation is that they fail to take into account equilibrium requirements at other spine levels. When those requirements are taken into account, then the predicted muscle recruitment patterns and spine loads can change (65), depending on the activity being considered. Another limitation is that they do not specifically address how muscle antagonism (111,138–140), whether voluntary or involuntary, can alter spine loading (185). A further limitation of such models is that they fail to take advantage of the inherent stiffness offered by the passive and active tissues that comprise the spine and trunk. Structural stiffness is an important parameter in defining the stability of a structure (70); recent models have considered how muscles may provide lumbar spine stability and hence make it less sensitive to unforeseen disturbances under load (33,63,69,82). Although these papers advance the field of spine modeling, we are not aware of any experimental evidence that a loss in spine stability ever actually occurs *in vivo* in the intact spine during stressful activities. Each nod of the head as an individual falls asleep in the upright posture is an example of a temporary loss, then recovery, of cervical spine stability through a momentary reduction in bending stiffness normally provided by the cervical muscles in the awake state.

Detailed discussions about various trunk muscle models and their use can be found in the literature (13,61,185,189,227–230,234,236).

Extension to Dynamic Performances

In tasks that are performed rapidly, the inertial forces and moments needed to accelerate body segments can become large compared to the forces and moments needed to equilibrate those segments in the same tasks performed slowly. In such dynamic performances, inertial loading needs to be accounted for in the computation of the net reaction. Dynamic performance of a task may also alter the calculation of the internal loads, if for no other reason than that there may be significant antagonistic muscle contraction. However, few studies of this latter phenomenon are available to guide biomechanical analyses.

To illustrate how inertial loading effects on net reactions can be calculated, consider the simple free-body models of upper-body sagittal rotation dynamics shown in Fig. 10. The model assumes that all body segments above the L-3 level are rotated about L-3 as a single rigid body, and the rotation angle is measured by θ. Those segments are represented as a block of mass m whose mass center lies distance l superior to L-3.

Problem

Given values $\dot{\theta}$ and $\ddot{\theta}$ for the angular velocity and acceleration of the block, calculate the net reaction components at L-3.

The reaction components can be divided into the horizontal reaction, H; the vertical re-

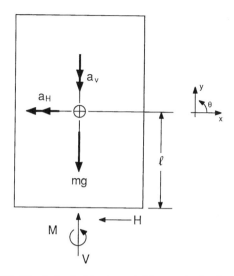

FIG. 10. A single-block model for analysis of upper body dynamics. The mass, *m,* of all body segments superior to the trunk level of interest is assumed to pivot as a single rigid body about the disk center. a_H and a_V are the components of the mass center acceleration. *H, V,* and *M* are the nonzero force and moment components of the net reaction.

action, *V;* and the trunk moment, *M.* In the course of calculating these quantities, knowledge of the horizontal and vertical components of the mass center acceleration, a_H and a_V, will be needed, along with the moment of inertia of the block, **I**, about the *z*-direction axis through its mass center.

The equations of plane rigid-body dynamics become

$$H = ma_H$$
$$V = m(g - a_V)$$
$$M = \mathbf{I}\ddot{\theta} \qquad (4)$$

The kinematic equations governing the mass center accelerations are

$$a_H = l\ddot{\theta}$$
$$a_V = l\dot{\theta}^2 \qquad (5)$$

To roughly assess the order of magnitude of the numbers involved, suppose that values for $\dot{\theta}$ and $\ddot{\theta}$ are chosen as the maximum angular velocity and angular acceleration that would occur during a sinusoidal oscillation with a

total excursion of 40° and a frequency of 1 Hz. Then, the maximum values of $\dot{\theta}$ and $\ddot{\theta}$ would be 2.19 rad/sec and 13.8 rad/sec². Suppose the block has a mass of 40 kg and a radius of gyration in the sagittal plane about L-3 of 0.289 m, so that its moment of inertia is 3.33 kgm². If we take *l* = 0.25 m and substitute the above numbers into equations 4 and 5, we obtain:

$$a_H = 3.45 \text{ m/sec}^2$$
$$a_V = 1.20 \text{ m/sec}^2$$
$$H = 138 \text{ N}$$
$$V = 344 \text{ N}$$
$$M = 45.5 \text{ Nm} \qquad (6)$$

Note that the centripetal acceleration causes the vertical reaction to be less than the weight of the upper body segments. The required inertial moment is on the order of one-fourth of typical maximum voluntary static trunk muscle strength and corresponds roughly to the moment required to support the upper body when the trunk is statically flexed at 30°. Dynamic performances of physical tasks clearly can load musculoskeletal structures heavily, even in the absence of externally applied loads. In fact, the strength of the muscles is what determines the largest linear and angular accelerations that can be produced.

Myoelectric-signal-enhanced biomechanical models have been used to assess the magnitudes of inertial load effects in dynamic performances. For example, in quasi-isometric trunk flexion–extension exertions to 60% of maximum voluntary strength, performed at 40 cycles per minute, inertial effects generally were responsible for less than 15% of the net lumbar trunk moment (268). Similarly, in rapid horizontal pulls that lifted a 20-kg mass, made in five different pull directions, magnitudes of the peak total moment these tasks imposed on the lumbar spine were approximately 30% to 60% higher than the total moment imposed when the mass was supported by a statically held pull in the same direction (264). Inertial effects accounted for approximately one-half of these increases; that is, 15% to 30%.

Inertial loading in lifting activities has also been analyzed by others (155). One study has shown that rapidly lifting a 50-N load can increase the L5–S1 moment, and hence strength requirements, by 87% over that required to simply hold it still in a given posture (274).

Deformable and Finite Element Models

Deformable element models are used to investigate how the configuration of a deformable structure is altered under conditions of loading and how those alterations are affected by the structural geometry and the mechanical properties of its constituents. The technique commonly used in such modeling is the direct stiffness method. A simple two-degree-of-freedom model illustrates the main ideas.

Consider the structure illustrated in Fig. 11A, a simple sagittal plane model of a spine motion segment. The foundation represents an inferior vertebra that is held fixed, and the block represents the segment's superior vertebra, which is movable. The passive flexion–extension resistance of the intervertebral disk is represented by the linear torsional spring of constant κ, and the longitudinal resistance of the disk and the ligamentous tissues of the posterior elements is represented by the linear spring of constant k.

If external force F_E and moment M_E are applied to this structure, point C displaces superiorly by amount z, and the vertebra rotates by amount θ. The torsional spring moment is $\kappa\theta$, and the linear spring force is $k(z + a\theta)$. A free-body analysis shows that vertical force and sagittal plane moment equilibrium of this structure are governed by two equations:

$$\begin{Bmatrix} F_E \\ M_E \end{Bmatrix} = \begin{bmatrix} k & ak \\ ak & (\kappa + \kappa a^2) \end{bmatrix} \begin{Bmatrix} z \\ \theta \end{Bmatrix} \qquad (7)$$

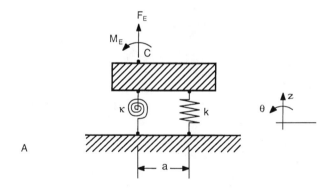

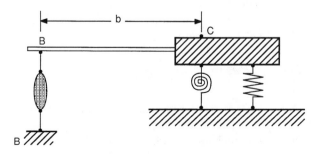

FIG. 11. Schematic diagram of model used to illustrate the ideas presented in the section Deformable and Finite Element Models.

If desired values of z and θ are given, equation 7 can be used to calculate the needed values of F_E and M_E. However, solution of the inverse problem is usually sought: F_E and M_E are given, and z and θ are sought.

Equation 7 can be inverted to obtain

$$\begin{Bmatrix} z \\ \theta \end{Bmatrix} = \frac{1}{k\kappa} \begin{bmatrix} (\kappa + ka^2) & -ak \\ -ak & k \end{bmatrix} \begin{Bmatrix} F_E \\ M_E \end{Bmatrix} \quad (8)$$

or, in more general symbols, as

$$\mathbf{D} = \mathbf{K}^{-1} F_E \quad (9)$$

where $\mathbf{D}$ is the vector of displacements and rotations, $\mathbf{K}^{-1}$ is the inverse of the stiffness matrix in equation 7, and F_E is the vector of applied forces and moments. Thus, given any set of values of F_E and M_E, the corresponding z and θ can be calculated.

Now suppose that posterior muscles contract so as to exert an inferior force P acting over moment arm b on the superior vertebra (Fig. 11B). This is statically equivalent to exerting a force $-P$ and a moment Pb at point C. Calling this muscle equivalent force and moment F_M and M_M, we have

$$\begin{Bmatrix} F_M \\ M_M \end{Bmatrix} = \begin{Bmatrix} -1 \\ b \end{Bmatrix} [P] \quad (10)$$

or, in more general symbols:

$$\mathbf{F}_M = \beta \mathbf{P}_M \quad (11)$$

where $\mathbf{F}_M$ is the vector of applied forces and moments, β is the matrix specifying the moment arms, and $\mathbf{P}_M$ is the vector of muscle contraction forces.

If the system behaves linearly, then the effects of the external and muscle-developed loads can be superposed, with the result

$$\mathbf{D} = \mathbf{K}^{-1}(\mathbf{F}_E + \beta \mathbf{P}_M) \quad (12)$$

where the vectors are the same as those defined in equations 9 and 11.

Problem

To make the model of Fig. 11 representative of a human lumbar motion segment, let a = 2 cm, M_E = 60 Nm/rad, and k = 104 N/cm.

1. What motions of the segment will occur if it must support a superincumbent body weight of 400 N acting 5 cm anterior of point C? (Answer: $z = -3.6$ mm, $\theta = 11.5°$)

2. What force does the linear spring develop, and what moment does the torsional spring develop? (Answer: 400 N, 12 Nm)

3. If the erector spinae muscles lie 6.5 cm posterior to point C, what force must they contract with to prevent flexion of the motion segment? How much does the combined loading displace the superior vertebra? (Answer: 356 N, $z = -0.76$ mm)

Equation 12 is quite general and can be used to construct deformable element models of the spine with hundreds of degrees of freedom and hundreds of deformable elements (14,32,101,231). With such models, the actions of each of the major trunk muscles can be examined (260). A main use of such models has been to investigate the biomechanics underlying the progression and correction of idiopathic scoliosis (24,66,67,108,235,264). For example, Closkey and Schultz (66) used a model of the spine and rib cage to study rib cage deformities in scoliosis. That model contained 119 rigid bodies and 503 deformable elements and had a total of 714 degrees of freedom (Fig. 12). The use of models this complex is justified only when simpler models do not capture the biomechanics essential to the phenomenon under study.

Finite element models of spine motion segments are a special class of deformable element models. They are useful for analyzing stress and pressure distributions within the spine, and Shirazi-Adl and co-workers provide recent examples of their use (239–243). Recent models have explored the poroelastic behavior of the intervertebral disk (133,238) as well as cancellous bone remodeling mechanisms in the vertebra (101).

SUMMARY

This chapter has summarized current theoretical and experimental knowledge of the biomechanics of the spine and trunk, both in

42. Bogduk, N., and Macintosh, J. E. (1984): The applied anatomy of the thoracolumbar fascia. *Spine,* 9:164–170.
43. Bogduk, N., Macintosh, J. E., and Hadfield, G. (1992): Anatomy and biomechanics of the psoas major. *Clin. Biomech.,* 7:109–119.
44. Bogduk, N., Macintosh, J. E., and Pearcy, M. J. (1992): A universal model of the lumbar back muscles in the upright position. *Spine,* 17:897–913.
45. Bradford, D. S., Swedenburg, S. M., Carpenter, R. J., Hofmeister, F., and Oegema, T. R. (1986): Facet joint changes after surgical excision of the nucleus pulposus of mature dogs. *Trans. Orthop. Res. Soc.,* 11:324.
46. Brailsford, J. F. (1929): Deformities of lumbosacral region of the spine. *Br. J. Surg.,* 16:562.
47. Brandner, M. E. (1970): Normal values of the vertebral body and intervertebral disc index during growth. *Am. J. Roentgenol.,* 110:618–627.
48. Brickley-Parsons, D., and Glimcher, M. (1983): Is the chemistry of collagen in intervertebral disks an expression of Wolff's law? A study in the human lumbar spine. *Spine,* 9:148–163.
49. Brinckmann, P. (1985): *Injury of the Annulus Fibrosus and Disc Protrusions. An in Vivo Investigation of Human Lumbar Motion Segments. Internal Report No. 22.* Orthopädische Universitätsklinik, Munster.
50. Brinckmann, P. (1994): Quantification of overload injuries to thoracolumbar vertebrae and discs in persons exposed to heavy physical exertions or vibration at the workplace. *Clin. Biomech.,* 9(Suppl. 1).
51. Brinckmann, P., Biggeman, M., and Hilweg, D. (1988): Fatigue fracture of human lumbar vertebrae. *Clin. Biomech. [Suppl. 1],* 3:1–23.
52. Brinckmann, P., Biggeman, M., and Hilweg, D. (1989): Prediction of the compressive strength of the human lumbar vertebrae. *Clin. Biomech. [Suppl. 2],* 4:1–27.
53. Brinckmann, P., Frobin, W., Hierholzer, E., and Horst, M. (1983): Deformation of the vertebral endplate under axial loading of the spine. *Spine,* 8:851–856.
54. Brinckmann, P., and Grootenboer, H. (1991): Change of disc height, radial disc bulge, and intradiscal pressure from discectomy. An *in vitro* investigation on human lumbar discs. *Spine,* 16:641–646.
55. Brinckmann, P., and Porter, R. W. (1994): A laboratory model of lumbar disc protrusion. Fissure and fragment. *Spine,* 19:228–235.
56. Brooks, S. V., and Faulkner, J. A. (1990): Contraction-induced injury: recovery of skeletal muscles in young and old mice. *Am. J. Physiol.,* 258:C436–C442.
57. Brooks, S. V., Zerba, E., and Faulkner, J. A. (1995): Injury to fibers after single stretches of passive and maximally stimulated muscles in mice. *J. Physiol. (Lond.),* 488:459–469.
58. Butler, D., Trafimow, J. H., and Andersson, G. B. J. (1990): Discs degenerate before facets. *Spine,* 15:111–113.
59. Carlsöo, S. (1961): The static muscle load in different work positions: An electromyographic study. *Kungl. Gymn. Centralinst.,* 1961:93–211.
60. Chaffin, D. B., and Ashton-Miller, J. A. (1991): Biomechanical aspects of low-back pain in the older worker. *Exp. Aging Res.,* 17:177–187.
61. Chaffin, D. B., and Erig, M. (1991): Three-dimensional biomechanical static strength prediction model sensitivity to postural and anthropometric inaccuracies. *IEEE Trans.,* 23:215–227.
62. Chaffin, D. B., Herrin, G., and Keyserling, M. (1978): Preemployment strength testing, an updated position. *J. Occup. Med.,* 20:403–8.
63. Cholewicki, J., and McGill, S. M. (1996): Mechanical stability of the *in vivo* lumbar spine: implications for injury and chronic low back pain. *Clin. Biomech.,* 11:1–15.
64. Clauser, C. E., McConville, J. T., and Toung, J. W. (1969): *Weight, Volume and Center of Mass of Segments of the Human Body.* Vol. AMRL-TR-69-70. Aerospace Medical Laboratories, Wright-Patterson Air Force Base, Ohio.
65. Close, R. I. (1972): Dynamic properties of mammalian skeletal muscles. *Physiol. Rev.,* 52:129–197.
66. Closkey, R. F., and Schultz, A. B. (1993): Rib cage deformities in scoliosis: spine morphology, rib cage stiffness, and tomography imaging. *J. Orthop. Res.,* 11:730–737.
67. Closkey, R. F., Schultz, A. B., and Luchies, C. L. (1992): A model for studies of the deformable rib cage. *J. Biomech.,* 25:529–539.
68. Cresswell, A., and Thorstensson, A. (1994): Changes in intra-abdominal pressure, trunk muscle activation and force during isokinetic lifting and lowering. *Eur. J. Appl. Physiol.,* 68:315–321.
69. Crisco, J. J., and Panjabi, M. M. (1990): Postural biomechanical stability and gross muscular architecture in the spine. In: *Multiple Muscle Systems: Biomechanics and Movement Organization,* edited by J. M. Winters and S. L.-Y. Woo, pp. 438–450. Springer-Verlag, New York.
70. Crisco, J. J., and Panjabi, M. M. (1991): The intersegmental and multisegmental muscles of the lumbar spine. A biomechanical model comparing lateral stabilizing potential. *Spine,* 16:793–799.
71. Crisco, J. J., Panjabi, M. M., and Dvorak, J. (1991): A model of the alar ligaments of the upper cervical spine in axial rotation. *J. Biomech.,* 24:607–614.
72. Crock, H. V., and Goldwasser, M. (1984): Anatomic studies of the circulation in the region of the vertebral endplate in adult greyhound dogs. *Spine,* 9:702–706.
73. Cummings, S. R., and Black, D. (1995): Bone mass measurements and risk of fracture in Caucasian women: A review of findings from prospective studies. *Am J. Med.,* 98:2A-24S–2A-28S.
74. Cyron, B. M., and Hutton, W. C. (1978): The fatigue strength of the lumbar neural arch in spondylolysis. *J. Bone Joint Surg.,* 60B:234–238.
75. Cyron, B. M., and Hutton, W. C. (1980): Articular tropism and the stability of the lumbar spine. *Spine,* 5:168–172.
76. Cyron, B. M., Hutton, W. C., and Troup, J. D. G. (1976): Spondylotic fractures. *J. Bone Joint Surg.,* 58-B:462–466.
77. Damkot, D. K., Pope, M. H., Lord, J., and Frymoyer, J. W. (1984): The relationship between work history, work environment and low-back pain in men. *Spine,* 9:395–399.
78. Davis, P. R. (1956): Variations of the human intraabdominal pressure during weight-lifting in different postures. *J. Anat. (Lond.),* 90:601.
79. Davis, P. R. (1985): Intratruncal pressure mechanisms. *Ergonomics,* 1:293–297.
80. DePuky, P. (1935): The physiological oscillations of the length of the body. *Acta Orthop. Scand.,* 6:338–347.
81. Deyo, R. A., and Tsui-Wu, Y. J. (1987): Descriptive epidemiology of low-back pain and its related medical care in the United States. *Spine,* 12:264–268.

82. Dietrich, M., Kedzior, K., and Zagrajek, T. (1990): Modeling of muscle action and stability of the human spine. In: *Multiple Muscle Systems: Biomechanics and Movement Organization*, edited by J. M. Winters and S. L.-Y. Woo, pp. 451–460. Springer-Verlag, New York.

83. Donisch, E. W., and Basmajian, J. V. (1972): Electromyography of deep back muscles in man. *Am. J. Anat.,* 133:25–36.

84. Drerup, B. (1985): Improvements in measuring vertebral rotation from the projections of the pedicles. *J. Biomech.,* 18:369–378.

85. Dunlop, R. B., Adams, M. A., and Hutton, W. C. (1984): Disc space narrowing and the lumbar facet joints. *J. Bone Joint Surg.,* 66B:706–710.

86. Dvorak, J., Panjabi, M. M., Novotny, J. E., and Antinnes, J. A. (1991): *In vivo* flexion/extension of the normal cervical spine. *J. Orthop. Res.,* 9:828–834.

87. Ecklund, J. A. E., and Corlett, E. N. (1984): Shrinkage as a measure of the effect of load on the spine. *Spine,* 9:189–194.

88. Eie, N., and Wehn, P. (1962): Measurements of the intra-abdominal pressure in relation to weight bearing of the lumbosacral spine. *J. Oslo City Hosp.,* 12:205–217.

89. Einkauf, D. K., Gohdes, M. L., Jensen, G. M., and Jewell, M. J. (1987): Changes in spinal mobility with increasing age in women. *Phys. Ther.,* 67:370–375.

90. El-Bohy, A. A., and King, A. I. (1986): Intervertebral disc and facet contact pressure in axial torsion. *Adv. Bioeng.,* 2:26–27.

91. Ericksen, M. F. (1978): Aging in the lumbar spine. II. L1 and L2. *Am. J. Phys. Anthropol.,* 48:241–246.

92. Eycleshymer, A. C., and Schoemaker, D. M. (1911): *A Cross-Section Anatomy.* Appleton-Century Crofts, New York.

93. Eyre, D. R., and Muir, H. (1976): Types I and II collagens in intervertebral disc. *Biochem. J.,* 157:267–270.

94. Farfan, H. F. (1973): *Mechanical Disorders of the Low Back*, pp. 33–35. Lea & Febiger, Philadelphia.

95. Farfan, H. F., Huberdeau, R. M., and Dubow, H. I. (1972): Lumbar intervertebral disc degeneration: the influence of geometrical features on the pattern of disc degeneration. *J. Bone Joint Surg.,* 54A:492–510.

96. Fiatarone, M. A., O'Neill, E. F., and Doyle Ryan, N. E. (1994): Exercise training and supplementation of physical frailty in very elderly people. *N. Engl. J. Med.,* 330:1769–1775.

97. Foster, D., John, D., Elliot, B., Ackland, T., and Fitch, K. (1989): Back injuries to fast bowlers in cricket: a prospective study. *Br. J. Sports Med.,* 23:150–154.

98. Fredickson, B. E., Baker, D., McHolick, W. J., Yuan, H. A., and Lubicky, J. P. (1984): The natural history of spondylolysis and spondylolisthesis. *J. Bone Joint Surg.,* 66A:699–707.

99. Gilsanz, V., Loro, M. L., Roe, T. F., Sayre, J., Gilsanz, R., and Schulz, E. E. (1995): Vertebral size in elderly women with osteoporosis. *Am. J. Clin. Invest.,* 95:2332–2337.

100. Goel, V. K., Clark, C. R., Galles, K., and Liu, Y. K. (1986): The biokinetics of occipito-atlantoaxial joint. *Adv. Bioeng.,* 2:42–43.

101. Goel, V. K., Ramirez, S. A., Kong, W., and Gilbertson, L. G. (1995): Cancellous bone Young's modulus variation within the vertebral body of a ligamentous lumbar spine—Application of bone adaptive remodeling concepts. *ASME J. Biomech. Eng.,* 117:266–271.

102. Gore, D. R., Sepic, S. B., and Gardner, G. M. (1986): Roentgenographic findings of the cervical spine in asymptomatic people. *Spine,* 11:521–524.

103. Granhed, H., Jonsson, R., and Hansson, T. (1987): The loads on the spine during extreme weight lifting. *Spine,* 12:146–149.

104. Greendale, G. A., Barret-Connor, E., Ingles, S., and Haile, R. (1995): Late physical and functional effects of osteoporotic fracture in women: The Rancho Bernado study. *J. Am. Geriatr. Soc.,* 43:955–961.

105. Grobler, L. J., Robertson, P. A., Novotny, J. E., and Pope, M. H. (1993): Etiology of spondylolisthesis: Assessment of the role played by lumbar facet joint morphology. *Spine,* 18:80–91.

106. Gunterberg, B., Romanus, B., and Stener, B. (1976): Pelvic strength after major amputation of the sacrum: an experimental study. *Acta Orthop. Scand.,* 47:635–642.

107. Gunzberg, R., Parkinson, R., and Moore, R. E. A. (1992): A cadaveric study comparing discography, MRI, histology and mechanical behaviour of the human lumbar disc. *Spine,* 17:417–423.

108. Haderspeck, K., and Schultz, A. (1981): Progression of idiopathic scoliosis. *Spine,* 6:447–455.

109. Hansson, T. B., Roos, B., and Nachemson, A. (1980): The bone mineral content and ultimate compression strength of lumbar vertebrae. *Spine,* 5:46–55.

110. Hellems, H. K., and Keats, T. E. (1971): Measurement of the normal lumbosacral angle. *Am. J. Roentgenol.,* 113:642–645.

111. Herzog, W., and Binding, P. (1992): Predictions of antagonistic muscle activity using non-linear optimization. *Math. Biosci.,* 111:217–229.

112. Heylings, D. J. A. (1978): Supraspinous and interspinous ligaments of the human lumbar spine. *J. Anat.,* 125:127–131.

113. Holm, S., Maroudas, A., Urban, J. P. G., Selstram, G., and Nachemson, A. (1981): Nutrition of the intervertebral disc: solute transport and mechanism. *Connect. Tissue Res.,* 8:101–119.

114. Holmes, A. D., Hukins, D. W. L., and Freemont, A. J. (1993): Endplate displacement during compression of lumbar-disc-vertebra segments and the mechanism of failure. *Spine,* 18:128–135.

115. Hormel, S. E., and Eyre, D. (1991): Collagen in the ageing human intervertebral disc: an increase in covalently bound fluoropheres and chromophores. *Biochim. Biophys. Acta,* 1078:243–250.

116. Hoshina, H. (1980): Spondylolysis in athletes. *Physician Sportsmed.,* 3:75–78.

117. Hukins, D. W. (1992): A simple model for the function of proteoglycans and collagen in the response to compression of the intervertebral disc. *Proc. R. Soc. (Lond.) Biol.,* 249:281–285.

118. Hutton, W. C., Cyron, B. M., and Stott, J. R. R. (1979): The compressive strength of lumbar vertebrae. *J. Anat.,* 129:753–758.

119. Ikai, M., and Fukunaga, J. (1968): Calculation of muscle strength per unit cross-sectional area of human muscle by means of ultrasonic measurement. *Int. Z. Angew. Physiol.,* 26:26–32.

120. Imamura, K., Ashida, H., Ishikawa, T., and Fujii, M. (1995): Human major psoas muscle and sacrospinalis muscle in relation to age: a study by computed tomography. *J. Gerontol.,* 38:678–681.

121. Jackson, A. B., Wiltse, L. L., and Cirincione, R. J.

(1976): Spondylolysis in the female gymnast. *Clin. Orthop. Rel. Res.,* 117:68–73.

122. Jakobs, T. J., Ashton-Miller, J. A., and Schultz, A. B. (1985): Trunk position sense in the frontal plane. *Exp. Neurol.,* 90:129–138.

123. Janevic, J. T., Ashton-Miller, J. A., and Schultz, A. B. (1991): Large compressive preloads decrease lumbar motion segment flexibilities. *J. Orthop. Res.,* 9:228–236.

124. Jensen, R. K. (1986): Body segment mass, radius and radius of gyration properties for children. *J. Biomech.,* 19:359–368.

125. Joyce, G. C., and Rack, M. H. (1969): Isotonic lengthening and shortening movements of cat soleus muscle. *J. Physiol. (Lond.),* 204:475–491.

126. Kawakami, Y., Nakazawa, K., Fukunaga, J., Nozaki, D., Miyashita, M., and Fukunaga, T. (1994): Specific tension of elbow flexor and extensor muscles based on magnetic resonance imaging. *Eur. J. Appl. Physiol.,* 68:139–147.

127. Keith, A. (1923): Man's posture: its evolution and disorders. *Br. Med. J.,* 1923:587–590.

128. Kelsey, J. L., Githens, P. B., O'Connor, T., et al. (1984): Acute prolapsed lumbar intervertebral disc. An epidemiological study with special reference to driving automobiles and cigarette smoking. *Spine,* 9:608–613.

129. King, A. I. (1984): A review of biomechanical models. *J. Biomech. Eng.,* 106:97–104.

130. Kishino, N. D., Mayer, T. G., Gatchel, R. J., et al. (1985): Quantification of lumbar function. Part 4: Isometric and isokinetic lifting simulation in normal subjects and low-back dysfunction patients. *Spine,* 10: 921–927.

131. Koeller, W., Muehlhaus, S., Meier, W., and Hartmann, F. (1986): Biomechanical properties of human intervertebral discs subjected to axial dynamic compression—influence of age and degeneration. *J. Biomech.,* 19:807–816.

132. Kottke, F. S., and Mundale, M. O. (1959): Range of mobility of the cervical spine. *Arch. Phys. Med.,* 40:379.

133. Laible, J. P., Pflaster, D. S., Krag, M. H., Simon, B. R., and Hayes, W. C. (1993): Poroelastic-swelling finite element model with application to the intervertebral disc. *Spine,* 18:659–670.

134. Langenberg, W. (1970): Morphologie, physiologischer querschnitt und kraft des m. erector spinae in lumbalbereich des menschen. *Z. Anat. Enwickl.-Gesch.,* 132: 158–190.

135. Lanier, R. R. (1939): The presacral vertebrae of American white and Negro males. *Am. J. Phys. Anthropol.,* 25:341–420.

136. Latham, J. M., Pearcy, M. J., Costi, J. J., et al. (1994): Mechanical consequences of annular tears and subsequent intervertebral disc degeneration. *Clin. Biomech.,* 9:211–219.

137. Lavender, S., Trafimow, J., Andersson, G. B. J., Mayer, R. S., and Chen, J. H. (1994): Trunk muscle activation. The effects of torso flexion, moment direction, and moment magnitude. *Spine,* 19:771–778.

138. Lavender, S. A., Tsuang, Y. H., and Andersson, G. B. J. (1993): Trunk muscle activation and cocontraction while resisting applied moments in a twisted posture. *Ergonomics,* 36:1145–1157.

139. Lavender, S. A., Tsuang, Y. H., Andersson, G. B. J., Hafezi, A., and Shin, C. C. (1992): Trunk muscle coactivation: The effects of moment direction and moment magnitude. *J. Orthop. Res.,* 10:691–700.

140. Lavender, S. A., Tsuang, Y. H., Hafezi, A., Andersson, G. B. J., Chaffin, D. B., and Hughes, R. E. (1992): Coactivation of the trunk muscles during asymmetric loading of the torso. *Hum. Factors,* 34:239–247.

141. Lipson, S.J., and Muir, H. (1981): Proteoglycans in experimental intervertebral disc degeneration. *Spine,* 6:194–210.

142. Lorenz, M., Patwardhan, A., and Vanderby, R. (1983): Load-bearing characteristics of lumbar facets in normal and surgically altered spinal segments. *Spine,* 8: 122–130.

143. Lucas, S. M., Ruff, R. L., and Binder, M. D. (1987): Specific tension measurements in single soleus and medial gastrocnemius muscle fibers of the cat. *Exp. Neurol.,* 95:142–154.

144. Macintosh, J. E., Bogduk, N., and Pearcy, M. J. (1993): The effects of flexion on the geometry and actions of the lumbar erector spinae. *Spine,* 18:884–893.

145. Macintosh, J. E., Pearcy, M. J., and Bogduk, N. (1995): The axial torque of the lumbar back muscles: torsion strength of the back muscles. *Aust. NZ J. Surg.,* 63: 205–212.

146. Magora, A. (1970): Investigation of the relation between low back pain and occupation. *Indust. Med.,* 39:504–510.

147. Mairiaux, P., Davis, P. R., Stubbs, D. A., and Baty, D. (1984): Relation between intra-abdominal pressure and lumbar moments when lifting weights in the erect posture. *Ergonomics,* 27:883–894.

148. Marchand, F., and Ahmed, A. M. (1990): Investigation of the laminate structure of the lumbar disc anulus. *Spine,* 15:402–410.

149. Martin, I. R., Krag, M. H., Seroussi, R., and Pope, M. S. (1986): A method for quantifying intradiscal deformation in response to load. *Adv. Bioeng. ASME,* 1986:24–25.

150. Mayer, T., Tencer, A. F., Kristoferson, S., and Mooney, V. (1984): Use of non-invasive techniques for quantification of spinal range-of-motion in normal subjects and chronic low-back dysfunction patients. *Spine,* 9:588–595.

151. Mazess, R. B. (1982): On aging bone loss. *Clin. Orthop.,* 165:239–252.

152. McBroom, R. J., Hayes, W. C., Edwards, W. T., Goldberg, R. P., and White, A. A. (1985): Prediction of vertebral body compressive fracture using quantitative computed tomography. *J. Bone Joint Surg.,* 67A:1206–1213.

153. McConville, J. T., Churchill, T. D., Clauser, C. E., and Cuzzi, J. (1980): *Anthropometric Relationships of Body and Body Segment Moment of Inertia. Vol. AFAMRL-TR-80-119.* Aerospace Medical Research Laboratories, Wright-Patterson Air Force Base, Ohio.

154. McCully, K. K., and Faulkner, J. A. (1986): Characteristics of lengthening contractions associated with injury to skeletal muscle fibers. *Am. J. Physiol.,* 61:293–299.

155. McGill, S. M. (1992): A myoelectrically based dynamic three-dimensional model to predict loads on the lumbar spine tissues during lateral bending. *J. Biomech.,* 25:395–414.

156. McGill, S. M., and Norman, R. W. (1986): Partitioning of the L4–L5 dynamic moment into disc, ligamentous, and muscular components during lifting. *Spine,* 11: 666–678.

157. McGill, S. M., Santaguida, L., and Stevens, J. (1993): Measurement of the trunk musculature from T5 to L5

using MRI scans of 15 young males corrected for muscle fiber orientation. *Clin. Biomech.,* 8:171–178.

158. McGlashen, K. M., Ashton-Miller, J. A., Green, M., and Schultz, A. B. (1991): Trunk positioning accuracy in the frontal and sagittal planes. *J. Orthop. Res.,* 9:576–583.

159. McGlashen, K. M., Ashton-Miller, J. A., Schultz, A. B., and Andersson, G. B. J. (1987): Load-displacement behavior of the human lumbosacral joint. *J. Orthop. Res.,* 5:488–496.

160. McNally, D. S., Adams, M. A., and Goodship, A. E. (1993): Can intervertebral disc prolapse be predicted by disc mechanics? *Spine,* 18:1525–1530.

161. McNeill, T., Warwick, D. N., Andersson, G. B. J., and Schultz, A. B. (1980): Trunk strength in attempted flexion, extension and lateral bending in healthy subjects and patients with low back disorders. *Spine,* 5:529–538.

162. Melrose, J., Ghosh, P., Taylor, T. K. F., et al. (1992): A longitudinal study of the matrix changes induced in the intervertebral disc by surgical damage to the annulus fibrosus. *J. Orthop. Res.,* 10:665–676.

163. Merritt, J. L., McLean, T. J., Erickson, R. P., and Offord, K. P. (1986): Measurement of trunk flexibility in normal subjects: reproducibility of three clinical methods. *Mayo Clin. Proc.,* 61:192–197.

164. Milne, J. S., and Lauder, I. J. (1974): Age effects in kyphosis and lordosis in adults. *Ann. Hum. Biol.,* 1: 327–337.

165. Moll, J. M. H., and Wright, V. (1971): Normal range of spinal mobility. *Ann. Rheum. Dis.,* 30:381.

166. Monkhouse, W. S., and Khalique, A. (1986): Variations in the composition of the human rectus sheath: a study of the anterior abdominal wall. *J. Anat.,* 145:61–66.

167. Moroney, S. P., Schultz, A. B., and Ashton-Miller, J. A. (1987): Analysis and measurement of neck loads. *J. Orthop. Res.,* 6:713–720.

168. Moroney, S. P., Schultz, A. B., and Ashton-Miller, J. A. (1988): Load-displacement properties of cervical spine motion segments. *J. Biomech.,* 21:769–779.

169. Morris, J. M., Benner, G., and Lucas, D. B. (1962): An electromyographic study of the intrinsic muscles of the back in man. *J. Anat. Lond.,* 96:509–520.

170. Morris, J. M., Lucas, D. B., and Bresler, B. (1961): Role of the trunk in stability of the spine. *J. Bone Joint Surg.,* 43(1):327–351.

171. Mundt, D. J., Kelsey, J. L., Golden, A. L., et al. (1993): An epidemiological study of non-occupational lifting as a risk factor for herniated lumbar intervertebral disc. *Spine,* 18:595–602.

172. Mundt, D. J., Kelsey, J. L., Golden, A. L., et al. (1993): An epidemiologic study of sports and weight lifting as possible risk factors for herniated lumbar and cervical discs. The Northeast Collaborative Group on Low Back Pain. *Am. J. Sports Med.,* 21:854–860.

173. Myers, B. S., McElhaney, J. H., Richardson, W. J., Nightingale, R. W., and Doherty, B. J. (1991): The influence of end condition on human cervical spine injury mechanisms. In: *Proceedings of the 35th Stapp Car Crash Conference 1991*, pp. 391–399. SAE Paper #912915.

174. Nachemson, A. (1960): Lumbar intradiscal pressure. Experimental studies of post-mortem material. *Acta Orthop. Scand. [Suppl.],* XLIII.

175. Nachemson, A., and Elfström, G. (1970): Intravital dynamic pressure measurements in lumbar discs. *Scand. J. Rehab. Med. Suppl.,* 1:1–40.

176. Nachemson, A., and Evans, J. (1968): Some mechanical properties of the third lumbar interlaminar ligament (ligamentum flavum). *J. Biomech.,* 1:211.

177. Nachemson, A., and Morris, J. M. (1964): *In vivo* measurements of intradiscal pressure. Discometry, a method for the determination of pressure in the lower lumbar discs. *J. Bone Joint Surg.,* 46A:1077–1092.

178. Nachemson, A. L. (1981): Disc pressure measurements. *Spine,* 6:94–99.

179. Nachemson, A. L. (1992): Newest knowledge of low back pain: A critical look. *Clin. Orthop.,* 279:8–20.

180. Nachemson, A. L., Andersson, G. B. J., and Schultz, A. B. (1986): Valsalva maneuver biomechanics—effects on lumbar trunk loads of elevated intraabdominal pressures. *Spine,* 11:476–479.

181. Nachemson, A. L., Schultz, A. B., and Berkson, M. H. (1979): Mechanical properties of human lumbar spine motion segments. Influences of age, sex, disc level and degeneration. *Spine,* 4:1–8.

182. Narici, M. V., Landoni, L., and Minetti, A. E. (1992): Assessment of human knee extensor muscles stress from *in vivo* physiological cross-sectional area and strength measurements. *Eur. J. Appl. Physiol.,* 65:438–444.

183. National Health Survey (1973): *Prevalence of Selected Impairments. Ser. 10, No. 87.* U.S. Department of Health, Education and Welfare, Washington, DC.

184. Nemeth, G., and Ohlsen, H. (1986): Moment arm lengths of trunk muscles to the lumbosacral joint obtained *in vivo* with computed tomography. *Spine,* 11:158–160.

185. Neumann, P., Nordwall, A., and Osvalder, A. L. (1995): Traumatic instability of the lumbar spine. A dynamic *in vitro* study of flexion–distraction injury. *Spine,* 20: 1111–1121.

186. Newton, M., Thow, M., Somerville, D., et al. (1993): Trunk strength testing with iso-machines. Part 2: Experimental evaluation of the Cybex II back testing system in normal subjects and patients with chronic low back pain. *Spine,* 18:812–824.

187. Newton, M., and Waddell, G. (1993): Trunk strength testing with iso-machines. Part 1: Review of a decade of scientific evidence. *Spine,* 18:801–811.

188. Noren, R., Trafimow, J., Andersson, G. B. J., and Huckman, M. S. (1991): The role of facet joint tropism and facet angle in disc degeneration. *Spine,* 16:530–532.

189. Nussbaum, M. A., Chaffin, D. B., and Martin, B. J. (1995): A back propagation neural network model of lumbar muscle recruitment during moderate static exertions. *J. Biomech.,* 28:1015–1024.

190. Nussbaum, M. A., Chaffin, D. B., and Rechtien, C. J. (1995): Muscle-lines-of-action affect predicted forces in optimization-based spine muscle modeling. *J. Biomech.,* 28:401–409.

191. Ogden, J. A. (1982): Postnatal development of the cervical spine. *Orthop. Trans.,* 6:89–90.

192. Olmarker, K., (1991): Spinal nerve root compression. Nutrition and function of the porcine cauda equina compressed in vivo. *Acta Orthop. Scand. Suppl.* 242:1–27.

192a.Ohshima, H., Urban, J.P.G., Bergel, D.H. (1995): Effect of static load on matrix synthesis rates in the intervertebral disc measured in vitro by a new perfusion technique. *J. Orthop. Res.* 13:22–29.

193. Ostgaard, H. C., Andersson, G. B. J., Schultz, A. B., and Ashton-Miller, J. A. (1993): Influence of some biomechanical factors on low-back pain in pregnancy. *Spine,* 18:61–65.

194. Osti, O. L., Vernon-Roberts, B., and Fraser, R. D. (1990): Annulus tears and intervertbral disc degeneration: an experimental study using an animal model. *Spine,* 15:762–767.

195. Panjabi, M. M., Brand, R. A., and White, A. A. (1976): Mechanical properties of the human thoracic spine. *J. Bone Joint Surg.,* 58A:642–652.

196. Panjabi, M. M., Dvorak, J., Crisco, J. J., Oda, T., Hillbrand, A., and Grob, D. (1991): Flexion, extension and lateral bending of the upper cervical spine in response to alar ligament transections. *J. Spinal Dis.,* 4:157–167.

197. Panjabi, M. M., Goel, V. K., and Takata, K. (1982): Physiologic strains in the lumbar spinal ligaments: an *in vitro* biomechanical study. *Spine,* 7:192–203.

198. Panjabi, M. M., Krag, M. H., and Chung, T. Q. (1984): Effects of disc injury on mechanical behavior of the human spine. *Spine,* 9:707–713.

199. Panjabi, M. M., Oxland, T. R., Takata, K., Goel, V., Duranceau, J., and Krag, M. (1993): Articular facets of the human spine. Quantitative three-dimensional anatomy. *Spine,* 18:1298–1310.

200. Panjabi, M. M., Oxland, T. R., Yamamoto, I., and Crisco, J. J. (1994): Mechanical behavior of the human lumbar and lumbosacral spine as shown by three-dimensional load–displacement curves. *J. Bone Joint Surg.,* 76:413–424.

201. Panjabi, M. M., White, A. A., and Johnson, R. M. (1975): Cervical spine mechanics as a function of transection of components. *J. Biomech.,* 8:327–336.

202. Panjabi, M. M., Yakata, K., and Goel, V. K. (1983): Kinematics of lumbar intervertebral foramen. *Spine,* 8:348–357.

203. Pauly, J. E. (1966): An electromyographic analysis of certain movements and exercises. *Anat. Rec.,* 155:223–234.

204. Pearcy, M. J., Portek, J., and Shepard, J. (1984): Three-dimensional x-ray analysis of normal measurement in the lumbar spine. *Spine,* 9:294–300.

205. Pearcy, M. J., and Tibrewal, S. B. (1984): Lumbar intervertebral disc and ligament deformations measured *in vivo. Clin. Orthop. Rel. Res.,* 191:281–286.

206. Pearcy, M. J., and Tibrewal, S. B. (1984): Axial rotation and lateral bending in the normal lumbar spine measured by three-dimensional radiography. *Spine,* 9:582–587.

207. Pfeiffer, M., Griss, M., and Franke, P. (1994): Degeneration model of the porcine lumbar motion segment: effects of various intradiscal procedures. *Eur. Spine J.,* 3:8–16.

208. Pintar, F. A., Sances, A., Yoganandan, N., Reinartz, J., Maiman, D. J., et al. (1990): Biodynamics of the total human cadaveric cervical spine. In: *Proceedings 34th Stapp Car Crash Conference,* SAE paper 902309. SAE, Warrendale, PA.

209. Pokras, R., and Kubishke, K. (1985): *Diagnosis-Related Groups Using Data from the National Hospital Discharge Survey: United States, 1982.* NCHS Advance Data 105, National Center for Health Statistics, Hyattsville, MD.

210. Pope, M. H., Andersson, G. B. J., Broman, H., Svensson, M., and Zetterberg, C. (1986): Electromyographic studies of the lumbar trunk musculature during the development of axial torques. *J. Orthop. Res.,* 4:288–297.

211. Portek, J., Pearcy, M. J., Reader, G. P., and Mowatt, A. G. (1983): Correlation between radiographic and clinical measurements of lumbar spine movement. *Br. J. Rheumatol.,* 22:197–205.

212. Porter, R. W., and Trailescu, I. F. (1991): Diurnal changes in straight leg raising. *Spine,* 15:103–106.

213. Postacchini, F., Lami, R., and Pugliese, O. (1991): Familial predisposition to discogenic low-back pain. An epidemiologic and immunologenetic study. *Spine,* 13: 1403–1406.

214. Pyka, G., Lindenberger, E., Charette, S., and Marcus, R. (1994): Muscle strength and fiber adaptations to year-long resistance training program in elderly men and women. *J. Gerontol. Med. Sci.,* 49:22–28.

215. Resch, A., Schneider, B., Bemecker, P., et al. (1995): Risk of vertebral fractures in men: Relationship to mineral density of the vertebral body. *Am. J. Radiol.,* 164:1447–1450.

216. Reuber, M., Schultz, A., Denis, F., and Spencer, D. (1982): Bulging of lumbar trunk intervertebral disks. *J. Biomech. Eng. Trans. ASME,* 104:187–192.

217. Richardson, J. K., Chung, T., Schultz, J.S., and Herevitz, E.A. (1997): A familial predisposition toward lumbar disc injury. *Spine* (In Press).

218. Rutkow, I. M. (1986): Orthopaedic operations in the United States, 1979 through 1983. *J. Bone Joint Surg.,* 68-A:716–719.

219. Saraste, H. (1984): *Spondylolysis and spondylolisthesis. Clinical and radiological relationships, and prognostic signs.* Ph.D. Dissertation, The Karolinska Hospital, Stockholm.

220. Sasaki, K. (1995): Magnetic resonance imaging findings of the lumbar root pathology in patients over 50 years old. *Eur. Spine J.,* 4:71–76.

221. Scholten, P. J., Schultz, A. B., Luchies, C. W., and Ashton-Miller, J. A. (1988): Motions and loads within the human pelvis: a biomechanical model study. *J. Orthop. Res.,* 6:840–850.

222. Scholten, P. J., and Veldhuizen, A. G. (1986): The bending stiffness of the trunk. *Spine,* 11:463–467.

223. Schultz, A. B. (1987): Biomechanics of the human spine and trunk. In: *Handbook of Bioengineering,* edited by R. Skalak and S. Chien, pp. 41.1–41.20. McGraw-Hill, New York.

224. Schultz, A. B. (1987): Loads on the lumbar spine. In: *The Lumbar Spine and Back Pain,* edited by I. V. Jayson, pp. 204–214. Churchill Livingstone, New York.

225. Schultz, A. B. (1991): The use of mathematical models for studies of scoliosis biomechanics. *Spine,* 16: 1211–1216.

226. Schultz, A. B., Alexander, N. B., and Ashton-Miller, J. A. (1993): Mobility biomechanics in young and old adults. In: *Sensorimotor Impairment in the Elderly,* edited by G. E. Stelmach and V. Homburg, pp. 169–174. Kluwer Academic Publishers, Boston.

227. Schultz, A. B., and Andersson, G. B. J. (1981): Analysis of loads on the lumbar spine. *Spine,* 6:76–82.

228. Schultz, A. B., Andersson, G. B. J., Haderspeck, K., Ortengren, R., Nordin, M., and Bjork, R. (1982): Analysis and measurement of lumbar trunk loads in tasks involving bends and twists. *J. Biomech.,* 15: 669–675.

229. Schultz, A. B., Andersson, G. B. J., Ortengren, R., Bjork, R., and Nordin, M. (1982): Analysis and quantitative myoelectric measurements of loads on the lumbar spine when holding weights in standing postures. *Spine,* 7:390–397.

230. Schultz, A. B., Andersson, G. B. J., Ortengren, R.,

Haderspeck, K., and Nachemson, A. (1982): Loads on the lumbar spine—validation of a biomechanical analysis by measurements of intradiscal pressures and myoelectric signals. *J. Bone Joint Surg.,* 64-A:713–720.

231. Schultz, A. B., Belytschko, T. B., and Andriacchi, T. P. (1973): Analog studies of forces in the human spine: mechanical properties and motion segment behavior. *J. Biomech.,* 6:373–383.

232. Schultz, A. B., Benson, D. R., and Hirsch, C. (1973): Force–deformation properties of human costo-sternal and costo-vertebral articulations. *J. Biomech.,* 7: 311–318.

233. Schultz, A. B., Benson, D. R., and Hirsch, C. (1973): Force–deformation properties of human ribs. *J. Biomech.,* 7:303–309.

234. Schultz, A. B., Cromwell, R., Warwick, D., and Andersson, G. B. J. (1987): Lumbar trunk muscle use in standing isometric heavy exertions. *J. Orthop. Res.,* 5: 320–329.

235. Schultz, A. B., Haderspeck, K., and Takashima, S. (1981): Correction of scoliosis by muscle stimulation: biomechanical analyses. *Spine,* 5:468–476.

236. Schultz, A. B., Haderspeck, K., Warwick, D., and Portillo, D. (1983): Use of lumbar trunk muscles in isometric performance of mechanically complex standing tasks. *J. Orthop. Res.,* 1:77–91.

237. Schultz, A. B., Warwick, D. N., Berkson, M. H., and Nachemson, A. L. (1979): Mechanical properties of human lumbar spine motion segments—Part 1: responses in flexion, extension, lateral bending, and torsion. *J. Biomech. Eng.,* 101:46–52.

238. Shirazi-Adl, A. (1992): Finite element simulation of changes in the fluid content of human lumbar discs: mechanical and clinical implications. *Spine,* 17:206–212.

239. Shirazi-Adl, A. (1994): Biomechanics of the lumbar spine in sagittal/lateral moments. *Spine,* 19:2407–2414.

240. Shirazi-Adl, A. (1994): Analysis of bone compliance on mechanics of a lumbar motion segment. *J. Biomech. Eng.* 116:488-492.

241. Shirazi-Adl, A., Ahmed, A. M., and Shrivastava, S. C. (1986): Mechanical response of a lumbar motion segment in axial torque alone and combined with compression. *Spine,* 11:914–927.

242. Shirazi-Adl, A., Ahmed, A. M., and Shrivastava, S. C. (1986): A finite element study of a lumbar motion segment subjected to pure sagittal plane moments. *J. Biomech.,* 19:331–350.

243. Shirazi-Adl, S. A., Shrivastava, S. C., and Ahmed, A. M. (1984): Stress analysis of the lumbar disc-body unit in compression—a three dimensional nonlinear finite element study. *Spine,* 9:120–134.

244. Sinaki, M., McPhee, M. C., Hodgson, S. F., Merritt, J. M., and Offord, K. P. (1986): Relationship between bone mineral density of spine and strength of back extensors in healthy postmenopausal women. *Mayo Clin. Proc.,* 61:116–122.

244a.Silva, M.J., Wang, C., Keaveny, T.M., and Hayes, W.C. (1994): Direct and computed tomographic thickness measurements of the human lumbar vertebral shell and endplate. *Bone* 15:409–414.

245. Sinkjaer, T., Toft, E., Andreassen, S., and Hornemann, B. C. (1988): Muscle stiffness in human ankle dorsiflexors: Intrinsic and reflex components. *J. Neurophysiol.,* 60:1110–1121.

246. Skaggs, D. L., Weidenbaum, M., Iatrides, J. C., Ratcliffe, A., and Mow, V. C. (1994): Regional variation in tensile properties and biochemical composition of the human anulus fibrosus. *Spine,* 19:1310–1319.

247. Skipor, A. F., Ashton-Miller, J. A., Spencer, D. L., and Schultz, A. B. (1985): Stiffness properties and geometry of lumbar spine posterior elements. *J. Biomech.,* 18:821–830.

248. Skogland, L. B., and Ashton-Miller, J. A. (1981): The length and proportions of the thoracolumbar spine in children with idiopathic scoliosis. *Acta Orthop. Scand.,* 51:779–789.

249. Slocum, L., and Terry, R. J. (1926): Influence of the sacrotuberous and sacrospinous ligaments in limiting movements of the sacroiliac joint. *JAMA,* 87:307–309.

250. Smith, S. S., Mayer, T. G., Gatchel, R. J., and Becker, T. J. (1985): Quantification of lumbar function. Part 1: Isometric and multispeed isokinetic trunk strength measures in sagittal and axial planes in normal subjects. *Spine,* 10:757–764.

251. Spencer, D. L. (1981): Intraosseous pressure in the lumbar spine. *Spine,* 6:159–161.

252. Spencer, D. L. (1990): Mechanisms of nerve root compression due to a herniated disc. In: *The Lumbar Spine,* edited by J. N. Weinstein, pp. 141–145. W. B. Saunders, Philadelphia.

253. Spencer, D. L., and Ashton-Miller, J. A. (1983): The mechanism of sciatic pain relief by chemonucleolysis. *Orthopedics,* 6:1600–1602.

254. Spencer, D. L., Ashton-Miller, J. A., and Bertolini, J. (1984): The effect of intervertebral disc narrowing on the contact force between the lumbar nerve root and a simulated disc protrusion. *Spine,* 9:422–426.

255. Spencer, D. L., Ashton-Miller, J. A., and Schultz, A. B. (1985): The effects of chemonucleolysis on the mechanical properties of the canine lumbar disc. *Spine,* 10:555–561.

256. Spencer, D. L., Irwin, G. S., and Ashton-Miller, J. A. (1983): Anatomy and significance of fixation of the lumbosacral nerve roots in sciatica. *Spine,* 8:672–679.

257. Stairmand, J. W., Holm, S., and Urban, J. P. (1991): Factors influencing oxygen concentration gradients in the intervertebral disc. A theoretical analysis. *Spine,* 16:444–449.

258. Stokes, I. A. F., and Greenapple, D. G. (1984): Surface strain on lumbar discs. *Trans. Orthop. Res. Soc.,* 9:253.

259. Stureson, B., Selvik, G., and Uden, A. (1989): Movements of the sacroiliac joints *in vivo:* a roentgen stereophotogrammetric analysis. *Spine,* 14:162–165.

260. Takashima, S. T., Singh, S. P., Haderspeck, K. A., and Schultz, A. B. (1979): A model for semi-quantitative studies of muscle actions. *J. Biomech.,* 12:929–939.

261. Tanaka, M., Nakahara, S., and Inoue, H. (1993): A pathological study of discs in the elderly. *Spine,* 18:1456–1462.

262. Tator, C. H., and Edmonds, V. E. (1984): National survey of spinal injuries in hockey players. *Can. Med. Assoc. J.,* 130:875–880.

263. Taylor, J. L., and McCloskey, D. I. (1990): Proprioceptive sensation in rotation of the trunk. *Exp. Brain Res.,* 81:413–416.

264. Thelen, D. G., Ashton-Miller, J. A., and Schultz, A. B. (1996): Lumbar trunk loads in rapid three-dimensional pulling tasks. *Spine* 21:605–613.

265. Thelen, D. G., Schultz, A. B., Alexander, J. A., and

Ashton-Miller, J. A. (1996): Effect of age on rapid ankle torque development. *J. Gerontol. Med. Sci.* 51A:M226–M232.

266. Thelen, D. G., Schultz, A. B., and Ashton-Miller, J. A. (1994): Quantitative interpretation of lumbar muscle myoelectric signals during rapid cyclic attempted trunk flexions and extensions. *J. Biomech.,* 27:157–167.

267. Thelen, D. G., Schultz, A. B., and Ashton-Miller, J. A. (1995): Co-contraction of lumbar muscles during the development of time-varying triaxial moments. *J. Orthop. Res.,* 13:390–398.

268. Thelen, D. G., Schultz, A. B., Fassois, S. D., and Ashton-Miller, J. A. (1994): Identification of dynamic myoelectric signal-to-force models during isometric lumbar muscle contractions. *J. Biomech.,* 27:907–919.

269. Tkaczuk, H. (1968): Tensile properties of human lumbar longitudinal ligaments. *Acta Orthop. Scand. [Suppl.],* 115.

270. Tracy, M. F., Gibson, M. J., Szypryt, E. P., Rutherford, A., and Corlett, E. N. (1993): The geometry of the muscles of the lumbar spine determined by magnetic resonance imaging. *Spine,* 14:186–193.

271. Troup, J. D. G., Leskinen, T. P. J., Stalhammar, H. R., and Kuorinka, I. A. A. (1983): A comparison of intraabdominal pressure increases, hip torque, and lumbar vertebral compression in different lifting techniques. *Hum. Factors,* 25:517–525.

272. Troup, J. G. (1976): Mechanical factors in spondylolisthesis and spondylolysis. *Clin. Orthop. Rel. Res.,* 117: 59–67.

273. Tsuang, Y. H., Novak, G. J., Schipplein, O. D., Hafezi, A., Trafimow, J. H., and Andersson, G. B. J. (1993): Trunk muscle geometry and centroid location when twisting. *J. Biomech.,* 26:537–546.

274. Tsuang, Y. H., Schipplein, O. D., Trafimow, J. H., and Andersson, G. B. J. (1992): Influence of body segment dynamics on loads at the lumbar spine during lifting. *Ergonomics,* 35:437–444.

275. Tveit, P., Daggfeldt, K., Hetland, S., and Thorstensson, A. (1994): Erector spinae lever arm length variations with changes in spinal curvature. *Spine,* 19: 199–204.

276. Urban, J. P. G., Holm, S., and Maroudas, A. (1978): Diffusion of small solutes into the intervertebral disk: An *in vivo* study. *Biorheology,* 15:203–223.

277. Urban, J. P. G., and McMullin, J. F. (1986): Swelling pressure of the intervertebral disc: Influence of proteoglycan and collagen contents. *Biorheology,* 22: 145–157.

278. Van Schaik, J. P. J., Verbiest, H., and Van Schaik, F. D. J. (1985): The orientation of laminae and facet joints in the lower lumbar spine. *Spine,* 10:59–63.

279. Varlotta, G. P., Brown, M. D., Kelsey, J. L., and Golden, A. L. (1991): Familial predisposition for herniation of a lumbar disc in patients who are less than twenty-one years old. *J. Bone Joint Surg.,* 73:124–128.

280. Videman, T., Battie, M. C., Manninen, H., Gill, K., Gibbons, L. E., and Fisher, L. D. (1995): Lifetime exercise and sport participation and disc degeneration: An MRI study in male identical twins. *Trans. Orthop. Res. Soc.,* 67–12.

281. Viitasalo, J. T., Era, P., Leskinen, P. A., and Heikkinen, E. (1985): Muscular strength profiles and anthropometry in random samples of men aged 31–35, 51–55, 71–75 years. *Ergonomics,* 28:1563–1574.

282. Vleeming, A., Volkers, A. C., Snijders, C. J., and Stoeckart, R. (1990): Relation between form and function in the sacroiliac joint. Part II: Biomechanical aspects. *Spine,* 15:133–136.

283. Vleeming, A., Volkers, A. C., Snijders, C. J., and Stoeckart, R. (1990): Relation between form and function of the sacroiliac joint. Part I. Anatomic aspects. *Spine,* 15:130–132.

284. Voutsinas, S. A., and MacEwan, G. D. (1986): Sagittal profiles of the spine. *Clin. Orthop. Rel. Res.,* 210: 235–242.

285. Wakano, K., Kasman, R., Chao, E. Y., and Bradford, D. S. (1983): Biochemical analysis of canine intervertebral disc after chymopapain injection. *Spine,* 8:59–68.

286. Walters, C. E., and Partridge, M. J. (1957): Electromyographic study of the differential action of the abdominal muscles during exercise. *Am. J. Phys. Med.,* 36:259–268.

287. Warren, G. L., Hayes, D. A., and Lowe, D. A. (1993): Mechanical factors in the initiation of eccentric contraction-induced injury in rat soleus muscle. *J. Physiol.,* 464:457–475.

288. Waters, R., and Morris, J. (1973): An *in vitro* study of normal and scoliotic interspinous ligaments. *J. Biomech.,* 6:343–348.

289. Weber, H. (1978): *Lumbar disc herniation. A prospective study of prognostic factors including a controlled trial.* Ph.D. Dissertation, University of Oslo.

290. Weidenbaum, M., Foster, R. J., Best, B. A., et al. (1992): Correlating magnetic resonance imaging with the biochemical content of the normal human intervertebral disc. *J. Orthop. Res.,* 10:552–561.

291. White, A. A., and Panjabi, M. M. (1978): *Clinical Biomechanics of the Spine,* p. 22. J. B. Lippincott, Philadelphia.

292. White, A. A., and Panjabi, M. M. (1978): The basic kinematics of the spine. *Spine,* 3:12.

293. Wilder, D. G., Pope, M. H., Seroussi, R. E., and Dimnet, J. (1987): Creep response of the statically and cyclically loaded lumbar motion segment. *Trans. Orthop. Res. Soc.,* 12:367.

294. Willner, S. (1983): Spine pantograph: a non-invasive anthropometric device for describing postures and asymmetries of the trunk. *J. Pediatr. Orthop.,* 3:245–249.

295. Willner, S., and Johnson, B. (1983): Thoracic kyphosis and lumbar lordosis during the growth period in children. *Acta Orthop. Scand.,* 72:873–878.

296. Wynne-Davies, R., and Scott, J. H. S. (1979): Inheritance and spondylolisthesis. A radiographic family survey. *J. Bone Joint Surg.,* 61B:301–305.

297. Yang, K. H., and King, A. I. (1984): Mechanism of facet load transmission as a hypothesis for low back pain. *Spine,* 9:557–565.

298. Yoganandan, N., Haffner, M., Maiman, D. J., et al. (1990): Epidemiology and injury biomechanics of motor vehicle related trauma to the spine. *SAE Trans.,* 98: 1790–1807.

299. Yoganandan, N., Larson, S. J., Pintar, F. A., Gallagher, M., Reinartz, J., and Droetz, K. (1994): Intravertebral pressure changes caused by spinal microtrauma. *Neurosurgery,* 35:415–421.

300. Yoganandan, N., Pintar, F. A., Sances, A., Reinartz, J., and Larson, S. J. (1991): Strength and kinematic response of dynamic cervical spine injuries. *Spine,* 16: 511–517.

Basic Orthopaedic Biomechanics, 2nd ed.,
edited by Van C. Mow and Wilson C. Hayes.
Lippincott–Raven Publishers, Philadelphia © 1997.

11

Biomechanics of Artificial Joints: The Hip

Rik Huiskes and Nico Verdonschot

*Department of Musculoskeletal Biomechanics, Institute of Orthopaedics, University of Nijmegen,
6500 HB Nijmegen, The Netherlands.*

TOTAL HIP REPLACEMENT

Development of Hip Replacement

Total hip replacement (THR) has become one of the major surgical advances of this century. At an estimated occurrence between 500,000 and 1 million operations per year (155), it is second only to dental reconstruction as an invasive treatment of body ailments. Its success rate as a satisfactory surgical therapy for serious disabilities or illnesses is probably surpassed only by removal of the appendix (W. H. Harris, *personal communication, 1987*).

Total hip replacement is an effective treatment for serious forms of osteoarthritis[1] and for disabling effects of rheumatoid arthritis, congenital deformities, and particular kinds of posttraumatic conditions. Osteoarthritis (OA) is the most frequent indication for THR, comprising about 65% of the total volume. According to an American study in 1981 (3), it is responsible for the majority of cases involving musculoskeletal discomfort and, second to cardiovascular conditions, is an important cause for complete or partial disabilities. About 17% of Americans have some form of arthritis (59,71,260). Ten percent of all Americans suffer from OA, half of them chronically.

The development and application of THR have achieved a tremendous reduction in disabilities, particularly in the older segment of the population. The economic effects of this surgical treatment on society as a whole in terms of savings in medical care, drugs, and disability aids and the reduction in sickness-related absence from jobs are significant (59,71,260). The personal effects on the happiness and life fulfillment of patients are overwhelming. The majority of patients receiving THR can hardly walk at all and suffer

---

[1]When the cause of degenerative joint disease is mechanically initiated, as is often the case, this disease is better referred to as osteoarthrosis.

serious continuous pain, day and night. A few
weeks after the operation, they will, with few
exceptions, be pain-free, able to function normally, and resume jobs and sometimes even
active sports. Complications will usually not
recur until after 10 to 20 years. When they do,
as a result of eventual wear or loosening, a revision operation is possible. At least 90% of
the patients live normal, pain-free lives for at
least 10 years after the operation (29,76,155).

The successful application of THR on a
large scale, which essentially evolved during
the last three decades, is an accomplishment of
scientific and technological developments in
orthopaedic surgery and bioengineering, in
particular from the scientific specialties of
biomaterials and biomechanics sciences. The
proliferation of applications started around
1960 with the introduction of two inventions
by Sir John Charnley (25,26). One was the
adoption of the "low-friction" principle,
whereby a relatively small metal femoral head
was made to rotate against a polyethylene acetabular cup. Another was the use of acrylic
cement (polymethylmethacrylate or PMMA)
as a filling material to accommodate uniform
load transfer between the smooth-shaped prosthesis and the irregular texture of the bone.
The PMMA, when introduced in a doughy
phase, interdigitates with the bone and cures to
form a solid but relatively flexible mantle between bone and prosthesis (Fig. 1). Polymethylmethacrylate is a relatively weak material, however, and long-term loosening of
prostheses has been attributed to its mechanical disintegration.

Efforts to improve the endurance of implant fixation have resulted in better cement-
ing techniques. Alternative prosthetic designs
have been aimed at replacing acrylic cement
with other means of fixation. Early noncemented prostheses were the press-fitted or
screwed-in types. Noncemented porous-
coated prostheses were introduced to provoke
bony ingrowth for improved fixation. Hydroxyapatite-coated hip prostheses (64–66,
121,175) are meant to form a firm biological
adhesive bond with bone (osseous integration). Some of these noncemented devices

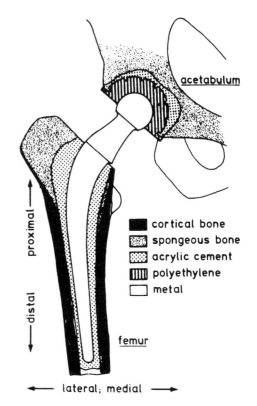

FIG. 1. Schematic section of a cemented
Charnley prosthesis. (From Huiskes, ref. 93,
with permission.)

have failed, but others are doing well in the
mid- to long term. Definite conclusions about
their ultimate clinical performances and about
the best fixation methods or designs require
longer-term studies. The noncemented prostheses are used predominantly in younger patients (<60 years), where it is assumed that
these prostheses eventually simplify a revision operation (120). Epidemiologic studies
show that for these younger patients, revision
surgery would probably be needed if they
were to receive a cemented prothesis.

Clinical Performance

The "quality" of a joint replacement depends on such clinical factors as medical complications the patient may suffer, presence of
residual pain, motion restrictions, and loosen-

ing of the components. Although the precise relationships are not always evident, the quality is basically determined by prosthetic design factors (materials, prosthetic shape, fixation concept, and surgical instruments), surgical factors (surgical skills and experience, including patient and device selection, and patient instruction), and patient factors (bone mechanical quality, general health condition, age, weight, and level of physical activity). The most frequent complication is long-term loosening unrelated to infection, which is usually called aseptic or mechanical loosening. Aseptic loosening is a gradual process (52,68,128,191,207) whereby the mechanical integrity of the implant–bone interface is lost, and a fibrous tissue is formed between the two surfaces. A gradual increase in thickness occurs with time. As a result, the patient develops pain and functional restrictions. Aseptic loosening is the limiting factor for the functional life span of THR reconstructions. Most of the clinical and bioengineering research and development performed aims at understanding its causes and postponing its occurrence.

The precise mechanism of aseptic loosening of cemented THR is not entirely certain, but several factors are known to contribute. Some of these affect the biological processes at the cement–bone junction directly. Wear particles from the cup–head articulation and other origins may migrate in the cement–bone interface. They provoke reactions from macrophage cells, which cause bone to resorb (88, 128,178,207). As an effect, a fibrous tissue layer is formed between cement and bone, reducing the integrity of the fixation. Repeated application of load on the hip will create relative motions between bone and cement, which are known to provoke further bone resorption and loosening (69). A similar result can occur in an early stage through resorption of interface bone after bone death. Interface bone death, or necrosis, can be caused by the mechanical rasping procedure during the operation (58), by thermal damage from the heat of polymerizing of acrylic cement (58,93,165), or by cell-toxic effects of residual monomer in the cement (58,257).

Another class of causative factors for aseptic loosening has mechanical origins (1,72,89, 130,142,170,220). The loads on the hip joint are relatively high and frequent, up to 1 million cycles per year. Eventually this may cause fatigue failure of the components and junctions in the THR reconstruction. In particular, acrylic cement (36) and its interfaces with bone and THR components are vulnerable to fatigue processes. Indirectly, mechanical forces also affect the biological processes in bone. Bone reacts to chronic overloading by bone formation, and to underloading by resorption, which is called strain-adaptive bone remodeling (13,116,126,229). In this way, the bone morphology and the integrity of the fixation may gradually change over time. This also affects the stresses in the materials and their strength.

Long-term follow-up studies in large patient groups have shown that the average life span of cemented THR lies somewhere between 10 and 20 years. Although individual variations are large, the average in a group of patients depends very much on prosthetic design and on the average age of the patient population at the time of the operation (2,79, 155). Younger patients have significantly shorter endurance expectations than older ones, probably as a result of higher physical activity levels, metabolic turnover rates, and biologic remodeling processes.

Problems associated with noncemented prostheses arise from three sources. The first concerns the interface fixation stability. The fixation relies on a good mechanical fit because no cement is used to fill the gaps between the prosthesis and the host bone. Thus, the dimensions and shape of the prosthetic components in relation to the host bone are more important than for cemented prostheses. In addition, more precise bone preparation techniques are required. The problem of producing a good fit has not been solved for the available contemporary prosthetic designs (4,9,148,171,176,187,206). As a result, the initial postoperative fixation (or initial stability) of the implants is usually far from ideal. The patients may subsequently suffer (often temporarily) from residual postoperative pain (midthigh pain) caused by relative motions of the implant during loading (50,255). These relative motions may also prevent bone ingrowth or osseous integration of the implant, thereby affecting the long-term stability of the device. The lack of adequate fit also leaves gaps at the implant–bone interface, which create routes for migrating wear debris, promoting long-term loosening.

Second, strain-adaptive bone remodeling phenomena affect the long-term postoperative behavior of noncemented joint replacements in particular. This is because these designs are usually relatively stiff, thereby affecting the strain patterns in bone more drastically than in the case of cemented replacements. This effect may be further amplified by the rigid interface formed by bone ingrowth or osseous integration. When this occurs, certain regions of the surrounding bone become understressed ("stress shielded" or "stress protected"), thus causing bone resorption to take place. The extent to which this mechanism affects the long-term clinical result is not known. However, certainly too much bone loss will eventually cause mechanical failure of the implant–bone structure. In addition, a weakened bone may create an unfavorable situation for revision surgery (53).

Third, prostheses that have been firmly fixed by bony ingrowth or by osseous integration are very difficult to remove, should it become necessary. Hence, it is not entirely certain that failed noncemented prostheses are more easily revised than failed cemented prostheses; this is often suggested as an advantage of the noncemented type.

To evaluate the quality of a hip prosthesis, relative to its potential for long-term endurance, survival rates are determined in patient series. Figure 2 shows an example of so-called survival-rate curves for two prosthetic types from the Swedish multicenter trials (155). The orthopaedic community in Sweden has developed a unique information system, the Swedish Register, for monitoring the long-term outcome of joint replacement. In this system, data on each THR procedure are

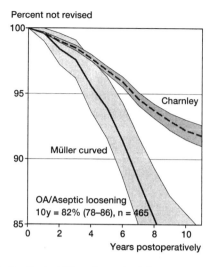

FIG. 2. Probability of survival (percentage not revised) of two cemented total hip replacements. The data are taken from the Swedish Register containing a total of 92,675 patients who received a THR between 1978 and 1990. The *shaded bands* give the 95% confidence intervals. (Adapted from Malchau et al., ref. 155.)

stored, including patient, surgical, and device-related information. Because virtually all surgeons contribute to providing the data, and each patient has a unique national identification number, all revisions are traceable and can be related to the specifications of the primary THR procedure. In this way, objective data can be obtained, whereby implant, patient, and surgical factors are correlated to prosthetic endurance with a high degree of statistical significance. This system has frequently enabled early detection of unsafe designs or provided information about the effectiveness of particular surgical procedures (76,77,79,155,225). It also gives feedback to individual orthopaedic centers about their relative performance. Similar follow-up studies in single or a restricted number of clinics have been less effective in discriminating causative factors for failures.

When revision is not taken as the indicator of failure, postoperative studies in patient series are less conclusive. Rating systems to score function and pain have been developed, but these mostly rely on patient interviews and are not objective (256). Longitudinal postoperative radiograms are another source of information on the quality of hip reconstructions. However, radiographic exposure procedures are not standardized; hence, morphologic and bone-density parameters tend to be variable. In addition, conventional radiograms are two-dimensional reductions of a three-dimensional reality. As a result, measurements based on their use tend to be imprecise (123,157).

In recent years, methods have been developed that allow for more precise determinations of prosthetic behavior and hence for earlier detection of problems. It has been shown that aseptic loosening of prosthetic components is virtually always preceded by migration (63,135,247). Roentgen stereophotogrammetric analysis (RSA) permits these migrations to be detected with an accuracy of some 100 μm (134,135,166,214). The use of this method, discussed in more detail in another section of this chapter, allows significant predictions of pending loosenings of THR even after 6 months postoperatively (135). Dual-energy X-ray absorptiometry (DEXA) is a new method to measure bone mass *in vivo*, with an accuracy of about 5%. This method can be used to detect loss of bone around a prosthesis and predict pending problems or assess the effectiveness of particular prostheses in their bone-preserving potential (13,28,56). Gait analysis, finally, is another method for objectively measuring the quality of THR and detecting problems in an early stage (81,174,183).

Biomechanics and the Innovation Cycle

The development of new prostheses is motivated not only by requests from the orthopaedic community but also by commercial considerations. Marketing a reasonably successful device, even for a small number of users, can be quite profitable. As a result, new types appear frequently, not necessarily providing for better quality reconstructions. Traditionally, new designs have often been developed through "trial and error," using the operating room as the laboratory and the patient as the experimental model. This was jus-

tified at a time when no satisfactory alternative existed, and often the new hip replacement did at least offer the patients adequate and safe treatment for a limited number of years. Today, the traditional time-tested cemented hip replacements provide safe and effective solutions for a long period of time, relative to which new devices must be tested (57). Ideas for new designs tend to be based on clinical research, in which particular problems are identified, or on experimental research with new concepts or materials for THR.

Whatever the origin, the new design should be tested preclinically before marketing to prevent unsafe devices from being tried in patients. These tests can be performed in animal models, laboratory bench tests, or computer-simulation models, depending on the particular failure scenarios investigated (102). Deficiencies in a design are not always detected in a preclinical test because new designs may create hitherto unknown problems. Hence, to prevent unsafe designs from being widely marketed, they should be tested in restricted clinical trials. Because endurance of THR is the most critical issue, and the average life span is already on the order of 10 to 20 years, the efficacy of clinical trials is not a trivial matter. Obviously, innovators and companies will be reluctant to postpone marketing for a decade; on the other hand, a clinical trial period of 2 years (as, for example, required by the FDA) is much too short to establish long-term safety and efficacy of a new prosthetic design. When objective and precise measuring techniques are applied, such as RSA, DEXA, or gait analysis, as mentioned above, these short-term trials may be more effective in detecting design deficiencies. Nevertheless, postmarketing surveillance, such as applied in the Swedish Register, is necessary to prevent unsafe marketed devices from creating a disaster in a large patient population.

Biomechanics research is intimately involved with virtually all activities in the innovation cycle. To understand clinical failure mechanisms of THR requires knowledge about the forces acting on the hip, the stresses they generate in bone and implant materials, and their effects on wear, damage accumulation, and bone remodeling. Biomechanics is important in the establishment of failure scenarios, which are required for effective preclinical testing (102). The development and validation of preclinical testing methods comprise another prominent area of biomechanics investigation, and, of course, biomechanicians are involved in designing new hip prostheses and surgical instruments. All these activities require basic information assessed in biomechanical studies, i.e., the evaluation of forces occurring in the joints and their related muscles in various functions, the study of motion characteristics of the joints, the assessment of geometric properties of the bones to which artificial components are to be connected, or the mechanical properties such as strength and elastic characteristics of bone and biomaterials involved.

This chapter on the biomechanics of THR emphasizes the analysis of load transfer from prosthesis to bone, its interaction with biological remodeling processes, and its effects on the mechanical behavior and endurance of hip reconstructions, both the cemented and the noncemented types. The principles of experimental design and analysis are emphasized, rather than the specifics of particular prostheses. Hence, the main purpose of this chapter is to acquaint the reader with the tools of research and development in this area. For illustrative purposes, some examples are also presented.

SOLID MECHANICS AND STRESS ANALYSIS

Some Principles of Solid Mechanics

In this section some definitions and principles of solid biomechanics are reviewed. For a more detailed discussion, the reader is referred to standard engineering textbooks (38,87,200,226).

Stress, Strain, and Hooke's Law

If a body is loaded, it deforms. Unless the body is regularly shaped (e.g., cube, bar, or beam), and the external load is evenly distributed and aligned with the geometry, these deformations produced in the body will not be uniform. The amount of deformation will vary throughout the body. To analyze the deformation, we select an infinitesimal cube of material inside the object and allow this cube to be stretched and compressed in the three edge directions. To quantify these deformations, we define a lineal strain along each edge, given as a change of length per original length (Fig. 3a). These three lineal strains also define the dilatation (change of volume per original volume; this is equal to the algebraic sum of the three lineal strains) of the cube. The lineal strains and dilatation depend on the applied loading and on the material that constitutes the object. We also allow the shape of the cube to distort in its three planes (Fig. 3b). These three angles are known as shear strains, and they also depend on the material and the external loading. These six variables completely describe the deformation of the tiny cube at any arbitrary point inside the body.

For a continuous body, load is transferred at every point inside the body. This implies that when we pass an imaginary plane through the body, the material on one side of the plane will exert a force on the material on the other side. These are internal forces, and they are transferred by chemical or physical bonds at the molecular level. Like the deformations, the magnitudes and orientations of these internal forces are not uniform but depend on the external loading, the shape of the object, and the intrinsic mechanical properties of the material

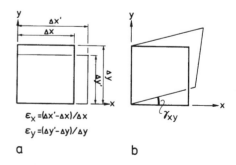

FIG. 3. Definitions of strain in the case of two-dimensional stress state. **(a)** direct strain; **(b)** shear strain. (From Huiskes, ref. 95, with permission.)

making up the object. To describe these internal forces, we must first define the concept of stress. Simply stated, stress is defined as force per unit area. For convenience, the areas we choose are the faces of the tiny cube described above (Fig. 4). On each face of the cube, the force vector may be arbitrarily oriented. This means that on each face of the cube the stress vector will also be arbitrarily oriented. This stress vector may be decomposed into a component perpendicular to the face of the cube (normal stress) and a component parallel to the face of the cube (shear stress). In general, the shear stress component will have two components, each parallel to an axis of the chosen coordinate system. Thus, a total of nine stress components (three normal stresses and six shear stresses) must be known to define the state of stress acting on the cube (Fig. 4). However, by conservation of angular momentum, the shear stresses are symmetric, i.e., $\tau_{xy} = \tau_{yx}$, $\tau_{yz} = \tau_{zy}$, $\tau_{zx} = \tau_{xz}$. Thus, only six independent stress components exist, three normal stress components (σ_x, σ_y, σ_z) and three shear stress components (τ_{xy}, τ_{yz}, τ_{zx}) (Fig. 4). We note that the normal stresses can be either tensile (positive) or compressive (negative). We also note that these stress values will vary with the orientation of the chosen cube (i.e., coordinate system) because the components of a vector will vary with the orientation of the chosen coordinate system.

Central to solid mechanics theory is the relationship between stresses and strains for the body. This relationship is given by a constitutive equation. The stiffness of the material depends on the intrinsic mechanical properties of the material, i.e., the coefficients of the constitutive equation or material constants. If this material is linearly elastic, the generalized Hooke's law may be applied (111). In this case, the six strain components are linearly related to the six stress components by a matrix of 36 elastic constants (of which 21 are independent) given by[2]

$$
\begin{bmatrix} \varepsilon_x \\ \varepsilon_y \\ \varepsilon_z \\ \gamma_{xy} \\ \gamma_{yz} \\ \gamma_{zx} \end{bmatrix} = \begin{bmatrix} S_{11} & S_{12} & S_{13} & S_{14} & S_{15} & S_{16} \\ S_{21} & S_{22} & S_{23} & S_{24} & S_{25} & S_{26} \\ S_{31} & S_{32} & S_{33} & S_{34} & S_{35} & S_{36} \\ S_{41} & S_{42} & S_{43} & S_{44} & S_{45} & S_{46} \\ S_{51} & S_{52} & S_{53} & S_{54} & S_{55} & S_{56} \\ S_{61} & S_{62} & S_{63} & S_{64} & S_{65} & S_{66} \end{bmatrix} \cdot \begin{bmatrix} \sigma_x \\ \sigma_y \\ \sigma_z \\ \tau_{xy} \\ \tau_{yz} \\ \tau_{zx} \end{bmatrix} \quad (1)
$$

This is a coupled set of six equations. It shows that a particular strain value may depend on all six stress values and vice versa. Irrespective of the kind of material considered, this matrix is always symmetric (i.e., $S_{ij} = S_{ji}$), which implies a maximum of 21 independent components. This set of six equations defines a completely anisotropic material if all these 21 elastic constants in the matrix are different. For most materials, some form of symmetry of the microstructure exists. If the material is orthotropic, all but the constants S_{ii}, S_{12}, S_{13}, and S_{23} reduce to zero, which leaves nine independent constants in the matrix. If the material is transversely isotropic, which means that the properties are equal for two of the three principal directions, the number of independent constants reduces to five. For the isotropic case, the number reduces to only two independent elastic constants. Most often, these are expressed in terms of the Young's modulus (or elastic modulus) E and Poisson's ratio ν. Other constants are commonly used as well, such as the Lame constants (λ, μ), modulus of rigidity or shear modulus (μ), and the

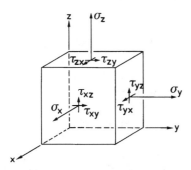

FIG. 4. Definition of the nine stress components relative to an infinitesimal cube in the material. Since $\tau_{zy} = \tau_{yz}$, $\tau_{xz} = \tau_{zx}$, and $\tau_{xy} = \tau_{yx}$, only six independent components remain to describe the three-dimensional stress state. (From Huiskes, ref. 95, with permission.)

---

[2]This equation is defined by matrix multiplication. For example, $\varepsilon_x = S_{11}\sigma_x + S_{12}\sigma_y + S_{13}\sigma_z + S_{14}\tau_{xy} + S_{15}\tau_{yz} + S_{16}\tau_{zx}$, etc.

bulk modulus (κ). These constants may be expressed in terms of E and v because only two constants are independent, and equation 1 may then be written as

$$\begin{bmatrix} \varepsilon_x \\ \varepsilon_y \\ \varepsilon_z \\ \gamma_{xy} \\ \gamma_{yz} \\ \gamma_{zx} \end{bmatrix} = \begin{bmatrix} 1/E & -v/E & -v/E & 0 & 0 & 0 \\ -v/E & 1/E & -v/E & 0 & 0 & 0 \\ -v/E & -v/E & 1/E & 0 & 0 & 0 \\ 0 & 0 & 0 & (2+2v)/E & 0 & 0 \\ 0 & 0 & 0 & 0 & (2+2v)/E & 0 \\ 0 & 0 & 0 & 0 & 0 & (2+2v)/E \end{bmatrix} \cdot \begin{bmatrix} \sigma_x \\ \sigma_y \\ \sigma_z \\ \tau_{xy} \\ \tau_{yz} \\ \tau_{zx} \end{bmatrix} \quad (2)$$

When the material is transversely isotropic, a total of five elastic constants are required (19, 193). For example, by approximation, cortical (haversian) bone is transversely isotropic. To describe cortical bone, a modulus is required for the longitudinal direction and another for the radial direction (the tangential direction has the same modulus as the radial one), along with two Poisson's ratios and a shear modulus.

We emphasize some important restrictions to linear elasticity theory and continuum mechanics. First, if a material is not linearly elastic, e.g., nonlinearly elastic, then Hooke's law does not apply. The material may also be plastic or viscoelastic in nature. For these types of material, the stress–strain laws are always much more complex. Biological materials can not, in general, be described by infinitesimal linear elasticity theory, although bone can, by reasonable approximation. Second, the definitions of stress and strain presume that the material is continuous. This implies that no matter how small a cube we have chosen, the properties in the cube are supposed to be identical to those of the material at a larger scale. This assumes that there are no imperfections or voids (discontinuities) in the material. For real materials, this is hardly ever true. Even metals have imperfections in their lattice structure and at grain boundaries. Plastics usually possess a certain degree of porosity, although the pore sizes are extremely small. Bone is essentially discontinuous, in particular trabecular bone. Hence, stress–strain relationships and the calculated stresses and strains are always approximations. The quality of these approximations ranges from very good (e.g., metal) to very rough (e.g., trabecular bone). The approach to a discontinuous material like bone is to designate a region in which

dimensions are large relative to the characteristic size of the microstructure of imperfections and only consider the calculated stresses and strains in that region as average.

Three- and Two-Dimensional and Uniaxial Stress States

If the characteristic features of a structure can be represented in a plane, and the external loads are also in that plane, then the stress state in the structure is two-dimensional. A two-dimensional problem may be described as a plane stress or a plane strain problem. In the plane-stress problem, the material is free to expand in the out-of-plane direction, and the normal stress in that direction is zero. This implies for equations 1 and 2 that when z is the out-of-plane direction, $\gamma_{yz} = \gamma_{zx} = 0$, and $\sigma_z = \tau_{yz} = \tau_{zx} = 0$. For the plane-strain case, the material is constrained in the out-of-plane direction, and the lineal strain in that direction is zero. This implies for equations 1 and 2 that $\varepsilon_z = \gamma_{yz} = \gamma_{zx} = 0$ and $\tau_{yz} = \tau_{zx} = 0$. In both of these cases, the stress state within the plane can be characterized by three stress variables (e.g., σ_x, σ_y, and $\tau_{xy} = \tau_{yx} = \tau$).

In the uniaxial stress state, only one independent stress component exists. This implies for equations 1 and 2 that, if x is the uniaxial direction, $\gamma_{xy} = \gamma_{yz} = \gamma_{zx} = 0$ and $\sigma_y = \sigma_z = \tau_{xy} = \tau_{yz} = \tau_{zx} = 0$. This state of stress occurs predominantly in long, slender bodies of regular prismatic shape (bars or columns), which are loaded externally at the end by axial tension or compression, transverse forces, or bending moments. This state of stress is most often used for tensile or compressive tests to determine the Young's modulus and Poisson's ratio of isotropic materials.

Principal Stresses and Stress Tensors

If we rotate the cube of Fig. 4 relative to a fixed coordinate system external to the object, the values of the stress components will change even though the stress state within the material remains the same. Thus, different components may describe the same stress state inside the material. At one particular orientation of the cube, all shear-stress components acting on the face of the cube will vanish. This orientation defines the principal directions for the state of stress at the cube inside the material. The associated normal stresses are known as the principal stresses. For any arbitrary state of stress, the principal stresses are the maximum and minimum stress at any point inside the object.

The state of stress is completely described by the six stress components. In its entirety, the state of stress is known as a stress tensor. Although the components may vary with the specific coordinate system chosen, the state of stress remains the same. In other words, the state of stress within an object does not depend on a specific chosen coordinate system (i.e., observer). It depends solely on the load-

ing, geometry, and material properties of the object. The simplest representations of a state of stress are either in the principal coordinate system or by the three principal normal stress components.

Bone prosthesis structures often require stress information about "interfaces," where different materials are connected. These interfaces do not always align with the external coordinate system, nor do they generally align with the principal stress directions. For that purpose, local coordinate systems at the point of interest can be introduced relative to which the interface normal and shear stresses are expressed. The three methods of stress representation (coordinate, principal, and interface stresses) are illustrated in Fig. 5 for a two-dimensional example.

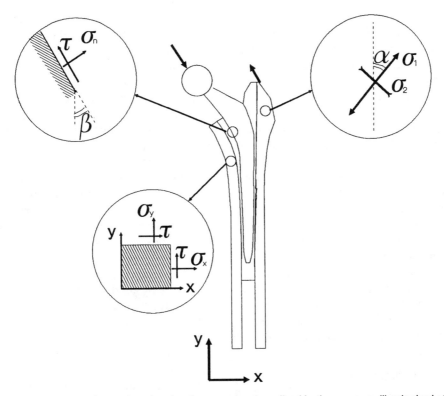

FIG. 5. The stress state in a point of a structure can be described in three ways: (i) principal stresses (σ_1, σ_2, and the principal-stress orientation α relative to the coordinate xy axes), (ii) coordinate stresses (σ_x, σ_y, and τ relative to a cube aligned with the coordinate axes), and (iii) interface stresses (compression/tension σ_n, normal to the interface, and shear τ, parallel to the interface, plus the orientation of the plane β). The principles of these representations are identical for three-dimensional stress states. One representation can directly and uniquely be converted to another by transformation of the coordinate system attitude.

Scalar Measures of Stress Intensity

The yield stress (or elastic limit) of a material is usually measured in uniaxial tensile and compressive or shear tests on material samples with simple geometric shapes. The question then is how to relate a two- or three-dimensional stress state, characterized by six stress components, to the yield stress data from uniaxial tests in order to estimate the probability of failure. For this purpose, an *equivalent* (or *effective*) *stress* is determined from a particular yield criterion. The von Mises yield criterion, for example, assumes that material will yield, i.e., deform plastically, when the distortion energy exceeds a certain value. The *von Mises stress* can be calculated from the equation

$$\sigma_{mi} = \left\{ \tfrac{1}{2}[(\sigma_1 - \sigma_2)^2 + (\sigma_1 - \sigma_3)^2 + (\sigma_2 - \sigma_3)^2] \right\}^{1/2} \qquad (3)$$

where σ_1, σ_2, and σ_3 are the principal stress values in the material point of interest. This von Mises equivalent stress value can simply be compared to stress values obtained from samples of the material tested in the laboratory in uniaxial tension or compression to estimate the probability of failure. It gives reasonable predictions for isotropic materials. It works less satisfactorily for anisotropic elastic materials (such as bone) or viscoelastic materials. Still, it is often used for these materials as well, to represent the six stress components in one generalized "stress intensity" factor, which greatly simplifies the interpretation and representation of results of stress analyses.

The *strain-energy density* (SED) also represents the stress state in a material but has not been directly related to a failure criterion. This quantity represents the elastic energy stored in the deformed material and can be calculated from the formula

$$U = \tfrac{1}{2}(\varepsilon_1 \sigma_1 + \varepsilon_2 \sigma_2 + \varepsilon_3 \sigma_3) \qquad (4)$$

where ε_1, ε_2, and ε_3 and σ_1, σ_2, and σ_3 are the principal strains and stresses, respectively. This form of SED is valid only for isotropic materials, where the directions of principal strains and principal stress are parallel. The SED function is commonly used to formulate nonlinearly elastic constitutive equations (hyperelastic materials). It is also used in strain-adaptive bone-remodeling theory.

Stress Analysis

Stress analysis in solid mechanics involves a particular structure with a given geometry made out of a particular material(s) with known elastic properties (i.e., Young's modulus and Poisson's ratio). The structure is loaded externally by forces and/or moments and is connected to the environment in a certain way. The objective of stress analysis may be to determine the stress and strain fields in the structure to see if the structure gives rise to excessive deformations or stresses that could cause mechanical failure.

Stress analysis may be conducted either numerically on a computer or with closed-form mathematical solutions. In the former case, a computer model is used, i.e., the finite-element method. In the latter case, the solution is obtained in explicit mathematical formulas. These closed-form solutions are available only for particular, regularly shaped structures such as prismatic bars and beams. If applicable, closed-form solutions are always to be preferred over numerical ones because, in addition to the actual numerical results, they also render insight into the relationships among structural parameters, material properties, geometric factors, loads, and stress–strain patterns (95). As a rule, all calculated stresses and strains should be experimentally verified. Strains acting at the surface of a structure may be determined experimentally, either directly with measurements or indirectly, using a laboratory model.

It is noted that the results of a stress analysis, whether experimental or analytic, depend very much on the model constructed to represent the structure. The accuracy of the stress and strain calculations depends very much on the realism of the model (i.e., geometry, constitutive equation for the material, material coefficients, loading conditions, and boundary conditions). Models are abstractions of reality, and they are used to simplify the actual problem. The essence of modeling is that each model must capture the salient characteristics of the problem appropriate to the needs of the situation. However, overly complex models are not necessarily better than simpler ones. There are no fixed rules for this modeling process. The question is never whether a model assumption is true in the real sense of the word (they almost never are) but whether a simplification is justified relative to the definition of the problem (107).

Finite-Element Analysis

The finite-element method (FEM) has become a widely used tool in orthopaedic biomechanics. It is a computer method suitable for determining stresses and strains at any given point inside a structure of arbitrary geometric and material complexity. A finite-element model relies on accurate constitutive representation of material characteristics (such as the elastic coefficients of generalized Hooke's law), geometric data, loading

characteristics, and boundary and interfacial conditions. The principles of FE analysis are described in many textbooks (e.g., 91,264). Attempts at more general introductions to FEM, particularly for orthopaedic biomechanics, have been published elsewhere (95,107,117,154). Only the basic principles and a few pitfalls are reviewed here. To develop a FEM model, the shape of the structure to be analyzed is divided into small elements. For three-dimensional analysis, elemental volumes of a particular shape (e.g., bricks) are used, and for a two-dimensional analysis, elemental areas of a particular shape (e.g., triangles or quadrilaterals) are used. Each element has nodal points, usually at the corners of the element. At each nodal point three (or two in the case of two-dimensional analysis) displacement components and three force components (two in a two-dimensional analysis) are identified.

As an illustrative example, consider a two-dimensional model with triangular elements, each with three nodal points (Fig. 6). The displacement vector **u** and force vector **f** at each

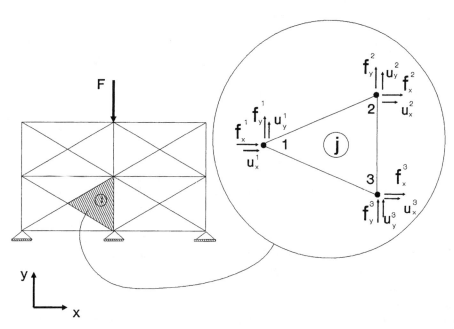

FIG. 6. A two-dimensional finite-element mesh and definition of nodal-point forces and nodal-point displacements.

nodal point i can be written in terms of their components:

$$\boldsymbol{u}^i = \begin{bmatrix} u_x^i \\ u_y^i \end{bmatrix} \quad \boldsymbol{f}^i = \begin{bmatrix} f_x^i \\ f_y^i \end{bmatrix} \quad (i = 1,2,3) \tag{5}$$

For the entire structure with n elements, these vectors at the jth element may be written as

$$\boldsymbol{u}^j = \begin{bmatrix} u^1 \\ u^2 \\ u^3 \end{bmatrix} = \begin{bmatrix} u_x^1 \\ u_y^1 \\ u_x^2 \\ u_y^2 \\ u_x^3 \\ u_y^3 \end{bmatrix} \quad \boldsymbol{f}^j = \begin{bmatrix} f_x^1 \\ f_y^1 \\ f_x^2 \\ f_y^2 \\ f_x^3 \\ f_y^3 \end{bmatrix} \quad (j = 1,...,n) \tag{6}$$

where n is the total number of elements in the mesh. When the material of the element is linearly elastic, and the deformations are small relative to the dimensions of the element, there is a linear relationship between the nodal point force and the nodal point displacement components, which may be written in vector notation as

$$\boldsymbol{f}^j = \mathbf{Q}^j \mathbf{u}^j \tag{7}$$

Here $\mathbf{Q}^j$ is called the "stiffness matrix" of the jth element and consists of 6×6 components. Let us assume for a moment that the values of all these 36 components are known for every one of the elements. The structure is then numerically "assembled," in the sense that all displacements and forces of the different elements belonging to the same nodal point are collected. Then one vector, $\mathbf{u}$, is formed in which all displacement components in all the nodal points are collected, and one vector, $\mathbf{f}$, is formed that contains all force components in all nodal points. Hence, we obtain an equation of the form

$$\mathbf{f} = \mathbf{Q}\,\mathbf{u} \tag{8}$$

where $\mathbf{Q}$ is the $m \times m$ "stiffness" matrix for the whole construction containing m^2 components, and m is the number of degrees of freedom in the model (usually $2n$ for a two-dimensional model or $3n$ if the model is three-dimensional). The value of each component is known from the assembling procedure. By Newton's third

law of action and reaction, many of the force components at nodal points are zero. Hence, the components of the nodal-point force vector $\mathbf{f}$ are either zero where no external force is applied, have a known value where external forces are applied, or are unknown where boundary constraints are applied. The components of the nodal point displacement vector $\mathbf{u}$ where the boundary conditions are applied are either unknown where the forces are prescribed or known where the displacements are prescribed. Hence, for each component (degree of freedom) at each nodal point, either the displacement is known or the force is known. In other words, equation 8 is a system of m linear, algebraic equations with m unknowns and hence can be solved to give the values of all displacements in all nodal points.

To determine the components of the stiffness matrices in equation 8, we must go back to the individual element and equation 7. We assume that the deformation in each element takes a specific form in such a way that the deformation within the element is determined by the relative displacements of the nodal points. For instance, the strain distribution in each element may be assumed to be uniform. This assumption makes possible the determination of the components of the element stiffness matrix from the volume of the element and its shape, elastic modulus, and Poisson's ratio. And it also makes it possible to determine the strain in each element from the nodal point displacements and subsequently the stress in the element from Hooke's law.

In developing the FE code as described above, we have made two important simplifications. First, we have limited the admissible deformation of each element to a uniform strain pattern (i.e., a linear displacement field) within the element. Second, we have assumed that all load transmission between elements is concentrated in the nodal points. Thus, all results obtained are approximate. In fact, the accuracy of the approximation depends on the kind of elements used and on the degree of mesh refinement. When the element density approaches infinity, the results converge to the exact solution.

Today, using the finite element method is much simpler than suggested above because most of the work is done by readily available computer codes. The art of FE analysis now is really concerned with the development of the FE model and the interpretation of its results rather than with the performance of the calculations. However, the development of an adequate FE model for a hip reconstruction is still not a trivial matter (107). Of course, building a three-dimensional anatomically realistic mesh is a lot more time-consuming and complicated than building a two-dimensional mesh. In the three-dimensional case there could be significant restrictions on the maximum number of elements and nodal points used, depending on the capacity of the computer available. This is more problematic in prosthetic analysis because joint reconstructions are composite structures. For example, some parts of the composites have very small dimensions (e.g., acrylic cement layers) and require small elements. As a consequence of mesh continuity requirements, the adjacent material also needs relatively small elements, which increases the total number of elements in the structure. Potential solutions to this problem are limited by requirements for the minimal element aspect ratio; a brick element, for instance, that is relatively thin is said to be distorted and to produce errors.

The sophistication of the element and the displacement field must also be considered. Different types of elements are available in the FE packages. These elements use different interpolation functions to represent the coordinates and displacements in the subsequent calculations of strains and stresses. These interpolation functions can be relatively simple, such as a bilinear function for a two-dimensional four-node element or a trilinear function for three-dimensional eight-node brick elements. The advantage of these simple elements is that the number of degrees of freedom is relatively low, which limits the computer costs. However, these elements may not be able to capture the strain and stress states that are generated in reality. For example, these relatively simple elements behave too

stiffly when they are exposed to a bending load. The reason for this is that the linear shear strain variation that is present in bending can not be described by the simple interpolation functions. In some FE codes this can be corrected to some extent by correcting the interpolation function. This procedure is called the assumed strain formulation. More complex elements have more complicated interpolation functions (two-dimensional eight-node elements and three-dimensional 20-node elements); they have quadratic interpolation functions and are more powerful to describe the true stress and strain distribution. If we use one element over the thickness of a substructure and a linear displacement field (i.e., constant strain element), then we will obtain constant stress and strain over that thickness. In reality, for such a structure, a strain gradient may exist such as that occurring in bending. If we want more detailed information, we must either use more elements or use a more sophisticated element with a quadratic displacement field (linear strain) that results in more nodal points per element. In both cases, the size of the computation problem increases. The number of nodal points or elements required for appropriate accuracy can be determined with so-called convergence tests (139).

When the mesh has been constructed, the computer code needs external loading characteristics, elastic constants for each element, and specifications for the boundary and composite interface conditions. This again is not a trivial step in the process of modeling THR reconstructions because, as discussed above, these characteristics tend to vary greatly in a patient population and over time, and in general they are not known precisely. Hence, in order to analyze some of the problems, again, simplifying approximations must be used.

Geometry and FE Mesh

The geometry or shape of the arthroplasty components is accounted for by the FE mesh itself. Conceptually, every detail of the structures can be taken into account by using sufficiently small elements, but in practice this is hardly feasible; hence, the problem must be schematized to some degree. The refinement to which the structure is described by the mesh depends on the kind of information required (107). Figure 7 shows a few FE meshes of THR structures of variable complexity. In Fig. 7A a so-called "anatomic" mesh of a femoral component is shown, a three-dimensional model aimed at a realistic geometric representation of the reconstruction. The model in Fig. 7B is also three-dimensional but is symmetric relative to the midfrontal plane of the prosthesis. Although the general features of the load-transfer mechanism are reproduced in both models, the "anatomic" one is able to show details that are lost in the symmetric one. Although it seems intuitively obvious that the "anatomic" model is the more desirable one, this is not always true. The question is always whether details are relevant relative to the purpose of the model (107). Sometimes we would rather dispose of the details in order to obtain a more generic picture.

A simplified alternative to a three-dimensional model is a two-dimensional one, representing the midfrontal plane only. Such a model is quite easily assembled. However, it ignores the 3-D elastic integrity of the bone. This can be restored by using a "side plate" (93). This is essentially a second 2-D FE model, superimposed over the first one, or "front plate." When these requirements are fulfilled, then this model reproduces the relevant stress patterns of a three-dimensional one in the midfrontal plane reasonably accurately (235). Evidently, the effects of out-of-plane loading (i.e., torsion) can not be studied with a two-dimensional model, and out-of-plane stresses (e.g., hoop stresses) can not be determined.

In initiating an FE analysis, it is not advisable to immediately start developing the most expensive and complex model. As in all scientific endeavors, it is imperative to stop and think first what it is one wishes to accomplish and tune the model to those requirements. This, of course, requires an understanding of the relationships between model features and potential results.

Voxel Element Meshes

Increasingly, FE meshes of bones and THR structures are produced on the basis of geometric assessments from serial computed-tomography (CT) scanning (Fig. 8A). The CT delivers a three-dimensional voxel mesh of density values from which the shape of the bone can be graphically reconstructed using contour detection algorithms. The graphic reconstruction then serves as a basis for the element mesh (116,131,138). Advantages of this procedure are that mesh generation can be automated to some extent and that the apparent density of the bone material, by approximation related to its elastic modulus, is evaluated as well. Apart from this latter advantage and the convenience of the nondestructive geometric assessment, the problem of adequate mesh generation in a three-dimensional volume remains. This problem can be solved with voxel-conversion methods (86,208,254).

In principle, each voxel from a CT scan can be converted directly into a cubic element. The cube corners provide the coordi-

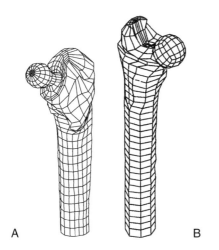

FIG. 7. Three-dimensional "anatomic" (**A**) and two-dimensional (**B**) finite-element models of femoral THA configurations.

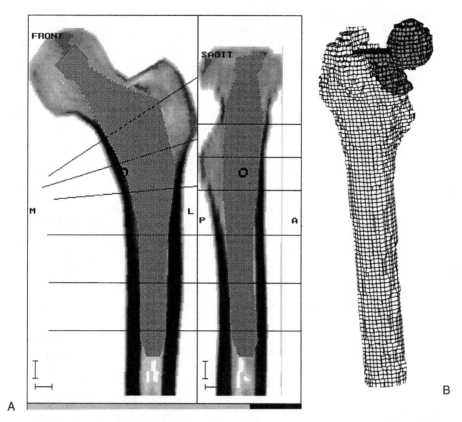

FIG. 8. (A) Example of a three-dimensional graphics computer program in which a CT-scanned bone can be imported, as well as the implant geometry. The implant can be moved relative to the bone in order to find the desired position. This is in fact an implantation-simulation procedure that can be done together with a surgeon. The finite-element mesh can be made directly from the geometric description. **(B)** Voxel model of an implanted femur. (Reproduced from 213a.)

nates of the nodal points, and the voxel density its elastic modulus. In fact, the whole mesh is available by the time the CT scan is made, ready for FEA. An example of such a mesh of a THR structure is shown in Fig. 8B. There are, however, disadvantages to this efficient procedure: the number of elements may be excessive, and the boundaries of the model are ragged instead of smooth. As was shown in comparative tests, the ragged boundaries hardly affect the mechanical behavior of a model at large. This implies that although the stress values calculated at the boundary are not dependable, those within the material are precise (85,125). The prob-

lem of excessive numbers of elements can be solved with alternative FE solution procedures that apply iterative optimization schemes. Examples are the element-by-element (EBE) procedure (84,92) and the row-by-row (RBR) procedure (231). The RBR procedure uses the fact that each element in the mesh has the same shape, dimension, and orientation, such that only a limited number of possible environments can exist. This makes the procedure much more efficient than EBE; hence, more elements can be used in the mesh. The RBR peocedure does require each element to have the same elastic constants, which is not the case for EBE.

Global Versus Local Mechanical Quantities

In many FE analyses of THR structures, local information about mechanical quantities is required. For example, one may need to evaluate the strength requirements of thin prosthetic coatings or study the stress environment of bone growing into pores. In such cases, the ratio between the typical volume to be studied and the dimensions of the whole THR structure may be on the order of 10^3. An adequate FE mesh for such a problem would imply too many elements for any computer. A traditional solution for this problem is to use FE models for different levels, applying the local nodal-point forces of a global model as boundary conditions for a local one. The precision of this method is questionable, however, because the stiffness characteristics of the local model are usually not equal to those of the corresponding volume in the global model (108). As a result, equal nodal-point forces produce different deformation patterns (nodal-point displacements). This problem can be solved by the application of homogenization theory (7,31,83,86,204).

In homogenization theory, a representative volume element (RVE) is produced from the stiffness characteristics of a local volume of interest, evaluated with an FE micromodel. The homogenized stiffness matrix of the RVE is substituted in the global mesh to determine its deformation characteristics, which then later serve as boundary conditions for an FE analysis of the local model, producing the local stresses and strains.

Loads

An FE analysis requires a numerical description of all external loads applied on the structure (point of application, magnitude, direction). These loads are usually variable and not always precisely known (12,14,15,34,46), so the question in FE analysis is often which approach to take in order to obtain useful information. A consideration that is always helpful is that FE analysis allows for easy parametric variation. Hence, the loads can be varied and the results studied in order to determine their relationships, and a "worst-case" situation can be defined. Often the worst-case (or typical-case) configuration is selected *a priori* from different possibilities. In such cases, it is advisable to investigate the sensitivity of the stress patterns to small deviations in the external loads. If different prosthetic designs are compared, different FE meshes are needed. Consequently, it is not trivial that the three-dimensional coordinates of the points where the external loads are applied are equal in all cases. Hence, the effects of different geometries on the stress and strain patterns are obscured by variations in load application location. This can be repaired by defining invariable points that are used to apply the external forces.

A set of three femoral loading cases can be considered that together represent average daily activities (Fig. 9; Table 1). Their magnitudes and directions have been chosen from telemetric measurements by Bergmann et al. (12) and Kotzar et al. (141) and are scaled for a person of 65 kg weight. The first two loading cases represent the peak joint forces that develop during the stance phase of normal walking (12,141), and the third loading case

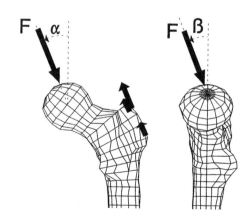

FIG. 9. The proximal part of a finite element model of a femoral bone. A set of three joint forces and three muscle forces can be selected, which represent typical daily loading configurations. Orientation is shown; values are listed in Table 1 (119,147).

TABLE 1. *Magnitudes and orientations of hip and muscle forces for three load cases (see Fig. 9)*

	Joint force	M. glut. max.	M. glut. med.	M. glut. min.
F_1 (N)	2132	637	637	214.5
α_1 (°)	23.4	39.9	24.6	28.4
β_1 (°)	5.7	43.0	24.8	28.4
F_2 (N)	1586	45.5	739	143
α_2 (°)	21.9	28.2	20.8	25.1
β_2 (°)	−4.6	24.3	10.5	1.9
F_3 (N)	1690	637	637	214.5
α_3 (°)	25	63.8	42.5	42.0
β_3 (°)	−15	62.0	57.7	55.1

represents the maximal joint load during stair climbing (141). The first loading case has the largest joint force (2132 N), whereas the third loading case has the largest out-of-plane component of this force. The insertions, orientations, and magnitudes of the corresponding forces in the three major muscles, the m. gluteus mimimus, the m. gluteus medius, and the m. gluteus maximus, have been taken from the work of Crowninshield and Brand (32) and Dostal and Andrews (49).

Hip-joint and muscle loads working at the acetabulum reconstruction during gait have been specified for FE analysis by Dalstra et al. (42), based on data from the same authors as mentioned above for the femur.

Figure 10 shows an example of the effects of variable loading in the hip joint during gait (12) on the bending stress patterns in a femoral THR structure (244). A worst-case load for the proximal stem would occur after 0.5 sec from the start of the stance phase. However, the distal stem stresses would reach a maximal value at 0.3 sec. This illustrates that a worst-case load for one part of the structure is not necessarily a worst case for another part.

Another approach to load selection is to use representative loading cases. This approach is especially useful when the effects of particular design features of a prosthesis are to be studied in a comparative analysis or when load-transfer mechanisms are to be studied. For instance, relative to femoral THR, the effects of the hip-joint force may be separated

into those resulting from the axial force, bending, and torsional components. The problem can then be analyzed for those three cases separately or for just the most important one. Finally, it is important to realize that most FE models of implant structures use infinitesimal linear elastic theory and that the surfaces are perfectly bonded at the interfaces. In these models, the principle of superposition may be used. Hence, the stress patterns that result from the application of the hip-joint force and the muscle forces together can be found from adding the results obtained from treating those forces separately.

Material Properties

In the FE model, each element must be assigned the appropriate elastic constants of the material. For an isotropic linearly elastic material, two material constants are required, e.g., Young's modulus and Poisson's ratio. This is the case for metallic implant materials. Acrylic cement and plastic components may be included in this category only by rough approximation (177). Cortical bone, by reasonable approximation, can be considered as linearly elastic and transversely isotropic, requiring five elastic constants for a complete description of its stress–strain relationship (19,193). The elastic relationship for cortical bone can also be simplified from transverse isotropy if the stresses and strains in the transverse and tangential directions are of lesser importance for the problem investigated (94).

Modeling cancellous bone is more complicated. To the first-order approximation, its elastic modulus can be expressed as a function of its porosity, measured by its apparent density (20). If a volume V (cm³) weighs w (g) without the fatty marrow, then the apparent density is defined by $\rho = w/V$ (g/cm³). The relationship between apparent density and the elastic modulus can be empirically defined by (20)

$$E = C\rho^\alpha \qquad (9)$$

with C and α being constants; α is somewhere between 2 and 3, probably closer to 2 (195). The elastic properties of cancellous

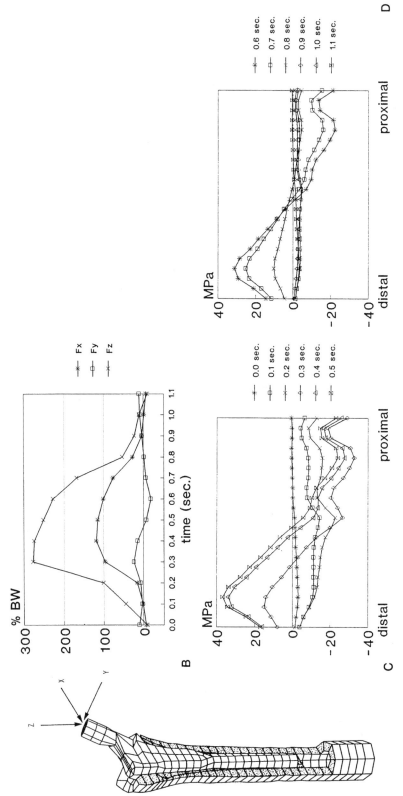

FIG. 10. (A) A finite-element model of a femoral stem–bone composite structure. **(B)** Hip joint forces determined from an *in vivo* instrumented prosthesis (12). **(C)** and **(D)** Distribution of the bending stresses at the medial side of the frontal plane of the prosthesis from 0 to 0.5 sec and from 0.6 to 1.1 sec (244).

TABLE 2. *Indicative values of Young's moduli and static strengths for most materials and interfaces used in THR reconstruction*

	Young's modulus	Static strength
CoCr alloy	200–220 GPa	800–1000 GPa under tension
Titanium	100–130 GPa	800–1500 GPa under tension
Acrylic cement (PMMA)	2–3 GPa	100 MPa under compression
		25–40 MPa under tension
UHMWPE	1 GPa	20–30 MPa under tension
Cortical bone	15–20 GPa	20–50 MPa under tension
		150–200 MPa under compression
Cancellous bone	500–1500 MPa	3–10 MPa under compression
Fibrous tissue	1 MPa	
Metal–acrylic cement interface		5–8 MPa under shear
		5–10 MPa under tension
Hydroxylapatite–bone interface		30–50 MPa under shear
Acrylic cement–bone interface		2–4 MPa under shear
		7–10 MPa under tension

bone also depend on the directionality of its structure, which can be the cause of its anisotropic behavior (78,227). The elastic constants of trabecular bone can be determined fully from measurements of its volume fraction, fabric, and degree of tissue mineralization (70,195,227,230,232). Of course, the elastic bone properties can be highly variable, depending on location and individual factors such as the degree of mineralization and osteoporosis (37).

To carry out an FE analysis, information about strength of materials is not needed. However, this information is required for the interpretation of results. In Table 2, indicative values for Young's moduli and the static strengths of the most important materials and interfaces used in THR are listed.

Nonlinear and Time-Dependent Materials

A bone–prosthesis structure can behave in a nonlinear elastic manner when one or more of its materials have nonlinear elastic properties, when deformations are large relative to the characteristic dimensions of the structure, or when its interfaces are not rigidly bonded (73,97,136,240). Examples of essentially nonlinear materials are collagenous tissues such as fibrous tissue membranes, articular cartilage, and ligaments. A finite deformation nonlinearity is illustrated in Fig. 11. Here a

post consisting of two materials, a relatively stiff one with elastic modulus E' and length l_0 and a relatively soft and thin one with modulus E and thickness d_0, is considered. The cross-sectional area of the post is A, and the post is loaded by a uniformly distributed compressive force F over the thin layer. By simple linear elastic theory in uniaxial compression theory, it can easily be shown that in the deformed state, the length of the rigid post will reduce to $l = l_0 - l_0 F/AE' = l_0(1 - F/AE')$, and the thickness of the layer will reduce to $d = d_0 - d_0 F/AE = d_0(1 - F/AE)$.

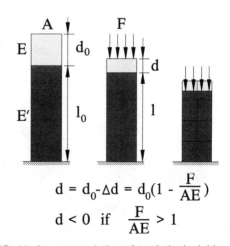

$$d = d_0 - \Delta d = d_0\left(1 - \frac{F}{AE}\right)$$

$$d < 0 \quad \text{if} \quad \frac{F}{AE} > 1$$

FIG. 11. A post consisting of a relatively rigid material (E') and a flexible layer (E) is compressed by a force F. If the ratio $F/AE > 1$, a linear analysis of the problem will predict a negative thickness of the soft layer.

Let us now assume that $A = 100$ mm^2, $F = 1000$ N, $E' = 100$ MPa, and $E = 5$ MPa. It follows that $l = 0.9l_0$, indicating a reduction in length of 10%. It also follows that $d = d_0 - 2d_0$ $0 = -d_0$, which implies a negative thickness of the soft thin layer! The reason for this unrealistic result is that the problem was treated as if it were linear and that infinitesimal strain assumptions remained valid. For finite deformation problems, the simple infinitesimal strain tensor must be replaced by finite deformation tensors, and an appropriate elastic constitutive law must be used. Constitutive laws for soft materials such as rubber and cartilage have been developed. A general feature of these laws is that they allow for the stiffness of the thin layer to gradually increase with increasing compressive load.

Similar problems occur with linear FE analyses of bone–prosthesis structures where thin layers of a low modulus exist next to more rigid materials (248). Thus, to analyze the fibrous tissue lining between bone and prostheses, a more complex FE code is required. If a structure behaves nonlinearly, the FE analysis must be performed in a stepwise fashion by increasing the external loads in small increments from zero until the desired end values are reached. The stiffness matrix in this algorithm is updated with every increment of load. Hence, instead of solving equation 8, one must solve

$$\Delta f = Q \, \Delta u \qquad (10)$$

for each increment of load (80,91,264).

In a linear analysis, the external load is applied in one step because the deformations are always linearly related to the magnitude of the load. In a nonlinear analysis, one in fact simulates a process of structural deformation by gradually applied external loads, which introduces a time factor. If materials behave in a time-dependent way, the rate of the process becomes a factor of significance as well. Examples of such materials are viscoelastic ones (e.g., biphasic interface soft tissues) or plastics susceptible to creep or cold flow (e.g., PMMA and polyethylene). The strategy for the solutions of these problems is similar to the above, in the sense that the process of deformation is simulated iteratively, updating the stiffness matrix in every iteration, depending on the time-development of material constitutive parameters (168,188,219,237)

Boundary and Interface Conditions

The boundary conditions for the FE model are imposed on the exterior surfaces of the object. The boundaries can be divided into free, loaded, and fixed boundaries. At a free boundary, no stress (or load) is transferred, and it is not constrained by a connecting structure. At a loaded boundary, external loads are applied. At a fixed boundary, no motion is allowed, or the motion is constrained by some surrounding structure. The last ones are usually those where the FE model is cut off from the environment with which it normally interacts. The characteristics of this interaction must be accounted for by introducing prescribed displacements in the appropriate nodal points. This is not always easily realized, and as a result, artifacts can be introduced in the stress patterns near those boundaries. This is not a problem as long as the boundary region is remote from the region of interest.

Some problems that boundaries sometimes may present are illustrated in the example of Fig. 12, where an FE analysis is applied to an acetabular THR component. The right side of Fig. 12 represents the case in which the cup is assumed to be loaded internally by a distributed force, representing its interaction with an artificial metallic femoral head. The resulting surface deformation is shown (exaggerated to make it visible). Evidently, this is not a realistic representation because the inner cup boundary would in reality be forced to conform itself to the spherical contour of the stiff metallic femoral head. This problem can be solved by including the metal head in the FE model (left side of Fig. 12) and allowing only compressive stress to be transferred at the head–cup connection as in a contact problem. To do this, the hip-joint load is applied to the stem, and the femoral head then transfers the load to the cup in such a way that the

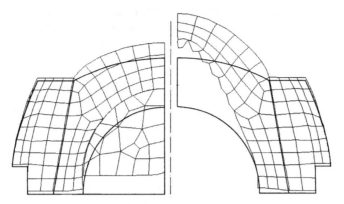

FIG. 12. Deformations determined by a finite-element model of an acetabular cup–bone composite structure (displacements are magnified to allow for visualization). When the femoral head is included in the model, the load transmission problem is a contact problem **(left).** In this case, the displacements at the surface of the cup are compatible. When the external force is applied directly on the inner surface of the cup with an assumed stress distribution, the resulting surface displacements may not be compatible with the form of the femoral head (109).

head is constrained to be in contact with the cup at all times.

At a connection (or interface) between two materials, which can be described as a surface, we can find stress transfer or relative motion, or a combination of both (Fig. 13). The stress transferred across the connecting surface can be represented by a normal stress (σ_n) perpendicular to the plane (tension or compression) and two shear-stress compo-

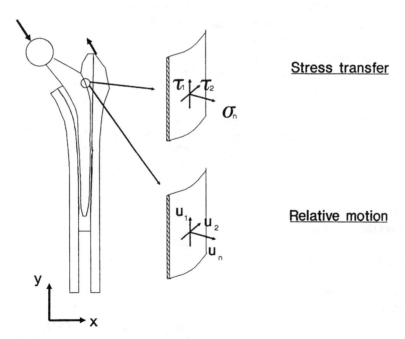

FIG. 13. Normal stress (σ_n) and shear stress (τ_1, τ_2) components transferred across a bonded interface. Normal (u_n) and tangential (u_1, u_2) displacement components are relative motions that may occur if the interface is unbonded.

nents (τ_1 and τ_2). The relative motions can also be characterized by three relative displacement components, u_n in the normal direction and u_1 and u_2 in the tangential directions. Various conditions at the boundary may now be written as follows:

- Bonded interfaces:

$$\sigma_n \neq 0,\ \tau_1 \neq 0,\ \tau_2 \neq 0,$$

$$u_n = u_1 = u_2 = 0 \qquad (11)$$

- Loose interfaces without friction:

$$\tau_1 = \tau_2 = 0,\ \sigma_n \leq 0\ \text{(i.e., } \sigma_n \text{ can only be compressive)}$$

$$u_n \geq 0\ \text{(i.e., } u_n \text{ can only be separation)},$$
$$u_1 \neq 0,\ u_2 \neq 0 \qquad (12)$$

- Loose interfaces with Coulomb friction:

$$\sigma_n \leq 0,\ (\tau_1{}^2 + \tau_2{}^2)^{1/2} \leq \mu|\sigma_n|,\ \text{where } \mu \text{ is the Coulomb coefficient of friction,}$$
$$u_n \geq 0,\ u_1 \neq 0,\ u_2 \neq 0 \qquad (13)$$

When interfaces are unbonded and hence loose without friction (equation 12) or loose with friction (equation 13), the problem becomes nonlinear and must be solved iteratively, using load increments. For this purpose, most FE packages use the so-called gap elements to account for separation and sliding of the surfaces. The load transfer from intramedullary implants (e.g., hip stems) is affected more dramatically by interface conditions than by any other structural parameter, in particular when comparing a fully bonded to a fully unbonded case (99).

STRESS TRANSFER IN COMPOSITE STRUCTURES

General Considerations

A bone–prosthesis structure is known as a composite structure. This implies that it consists of separate substructures with different elastic and geometric properties that are bonded to each other in some specified manner. The stress patterns in these composite structures are dependent on the bonding characteristics at the interfaces between the substructures and by the relative magnitudes of their elastic moduli.

The latter effect can be illustrated relative to the phenomenon of load sharing in a composite bar (Fig. 14A and B). Here, a tensile force F is transferred through a composite bar comprised of two bars bonded to each other. The two bars have different Young's moduli, E_1 and E_2, and cross-sectional areas A_1 and A_2. The quantity AE is known as the axial stiffness of a bar. When the loading is applied as shown, the individual bars of the composite will share in the load transfer from one to the other such that $F_1 + F_2 = F$. For this composite bar, the forces F_1 and F_2 are given by the ratio of axial stiffnesses:

$$F_1/F_2 = A_1E_1/A_2E_2 \qquad (14)$$

This formula shows that the bar with the higher axial stiffness will carry more load. We note that equation 14 is based on the assumption that the axial strains in the bars are equal, i.e., $\varepsilon_1 = \varepsilon_2 = \varepsilon$. Hence, from Hooke's law in uniaxial tension, $\sigma_1 = E_1\varepsilon$ and $\sigma_2 = E_2\varepsilon$, it follows that

$$\sigma_1/\sigma_2 = E_1/E_2 \qquad (15)$$

Equation 15 states that when a deformation (ε) is imposed on a composite bar, the material with higher elastic modulus will experience greater stresses. Similar formulas exist for the composite beam loaded transversely in bending or composite shafts loaded in torsion (95). For each case, the stiffer beam will carry a higher load.

The illustrative example of Fig. 14A and B is one of pure load sharing, because the external force F is applied on both bars simultaneously. If the force were only applied on bar 1, then load sharing would not occur in the segment of bar 1 to the right of bar 2 (Fig. 14C). Obviously, load sharing would take place only where bar 1 and bar 2 are bonded together. In this example, load transfer is via the shear stress developed at the interface between bar 1 and bar 2. In bar 1, in going from right to left, the load F_1 reduces from $F_1 = F$ to $F_1 =$

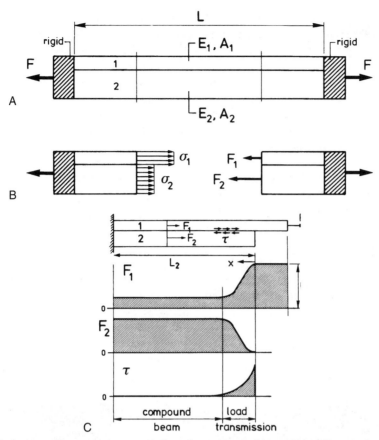

FIG. 14. (A) A composite structure consisting of two bonded bars with different elastic moduli and cross-sectional areas. The structure is uniformly stretched by an external axial force *F*. **(B)** The internal forces F_1 and F_2 differ by virtue of the different elastic moduli; the internal stresses $\sigma_1 = F_1/A_1$ and $\sigma_2 = F_2/A_2$ are also different. **(C)** Load transfer by means of shear stress τ at the interface between the two bars. The loads F_1 and F_2 inside the two bars and the shear-stress distribution τ at the interface are shown.(From Huiskes, ref. 95, with permission.)

$A_1E_1F/(A_1E_1 + A_2E_2)$, and in bar 2, the load F_2 increases from $F_2 = 0$ to $F_2 = A_2E_2F/(A_1E_1 + A_2E_2)$). This load transfer mechanism between the two bars is important, because the shear stresses it produces may cause the bond to fail at the interface.

Clearly, the total amount of load transferred from bar 1 to bar 2 must equal

$$F_2 = A_2E_2F/(A_1E_1 + A_2E_2) \qquad (16)$$

This force must act over the available area for the bar, L_2d_2, at the interface. Here, L_2 is the length of the bar, and d_2 its depth (in the perpendicular direction). Although the average shear stress over the length L_2 would be $\tau_{av} =$ F_2/L_2d_2, the actual maximal stress is much higher because τ is far from uniform, with a peak value at L_2, where bar 2 begins to carry load. The actual shear-stress pattern $\tau(z)$ can be determined from a shear-lag distribution function given by

$$\tau(z) = \lambda F_2 e^{-\lambda z}/d_2 \qquad (17)$$

where λ is a structural parameter depending on the elastic moduli and the cross-sectional areas of the two bars (93). Again, similar formulas exist for beams in bending and shafts in torsion (93,95,96).

To review some basic aspects of compressive load transfer in composite structures, let us consider a very simple model of a solid layer (prosthesis) fixed to a substrate (bone) (Fig. 15). We assume both materials, separately, to have uniform elastic properties and that the top layer is rigidly bonded to the substrate. Figure 15 presents von Mises stress patterns in materials for the case where the prosthesis is loaded by a single point force F. Figure 15A presents the case for which the prosthesis has the same elastic properties as bone ("isoelastic material"), whereas in Fig. 15B, the prosthesis is made out of a metal, say titanium, that is much stiffer than bone. From these results, we note the following characteristics:

1. The stresses are essentially nonuniform, concentrated predominantly in a central band in the structure, directly under the applied load.

2. When the moduli of the two materials are equal (Fig. 15A), the stresses are continuous over the interface; when the materials are different (Fig. 15B), the stresses are discontinuous over the interface.

3. The stress patterns are more uniformly distributed for the case of the stiff prosthesis (Fig. 15B) than in the case of the softer prosthesis (Fig. 15A). As a result, the stress magnitudes are higher for the case of the prosthesis made of softer material.

The normal (compressive) stress σ_y at the interfaces in Fig. 15 must balance the applied force F in the y direction. It would be immediately obvious from a free-body diagram of the prosthesis that the average compressive interface stress $\bar{\sigma}_y$ equals F/Ld, where L is the length and d the width of the elastic layer. The *actual* stress, σ_y, is nonuniform and must also

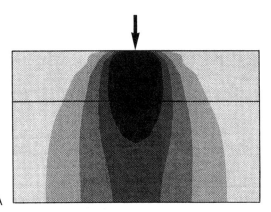

A

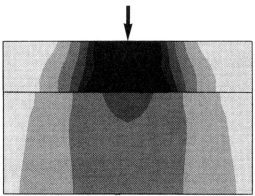

B

C

FIG. 15. Stress distribution calculated from a simple finite-element model of an elastic layer resting on an elastic foundation subject to a force F. **(A)** The von Mises stress distribution (equation 3) is shown for the case in which the top layer (prosthesis) has the same elastic properties as the foundation (bone). **(B)** The von Mises stress distribution for the case in which the prosthesis is made out of a material (e.g., titanium) much stiffer than the foundation (bone). **(C)** Load transfer through a plate on a flexible foundation. In addition to compressive stress developed at the interface as a direct effect of load transfer, shear stresses also develop. The load also created bending of the plate, with compression on one side and tension on the other side of the neutral plane (n.p.) (Adapted from ref. [97a], with permission.)

satisfy the equilibrium condition. Thus, a simple relationship exists relating the average stress, $\bar{\sigma}_y$, and the actual stress:

$$\bar{\sigma}_y L d = d \int_0^L \sigma_y dx = F \qquad (18)$$

We note that although the average stress may be used in certain situations, when suspected stress concentrations exist in the composite structure, the average stress should not be taken as representative of the maximal stress value. Equation 18 also shows that since the stress distribution σ_y must always balance the applied load F, a composite structure that leads to a narrower load distribution (Fig. 15A), when compared to that in Fig. 15B, has a higher maximal value. This demonstrates that our intuitive expectation that a material with similar elastic properties to bone would be ideal for implants in fact may not be true. In general, the stress patterns in a surface-fixation structure depend not only on the articular loading characteristics (magnitude, direction, contact location, and contact area size) but also the flexural rigidity (elastic moduli and dimensions) of the component, the elastic characteristics of the supporting bone, and the bonding characteristics.

This illustrates that the load-transfer and load-sharing mechanisms in composite structures can be complex, even in relatively simple regular structures. In general, stresses within a structure cannot simply be determined by dividing the load to be transferred by the area available for load transfer. As a rule, the stresses are not uniform over a particular area, and peak values are bound to occur, depending on the geometry and the material characteristics of the separate components in the composite. High values of stresses generally occur in structures with notches, sharp corners, and holes. These high values are known as stress concentrations.

Very often, stresses in composite structures are generated not as a direct effect of load sharing or load transfer but as an indirect effect of deformational variations caused by differences in elastic moduli (Fig. 15C). Because of the compressive force, compressive stresses will arise at the interface as direct effects of the load transfer mechanism. However, high shear stresses at the interface may also arise as an indirect effect. This is caused by the difference in lateral displacements of the plate and the foundation. If the elastic foundation has a lower elastic modulus than the plate, it will tend to expand more in the lateral direction. This expansion is resisted by the shear stresses developed at the interface. Another mechanism occurs as well. The external load causes the plate to deform in bending. Hence, we find a "neutral plane" (n.p.) where the bending stress in the plate is zero. Above it, compression occurs, and under it, tension. These three mechanisms are, of course, interrelated and dependent on the precise characteristics of the structure. For instance, if the plate is relatively stiff, it deforms less, which will also affect the interface stress distribution.

In the above example, we assumed that the stiffness characteristics of the elastic foundation (i.e., bone) are uniform. This, however, is hardly ever the case in prosthetic composite structures. The stiffness S of a layer of material through which load is to be transferred (e.g., cement or cancellous bone), in terms of the ratio between normal stress (σ_n) and deflection (δ), depends on its Young's modulus (E) and its thickness (t): $S = \sigma_n/\delta = E/t$ (i.e., this is Hooke's law for uniaxial compression). Hence, from the surface, a nonuniform layer bonded to a rigid substrate would appear stiff if either its elastic modulus is high and/or its thickness is relatively small. These stiff parts of the layer (high E or small t) would tend to develop higher stresses and thereby carry more loads than the softer regions. This concept is illustrated in Fig. 16A. This figure shows graphic representations of stresses calculated from finite-element models used to study the effects of prosthetic femoral stem placement in the medullary canal. Clearly, the thin bony regions develop more stress than the thick regions. When the stem is more centrally placed, the layer thickness is more uniform (Fig. 16B), and thus, no stress concentrations are developed.

Stress transfer in composite structures is very much affected by the bonding characteris-

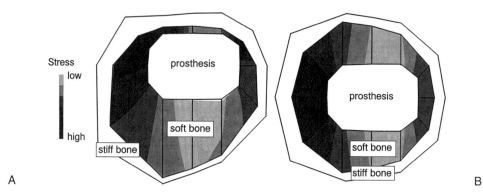

FIG. 16. The von Mises stress distributions in the trabecular bone at a cross section of a proximal femur with a noncemented bonded stem: **(A)** determined from a three-dimensional anatomic finite-element model and **(B)** determined in a three-dimensional symmetric finite-element model (235).

tics at the interface. The frictional and adhesive characteristics of the surfaces are important factors. The orientation of the interface relative to the dominant direction of loading is also important. So are surface microstructures and textures important. If the interface is smooth, unbonded, and lubricated, then no shear stress will be developed no matter how large the disparity in the lateral displacement. The difference between bonded (adhesive) and unbonded (lubricated) interfaces can be most simply seen for uniaxial loading (Fig. 17). For the unbonded or lubricated case (right), only compressive stress is developed in the material; the material is in a state of uniaxial compression. For the bonded or perfectly adhesive case (left), shear stresses are developed at the interface as

well. The compressive stresses at the interface are sufficient to balance the external force. The shear stresses merely develop as a secondary effect, and they must balance themselves.

This is no longer true when the interface is not perpendicular to the applied force. Figure 18 depicts a cone-shaped object (implant) inserted into a tubular structure (bone) where the interface is bonded by cement or by some other mechanism. In this case, the applied force will create compressive and shear stresses along the interface. If the cone angle is relatively small, as is the case with most hip prostheses, the magnitude of the shear stress developed will be much greater than the compressive stress. This load transfer would occur predominantly by the shear stress, as shown in

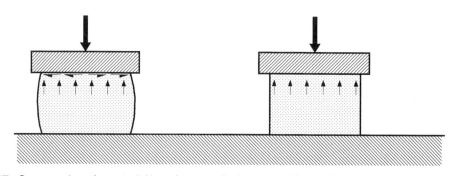

FIG. 17. Compression of a material by a force applied onto an adhesive interface will create both compression and shear at the interface **(left).** When the interface is unbonded and lubricated, it can slide without friction at the interface. In this case, only compressive stresses occur **(right).**

Fig. 18. When the interface is unbonded and lubricated (e.g., by body fluids at the bone surface), shear stress at the interface can no longer exist or is minimal. To develop a significant reaction force to equilibrate the applied load (Fig. 18), the cone-shaped prosthesis must subside into the tubular bone to create a significant compressive stress at the interface. Again because of the small cone angle, a very large compressive stress must be developed at the interface to generate a sufficient amount of force to equilibrate the applied load. In this process, a tensile hoop stress must be developed in the bone to prevent expansion.

The basic concepts discussed above are of importance for any composite implant structure. In the next two sections, the intramedullary stem fixation of the femoral component in THR and the acetabular cup fixation are considered in more detail.

Intramedullary Stem Fixation

The principles of load transfer in intramedullary fixation are based on load sharing, similar to the principles in Fig. 14. As a simplified model, we choose a metal rod (the stem) fixed in a tubular bone. The stem is loaded by an axial force (Fig. 19A) that must be transferred to the bone. Again, the load transfer between the stem and the bone is realized by shear stresses at the interfaces. In

fact, a free-body diagram of the stem would indicate that these shear stresses must balance the external load; hence, the average shear stress times the surface area of the stem equals the axial force. But again, these shear stresses are not uniformly distributed; rather, stress concentrations occur on the distal and the proximal sides. This is illustrated in Fig. 19A, together with the load-sharing patterns in the stem and the bone.

When the stem is loaded in bending (Fig. 19B), a very similar load-transfer mechanism occurs. This time, however, the bending moment is to be transferred from the stem to the bone via interface stresses (tension, compression, and tangential shear) to effectuate this moment transfer. These stresses are again nonuniform and are concentrated mainly at the proximal and distal sides.

The graphs of Fig. 19 illustrate the most important basic principles of load transfer in intramedullary fixation of artificial joints (93,95,96):

1. The structure can be divided into three regions, a middle region where load sharing occurs and two load-transfer regions on the proximal and distal sides.

2. In the middle region, pure load sharing occurs, whereby the stem carries $\varepsilon_n \times 100\%$ of the axial force or $\varepsilon_t \times 100\%$ of the bending moment. Here, ε_n and ε_t are relative axial and flexural rigidities defined as:

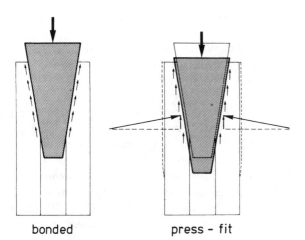

bonded   press - fit

FIG. 18. Load transfer via a straight-tapered cone pushed into a cylindrical counterpart. **(Left)** The shear stress at the bonded interface can equilibrate the applied force. **(Right)** At a smooth, press-fitted interface, equilibrium relies on the vertical component of compressive interface stress. For slightly tapered cones, a significant amount of subsidence must occur in order for the compressive stress required for equilibrium to develop. (From Huiskes, ref. 99, with permission.)

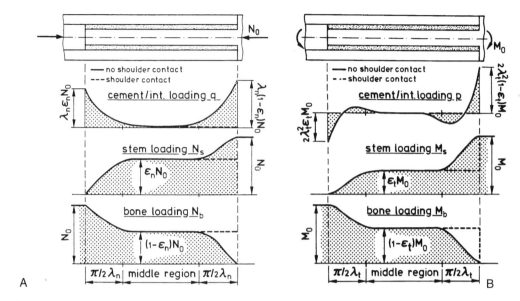

FIG. 19. The load-transfer characteristics in a simple model of a straight stem cemented in tubular bone with and without shoulder contact **(A)** Axial loading. **(B)** Bending. In both drawings, left is distal, right proximal. From top to bottom: **(A)** distributions of shear loading, and **(B)** the bending moment in the stem; and **(A)** the axial force, and **(B)** the bending moment in the bone. (From Huiskes, ref. 96, with permission.)

$$\varepsilon_n = A_s E_s/(A_s E_s + A_b E_b) \qquad (19)$$

$$\varepsilon_t = I_s E_s/(I_s E_s + I_b E_b) \qquad (20)$$

where E, A, and I are the elastic moduli, the cross-sectional areas, and the second moments of inertia of the stem (s) and the bone (b).

3. The load carried by the stem and the bone is normally carried by the bone alone; hence, the bone is stress-shielded by the stem. The higher ε_n and ε_t are, the higher is the percentage of load that is carried by the stem, and the more extensive the stress-shielding effect.

4. The higher the percentage of load carried by the stem in the middle region, the less is transferred proximally and the more distally, and vice versa. As can be seen in Fig. 19, the proximal load transfer is proportional to $(1 - \varepsilon_n)$ and $(1 - \varepsilon_t)$, and the distal load transfer to ε_n and ε_t, respectively. Hence, the stiffer the stem, the higher the distal interface stresses; the more flexible the stem, the higher the proximal interface stresses.

5. The length of the distal and proximal load-transfer regions and the peak interface loads on the distal and proximal sides depend on the parameters λ_n and λ_t, the fixation exponents for axial and transverse loading (93,95,96). These parameters depend not only on the axial and flexural rigidities of the stem and the bone but also, and most predominantly, on the elastic modulus and the thickness of an intermediate layer (e.g., acrylic cement or cancellous bone). A stiff intermediate layer (i.e., high modulus and/or thin layer) reduces the length of the load-transfer regions and thus increases the gradients in the interface loads.

6. The peak interface stresses do not necessarily reduce when the stem is made longer. Here again, the notion "stress is load per available area" is misleading. When the stem is made longer, the load-transfer regions merely shift further apart, and nothing else changes. It is only when the stem is made short (less than π/λ_n or π/λ_t) (Fig. 19), which makes the middle region disappear, that a fur-

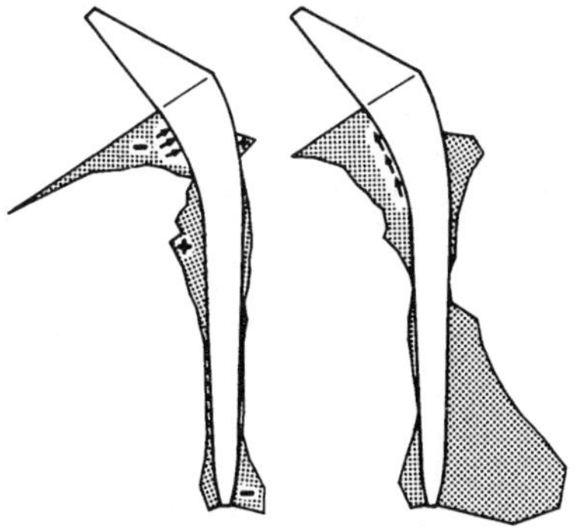

FIG. 20. Distribution of tensile, compressive, and shear stresses at a stem–cement interface for a loaded cemented THA stem from a two-dimensional finite-element model. **(Left)** Stress normal to the interface (tension–compression). **(Right)** Shear stress. (From Huiskes, ref. 99, with permission.)

ther reduction in length starts to affect the interface stresses.

7. If a collar on the proximal stem is bonded to the proximal bone (Fig. 19), the proximal load-transfer region is bypassed. Hence, conceptually, no load is transferred on the proximal side over the interfaces.

The above considerations are basic principles derived from a simplified, generalized model (93) and in fact are very helpful as baseline information for prosthetic design. In reality, of course, the load-transfer mechanism and the stress patterns are much more complex. Loads do not occur as isolated axial compression or bending, stems are usually not straight, interfaces are not always rigidly bonded, and bone has more complex properties and shapes than in this model. However, awareness of these basic phenomena facilitates the interpretation of more realistic, and complicated, analyses. If we formulate the conceptual analytic model of Fig. 19 in an FE model, we see the basic principles reflected in the results (93). We can recognize the proximal and distal load-transfer regions in the interface shear stresses and in the bone-bending stresses. The middle region of load sharing is obvious as well. Such an analysis also confirms that the ratios of proximal to distal interface stress transfer and of middle region load sharing both change when a more flexible stem material (metal versus isoelastic) is used.

In the case of a more realistically tapered stem in an "anatomic" bone model, these basic principles are less obvious, but still recognizable, as illustrated in Figs. 20 (99) and 21 (240). The interface stress patterns in the two-dimensional (Fig. 20) and three-dimensional FE models (Fig. 21) clearly demonstrate the proximal and distal stress-concentration regions. The ratio between proximal and distal stresses in these "anatomic" cases is regulated not just by the stiffness of the stem but also by the prominence of the taper shape. The stronger the distal taper of the stem, the more the distal stresses are reduced (93). Hence, although the principles of the load-transfer mechanism remain intact, the actual stress patterns are affected by stem design (112).

The rigidity of the stem is an important design parameter, as it affects both the bone stresses (which may provoke bone resorption) and the interface stresses (which may provoke interface loosening). Using the same stem design, we obtain less abnormal bone

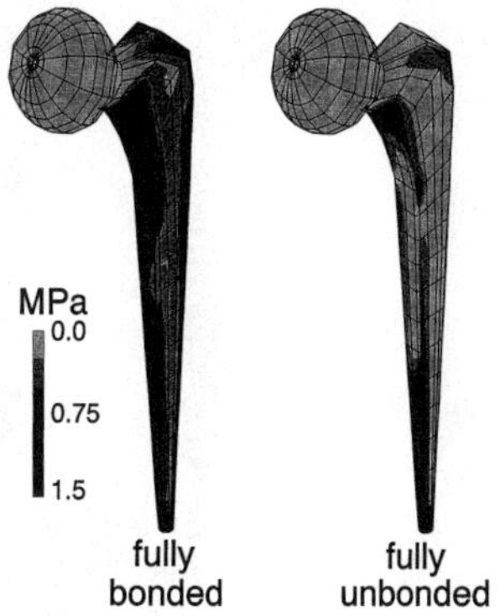

FIG. 21. Shear stresses at the stem–cement interface generated by stems that are either fully bonded **(left)** or unbonded **(right)** to the cement mantle, calculated with a CT-based three-dimensional finite-element model. (From Verdonschot and Huiskes, ref. 241, with permission.)

stresses but higher proximal interface stresses when a flexible (isoelastic) material is used instead of a metal. We see that confirmed in a three-dimensional FE study (116). In view of the potential problems of bone resorption and interface loosening, this principle presents incompatible design goals for which a compromise must be sought. Noncemented stems tend to be medullary-canal filling and much thicker, hence stiffer, than cemented ones. This means that stress shielding is more of a problem in noncemented THR, whereas proximal cement and interface stresses are more of a concern in the cemented ones.

Many designers do not realize, however, that the governing parameter for the load-sharing ratio between stem and bone is not the stem rigidity but the ratio between stem rigidity and bone rigidity (13,93,105). The basis for this relationship was shown in equations 19 and 20. It was found both clinically and analytically that long-term adaptive bone resorption around hip stems, as a result of stress shielding, is highly sensitive for initial bone rigidity (55,101,104,116). These results sug-

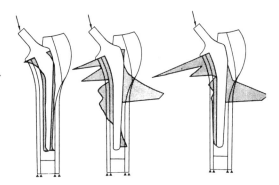

FIG. 23. Normal stresses in the cement at the stem–cement interface assuming bonded interface conditions **(left),** frictionless unbonded conditions **(middle),** and frictionless unbonded conditions with fibrous-tissue interposition **(right)** at the cement–bone interface. (Adapted from Weinans et al., ref. 248.)

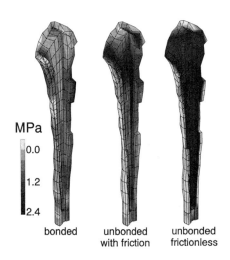

FIG. 22. Tensile stress distribution in the cement mantle assuming bonded or unbonded (frictionless and frictional) stem–cement interface conditions. Only the anterior half of the cement mantle is shown. (Adapted from Verdonschot and Huiskes, ref. 240.)

gest that, in the above relationship, the bone stiffness plays a more important role in load transfer than the stem stiffness because the former is more highly variable than the latter in a patient population. Hence, bone stiffness, as dependent on density and thickness, is a significant "design" parameter.

Another set of parameters that play an important role for the load-transfer mechanism are the mechanical characteristics of bonds between the different materials. Above (Fig. 18), we have seen that an unbonded, conically shaped stem has a different load-transfer mechanism than a bonded one. An unbonded, frictionless cone pushed in a tube must subside to create enough compressive interface stress for equilibrium, which also produces excessive tensile hoop stress in the tube. Cemented stems in THR tend to become debonded from the cement early postoperatively (127). Figure 22 illustrates the effects of debonding on cement stresses, as determined in a three-dimensional FE analysis. We see dramatic increases in cement stresses from a bonded (Fig. 22, left) to a debonded, frictionless configuration (Fig. 22, right). If we do assume friction to occur (Fig. 22, middle), the cement stresses are still higher than those in the bonded case, but not that much higher. Evidently, the bonding and friction conditions are very important for the cement stresses and the probability of cement failure (73,160,240).

Another effect of similar consequences is that of cement–bone interface loosening, resorption, and fibrous-tissue interposition. Figure 23 shows an example of that, as determined in a two-dimensional FE model, applying nonlinear interface conditions to model the effects of loosening and a nonlinear constitutive description of a 1-mm-thick fibrous tissue membrane (248). As evident from Fig. 23, the load-transfer mechanism (as represented by stem–cement interface normal stresses) changes drastically from a bonded to a (frictionless) debonded cement–bone interface and then again somewhat from a debonded interface to one with the fibrous membrane interposed. The most drastic effect, however, is caused by debonding.

The stem–bone bonding conditions also play important roles in the load-transfer mechanism of noncemented THR, particularly concerning interface stresses and relative motions (17,67,136). These conditions depend largely on the precision of fit of the stem and on the extent and location of ingrowth coatings. Where debonding from the bone and friction are concerned, similar relationships occur in the load-transfer mechanism as for stem debonding from cement (160,240). An important difference is, of course, that cemented stems are bonded best in the beginning, whereas noncemented ones become bonded only later on. During the ingrowth period, stem design and interface-stress transfer play important roles for the ingrowth process (105). For noncoated, press-fitted stems, the interface coefficient of friction is very important for the eventual fixation characteristics, as these stems tend to sink in the bone and find fixation later. In this process, proximal load transfer may shift to distal, with stress shielding and bone resorption as a result (229).

Usually, a noncemented stem is not fully coated for bone ingrowth, but only proximally. The reason for that is twofold. First, this is thought to promote proximal stress transfer rather than distal stress transfer, so

stress shielding and adaptive bone resorption would be reduced. This can be confirmed in FE analyses, but the effect is not as pronounced as sometimes expected when the distal stem is still in (compressive stress-transferring) contact with the bone (119,253). Second, it facilitates a possible revision operation. Full coatings are sometimes preferred because they are thought to enhance the extent of ingrowth, thereby reducing the probability of interface debonding. This thought is partly based on the idea that interface stresses reduce when the contact area is increased. As we have seen above, however, one must be very careful with the notion that stress is force per unit area. If we compare the interface stresses for the same prosthesis in the same bone, coated fully, proximally and with 5 proximal bands, we find that the differences in maximal values are very small (119; Fig. 24). The reason, again, is that all parts of the interfaces do not participate equally in stress transfer. So ingrowth at mechanically strategic locations is more important than the total area it occupies.

Acetabular Cup Fixation

The acetabulum is structurally more complex than the femur and does not easily lend itself to reduction to a simpler geometry, which would make it accessible for conceptual analytic studies, in the same way as composite beam theory provided the basis for the femoral reconstruction. In addition, in comparison to the femoral reconstruction, far fewer stress analyses have been conducted. Some strain gauge experiments to study the effects of cup fixation on acetabular surface stress transfer have been reported (40,60,124, 152,184,196). Finite-element analyses of the acetabular reconstruction were conducted, using two-dimensional (21,192,233), axisymmetric (98,179), or three-dimensional models (42,149,194). In addition, the stresses in the polyethylene (PE) liner were analyzed, particularly with regard to friction, wear, and PE failure prospects (10). Some generic information is discussed here, mostly as it resulted

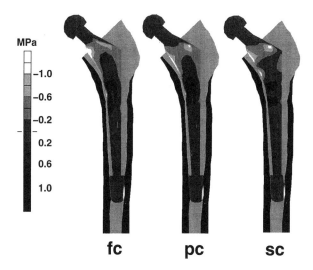

FIG. 24. Normal stress distributions at the implant–bone interface for different coating configurations, shown as shades on the stem surface. High tensile stresses (positive) are white, and high compressive stresses black; zero stress is a medium gray shade. (fc, fully coated; pc, proximally coated; sc, proximally stripe coated). (Adapted from Huiskes, and Van Rietbergen, ref. 119).

from our own three-dimensional FE model (39,41–43).

The hip-joint force is introduced by the contact between femoral head and PE liner and varies greatly in magnitude and orientation during gait. The stresses in the pelvis reach a maximum at the beginning of the single-leg stance phase (41). The distribution of the stresses over the articulating surface of the PE liner depends on its stiffness characteristics, which are determined by the PE thickness and whether or not a metal backing is present (10,43). A thicker PE liner distributes stress

better and reduces the peak value. This mechanism is similar to what was discussed relative to Fig. 15. At the time of heel strike, when the force is maximal, the superior-anterior rim is the high-stress location. From the liner the stress is then distributed to the bone, through the cement (if a cemented cup is used) and the metal backing (if present). The stress-transfer mechanism here again depends mostly on the rigidity of the structure. Metal backing, providing a higher stiffness, tends to distribute stress better over the cement and the subchondral bone. This was originally thought to be its

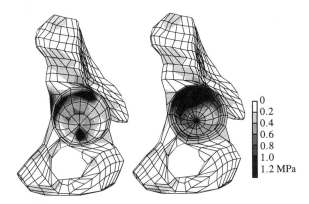

FIG. 25. Distributions of the Von Mises stresses in the trabecular bone of a normal bone **(left)** and a pelvic bone with a cemented non-backed cup **(right)**. (Reproduced from Dalstra and Huiskes, ref. 43.)

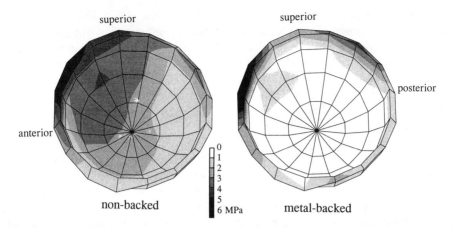

FIG. 26. Von Mises stresses in the cement mantle for a nonbacked polyethylene cup **(left)** and a metal-backed cup **(right)**. (From Dalstra, ref. 39, with permission.)

greatest mechanical advantage (35). However, three-dimensional FE analysis has shown that it does provide cement and interface stress concentrations at the rim of the fixation (Fig. 26). As an effect, the maximal cement and bone interface stress peaks of the metal-backed cup surpass those of a nonbacked one, providing higher failure probabilities. This is a result of the fact that the bone rim and the metal backing are both stiff relative to their environments in the structure.

The stress transfer to the subchondral trabecular bone differs between an intact and the reconstructed case (Fig. 25). Whereas in the intact acetabulum the stresses are well distributed, in the reconstructed case they are concentrated in the anterior-superior region (39). It is also clear that stress shielding in the acetabular bone does occur, particularly in the dome region. This region is also the one where bone resorption is often seen (185), which is usually attributed to a loosening process. The stress patterns, however, do suggest that it might be a result of mechanical disuse, similar to what occurs in the femur. Further away from the cup in the cortical shells, there is very little difference between the stress patterns of the intact and reconstructed cases. The consequence of this is that little information about the local stresses in and around the implant can be obtained from

experiments involving strain gauges on the external bone surfaces. The strains here are simply not very sensitive to the design and fixation characteristics of the cup.

DESIGN ASSESSMENT AND DEVELOPMENT

In the first section of this chapter, we discussed the performance and endurance of THR and summarized what is known about failure mechanisms. It was argued that biomechanics is important in all activities of the innovation cycle. This is particularly so for design and design assessment of new prostheses, in which the engineering task is substantial (102,103). In order to rationalize the design process, five questions must always be addressed: (a) What clinical problem creates a traditional design? (b) How does this problem relate to the design characteristics? (c) What innovative feature would improve the design? (d) Does this feature indeed solve the clinical problem? (e) Will this innovative design cause another clinical problem, worse than the original one? To answer these questions is not an easy task, first because patient factors (both biological and functional ones) and surgical factors (technical feasibilities and skills) can hold many surprises in waiting. Second, although a clinical problem may be well documented, its cause in terms of precise failure mechanisms often remains obscure. Third, engineering design goals in THR tend to be incompatible; i.e., what prevents one failure mechanism often promotes another (102,103). In this section a few biomechanical methods are discussed that are useful to analyze these questions and problems.

Failure Scenarios and Design Assessment

It is essential that new designs for THR be preclinically tested before they are applied in patients and clinically tested before they reach the market. This seems trivial, but in the orthopaedic trial-and-error culture, this is not always evident (102,156). It is also not easily realized because of two principal problems. First, the endurance of a THR design can only be established in fact in long-term clinical trials with large patient series, using sophisticated actuarial methods (79,155). Conventional methods of THR performance assessment, such as radiography and patient interviews, are notoriously imprecise and subjective. However, new clinical methods have been developed in the recent past that enable more precise assessment of THR performance within a reasonable time period. The most powerful of these is roentgen stereophotogrammetric analysis (RSA) (212), which allows precise evaluations of three-dimensional relative displacements of the implant relative to the bone in the course of time.

It is known that the extent of these motions is correlated with endurance of the THR. With RSA, these migrations can be detected in an early stage. This method is discussed separately below. A less sensitive method with the same purpose, but more easily conducted, is digital radiography (63,123,157,247). Digitizing radiographs makes them accessible for computer-graphics evaluations, which improves the precision and the objectivity of radiographic measurements. Another radiographic method with high precision is dual-energy X-ray absorptiometry (DEXA), useful to determine the development of bone density in the course of time (13,28,56,189). Whether a particular prosthetic design provokes excessive bone resorption can be checked early postoperatively with this method. It is also useful in laboratory studies with postmortem bones (56). A fourth clinical evaluation method sensitive to THR performance in an early stage is gait analysis (81,174,183).

The second problem in design confirmation of innovative THR components is the difficulty of defining valid preclinical tests. In order to preclinically check a prosthetic design in a laboratory or computer-simulation test, one has to know what to test for. Because failure mechanisms are not always well understood, the design of valid testing methods is not trivial. In order to facilitate that, we propose the application of failure scenarios to which testing methods can be tailored (102). A failure scenario is a paradigm of a failure mechanism. It is a course of events that does or does not occur but is always latent. Preclinical tests can be designed to establish how sensitive a THR prosthesis is for a particular failure scenario.

In an example of a definite failure scenario for cemented THR stems, it is proposed that, as a result of the weakness of the metal–cement bond, debonding is likely to occur early postoperatively. This promotes, on the one hand, stem subsidence in cement, cement stress increase, and crack formation (compare discussion in relation to Fig. 22). On the other hand, the debonded stem will rub against the cement and produce wear particles. Both mechanisms in this scenario are likely to cause cement–bone interface resorption and clinical failure of the reconstruction. Questions to be answered relative to this scenario, for the assessment of a new prosthesis, are: Will the stem easily debond? If debonded, to what extent does it increase cement stresses and the probability of failure? If debonded, what metal–cement relative motions does it produce, and will these promote excessive production of wear particles? As described later below, laboratory and computer-simulation methods are now available to analyze these questions for preclinically testing new designs.

The above specified failure scenario is a mixture of two generic scenarios for long-term aseptic (noninfected) loosening, out of a total of six proposed (102). The first of these is the *accumulated-damage* scenario. This is based on gradual accumulation of mechanical damage in materials and interfaces from repetitive dynamic loading. The damaging process eventually proliferates to disruption of the implant from the bone, interface micromotion, bone resorption and fibrous interposition, and finally, gross loosening. As a generic scenario, it is certainly relevant not only for cemented stems, as in the above example, but also for cemented acetabular cups and for noncemented components of both sides (e.g., it may lead to disruption of prosthetic coatings). The fact that cemented stems are more sensitive than other types of components for this scenario is not the issue here. The whole point of failure scenarios is how easily they could be provoked by a new design.

The second, also involved in the above example, is the *particulate-reaction* scenario. Wear particles from articulating surfaces, debonded interfaces, or modular-component connections can migrate into the cement–bone (cemented) or implant–bone (noncemented) interfaces. These small particles activate microphages at the interface into inflammatory responses of local bone resorption (lysis), thereby gradually debonding cement and bone (5,47,207). Eventually, this process produces relative interface motions and proliferates to gross loosening in much the same way as the final stage of the accumulated-damage scenario described above. This means that one can usually not discriminate between these two scenarios by studying radiograms or retrieved specimens, because the eventual results are the same. The elements of the particulate-reaction scenario include, besides wear-particle production, particle transport and biological bone reactions. Although the latter is a patient rather than an implant design factor, the characteristics of wear particles in terms of material, size, and shape are certainly relevant for this scenario (159,213). This could be tested preclinically. The same is true for the potential

of a design, and its inherent fixation method, to produce excessive wear particles and provoke transportation to the implant–bone interface.

The next, valid for noncemented components only, is the *failed-bonding* scenario. This implies that ingrowth or osseus integration does not occur because of gaps and relative motions at the implant–bone interface (54,205,216). The biological bonding or ingrowth processes require a certain quiescence at the interface to succeed. If relative motions occur beyond some 150 μm (186), ingrowth will be prevented, and motions will be enhanced, provoking bone resorption, fibrous-tissue formation, and eventually, loosening. The elements of this scenario are initial fit, osseus induction (the capacity of a coating material to induce bony adhesion and fill gaps), initial relative interface motions, and interface motion-induced bone resorption. Methods to test for the latter biomechanical interface phenomena are discussed below. Where fit is concerned, preclinical tests can be performed in series of postmortem bones (171,172,206). This seems rather trivial, but tests like this are hardly ever reported.

The *stress-shielding* scenario particularly involves the bone around the femoral stem. Because the bone is stress-shielded by the stem, the bone stresses are subnormal (see Fig. 19). In accordance with Wolff's law (198,258), resorption develops. Although this does not automatically lead to prosthetic loosening, it may enhance bone or stem fracture and complicate a possible revision operation. The potential of a particular stem design to provoke excessive bone resorption can now be preclinically tested with computer-simulation methods with good accuracy, as discussed below.

A fifth model is the *stress-bypass* scenario. This is similar to the stress-shielding scenario but develops through another route, when proximal load transfer in the noncemented femoral THR is bypassed in favor of distal load transfer. As a result, the proximal bone is again understressed. Its cause can be inadequate proximal fit, either initially as an effect of inadequate fit or bone preparation, or gradually postoperatively as an effect of stem subsidence (229).

The final one proposed until now is the *destructive-wear* scenario, which implies that articulating surfaces or modular–component connections (e.g., cone connections between metal head and stem of the femoral component, or connections between PE liner and metal backing in the acetabulum) simply wear out, to the extent that mechanical integrity can no longer be maintained (203). The sensitivity of a design for this scenario can be preclinically tested in hip simulators (162,203).

It must be noted that whether or not an innovative design will be successful can not be determined preclinically with certainty. This also depends on patient and surgical factors independent of design. In addition, new materials or shapes may introduce failure mechanisms hitherto unknown. In this respect, the scenarios discussed above may not be complete or sufficiently detailed. Further research will have to provide more certainty. In any case, preclinical testing can only provide a first sieve for unsafe devices.

Roentgen Stereophotogrammetric Analysis

Roentgen stereophotogrammetric analysis (RSA) was developed by the late Dr. Goran Selvik (212). The method is based on the principle that three-dimensional coordinates can be reconstructed from two radiographic images (Fig. 27A). To be able to determine the three-dimensional position of a point in space, the space has to be defined in the so-called laboratory coordinate system. When the positions of the two X-ray foci and the radiographic plates are known, the position of an object point can be reconstructed by calculating the intersection of the X-ray beams. The laboratory coordinate system is determined by a calibration cage. To this cage, markers made out of a high-density material (tantalum) have been attached, and their relative positions are accurately measured. Within the calibration cage, two planes with markers can be distinguished. The plane closer to the foci contains the "control markers" and is

called the "control plane." The plane closer to the radiographic films contains the "fiducial markers" and is called the "fiducial plane." The fiducial markers are used to define the laboratory coordinate system, whereas the control points are used to calculate the positions of the two foci.

If we want to determine the three-dimensional coordinates of an object point somewhere in the calibration cage, we obtain two images. Both images have a two-dimensional local coordinate system (x', y'). The relationship between the global coordinates (x, y) of the fiducial markers and those on the images (x', y') can be determined using the Hallert transformation (212):

$$x = \frac{a_1 \cdot x' + b_1 \cdot y' + d_1}{a_4 \cdot x' + b_4 \cdot y' + 1} \quad \text{and}$$

$$y = \frac{a_2 \cdot x' + b_2 \cdot y' + d_2}{a_4 \cdot x' + b_4 \cdot y' + 1} \quad (21)$$

These relations have four unknown variables (a_1, b_1, d_1, a_2, b_2, d_2, a_4, b_4), which depend on the position and orientation of the fiducial plane relative to the radiographic films and on the positions of the two foci. If four fiducial markers of the calibration cage are projected on both X-ray films, the eight measuring points can be used to solve the eight unknown variables in equation 21. After this procedure, the (imaginary) projection of an object point in the fiducial plane can be calculated. Subsequently, the positions of the foci can now be reconstructed by using the control coordinates of the calibration cage and the calculated projections of these points in the fiducial plane. After this procedure, the three-dimensional position of any point in space, provided that it is projected on both radiographic films, can be reconstructed by calculation of the intersection of the two lines between the foci and the projection of the object point on the (x, y) fiducial plane. Once the coordinates of the foci are determined and remain steady with respect to the fiducial plane, the control plane becomes redundant for the duration of a measurement session. For that reason, a "reference plate" with markers is commonly added to the configuration, to represent the fiducial plane after calibration (212). This implies that the calibration cage can be removed, and the object no longer needs to be positioned within its constraints. Because of measuring errors, the two lines do not usually intersect mathematically, which leads to inaccuracies in the results. The accuracy can be improved by using a redundant system of fiducial and control markers (for example, nine of each). A computer program (X-RAY; 212) is used to determine the most probable intersection point by mathematical optimization. In addition, the program provides information about the accuracy of the measurements, based on the standard deviations of the redundant system. With this technique, the three-dimensional coordinates of an object point can be reconstructed with an accuracy of about 25 μm (212).

Usually, one is interested in the position of a rigid body (prosthesis) relative to another one (bone), and how this changes in time. The position of each of these rigid bodies can be determined from at least three marked points in the bodies. When two or more pairs of radiographs in a particular time sequence are available, the migration of one rigid body rel-

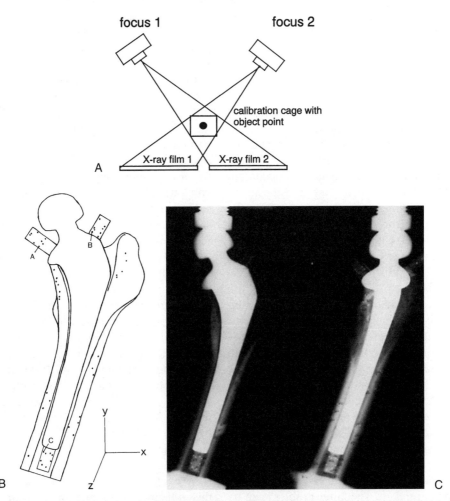

FIG. 27. For the RSA analysis, the bone and stem with attached acrylic posts are provided with tantalum pellets. **(A)** The projections of the calibration cage markers and object point on two radiographic films. **(B)** Schematic. **(C)** Double X-rays.

ative to the other over time can be determined in terms of three rotations and three translations (212). To minimize errors, more than three markers should be used, particularly when it is expected that the bodies do not behave as ideally rigid. A computer program (KINEMA; 212) is used to determine the relative kinematics of the two rigid bodies. In addition to the information about the measuring errors produced by X-RAY, the computer program KINEMA provides information about the rigidity of the bodies. For this purpose, the program calculates the distances between the marker points in the rigid body. If the body is ideally rigid, these distances are constant in time. If this is not the case, the body does not behave as a rigid one, meaning that the body is very flexible or that one marker may have come loose.

An experimental setup to measure relative motion (migration) of a femoral component of a THR requires, apart from a testing machine, two X-ray tubes, specially prepared X-ray cassettes with optimally flat films, tantalum pellets to mark the bone and the prosthesis, and a calibration cage. Figure 27B shows the arrangements of the tantalum pellets in bone, cement, and prosthesis. In order to minimize measurement errors, the scattering of the pellets should be optimal. The scattering can be quantified using a condition number as defined by Söderqvist and Wedin (217). It is possible to use clear markings on the prosthetic components for the RSA measurements, such as the metal ring in the PE cup, the prosthetic tip, the center of the prosthetic head, or the collar of the prosthesis. In an experimental setup one could come close to the optimal scattering of the pellets. However, under *in vivo* conditions the surgeon has a limited region where the pellets can be inserted (only the proximal femur); some pellets may migrate as a result of bone remodeling; and the images of the pellets may not always be visible on the radiograph as they are obscured by the image of the metal implant. The latter problem can be minimized by standardizing the way in which the pellets are inserted and the radi-

ographs are made. Figure 27C shows the radiographic pair of the specimen. First, all markers must be identified and numbered, and then digitized. The digitizer must have a high resolution (about 5 μm). The identification and digitization procedures are time consuming but can be automated.

The RSA system was originally developed as a method to accurately determine three-dimensional motion patterns between bone segments, such as in human joints. In addition to this application, the method has been used in studies concerning bone growth, the stability of joints, bone fractures and spinal segments, volume measurements, and fixation of prostheses (133). With respect to joint reconstructions, the method was applied to study permanent displacements (migration) and induced relative motions between prosthetic components and bone *in vivo* (135,167,201,215). These studies have shown that early excessive migration of components is correlated with early revision and that the RSA technique has appropriate sensitivity to detect these early micromotions (Fig. 28). Kärrholm et al. (135) could identify a migration threshold by 6 months, beyond which there was an increased risk of subsequent revision.

The advantage of RSA is that it can provide significant information about the quality of THR designs early postoperatively (6 to 24 months). The RSA technique is very precise and dependable, and it provides real three-dimensional relative motions between two segments, which are impossible to obtain with other techniques. On the negative side, the evaluation tends to be rather tedious and time consuming. In addition, the technique is suitable for quasistatic loading only, because radiographs must be made after each load increment. In the near future, dynamic RSA studies will be possible as the techniques for synchronization of the roentgen cameras are developed and high-speed film exchangers become available. Using this dynamic technique in addition to the quasistatic one will make the RSA technique even more effective as an *in vivo* tool

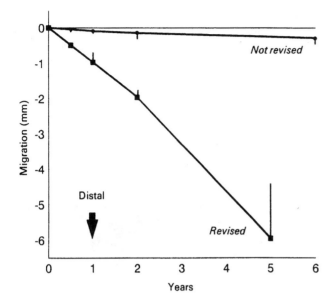

FIG. 28. *In vivo* proximal/distal migration (mm) of the center of the femoral head (mean and standard error) determined with RSA techniques in a series of 80 cemented THR reconstructions. The reconstructions that were revised within 6 years because of failure, and those that were not, could be discriminated significantly within 1 year postoperatively by using RSA. (From Kärrholm and Snorrason, ref. 135, with permission.)

to analyze failure processes in THR reconstructions.

Laboratory Bench Tests

Laboratory experiments to investigate or preclinicallly test the mechanical behavior of THR reconstructions can grossly be divided into two types. The first type aims at determining the relative motions of the components under (dynamic) loading (17,158,209–211,223, 224,246). As discussed earlier, the amount of micromotion between implant and bone is a critical factor in the fixation mechanism of cementless prostheses. These implants require minimal motions at the implant–bone interface to allow bony ingrowth into porous surfaces or bonding to hydroxylapatite coatings (186). High relative motions may also cause bone to resorb at the interface and create a fibrous-tissue membrane (114,181,251). Hence, it is important for noncemented stems to have adequate "initial stability," which can be tested in laboratory bench tests. Laboratory micromotion analyses can also be applied to cemented THR reconstruction (17,158,246). These analyses are meant to test whether micromotions between the stem and the cement mantle are produced when the structure is dy-

namically loaded. The detection of relative motions would indicate that the stems had debonded from the cement mantles, thereby giving rise to the accumulated-damage and particulate-reaction failure scenarios.

In a laboratory micromotion analysis, the structure is (dynamically) loaded, and the motions of the components are recorded. The (micro)motions can be measured experimentally, for instance, by providing the prosthesis with sensors that measure the displacements at one or more points of the prosthesis, relative to the bone (209,210,223,224,246). Sometimes only particular motion components are measured, for instance, subsidence in axial or rotation in torsional loading of femoral stems. A complete evaluation of prosthetic motions is not trivial. The rigid-body motion of a prosthetic component relative to the bone can be described by three translations of a chosen base point (e.g., superior–inferior subsidence, AP translation, and medial-lateral translation) and three rotations about mutually perpendicular axes (e.g., axial rotation, flexion, and varus–valgus rotation). In order to determine these six rigid-body motions, at least six relative displacements of three points must be determined (e.g., the x, y, and z displacement of one point, the x and y displacements of a second point, and the z displacement of a third point). An additional complication is that some prosthetic components undergo nonnegligible deformations when loaded, for instance, the bending of a hip stem. Hence, the prosthesis does not always behave as a rigid body, which requires additional displacement sensors in particular regions far removed from the base point.

Figure 29A shows an example of an experimental setup (209) in which three rigid-body translations and one (axial) rigid-body rotation are measured in addition to four local relative interface motions at the proximal and distal ends of the hip stem. The load can be applied dynamically, and the sensors allow for continuous data sampling. When tests of this kind are conducted, the displacements must

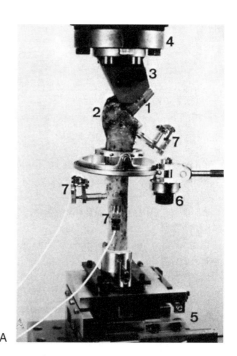

FIG. 29. **(A)** An experimental setup for direct measurements of motion of a prosthesis implanted in bone: (1) prosthesis, (2) bone specimen, (3) clamping flanges, (4) load cell, (5) an *xy* translation table that allows measurement of horizontal motion and transmits axial and torsional loads, (6) rotation transducer, and (7) interface transducers for measurement of local prosthetic motion. (From Schneider, ref. 209, with permission.) **(B)** Femur specimen with 100 strain-gauge rosettes for strain analysis on the periosteal bone. (Reprinted from ref. [106], with permission.)

A

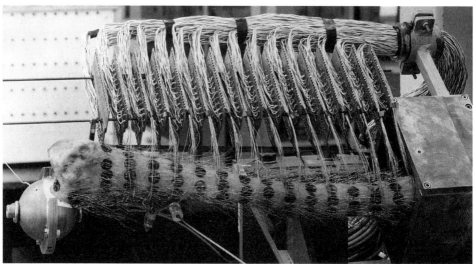

B

be divided into permanent ones, representing a setting process or migration of the prosthesis, and recoverable ones, which are the true repetitive relative motions occurring under dynamic loading.

The loads in laboratory bench tests are usually simplified. Muscle forces are often absent (e.g., 209,246) or restricted to the representation of the abductor muscles only (e.g., 18,158). In the latter case, a strap is usually attached to the greater trochanter and connected to the loading rig. A problem may arise when different prosthetic designs are tested. Ideally, the positions where the loads are applied should be the same in all cases. However, because of the different prosthetic shapes and implantation procedures, the position of load application may vary considerably (e.g., as a consequence of different offsets). This can affect the local loading conditions considerably (a smaller offset results in reduction of the bending moment) and obscures the interpretation of the results obtained with the various designs.

Laboratory studies with series of cadaver femurs are hampered by the variety in geometric and mechanical properties of human femurs. To overcome this problem, synthetic composite femurs can be used. It has been shown that the mechanical properties of these femurs, such as their bending stiffness, are similar to those of bones (163). This indicates that the cortical bone is adequately represented. However, the inner side of the synthetic bone consists of a foamy substance, and there is no intramedullary canal. Hence, the interior of the bone is not adequately represented, and one should be aware of these weaknesses when selecting this type of bone for experiments.

The second type of laboratory bench tests are the ones that focus on stress analysis in the bone–implant composite (42,48,60,62,90,106, 129,150,173,197). These studies are usually applied on laboratory models, using bone specimens or bone substitutes. In all cases, deformations are actually measured and then either visually interpreted or used to calculate the stresses utilizing elasticity theory. The common methods used to measure deformations in biomechanics are strain-gauge analysis, holography, photoelastic analysis (with photoelastic models, coatings, or films), and thermography.

The most popular method is strain-gauge analysis whereby an electrical gauge is glued to a free surface of an object (38). The gauge contains one or more electrical filaments, which deform with the surface to which they are attached. A strain gauge works on the principle that a deformation of the filament is proportional to a change in its electrical resistance; thus, the strain of the material at the point where the gauge is applied can be measured by simply measuring the difference in electrical resistance. Because the filament is a lineal element, a strain gauge can measure strain in only one direction. To determine the complete strain state (two lineal strains and one shear strain) at a free surface, a strain-gauge rosette can be used. A rosette contains three filaments (usually oriented at $30°$ or $45°$ from each other) that measure three lineal strains at the point of application. These three lineal strains may be used to calculate the complete strain state as well as the principal strain values and principal directions. When the elastic properties of the object are known, the stresses can be calculated using the generalized Hooke's law.

In biomechanics, strain gauges have been applied mostly to assess deformation patterns at periosteal bone surfaces (48,60,62,106, 150,173). In an example of this procedure (Fig. 29B), 100 rosette strain gauges have been glued to the surface of the femur, and these gauges are used to assess strain patterns in the bone before and after prosthetic fixation. Strain gauges applied for this purpose have some limitations, however. First, the deformation patterns, and therefore stress patterns, at the outside bone surface are not very sensitive to the details of stress transfer far away within the structure at implant–bone interfaces. Further, from the surface measurements, no information exists about the stress state within the structure. Hence, this method lacks the required sensitivity for artificial-joint design. Second, strains are obtained in a particular region of finite dimensions. The number of spots to be sampled is limited by space, instrumentation, and cost restrictions. Hence, to obtain a good representation of the stress patterns, one must either know *a priori* where the values of interest might occur or have a method of interpolating the data. For example, diaphyses of long bones, such as the femur, behave in accordance with beam theory (94,106); hence, this theory can be used to interpolate strain values measured from a limited number of locations. Strain gauges have also been applied on the surface of prosthetic components (124) and have even been enclosed in acrylic cement (33). In the latter case, strain within the material is measured. It is uncertain as yet, however, whether this method possesses sufficient accuracy (61).

Continuous strain patterns on the outside surface of bone specimens can be visualized by using photoelastic coatings (263). The deformations in the coating, which is thin and flexible, follow precisely those of the bone surface and can be visualized as optical fringe patterns when viewed under polarized light. Photoelastic coatings have the same limitations as strain gauges because information is obtained only about the outside surface of the bone. They have an additional disadvantage of being difficult to quantify accurately. However, they do give continuous strain patterns that provide easy qualitative interpretation. Methods with similar results, advantages, and limitations are holography and thermography. These methods also display continuous deformation patterns on the outside surface of structures. Holography has been used to provide very accurate measurements of deformation, whereas thermography usually provides rough qualitative pictures of the deformation field. These methods have been occasionally used in this area of biomechanics (140).

A method suitable for the assessment of strain patterns inside materials is three-dimensional photoelasticity (51). In this case, a laboratory model of the structure to be analyzed must be constructed from a birefringent plastic. When this model is loaded and viewed under polarized light, optical fringes develop representing the deformation patterns in the plastic material. In the three-dimensional model, the deformation patterns in the plastic material are "frozen in" by heating the model in the deformed state and physically slicing it when it has cooled off. An important limitation of three-dimensional photoelastic analysis is the requirement for building a physical model of the structure with correct properties of the components of the composite structure. This is often impossible because the birefringent plastics are available only in a relatively narrow range of elastic moduli. Thus, at present, this method is rarely used. In addition, the required information can be obtained more easily using FE analysis.

Computer-Simulation Analysis

Computer-simulation methods are useful for the purpose of research in THR, preclinical testing, and design. Particularly in the last decade, their applicabilities were improved tremendously through research and developments in computer hardware (117). As tools of research of failure processes, computer-simulation models are conceptually similar to others, such as laboratory models, *in vitro* culture models, animal models, and clinical models. In any investigation, one must consider closeness to reality of the model used versus experimental control. A patient is very real, but when one is used for investigative purposes as a clinical model, there is very little control over the experimental parameters. Conversely, a computer simulation provides virtually absolute experimental control but is remote from reality. Other models can be positioned between these two extremes. In using computer-simulation models one can investigate pure cause–effect relationships for well-defined sets of parameters. A single parameter can be varied to estimate its role in a particular process. Another advantage is that computer simulation is relatively cheap. For example, THR designs can be tested directly from the drawing board; no prototypes are required. These advantages can be exploited and weighted against the limitations of remoteness from reality.

Creep in Acrylic Cement

Creep of a material is defined as the time-dependent deformation of a material under constant loading conditions. Significant creep may occur in plastic materials such as acrylic cement and polyethylene. In this paragraph we show how cement creep can be simulated using FE techniques.

The constitutive theory used in a creep simulation is based on the same concepts as used in the flow theory of plasticity. It is assumed that the total strain is composed of an elastic and a creep strain. The next paragraph describes how the creep properties of bone cement can be implemented in an FE model.

The stress state in the cement mantle around femoral hip implants is typically three-dimensional. Hence, three principal stress components and the principal stress orientations determine the local stress state. Experimental creep data are based on uniaxial tests, which consider the presence of only one stress component (27,236,237). For this reason, the uniaxial creep laws can not be applied directly to structures with three-dimensional stress states. The solution for this problem is to define an equivalent stress, which relates the three-dimensional stress state to the uniaxial one and can be used in the creep laws. We selected the Von Mises stress as the equivalent stress, in accordance with what is usually used in creep simulations (80).

Another problem that obstructs the direct use of the creep laws is the fact that these were determined assuming stress conditions that were either purely static (27) or cyclic dynamic (236,237). Assuming bonded or frictionless unbonded stem–cement interface conditions, the stress state is purely dynamic, and the creep laws determined under cyclic dynamic stress conditions can be applied. However, when the stem–cement interface is assumed to be unbonded, and friction occurs, the stress state is neither purely static nor cyclic dynamic (Fig. 30). Because of frictional forces at the interface, the stresses are not completely released after unloading (240). Therefore, the local Von

Mises stress level is divided into a static residual stress (σ_{res}) and a dynamic (cyclic) one (σ_{dyn}). Obviously, the Von Mises stress level at full loading (σ_{vm}) will be affected by the creep process and is a function of the number of loading cycles (N), according to

$$\sigma_{vm}(N) = \sigma_{dyn}(N) + \sigma_{res}(N) \quad (22)$$

The ratio (R) of the Von Mises stress levels in the cement in the unloaded and loaded conditions can be determined before the actual creep simulation by loading and subsequently unloading the structure. Hence, the ratio (R) is assumed to remain constant during the whole creep process and is described by

$$R = \frac{\sigma_{vm}^{unloaded}}{\sigma_{vm}^{loaded}} \, , \quad (23)$$

which produces

$$\sigma_{res}(N) = R\sigma_{vm}(N) \quad (24)$$

and

$$\sigma_{dyn}(N) = (1 - R)\,\sigma_{vm}(N) \quad (25)$$

For the case of the bonded stem–cement interface conditions, σ_{res} and R are zero.

Similar to the application of the Boltzmann principle, which can be used for linear viscoelastic materials (262), the total creep strain

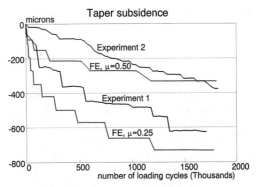

FIG. 30. Subsidence patterns of an unbonded taper within the cement mantle caused by cement creep, assuming friction coefficients (μ) of 0.25 and 0.5, shown together with experimental results. (From Verdonschot and Huiskes, ref. 239, with permission.)

can be expressed by superimposing the creep strains caused by the residual load and those by the dynamic loads, as

$$\epsilon^c(N,\sigma_{vm},R) = \epsilon^c_{dyn}(N,\sigma_{dyn}) + \epsilon^c_{res}(N,\sigma_{res}) \quad (26)$$

To determine the creep strain attributable to the residual stress component, the creep law determined by Chwirut (27),

$$\epsilon^c_{stat} = 1.798 \; 10^{-6} \; N^{0.283}\sigma^{1.858}_{res} \quad (27)$$

was used, where N is the number of loading cycles, and σ_{res} the residual stress level (in megapascals). In this formula, the original time variable (27) must be transformed to the number of loading cycles for the frequency of 1 Hz we applied. To determine the creep strain caused by the dynamic stress amplitude, two creep laws are available. The first one describes the creep strain under dynamic tensile loading (236), whereas the second one was established for dynamic compressive loading conditions (237). The creep strains related to the dynamic stress amplitude can be calculated using one of these laws, depending on whether the local maximal principal stress (σ_{prmax}) was tensile or compressive. Hence,

$$\epsilon^c_{dyn} = 7.985 \; 10^{-7} \; N^{0.4113} \; \sigma^{1.9063}_{dyn} \; N^{-0.116 \log\sigma_{dyn}},$$
$$if \; \sigma_{prmax} > 0, \quad (28a)$$

$$\epsilon^c_{dyn} = 1.225 \; 10^{-5} \; N^{0.314} \; 10^{0.033\sigma_{dyn}},$$
$$if \; \sigma_{prmax} < 0, \quad (28b)$$

where N is the number of loading cycles, and σ_{dyn} is the dynamic stress amplitude (in megapascals).

As the creep process develops, the stress levels in the structure change. Hence, an incremental procedure is required, for which incremental creep strains can be calculated, using an appropriate time step. The value of the time step is defined by the ratio of the creep strain increment permitted to the elastic strain. This ratio has a maximal value of 0.05 and ensures that the creep strain increments are small relative to the elastic strains; hence,

$$\Delta\epsilon^c/\epsilon^{el} < 0.05 \quad (29)$$

The creep-strain increment can then be used in the FE code to calculate the various

three-dimensional creep-strain components ($\Delta\epsilon^c_{ij}$), using a flow rule that identifies how the Von Mises stress is affected by the various stress components:

$$\Delta\epsilon^c_{ij} = \Delta\epsilon^c \frac{\partial\sigma_{vm}}{\partial\sigma_{ij}} \quad (30)$$

From the creep-strain components and the stiffness matrix, a nodal force vector is calculated, which is subtracted from the force vector already present. Then a new FE iteration is performed with the modified force vector.

The first example to which the theory was applied is an axisymmetric structure consisting of a metal taper in a cement mantle (239). Figure 30 shows the subsidence of the taper within the cement mantle produced by the creep simulation and obtained with laboratory experiments. The subsidence pattern of the tapers was not continuous but had a stepwise appearance as a result of stick–slip mechanisms at the interface. Changing the coefficient of friction from 0.25 to 0.5 led to a significant reduction in subsidence.

When the method is applied to a three-dimensional FE model of a cemented femoral THR (242), it can be shown that creep of acrylic cement indeed has a stress-relaxing effect in the cement mantle, particularly at the exterior side (Fig. 31). At the interior side, however, cement stresses are not reduced significantly, resulting in maximal cement stresses that are virtually constant in time.

Accumulated Damage Analysis

The accumulated-damage failure scenario is one of the most prominent ones in cemented THR, particularly where the femoral component is concerned. As described above, this scenario involves the accumulation of mechanical damage in materials and interfaces caused by repetitive dynamic loading, eventually resulting in gross loosening. When the theory of continuum damage mechanics (CDM) is combined with FE techniques, the process of damage accumulation can be simulated (238,239). In this section, a method is described for ways the

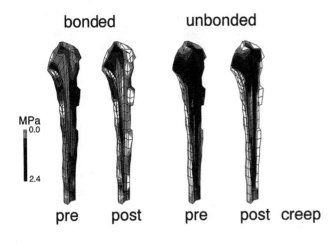

FIG. 31. Tensile stress distributions in the cement mantle (only the anterior part of the cement mantle is shown) before and after the simulation of cement creep, assuming either bonded or frictional unbonded stem–cement interface conditions. (From Verdonschot and Huiskes, ref. 242, with permission.)

theory of CDM can be implemented in FE simulations.

When a material is dynamically loaded, microcracks may be initiated. When this occurs, the material is damaged. The amount of damage accumulated in a material can be measured by a reduction in stiffness, strength, or residual lifetime (23,24). Assuming constant environmental conditions, the amount of damage depends on the applied load and the number of loading cycles. Consider, for the sake of simplicity, the one-dimensional case, where damage can be described with a scalar variable. When only the load level is varied during the damage process, the amount of damage (D) becomes a function of the number of cycles (n) and the load level (S):

$$D = F(n,S) = f(n/N) \qquad (31)$$

with the restrictions: $D = 0.0$ when $n = 0$, and $D = 1.0$ when $n = N$, where N is the number of cycles to failure for constant-amplitude loading in a fatigue bench test of the same material. In these tests, specimens are exposed to a dynamic load with a constant load level, and the number of cycles to failure is recorded. Repeating these tests with different load levels allows the relationship between load level (S) and the number of cycles to failure (N) to be determined. Results of fatigue tests are often presented as S–N curves.

The function $f(n/N)$ in equation 31, which is called the damage rule, defines the rela-

tionship between the amount of damage and the ratio of number of cycles of loading to number of cycles to failure. In the analyses, a linear cumulative damage rule is chosen, which is called the "Palmgren–Miner" rule (164). This damage rule, which itself is stress-independent, states that the damage is a linear function of the number of cycles of operations (n):

$$D = f(n/N) = n/N \qquad (32)$$

The rate of microcrack development in acrylic bone cement can be determined with fatigue experiments (44,143). These experiments provide a relationship between the stress amplitude σ and the number of cycles to failure N at that stress level, according to (44)

$$\log N = 4.68 - \log \sigma + 8.77 \qquad (33)$$

In reality, structures are often exposed to dynamic loads in which the load level varies in time. The damage sum accumulated during fatigue loading for a number of cycles of n_i at load levels S_i can be written as (122):

$$D = \sum_{i=1}^{m} \Delta D_i \qquad (34)$$

where ΔD_i represents the amount of damage accumulation during fatigue at load level S_i, and m is the number of load levels.

Because of the elastic relationship between stresses and strains, the amount of damage in an element can be coupled to the elastic properties (151). However, when the material is brittle, it can be assumed that the damage and the stiffness of the cement material are uncoupled. This means that the elastic properties of the cement are assumed constant until the damage is complete ($D = 1.0$). In the two- and three-dimensional cases, the damage (D) becomes a tensor. Because of cyclic loading in a particular direction, the material can be completely damaged in one direction, whereas it may be unaffected in another one. Perpendicular to the damage directions (the crack direction), the material loses its stiffness, resulting in anisotropic postdamage material behavior. In most FE codes, material anisotropy can be fed into the FE program. However, one may also use cracking options, which are available in some FE packages to simulate the postcracking material behavior. The stress patterns in the cement mantle change when the cement cracks locally. Hence, after creation of a cement crack, a new FE iteration is required to calculate the new stress distribution, resulting in an iterative FE simulation of the accumulation of damage in the cement mantle (Fig. 32).

Application of this method to an FE model of a cemented femoral THR reconstruction facilitates the analysis of parametric effects and the mechanisms involved during the damage accumulation process in THR reconstructions. An important mechanism is shown in Fig. 33. This figure shows that the accumulation of cement cracks does not result in an increase of cement stresses, as one might expect. On the contrary, tensile stresses are released after the material has cracked and lost its stiffness in the tensile hoop direction.

It should be realized that the method of accumulated damage as described in this paragraph has not been extensively validated as yet. Hence, this method can be used only to provide insight in the mechanisms involved in cement failure. It can determine the time-dependent effects of parametric variations only on a qualitative and relative basis.

Debonding and Micromotion

Loosening of THR components is often accompanied by disruption or noningrowth of interfaces. Finite-element studies have considered the interface debonding and micromotion processes (73,136,147,153,199,241,245,248).

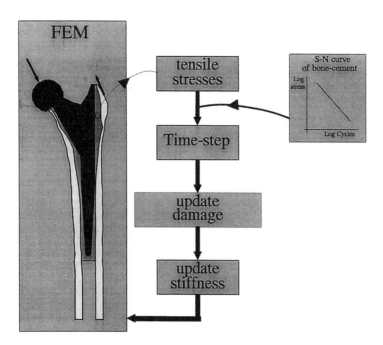

FIG. 32. Iteration scheme of the accumulative damage simulation in the cement mantle.

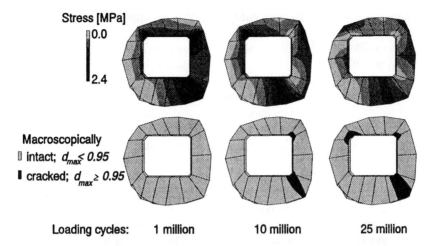

Stress [MPa]
0.0

2.4

Macroscopically
intact; $d_{max} \leq 0.95$
cracked; $d_{max} \geq 0.95$

Loading cycles: 1 million   10 million   25 million

FIG. 33. The stress distribution **(top)** and crack distribution **(bottom)** in a transverse cross section of the cement mantle in the finite-element model at various times (from left to right) in the damage process. Stem–cement interface conditions were assumed as unbonded, with a friction coefficient of $\mu = 0.25$. (From Verdonschot and Huiskes, ref. 243, with permission.)

Clinically, debonding of the stem–cement interface does occur, if not immediately postoperatively, then most certainly after long-term dynamic loading (74,103,127). Debonding of the stem–cement interface is governed by the stresses relative to the fatigue strength of the stem–cement interfacial bond. There are, however, little data about the fatigue strength of the interface reported in the literature. This makes it impossible to simulate the debonding process in a realistic time frame. However, if we assume that debonding does occur, we can determine where debonding is most likely to be initiated and how it progresses. To determine where local debonding will occur, a multiaxial Hoffman's failure index (82) can be used. Hoffman used this index to determine material failure exposed to a multiaxial stress situation. The same procedure was successfully applied by Stone et al. (221) to establish failure of cancellous bone. Weinans et al. (251) incorporated this index in a finite-element model simulating the process of prosthesis–bone disruption. The failure index (*FI*) can be defined as

$$FI = \frac{1}{S_t S_c}\sigma^2 + (\frac{1}{S_t} - \frac{1}{S_c})\sigma + \frac{1}{S_s^2}\tau^2$$

where bonded,   (35a)

and

$$FI = 0 \quad \text{where debonded} \qquad (35b)$$

where $S_t = 8$ MPa is the tensile strength of the metal–cement interface (137), $S_c = 70$ MPa is the compressive strength of the interface (the compressive strength of acrylic cement according to Saha and Pal [202]), $S_s = 6$ MPa is the shear strength of the interface (6,8,190, 222), and σ the normal and τ the shear stress at the interface. When *FI* has a value equal to 1.0, the stress situation at the interface equals that of the static interfacial strength. Hence, a value of *FI* beyond 1.0 indicates immediate failure. A lower value would indicate that no immediate static interface failure can be expected. For a particular value of the shear stress, *FI* is higher for tensile stresses than for compressive ones. Hence, a combination of shear and tension is assumed to be more harmful to the interfacial bond than shear in combination with compression. The debonding process requires an iterative FE simulation, starting with a completely bonded stem–cement interface. In every increment, the maximal *FI* is calculated, and the interface is debonded at that location. This change in local interface condition will affect the interface stresses elsewhere in the structure and requires a new FE iteration to calculate these changes. This procedure is repeated until the whole interface is debonded.

When this method is applied to a three-dimensional FE model of a cemented femoral THR, the debonding process can be simulated (Fig. 34). In this model, debonding started in the distal and proximal regions. These regions expanded until the whole interface was debonded.

Stem–cement debonding not only elevates the cement stresses, thereby intensifying the accumulated-damage failure scenario as demonstrated previously, but it also allows the stem to move relative to the cement mantle. Depending on the roughness and the relative motions, this can lead to the production of metal and acrylic cement wear products, which promote the particulate-reaction failure scenario. Finite-element models can be used to determine the micromotions at the debonded interface (240). A result of this type of analysis is depicted in Fig. 35. The cyclic slip at the stem–cement interface is shown under dynamic loaded (stance-phase loading) and unloaded (swing-phase) conditions. It is clear that friction (and surface roughness) does affect these motions considerably. Assuming no friction at the interface, a cyclic slip at the inter-

face is generated in the range of 200 μm (Fig. 35). After load release, the stem returns to its original position. In any consecutive load cycle, this behavior is repeated. When friction is assumed, the stem sticks to the cement mantle after the first loading cycle, which leads to a considerable reduction of the micromotions at the stem–cement interface (Fig. 35).

According to the failed-bonding scenario, large gaps and relative motions between the implant and the bone play a dominant role in the failure process of noncemented components (102). High cyclic micromotions can be generated because of the lack of mechanical stability and may prevent the bone from growing into the surface of the implant. Finite-element computer simulations have been utilized to analyze this problem (136,147,199,245,248). An example of such an analysis is shown in Fig. 36. The analysis is performed with a two-dimensional side-plated FE model using three different loading modes (147). The analysis shows that implant–bone motions are clearly affected by interface friction and material stiffness properties. If the stem is made of a material that has a similar stiffness to cortical bone (an "isoelastic" material), higher micromotions are produced as compared to the cases with a stiffer titanium implant. A limitation of these

Debonded sites at the stem-cement interface

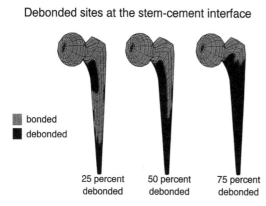

bonded
debonded

25 percent debonded   50 percent debonded   75 percent debonded

FIG. 34. Sites of stem–cement debonding at various stages in a debonding process during dynamic loading. (Adapted from Verdonschot and Huiskes, ref. 241.)

Cyclic slip at the stem/cement interface

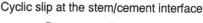

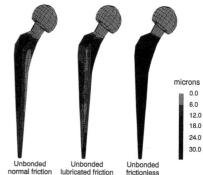

microns
0.0
6.0
12.0
18.0
24.0
30.0

Unbonded normal friction   Unbonded lubricated friction   Unbonded frictionless

FIG. 35. Cyclic micromotion patterns between the stem and the cement, assuming friction coefficients of 0.25, 0.05, and 0.0 (from left to right). (From Verdonschot and Huiskes, ref. 240, with permission.)

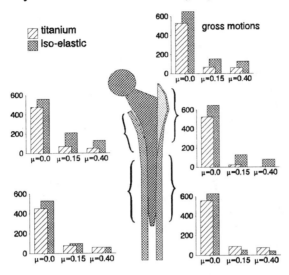

FIG. 36. Amplitudes of the cyclic movements along the implant–bone interface for two values of the prosthetic Young's modulus and three values of the coefficient of friction between bone and implant. (Adapted from Kuiper and Huiskes, ref. 147.)

FE micromotion studies is that they do not usually consider the mismatch of the shape of the implant and the bone cavity created by the surgeon. Hence, these studies only consider the stability of the implant assuming a perfect fit. Although this is a serious limitation, they can provide important information about the inherent stability of the implant, depending on shape, material properties, and interface characteristics, and thus provide the possibility of testing this at a preclinical stage, before patients are put at risk.

Motion-Induced Interface Resorption

Bone resorption and fibrous tissue formation between implants and bone are important determinants for clinical loosening. They can be the result of reactions to wear particles but can also be induced by relative motions between implant and bone (16,180,182,188,216). A conceptual scheme for such a process is shown in Fig. 37. Relative motions in a local interface region are

the effects of external joint and muscle loads in combination with the structural and bonding characteristics of the THR reconstruction as a whole. It is assumed that if these local motions exceed 150 μm, bone ingrowth or osseus integration does not occur, and fibrous tissue starts to develop (186,216). The motion-induced interface resorption paradigm now implies that the repetitive deformations in that fibrous membrane are the driving forces for its growth (Fig. 37). Which mechanical signal derived from the tissue deformation would in fact stimulate the cells in the tissues, we do not know.

For a first conceptual analysis of this process, we assumed that the growth rate of the tissue membrane is proportional to the strain in the tissue; hence,

$$db/dt = c_{ij}\varepsilon_{ij} \qquad (36)$$

where $b(t)$ is the actual tissue thickness, and ε_{ij} is the strain tensor (Fig. 38). For the purpose of the computer simulation in conjunc-

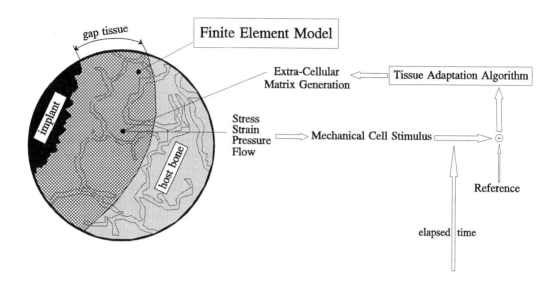

FIG. 37. A conceptual scheme for bone resorption and fibrous-tissue formation around implants.

tion with an FE model, we reduced this feedback relationship to the iterative formula

$$\Delta b = (c'\Delta u_n/b + c''\Delta u_p/b)\Delta t \qquad (37)$$

where c' and c'' are constants, and Δu_n and Δu_p are the overall elastic displacements of the implant relative to bone in normal and tangential directions (Fig. 38A). This relationship is for a plane-strain state and assumes that the fibrous layer is relatively thin (248). For the purpose of FE analysis, we modeled the fibrous tissue as a nonlinear elastic material with negligible resistance against shear and tension (251).

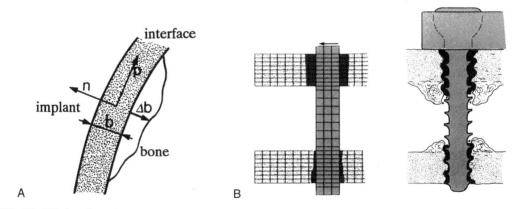

FIG. 38. (A) Interface layer with implant at the left and bone at the right. The coordinates n and p are taken parallel and normal to the interface. The thickness and growth of the interface are expressed by b and Δb, respectively. (From Weinans et al., ref. 251, with permission.) **(B)** *Left:* Simulation of the resorption process around a bone screw. The resorbed bone is indicated in black. (Reproduced from [251].) *Right:* The general resorption pattern around the bone screw fixations with fibrous tissue indicated in black. (Adapted from [180].)

This model was used to simulate loosening processes of a number of implant configurations (251). It concerns a screw used in fracture fixation with bone plates, which gradually loosens as an effect of repetitive transverse forces (182). The simulation model is able to predict the typical resorption patterns around the screw in both bone-cortex regions it penetrated (Fig. 38B). Similarly, the typical resorption patterns of femoral-head surface replacements (65) could be predicted in this way (249).

This model is very simple indeed. It neglects the three-dimensional viscoelastic properties of the fibrous tissue, important in relation to the dynamic character of the load, and the mechanical signal for the bone-resorbing cells in the membrane is not specified (Fig. 37). The first results, however, are promising. To develop this model further, biphasic theory (168) was used in FE analyses of mechanical variables during fibrous-tissue differentiation in periimplant tissues (188). In a well-controlled animal experimental model (216), the differentiation of tissue from fibrous to cartilaginous and eventually to bone could be explained as the effects of mechanical stimuli, such as strain, hydrostatic pressure, and fluid flow. It is ex-pected that these results can be used to develop a valid computer-simulation model to predict implant loosening processes as effects of dynamic loads.

Strain-Adaptive Bone Remodeling Analysis

The ability of bone to form optimal structures to support loads and to adapt structurally to changing loads has been qualitatively described by Wolff's law (198,258). The ability implies that bone must have some internal sensors to detect stresses and strains. It also implies that bone must possess a mechanochemical transduction mechanism to translate these mechanical signals to biochemical ones at the cellular level. Figure 39 shows the chain of events generally assumed for Wolff's law. A local change in mechanical signal is sensed by the bone and is translated by an as yet unknown transducer to a chemical remodeling potential. When this potential is integrated with genetic, hormonal, and metabolic factors, a remodeling signal is generated for modulating osteoblast and osteoclast activities, causing a net increase or decrease of bone mass. This entire process is known as the strain-adaptive remodeling paradigm.

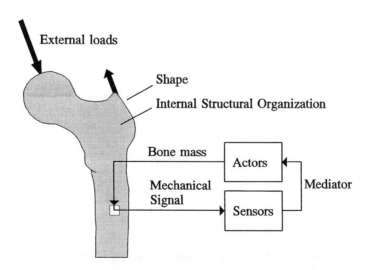

FIG. 39. A hypothesis for the mechanisms of Wolff's law.

In recent years, a number of strain-adaptive bone-remodeling theories have been formulated (22,30,75,110). These theories are mathematical descriptions of the process depicted in Fig. 39, thus providing a quantitative formulation of Wolff's law. The theories assume a relationship between local, strain-related variables and the net change of bone mass. Such variables are called remodeling signals, and the relationships are called remodeling rules. These rules are written as mathematical statements and are combined with an FE model of the bone or the bone–prosthesis structure. Thus, computer simulations of these strain-adaptive bone remodeling processes may be achieved numerically. These models have been used to explain the density patterns and trabecular architectures of bones as effects of their external loads (11,22,169,250). Similar models have also been applied to predict long-term bone remodeling around prostheses, to evaluate the consequences of stress shielding, and to preclinically test THR stem designs (113,116,119,249,253). The theory used for these computer-simulation analyses is briefly summarized in this section.

We assume that the bone cells react to a mechanical signal S, which is the local expression of the bone deformation patterns

caused by the external load. The distribution of S is calculated in an FE model of the bone with prosthesis. The signal value is compared to a target value S_{ref}, taking into account a threshold level s. Hence, the target signal value range is

$$(1 - s)S_{ref} \leq S \leq (1 + s)S_{ref} \qquad (38)$$

where s is expressed as a fraction. S_{ref} is the local signal value for the normal bone under remodeling equilibrium. The distribution of S_{ref} is also determined in an FE model representing these conditions. If the signal exceeds the target range, then net bone mass M is added ($dM/dt > 0$); if it is below the target range, bone is removed ($dM/dt < 0$), as illustrated in Fig. 40. The adaptive process in the operated femur can then be expressed in the rate of net bone turnover

$$dM/dt = \tau A(\rho)[S - (1 - s)S_{ref}]$$
$$\text{if } S \leq (1 - s)S_{ref}$$

$$dM/dt = 0$$
$$\text{if } (1 - s)S_{ref} < S < (1 + s)S_{ref}$$

$$dM/dt = \tau A(\rho)[S - (1 + s)S_{ref}]$$
$$\text{if } S \geq (1 + s)S_{ref}$$

$$0.01 \geq \rho \geq 1.73 \text{ gr/cm}^3 \qquad (39)$$

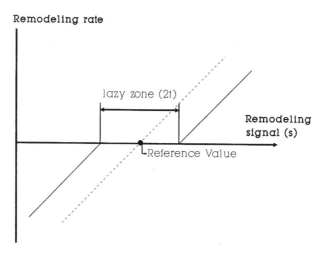

FIG. 40. Relationship between remodeling rate and remodeling signal, with *(solid lines)* and without *(dotted lines)* a lazy zone (110).

where τ is a time constant expressed in grams per millimeters^2[joules/gram]/month, ρ is the apparent density of the bone (in g/cm^3), with a maximal value of 1.73, $A(\rho)$ is the free surface available for remodeling at the periosteum or in the internal bone structure, and s represents the threshold level. The time t is given in units of months.

In the simulation, remodeling takes place within the bone (internal remodeling, a change in apparent density ρ) and at its periosteal surface (external or surface remodeling, a change in shape). The rate of net bone turnover dM/dt can now be expressed as a rate of change of the external (periosteal) geometry, dx/dt, by

$$dM/dt = \rho A(dx/dt) \qquad (40)$$

with A the external surface area at which the rate of mass change dM/dt takes place (the external face of the element concerned) and x a characteristic surface coordinate, perpendicular to the periosteal surface. For the adaptation of the internal bone mass as a result of porosity changes we use

$$dM/dt = V(d\rho/dt) \qquad (41)$$

with V the volume in which the bone mass change takes place (the volume of the element

concerned) and $d\rho/dt$ the rate of change in apparent density. Equation 39 can now be written in terms of dx/dt for surface remodeling and in terms of $d\rho/dt$ for internal remodeling. If we substitute this in equation 39, the proportionality parameters τ/ρ and $\tau A/V$ appear, which regulate the rates of the remodeling processes at the surface and internally, respectively. In the latter location, $A(\rho)$ is the pore surface in the bone, which can be expressed in the apparent density ρ by using a theory of Martin (161).

For the mechanical signal S we take the average elastic energy per unit of mass (joules/gram) from a series of m external loading configurations, each consisting of joint and muscle forces; hence,

$$S = \frac{1}{m} \sum_{i=1}^{m} \frac{U_i}{\rho} \qquad (42)$$

where U_i is the strain-energy density (see equation 4) for loading case i. The distribution of S_{ref} is determined accordingly in an FE model of the intact (preoperative) bone. The distribution of the actual signal S in the THR is updated iteratively. The external loading configurations are always assumed identical before and after the operation. Through forward Euler integration, the equations can be

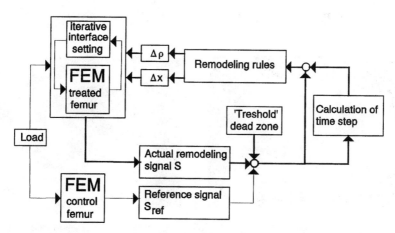

FIG. 41. Schematic representation of the iterative computer simulation model of bone remodeling around implants. (Adapted from Weinans et al., ref. 252.)

solved iteratively to find the new coordinates of the surface nodes and new apparent density values in the integration points after every iterative step. In the computer program, the integration is carried out in steps of $\tau\Delta t$, which represents the proceeding of the processes at an arbitrary computer time scale. The time step in the integration process is variable and determined in each iterative step such that the maximal density change in the integration point where the maximal rate of density change occurs will not exceed $\frac{1}{2}\rho_{max}$ ($= 0.865$ g/cm^3) (229). The iterative simulation process is depicted in Fig. 41.

The value of the threshold s was determined experimentally for dogs as $s = 0.35$. The time constant τ was empirically determined in the same study as $\tau = 130$ g/[mm^2(J/g)month] to have the time t given in units of 1 month (252).

For humans the threshold level is taken as $s = 0.75$ (116). A realistic time constant is not known for this case.

The simulation model presented above was validated with respect to six series of animal experiments with THR in dogs (118,229,252). In each series different stem materials and coating conditions were applied. The cortical bone areas and medullary bone densities were measured postmortem 6 months and 2 years postoperatively and compared to the predictions of the simulation model. As shown in Fig. 42, the predictions by the model and the actual morphology found in the dogs were very similar, even in detail. When the predictions of overall bone remodeling were compared per series to the experimental averages and standard deviations, significant correspondence was obtained, as shown for one series in Fig. 43.

Left   **Right**

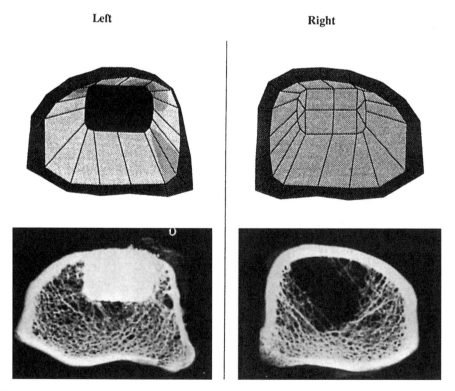

FIG. 42. Animal experimental results (2 years' follow-up) of bone remodeling in canine femurs with fully bonded prostheses compared with the prediction using the remodeling simulation. The **left** femur is the treated case, and the **right** is the control. (Adapted from Van Rietbergen et al. [229].)

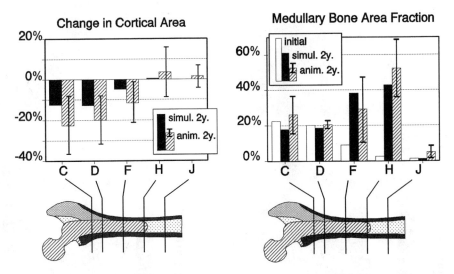

FIG. 43. A comparison between 2-year experimental results in animals and those of the simulation for the uncoated-stem series. The predicted CBA and MBAF are within the 95% confidence interval of the experimental values. (Adapted from Van Rietbergen et al., ref. 229.)

In regard to human configurations, we have hitherto only used internal remodeling because in humans cortical porosis is the main mechanism of bone loss. Figure 44 shows an example of predicted long-term bone loss around a titanium stem in THR. These results were verified relative to mean bone resorption values measured in a series of retrieved THR bone specimens (55,101,104). One-to-one validation relative to the individual patients in this series is in progress.

The computer simulation method discussed here is now used routinely to test prosthetic designs preclinically relative to the stress-shielding failure scenario, on a relative basis, always comparing one configuration with another (116,119,228,249,253).

Numerical Design Optimization

It is evident from the discussion of failure scenarios that many design goals in THR are incompatible. In order to improve fit of noncemented prostheses, modular components to be assembled at the operating table are useful. However, modularity implies more connections subject to wear. Hence, to prevent the failed-bonding failure scenario,

components should be modular, but to prevent the particulate-reaction scenario, they should be monoblocs. They can not be both at the same time, so sensible compromises will have to be found. There are many examples of incompatible design goals in THR (102). In an earlier section, we discussed the effects of femoral stem stiffness on bone and interface stresses. Basically, when the stiffness of the stem increases, the interface stresses reduce, but stress shielding increases. So a rigid stem promotes the stress-shielding scenario, and a flexible one promotes both the failed-bonding and the accumulated-damage scenarios. This is another notorious incompatibility in THR design goals, and again sensible compromises are indicated. To assist the designer in finding the best compromise available, numerical design optimization, using FE models, can be a useful tool (39,45,111,112,144–146,261).

The usual approach to FE analysis is to take a particular design (shape and material properties) and determine the stress patterns within the structure under specified loads. In optimization analysis, this procedure is conceptually reversed in that a desired stress pattern in a THR structure is specified and the

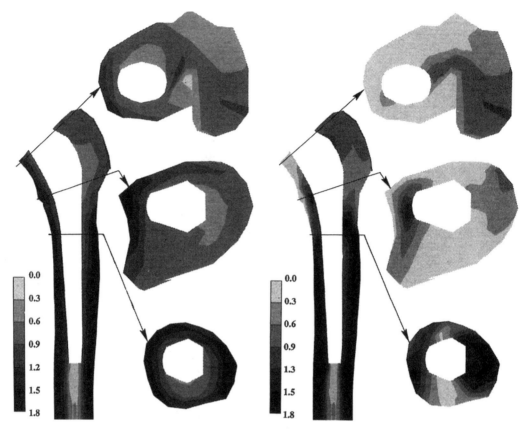

FIG. 44. Immediate postoperative density distribution, as based on CT scan **(left),** and density distribution after long-term remodeling simulation **(right).** (From Huiskes, ref. 101, with permission.)

design characteristics by which it is realized are determined. As in the computer simulations discussed above, this is accomplished in an iterative procedure (Fig. 45). The process is started with an initial design for which the stresses, strains, or other mechanical variables (e.g., strain-energy density, SED) are determined from the initial FE model. If the stress distributions deviate from the desired ones, the shape or material

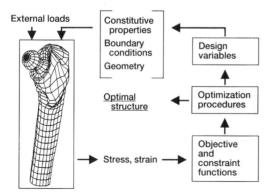

FIG. 45. A general scheme for iterative optimization in combination with a FE-model. (Reproduced from [102]).

characteristics of the design are adapted in such a way that the stresses and strains are changed toward the specified values. This iterative process is repeated until the desired stress patterns are approximated as closely as possible or within a specified range of error. The way in which the shape of the prosthesis is adapted in each iteration is determined by a search procedure that determines the search direction. Experience shows that it is an exception, rather than a rule, that the desired stress and strain distributions are realized precisely by the final design. One must be satisfied with a reasonable approximation of the desired stress and strain distributions.

An optimization process is conducted relative to particular criteria, for instance, minimal stress shielding, minimal interface tension, or minimal cement stress. These criteria are written in mathematical forms as *objective functions* to be minimized. In the optimization procedure, the values of these objective functions are minimized by the particular design characteristics evolved from the iterative process. Hence, these characteristics are "optimal" only relative to the particular objective function selected. This means the criteria must be defined very carefully by the pros-

thesis designer. This optimization procedure must also include a check against unrealistic properties. For example, the stem of a femoral prosthesis cannot be bigger than the bone into which it is to be fixed. Or the elastic modulus of a material must fit into the range of what can be actually produced. For this reason, certain *boundary constraints* are required for use in the optimization procedure. Finally, the design variations considered in a particular prosthesis are limited to a particular, limited number of dimensional or material parameters, called *design variables*, for instance, parameters that define length or cross-sectional shape of a femoral stem or the parameters of a function that describe the allowable elastic modulus distribution field in a structure. The values of the selected design variables are varied in the process, but all other parameters remain fixed.

As an illustration (Fig. 46), an optimization procedure is applied to optimize the design of a "metal-backed" acetabular cup (100,115). Previous FEM analysis has shown that a metal-backed polyethylene acetabular cup reduces some cement and cement–bone interface stresses (179). However, it was also found that this metal backing tends to in-

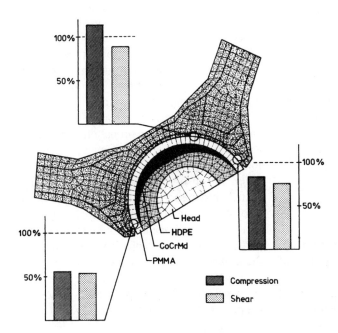

FIG. 46. Compressive and shear-stress values at the cement–bone interface in an acetabular reconstruction for an "optimized" metal-backed shell normalized against the uniform-thickness case (100%) (100,115).

crease interface shear stresses near the edges of the cup (43,109), as discussed in an earlier section. Hence, the question posed was whether a metal-backing shape could be found that would minimize the cement and interface stresses over the whole cup.

The solution procedure was based on a two-dimensional FE model with nonuniform bone properties (179). Other conditions simulated by the FE model included the complete removal of the subchondral bone layer, a uniform cement-layer thickness of 3 mm, a femoral head diameter of 28 mm, and a unit hip-joint force in a direction corresponding to the maximal force during the stance phase of gait. The metal backing shell was assumed to be made out of CoCrMd. A maximal shell thickness of 5 mm and a minimal thickness of zero were taken as boundary constraints in the optimization procedure. Three design variables were used: the thickness of the shell at the dome of the cup, the thickness at the lateral edge, and the thickness at the medial edge. The objective function was the sum of the strain-energy density function for all nodal points at the cement elements. In this sense, the minimization procedure seeks a solution in which minimal load-transfer stresses would occur at the cement–bone interface. The mathematical formulation of the problem may be described as follows:

Design variables:

$$\mathbf{v} = (t_l, t_d, t_m) \qquad (43)$$

where t_l = lateral shell thickness, t_d = shell thickness at the dome, t_m = medial shell thickness (linear interpolation between).

Boundary constraints:

$$0 < t_l \leq 5, \, 0 < t_d \leq 5, \, 0 < t_m \leq 5 \qquad (44)$$

Objective function:

$$F(\mathbf{v}) = \sum_{k=1}^{n} [U_k(\mathbf{v})]^p \qquad (45)$$

where U_k is the strain-energy density at nodal point k of the cement, n is the total number of nodal points, and p is an exponent.

Figure 46 shows the resulting optimal shape of the metal shell and the maximal ce-

ment/bone interface stress values (compression and shear) relative to those found for a shell of 2-mm uniform thickness. The optimal inner contour of the shell tends to make it as thick as possible at the cup dome (the maximal value of 5 mm) and as thin as possible at the cup edges. The reductions of stress compared to the case of the uniform shell thickness are on the order of about 15% at the medial and about 45% at the lateral side. At the cranial side, above the hip-joint load, the compressive stress is slightly higher, and shear is slightly lower, than in the case of a uniformly thick metal backing.

A similar optimization procedure applied to a cemented stem produced a typical shape, with a taper at the proximal/medial side, a belly-shaped middle region, and a strongly tapered distal end. Relative to a conventional femoral stem design, cement and interface stress reductions of 30% to 70% could be obtained with this optimized shape (111,112).

For FE analysis of structures, parametric studies require selected design parameters that depend on the intuition and experience of the designer. For optimization analysis, the selection is automated, and the search for the optimal parameters is defined with respect to assumed physical and geometric constraints and criteria. Thus, FE integrated optimization can be a powerful tool in the prosthesis design process. These concepts are obviously not limited to shape optimization but can also be applied to optimization of material properties and boundary conditions, taking adaptive bone remodeling into account.

For this purpose, optimization studies were conducted in which the probability of mechanical interface failure of a cemented stem was formulated mathematically as an objective criterion for an optimization analysis. The integrated elastic energy in the bone was used for a constraint function, in the sense that the maximal amount of bone loss would be limited to a particular maximum value. To accomplish that, the elastic modulus distribution of the stem material was varied between zero and a maximum of 100 GPa. The parameters describing the potential modulus distribution were used as

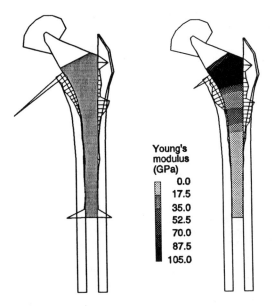

FIG. 47. The stem stiffness distribution before **(left)** and after **(right)** an optimization procedure. (Adapted from Kuiper and Huiskes, ref. 145.)

Young's modulus (GPa)
0.0
17.5
35.0
52.5
70.0
87.5
105.0

the design variables. Analyses were conducted in two- and three-dimensional models (144–146). Figure 47 shows an example of a configuration obtained in which the stem elastic modulus varies from high proximally to low distally. Compared to a full titanium stem (modulus 115 GPa), the amount of bone resorption predicted would reduce from 26% to 7.5%. This would also be realized by an "isoelastic" stem with a uniform modulus of 36 GPa, but for such a stem the peak interface stress would be a factor of three higher than for the optimized design. Evidently, it is questionable whether a material distribution as in Fig. 47 could actually be produced, so the matter is presently rather academic. However, these results illustrate that in principle, solutions for incompatible design goals are to be found with numerical optimization methods.

REFERENCES

1. Ahmed, A. M., Raab, S., and Miller, J. E. (1984): Metal–cement interface strength in cemented stem fixation. *J. Orthop. Res.,* 2:105–118.
2. Ahnfelt, L., Herberts, P., Malchau, H., and Andersson, G. B. J. (1990): Prognosis of total hip replacement. *Acta Orthop. Scand. [Suppl.],* 238.
3. American Academy of Orthopaedic Surgeons (1981): *Musculoskeletal System Research, Current and Future Research Needs.* AAOS Publication TFR-81, Chicago.
4. Amstutz, H. C., Nasser, S., More, R. C., and Kabo, J. M. (1989): The anthropometric total hip femoral prosthesis. Preliminary clinical and roentgenographic findings of exact-fit cementless application. *Clin. Orthop.,* 242:104–119.
5. Amstutz, H. C., Campbell, P., Kossovsky, N., and Clarke, I. C. (1992): Mechanism and clinical significance of wear debris-induced osteolysis. *Clin. Orthop.,* 276:7–18.
6. Arroyo, N. A., and Stark, C. F. (1987): The effect of textures, surface finish and precoating on the strength of bone cement/stem interfaces. *Proc. Soc. Biomat.,* 13:218.
7. Bakhvalov, and Panasenko (1989): *Homogenisation: Averaging Process in Periodic Media.* Kluwer Academic Publisher, Dordrecht.
8. Barb, W., Park, J. B., Kenner, G. H., and Recum, A. F. (1982): Intramedullary fixation of artificial hip joints with bone cement-precoated implants. Interfacial strengths. *J. Biomed. Mater. Res.,* 16:447–458.
9. Bargar, W. L. (1989): Shape the implant to the patient. A rationale for the use of custom-fit cementless total hip implants. *Clin. Orthop.,* 249:73–78.
10. Bartel, D. L., Bickness, V. L., and Wright, T. J. (1986): The effect of conformity, thickness, and material on stresses in ultra-high molecular weight components for total joint replacement. *J. Bone Joint Surg.,* 68-Am:1041–1051.
11. Beaupré, G. S., Orr, T. E., and Carter, D. R. (1990): An approach for time-dependent bone modeling and remodeling—application: a preliminary remodeling simulation. *J. Orthop. Res.,* 8:662–670.
12. Bergmann, G., Graichen, F., and Rohlmann, A. (1993): Hip joint loading during walking and running, measured in two patients. *J. Biomech.,* 26:969–990.
13. Bobyn, J. D., Mortimer, E. S., Glassman, A. H., Engh, C. A., Miller, J. E., and Brooks, C. E. (1992): Producing and avoiding stress shielding. Laboratory and clinical observations of noncemented total hip arthroplasty. *Clin. Orthop.,* 274:79–96.
14. Brand, R. A., and Pedersen, D. R. (1984): Computer modeling of surgery and a consideration of the mechanical effects of proximal femoral osteotomies. In: *The Hip,* edited by R. B. Welch, pp. 193–210. C. V. Mosby, St. Louis.
15. Brand, R. A., Pedersen, D. R., Davy, D. T., Kotzar, G. M., Heiple, K. G., and Goldberg, V. M. (1994): Comparison of hip force calculations and measurements in the same patient. *J. Arthropol.,* 9:45–51.
16. Brunski, J. B., Aquilante, F. M., Pollack, S. R., Korostoff, E., and Trachtenberg, E. I. (1979): The influence of functonal use of endosseous dental implants on tissue–implant interface. I. Histological aspects. *J. Dent. Res.,* 10:1953–1969.
17. Burke, D. W., O'Connor, D. O., Zalenski, E. B., Jasty, M., and Harris, W. H. (1991): Micromotion of cement and uncemented femoral components. *J. Bone Joint Surg.,* 73-B:22–37.
18. Carlsson, L., Albrektsson, B., and Freeman, M. A. R.

(1988): Femoral neck retention in hip arthroplasty. *Acta Orthop. Scand.,* 59:6–8.

19. Carter, D. R. (1978): Anisotropic analysis of strain rosette information from cortical bone. *J. Biomech.,* 11:199–202.

20. Carter, D. R., and Hayes, W. C. (1977): The behavior of bone as a two-phase porous structure. *J. Bone Joint Surg.,* 59-A:954–962.

21. Carter, D. R., Vasu, R., and Harris, W. H. (1982): Stress distributions in the acetabular region—II: effects of cement thickness and metal backing of the total hip acetabular component. *J. Biomech.,* 15:165–170.

22. Carter, D. R., Fyhrie, D. P., and Whalen, R. T. (1987): Trabecular bone density and loading history: regulation of connective tissue biology by mechanical energy. *J. Biomech.,* 20:785–794.

23. Chaboche, J. L. (1988): Continuum damage mechanics: Part I—General concepts. *J. Appl. Mech.,* 55:59–64.

24. Chaboche, J. L. (1988): Continuum damage mechanics: Part II—Damage growth, crack initiation, and crack growth. *J. Appl. Mech.,* 55:65–72.

25. Charnley, J. (1970): *Acrylic Cement in Orthopaedic Surgery.* E. and S. Livingstone; Edinburgh.

26. Charnley, J. (1978): *Low Friction Arthroplasty of the Hip.* Springer Verlag, New York.

27. Chwirut, D. J. (1984): Long-term compressive creep deformation and damage in acrylic bone cements. *J. Biomed. Mater. Res.,* 18:25–37.

28. Cohen, B., and Rushton, N. (1995): Accuracy of DEXA measurement of bone mineral density after total hip arthroplasty. *J. Bone Joint Surg.,* 77-Br:479--483.

29. Concensus Development Panel (1982): *Total Hip Replacement in the United States.* Report of Concensus Conference, NIH, 1-3 March 1982, Bethesda, MD. *JAMA,* 248:1817–1821.

30. Cowin, S. C., and Hegedus, D. H. (1976): Bone remodeling I: theory of adaptive elasticty. *J. Elasticity,* 6:313–326.

31. Crolet, J. M., Aoubiza, B., and Meunier, A. (1993): Compact bone: numerical simulation of mechanical characteristics. *J. Biomech.,* 26:677–689.

32. Crowninshield, R. D., and Brand, R. A. (1981): A physiologically based criterion of muscle force prediction in locomotion. *J. Biomech.,* 14:793–801.

33. Crowninshield, R. D., and Tolbert, J. R. (1983): Cement strain measurement surrounding loose and well-fixed femoral component stems. *J. Biomed. Mater. Res.,* 17:819–828.

34. Crowninshield, R. D., Johnston, R. C., and Andrews, J. G. (1978): A biomechanical investigation of the human hip. *J. Biomech.,* 11:75–86

35. Crowninshield, R. D., Brand, R. A., and Pedersen, D. R. (1983): A stress analysis of acetabular reconstruction in protrusio acetabuli. *J. Bone Joint Surg.,* 65-Am: 495–499.

36. Culleton, T. P., Prendergast, P. J., and Taylor, D. (1993): Fatigue failure in the cement mantle of an artificial joint. *Clin. Mater.,* 12:95–102.

37. Currey, J. (1984): *The Mechanical Adaptations of Bone.* Princeton University Press, Guildford, UK.

38. Dally, J. W., and Riley, W. F. (1965): *Experimental Stress Analysis.* McGraw-Hill, New York.

39. Dalstra M. (1993): *Biomechanical aspects of the pelvic bone and design criteria for acetabular prostheses.* Ph.D. thesis, Nijmegen University, The Netherlands.

40. Dalstra, M., and Huiskes, R. (1994): Prestresses around the acetabulum generated by screwed cups. *Clin. Mater.,* 16:145–154.

41. Dalstra, M., and Huiskes, R. (1995): Load transfer across the pelvic bone. *J. Biomech.,* 28:715–724.

42. Dalstra, M., Huiskes, R., and Van Erning, L. (1995): Development and validation of a three-dimensional finite element model of the pelvic bone. *J. Biomech. Eng.,* 117:272–278.

43. Dalstra, M., and Huiskes, R. (1997): The effects of total hip replacement on pelvic load transfer. *J. Orthop. Res.* (in press).

44. Davies, J. P., Burke, D. W., O'Connor, D. O., and Harris, W. H. (1987): Comparison of the fatigue characteristics of centrifuged and uncentrifuged Simplex P bone cement. *J. Orthop. Res.,* 5:366–371.

45. Davy, D. T., and Katoozian, H. (1994): Three-dimensional shape optimization of femoral components of hip prostheses with frictional interfaces. *Trans. ORS,* 40:223.

46. Davy, D. T., Kotzar, G. M., Brown, R. H., Heiple, K. G., Goldberg, V. M., Heiple, K. G., Jr., Berilla, J., and Burstein, A. H. (1988): Telemetric force measurements across the hip after total arthroplasty. *J. Bone Joint Surg.,* 70-Am:45–50.

47. DiCarlo, E. F., and Bullough, P. G. (1992): The biological responses to orthopaedic implants and their wear debris. *Clin. Mater.,* 9:235–260.

48. Diegel, P. D., Daniels, A. U., and Dunn, H. K. (1989): Initial effect of collarless stem stiffness on femoral bone strain. *J. Arthroplasty,* 4:173–179.

49. Dostal, W. F., and Andrews, J. F. (1981): A three dimensional biomechanical model of hip musculature. *J. Biomech.,* 14:802–881.

50. Duparc, J., and Massin, P. (1992): Results of 203 total hip replacements using a smooth, cementless femoral component. *J. Bone Joint Surg.,* 74-Br:251–256.

51. Durelli, A. J. (1977): The difficult choice: evaluation of methods used to determine experimentally displacements, strains and stresses. *Appl. Mech. Rev.,* 30(9): 1167–1174.

52. Eftekar, M. S., Doty, S. B., Johnston, A. D., and Parisien, M. V. (1985): Prosthetic synovitis. In: *The Hip,* edited by R. H. Fitzgerald, pp. 169–183. C. V. Mosby, St. Louis.

53. Engh, C. A., and Bobyn, J. D. (1988): The influence of stem size and extent of porous coating on femoral bone resorption after primary cementless hip arthroplasty. *Clin. Orthop.,* 231:7–28.

54. Engh, C. A., and Massin, P. (1989): Cementless total hip replacement using the AML stem. 0–10 year results using a survivorship analysis. *Nippon Seikeigeka Gakkai Zasshi,* 63:653–666.

55. Engh, C. A., McGovern, T. F., Bobyn, J. D., and Harris, W. H. (1992): A quantitative evaluation of periprosthetic bone-remodeling after cementless total hip arthroplasty. *J. Bone Joint Surg.,* 74-Am:1009–1020.

56. Engh, C. A., Hooten, J. P., Jr., Zettl-Schaffer, K. F., Ghaffarpour, M., McGovern, T. F., Macalino, G. E., and Zicat, B. A. (1994): Porous-coated total hip replacement. *Clin. Orthop.,* 298:89–96.

57. Faro, L. M., and Huiskes, R. (1992): Quality assurance of joint replacement. Legal regulation and medical judgement. *Acta Orthop. Scand. [Suppl.],* 250:1–33.

58. Feith, R. (1975): Side-effects of acrylic cement, implanted into bone. *Acta Orthop. Scand. [Suppl.],* 161.

59. Felts, W., and Yelin, E. (1989): The economic impact of the rheumatic diseases in the United States. *J Rheumatol.,* 16:867–884.

60. Finlay, J. B., Bourne, R. B., Landsberg, R. P. D., and Andreae, P. (1986): Pelvic stresses *in vitro*—I. Malsizing of endoprostheses. *J. Biomech.,* 19:703–714.

61. Finlay, J. B., and Bourne, R. B. (1989): Potential reinforcement-errors from the use of foil strain-gauges. *Trans. Orthop. Res. Soc.,* 14:491.

62. Finlay, J. B., Rorabeck, C. H., Bourne, R. B., and Tew, W. M. (1989): *In vitro* analysis of proximal femoral strains using PCA femoral implants and a hip-abductor muscle simulator. *J. Arthroplasty,* 4:335–345.

63. Freeman, M. A. R., and Plante-Bordeneuve, P. (1994): Early migration and late aseptic failure of proximal femoral prostheses. *J. Bone Joint Surg.,* 76-Br:432–438.

64. Furlong, R. (1993): Six years use of the unmodified Furlong hydroxyapatite ceramic coated total hip replacement. *Acta Orthop. Belg.,* 59(Suppl. 1):323–325.

65. Geesink, R. G. T., Groot, K. de, and Klein, C. P. A. T. (1987): Chemical implant fixation using hydroxyl-apatite coatings. *Clin. Orthop.,* 225:147–170.

66. Geesink, R. G., and Hoefnagels, N. H. (1995): Six-year results of hydroxyapatite-coated total hip replacement. *J. Bone Joint Surg.,* 77-Br:534–547.

67. Gilbert, J. L., Blommfield, R. S., Lautenschlager, E. P., and Wixson, R. L. (1992): A computer-based biomechanical analysis of the three-dimensional motion of cementless hip prostheses. *J. Biomech.,* 25:329–340.

68. Goldring, S. R., Schiller, A. L., Roelke, M., Rourke, C. M., O'Neill, D. A., and Harris, W. H. (1983): The synovial-like membrane at the bone–cement interface in loose total hip replacements and its proposed role in bone lysis. *J. Bone Joint Surg.,* 65A:575–583.

69. Goodman, S. B., Aspenberg, P., Song, Y., Regual, D., Doshi, A., and Lidgren. L. (1994): Effects of intermittent micromotion versus polymer particles on tissue ingrowth: experiment using a micromotion chamber implanted in rabbits. *J. Appl. Biomater.,* 5:117–123.

70. Goulet, R. W., Goldstein, S. A., Ciarelli, M. J., Kuhn, J. L., Brown, M. B., and Feldkamp, L. A. (1994): The relationship between the structural and orthogonal compressive properties of trabecular bone. *J. Biomech.,* 27:375–389.

71. Grazier, K. L., Holbrook, T. L., Kelsey, J. L., and Stauffer, R. N. (1984): *The Frequency of Occurence, Impact and Cost of Musculoskeletal Conditions in the United States.* American Academy of Orthopaedic Surgeons, Chicago.

72. Gruen, T. A., McNeic, G. M., and Amstutz, H. C. (1979): "Modes of failure" of cemented stem-type femoral components: A radiographic analysis of loosening. *Clin. Orthop.,* 141:17–23.

73. Harrigan, T., and Harris, W. H. (1991): A three-dimensional non-linear finite element study of the effect of cement-prosthesis debonding in cemented femoral total hip components. *J. Biomech.,* 24:1047–1058.

74. Harris, W. H. (1992): Is it advantageous to strengthen the cement–metal interface and use a collar for cemented femoral components of total hip replacement? *Clin. Orthop.,* 285:67–72.

75. Hart, R. T., Davy, D. T., and Heiple, K. G. (1984): A computational method of stress analysis of adaptive elastic materials with a view toward application in strain induced remodeling. *J. Biomech. Eng.,* 106:342–350.

76. Havelin, L. I., Espehaug, B., Vollset, S. E., and Engesaeter, L. B. (1995): The effect of the type of cement on early revision of Charnley total hip prostheses. A review of eight thousand five hundred and seventy-nine primary arthroplasties from the Norwegian Arthroplasty Register. *J. Bone Joint Surg.,* 77-Am:1543–1550.

77. Havelin, L. I., Espehaug, B., Vollset, S. E., and Engesaeter, L. B. (1995): Early aseptic loosening of uncemented femoral components in primary total hip replacement. A review based on the Norwegian Arthroplasty Register. *J. Bone Joint Surg.,* 77-Br:11–17.

78. Hayes, W. C., and Snyder, B. (1981): Toward a quantitative formulation of Wolff's law in trabecular bone. In: *Mechanical Properties of Bone,* edited by S. C. Cowin, pp. 43–69. American Society of Mechanical Engineers, New York.

79. Herberts, P., Ahnfelt, L., Malchau, H., Strömberg, C., and Andersson, G. B. J. (1989): Multicenter clinical trials and their value in assessing total joint arthroplasty. *Clin. Orthop.,* 249:48–55.

80. Hinton, E. (1992): *NAFEMS Introduction to Nonlinear Finite Element Analysis.* Bell and Bain, Glasgow.

81. Hodge, W. A., Andriacchi, T. P., and Galante, J. O. (1991): A relationship between stem orientation and function following total hip arthroplasty. *J. Arthopl.,* 6:229–235.

82. Hoffman, O. (1967): The brittle strength of orthotropic materials. *J. Comp. Mater.,* 1:200–206.

83. Hollister, S. J., Fyhrie, D. P., Jepsen, K. J., and Goldstein, S. A. (1991): Application of homogenization theory to the study of trabecular bone mechanics. *J. Biomech.,* 24:825–839.

84. Hollister, S. J., and Kikuchi, N. (1992): Direct analysis of trabecular bone stiffness and tissue level mechanics using an element-by-element homogenization method. *Trans. ORS,* 38:559.

85. Hollister, S. J., Brennan, J. M., and Kikuchi, N. (1992): Homogenization sampling analysis of trabecular bone microstructural mechanics. In: *Recent Advances in Computer Methods in Biomechanics and Biomedical Engineering,* edited by J. Middleton, G. N. Pande, and K. R. Williams, pp. 308–317. Books & Journals Int. LTD, Swansea.

86. Hollister, S. J., Brennan, J. M., and Kikuchi, N. (1994): A homogenization sampling prodedure for calculating trabecular bone effective stiffness and tissue level stress. *J. Biomech.,* 27:433–444.

87. Holman, J. P. (1978): *Experimental Methods for Engineers,* 3rd ed. McGraw-Hill Kogakusha, Tokyo.

88. Horikoshi, M., Macaulay, W., Booth, R. E., Crossett, L. S., and Rubash, H. E. (1994): Comparison of interface membranes obtained from failed cemented and cementless hip and knee prostheses. *Clin. Orthop.,* 309:69–87.

89. Horowitz, S. M., Doty, S. B., Lane, J. M., and Burstein, A. H. (1993): Studies of the mechanism by which the mechanical failure of polymethylmethacrylate leads to bone resorption. *J. Bone Joint Surg.,* 75-Am:802–813.

90. Hua, J., and Walker, P. S. (1995): Closeness of fit of uncemented stems improves the strain distribution in the femur. *J. Orthop. Res.,* 13:339–346.

91. Hughes, T. J. R. (1987): *The Finite Element Method; Linear Static and Dynamic Finite Element Analysis.* Prentice-Hall, Englewood Cliffs, NJ.

92. Hughes, J. R., Ferencz, R. M., and Hallquist, J. O. (1987): Large-scale vectorized implicit calculations in

solid mechancs on a cray S-MP/48 utilizing EBE pre-conditioned conjugate gradients. *Comp. Meth. Appl. Mech. Eng.,* 61:215–248.

93. Huiskes, R. (1980): Some fundamental aspects of human-joint replacement. *Acta Orthop. Scand. [Suppl.],* 185.

94. Huiskes, R. (1982): On the modelling of long bones in structural analyses. *J. Biomech.,* 15:65–69.

95. Huiskes, R. (1984): Principles and methods of solid biomechanics. In: *Functional Behavior of Orthopaedic Materials. Vol. I: Fundamentals,* edited by P. Ducheyne and G. Hastings, pp. 51–98. CRC-Press, Boca Raton, FL.

96. Huiskes, R. (1984): Design, fixation, and stress analysis of permanent orthopedic implants: the hip joint. In: *Functional Behavior of Biomaterials. Vol. II: Applications,* edited by P. Ducheyne and G. Hastings, pp. 121–162. CRC-Press, Boca Raton, FL.

97. Huskes, R., (1985): Properties of the stem–cement interface and artificial hip-joint failure. In: *The Bone–Implant Interface,* edited by J. L. Lewis and J. O. Galante, pp. 86–101. American Academy of Orthopaedic Surgeons, Chicago.

97a.Huiskes, R., Strens, P.H.G.E., Heck, J. van, and Slooff, T.J. (1985) Interface stresses in the resurfaced hip. *Acta Orthop. Scand.,* 56, pp. 474–478.

98. Huiskes, R. (1987): Finite element analysis of acetabular reconstruction. *Acta Orthop. Scand.,* 58:620–625.

99. Huiskes, R. (1990): The various stress patterns of press-fit, ingrown and cemented femoral stems. *Clin. Orthop.* 261:27–38.

100. Huiskes, R. (1991): New approaches to cemented hip-prosthetic design. In: *Safety of Implants,* edited by G. Buchorn and H. G. Willert, pp. 227–236. Hans Huber Verlag, Bern.

101. Huiskes, R. (1993): Stress shielding and bone resorption in THA: clinical versus computer-simulation studies. *Acta Orthop. Belg.,* 59(Suppl. 1):118–129.

102. Huiskes, R. (1993): Failed innovation in total hip replacement. *Acta Orthop. Scand.,* 64:699–716.

103. Huiskes, R. (1993): Mechanical failure in total hip arthroplasty with cement. *Curr. Orthop.,* 7:239–247.

104. Huiskes, R. (1995): Bone remodeling around implants can be explained as an effect of mechanical adaptiation. In: *Total Hip Revision Surgery,* edited by J. O. Galante, A. G. Rosenberg, and J. J. Gallaghan, pp. 159–171. Raven Press, Ltd., New York.

105. Huiskes, R. (1996): Biomechanics of noncemented total hip arthroplasty. *Curr. Orthop.* 7:32–37.

106. Huiskes, R., Janssen, J. D., and Slooff, T. J. (1981): A detailed comparison of experimental and theoretical stress-analyses of a human femur. In: *Mechanical Properties of Bone,* edited by S. C. Cowin, pp. 211–234. The American Society of Mechanical Engineers, New York.

107. Huiskes, R., and Chao, E. Y. S. (1983): A survey of finite element methods in orthopaedic biomechanics. *J. Biomech.,* 16:385–409.

108. Huiskes, R., and Nunamaker, D. (1984): Local stresses and bone adaptation around orthopaedic implants. *Calcif. Tissue Int.,* 36:S110–S117.

109. Huiskes, R., and Slooff, T. J. (1987): Stress transfer across the hip joint in reconstructed acetabuli. In: *Biomechanics: Basic and Applied Research,* edited by G.

Bergmann, R. Koelbel, and A. Rohlmann, pp. 333–340. Martinus Nijhoff, Dordrecht.

110. Huiskes, R., Weinans, H., Grootenboer, H. J., Dalstra, M., Fudala, B., and Slooff, T. J. (1987): Adaptive bone-remodeling theory applied to prosthetic-design analysis. *J. Biomech.,* 20(11/12):1135–1150.

111. Huiskes, R., and Boeklagen, R. (1988): The application of numerical shape optimization to artificial joint design. In: *Computational Methods in Bioengineering,* edited by R. L. Spilker and B. R. Simon, pp. 185–198. The American Society of Mechanical Engineers, New York.

112. Huiskes, R., and Boeklagen, R. (1989): Mathematical shape optimization of hip-prosthesis design. *J. Biomechanics,* 22:793–804.

113. Huiskes, R., Weinans, H., and Dalstra, M. (1989): Adaptive bone remodeling and biomechanical design considerations for noncemented total hip arthroplasty. *Orthopedics,* 12:1255–1267.

114. Huiskes, R., Strens, P. Vroemen, W., and Slooff, T. J. (1990): Post-loosening mechanical behavior of femoral resurfacing prostheses. *Clin. Mater.,* 6:37–55.

115. Huiskes, R., Venne, R. van der, and Spierings, P. T. J. (1990): Numeral shape optimization applied to cemented acetabular-cup design in THA. *Proc. Ann. Meet. ORS,* 255.

116. Huiskes, R., Weinans, H., and Van Rietbergen, B. (1992): The relationship between stress shielding and bone resoption around total hip stems and the effects of flexible materials. *Clin. Orthop.,* 272:124–134.

117. Huiskes, R., and Hollister, S. J. (1993): From structure to process, from organ to cell: recent developments of FE-analysis in orthopaedic biomechancics. *J. Biomech. Eng.,* 115:520–527.

118. Huiskes, R., Van Rietbergen, B., Weinans, H., Sumner, D. R., Turner, T., and Galante, J. O. (1994): Validation of strain-adaptive bone-remodeling simulation models. *World Cong. Biomech.,* 2:57.

119. Huiskes, R., and Van Rietbergen, B. (1995): Preclinical testing of total hip stems; The effects of coating placement. *Clin. Orthop.,* 319:64–76.

120. Hungerford, D. S., Hedley, A., Habermann, E. T., Borden, L. S., and Kenna, R. V. (1984): *Total Hip Arthroplasty: A New Approach.* University Park Press, Baltimore.

121. Huracek, J., and Spirig, P. (1994): The effect of hydroxyapatite coating on the fixation of hip prostheses. A comparison of clinical and radiographic results of hip replacement in a matched-pair study. *Arch. Orthop. Trauma Surg.,* 113:72–77.

122. Hwang, W., and Han, K. S. (1986): Cumulative damage models and multi-stress fatigue life prediction. *J. Comp. Mater.,* 20:125–153.

123. Ilchmann, T., Franzén, H., Mjöberg, G., and Wingstrand, H. (1992): Measurement accuracy in acetabular cup migration. A comparison of four radiologic methods versus roentgen stereo-grammetric analysis. *J. Arthroplasty,* 7:121–127.

124. Jacob, H. A. C., and Huggler, A. H. (1980): An investigation into biomechanical causes of prosthesis stem loosening within the proximal end of the human femur. *J. Biomech.,* 13:159–171.

125. Jacobs, C. R., Mandell, J. A., and Beaupré, G. S. (1993): A comparative study of automatic finite ele-

ment mesh generation techniques in orthopaedic biomechanics. *ASME,* 24:512–514.

126. Jacobs, J. J., Galante, J. O. and Sumner, D. R. (1992): Local response to biomaterials: bone loss in cementless femoral stems. *Instr. Course Lect.,* 41:119–125.

127. Jasty, M., Maloney, W. J., Bragdon, C. R., O'Connor, D. O., Haire, T., and Harris, W. H. (1991): The initiation of failure in cemented femoral components of hip arthroplasties. *J. Bone Joint Surg.,* 73-Br:551–558.

128. Jasty, M., Jiranek, W., and Harris, W. H. (1992): Acrylic fragmentation in total hip replacements and its biological consequences. *Clin. Orthop.,* 285:116–128.

129. Jasty, M., O'Connor, D. O., Henshaw, R. M., Harrigan, T. P., and Harris, W. H. (1994): Fit of the uncemented femoral components and the use of cement influence the strain transfer to the femoral cortex. *J. Orthop. Res.,* 12:648–656.

130. Johnston, R. C. (1987): The case for cemented hips. *Iowa Orthop. J.,* 6:60–64.

131. Kang, Y. K., Park, H. C., Youm, Y., Lee, I. K., Ahn, M. H., and Ihn, J. C. (1993): Three dimensional shape reconstruction and finite element analysis of femur before and after the cementless type of total hip replacement. *J. Biomed. Eng.,* 15:497–504.

132. Kaplan, E. L., and Meier, P. (1958): Nonparametric estimation from incomplete observations *Am. Stat. Assoc. J.,* 54:457–557.

133. Kärrholm, J. (1989): Roentgen stereophotogrammetry. Review of orthopaedic applications. *Acta Orthop. Scand.,* 60:491–503.

134. Kärrholm, J., and Snorrason, F. (1992): Migration of porous coated acetabular prostheses fixed with screws. *J. Orthop. Res.,* 10:826–835.

135. Kärrholm, J., Borssén, B., Löwenhielm, G., and Snorrason, F. (1994): Does early micromotion of femoral stem prostheses matter? *J. Bone Joint Surg.,* 76-Br:912–917.

136. Keaveny, T. M., and Bartel, D. L. (1993): Effects of porous coating and collar support on early load transfer for a cementless hip prosthesis. *J. Biomech.,* 26: 1205–1216.

137. Keller, J. C., Lautenschlager, E. P., Marshall, G. W., Meyer, P. R. (1980): Factors affecting surgical alloy/bone cement interface adhesion. *J. Biomed. Mater. Res.,* 14:1639–1651.

138. Keyak, J. H., Meagher, J. M., Skinner, H. B., and Mote, C. D., Jr. (1990): Automated three-dimensional finite element modelling of bone: a new method. *J. Biomed. Eng.,* 12:389–397.

139. Keyak, J. H., and Skinner, H. B. (1992): Three-dimensional finite element modelling of bone: effects of element size. *J. Biomed. Eng.,* 14:483–489.

140. Kohles, S. S., Vanderby, R., Manley, P. M., Belloli, D. M., Sandar, B. I., and McBeath, A. A. (1989): A comparison of strain gage analysis to differential infraved thermography in the proximal canine femur. *Trans. Orthop. Res. Soc.,* 14:490.

141. Kotzar, G. M., Davy, D. T., Goldberg, V. M., Heiple, K. G., Berilla, J., Heiple, K. G., Jr., Brown, R. H., and Burstein, A. H. (1991): Telemetrized *in vivo* hip joint force data: a report on two patients after total hip surgery. *J. Orthop. Res.,* 9:621–633.

142. Krause, W. R., Krug, W., and Miller, J. (1982): Strength of the cement-bone interface. *Clin. Orthop.,* 163: 290–299

143. Krause, W. R., Mathis, R. S., and Grimes, L. W. (1988): Fatigue properties of acrylic bone cement: S-N, P-N, and P-S-N data. *J. Biomed. Mater. Res.,* 22:221–244.

144. Kuiper, J. H., and Huiskes, R. (1992): Numerical optimization of hip-prosthetic material. *Recent Advances in Computer Methods in Biomechanics and Biomedical Engineering,* edited by J. Middleton, G. N. Pande, and K. R. Williams, pp. 76–84. Books & Journals Int., Swansea, UK.

145. Kuiper, J. H., and Huiskes, R. (1997): Mathematical optimization of elastic properties—Application to cementless hip stem design. *J Biomech. Eng.,* 14:36–43.

146. Kuiper, J. H., and Huiskes, R. (1997): The predictive value of stress shielding for quantification of adaptive resorption around hip replacements. *J. Biomech. Eng.* (in press).

147. Kuiper, J. H., and Huiskes, R. (1996): Friction and stem stiffness affect dynamic interface motion in total hip replacement. *J. Orthop. Res.* 14:36–43.

148. Kwong, L. M., O'Connor, D. O., Sedlacek, R. C., Krushell, R. J., Maloney, W. J., and Harris, W. H. (1994): A quantitative *in vitro* assessment of fit and screw fixation on the stability of a cementless hemispherical acetabular component. *J. Arthroplasty,* 9:163–170.

149. Landjerit, B., Jacquard-Simon, N., Thourot, M., Massin, P. H. (1992): Physiological loadings on human pelvis: a comparison between numerical and experimental simulations. *Proc. Eur. Soc. Biomech.,* 8:195.

150. Lanyon, L. E., Paul, I. L., and Rubin, C. T. (1981): *In vivo* strain measurements from bone and prosthesis following total hip replacements. *J. Bone Joint Surg.,* 63A:989–994.

151. Lemaitre, J. (1984): How to use damage mechanics. *Nucl. Eng. Design,* 80:233–245.

152. Lionberger, D., Walker, P. S., and Granholm, J. (1985): Effects of prosthetic acetabular replacement on strains in the pelvis. *J. Orthop. Res.,* 3:372–379.

153. Lu, Z., Ebramzadeh, E., and Sarmiento, A. (1993): The effect of failure of the cement interfaces on gross loosening of cemented total hip femoral components. *Trans. ORS,* 39:519.

154. Mackerle, J. (1992): Finite and boundary element methods in biomechanics: A bibliography. *Eng. Comput.,* 9:403–435.

155. Malchau, H., Herberts, P., and Ahnfelt, L. (1993): Prognosis of total hip replacement in Sweden. Follow-up of 92,675 operations performed 1978–1990. *Acta Orthop Scand.,* 64:497–506.

156. Malchau, H. (1995): *On the importance of stepwise introduction of new hip implant technolgy.* Ph.D. thesis, Göteborg University, Sweden.

157. Malchau, H., Kärrholm, J., Wang, Y. X., and Herberts, P. (1995): Accuracy of migration analysis in hip arthroplasty. *Acta Orthop. Scand.,* 66:418–424.

158. Maloney, W. J., Jasty, M., Burke, D. W., O'Connor, D. O., Zalenski, E. B., Bragdon, C., and Harris, W. H. (1989): Biomechanical and histologic investigation of cemented total hip arthroplasties. A study of autopsy-retrieved femurs after *in vivo* cycling. *Clin. Orthop.,* 249:129–140.

159. Maloney, W. J., Smith, R. L., Schmalzried, T. P., Chiba, J., Huene, D., and Rubash, H. (1995): Isolation and characterization of wear particles generated in patients

who have had failure of a hip arthroplasty without cement. *J. Bone Joint Surg.*, 77-Am:1201–1210.

160. Mann, K. A., Bartel, D. L., Wright, T. M., and Burstein,
A. H. (1995): Coulomb frictional interfaces in modeling cemented total hip replacements: a more realistic
model. *J. Biomech.*, 28:1067–1078.

161. Martin, R. B. (1972): The effects of geometric feedback in the development of osteoporosis. *J. Biomech.*,
5:447–455.

162. McKellop, H., Campbeel P., Park S.H., Schmalzried
T.P., Grigoris P., Amstutz H.C., Sarmiento A. (1995)
The origin of submicron polyethylene wear debris in
total hip arthroplasty. *Clin. Orthop.*, 311: 3–20.

163. McNamara BP, Cristofolini L, Toni A, and Tayor D
(1995): Evaluation of experimental and finite element
models of synthetic and cadaveric femora for pre-clinical design-analysis. *Clin. Mater.*, 17:131–140.

164. Miner, M. A. (1945): Cumulative damage in fatigue. *J.
Appl. Mech.*, 159–164.

165. Mjöberg, B. (1986): Loosening of the cemented hip
prosthesis. The importance of heat injury. *Acta Orthop.
Scand. [Suppl.]*, 221.

166. Mjöberg, B. (1991): Fixation and loosening of hip prostheses. A review. *Acta Orthop. Scand.*, 62:500–508.

167. Mjöberg, B., Hanson, L. I., and Selvik, G. (1984): Instability, migration and laxity of total hip prostheses. A
röntgen stereophotogrammetric study. *Acta Orthop.
Scand.*, 55:504–506.

168. Mow, V. C., Ateshian, G. A., and Spilker, R. L. (1993):
Biomechanics of diathrodial joints: a review of twenty
years of progress. *J. Biomech. Eng.*, 115:460–467.

169. Mullender, M. G., and Huiskes, R. (1995): Proposal for
the regulatory mechanism of Wolff's Law. *J. Orthop.
Res.*, 13:503–512.

170. NIH (1995): Total hip replacement. NIH Consensus
Development Panel on Total Hip Replacement. *NIH
Concen. Conf.*, 273:1950–1956.

171. Noble, P. C., Alexander, J. W., Granberry, M. L., et al.
(1988): *The myth of "press-fit" in the proximal femur.*
Scientific Exhibit, 55th AAOS, Atlanta GA, February
4–9.

172. Noble, P. C., Alexander, J. W., Lindahl, L. J., Yew, D. T.,
Granberry, W. M., and Tullos, H. S. (1988): The
anatomic basis of femoral component design. *Clin. Orthop.*, 235:148–165.

173. Oh, I., and Harris, W. H. (1978): Proximal strain distribution in the loaded femur. *J. Bone Joint Surg.*,
60A:75–85.

174. Olsson, E. (1986): Gait analysis in hip and knee
surgery. *Scand. J. Rehabil. Med. Suppl.*, 15:1–55.

175. Osborn, J. F. (1987): The biological behavior of the hydroxyapatite ceramic coating on a titanium stem of a
hip prosthesis. *Biomed. Technol.*, 32:177–183.

176. Otani, T., Whiteside, L. A., White, S. E., and McCarthy,
D. S. (1995): Reaming technique of the femoral diaphysis in cementless total hip arthroplasty. *Clin. Orthop.*,
311:210–221.

177. Pal, S., and Saha, S. (1982): Stress relaxation and creep
behaviour of normal and carbon fibre reinforced
acrylic bone cement. *Biomaterials*, 3:93–95.

178. Pazzaglia, U. E. (1990): Pathology of the bone–cement
interface in loosening of total hip replacement. *Arch.
Orthop. Trauma Surg.*, 109:83–88.

179. Pedersen, D. R., Crowninshield, R. D., Brand, R. A.,
and Johnston, R.C. (1982): An axial symmetric model

of acetabular components in total hip arthroplasty. *J.
Biomech.*, 15:305–315.

180. Perren, S. M. (1983): Induction der Knochenresorptio
bei Prothesenlockerung. In: *Die Zementlose Fixation
von Hüftendoprothesen,* edited by E. Morcher, pp.
38–40. Springer Verlag, Berlin.

181. Perren, S. M., Ganz, R., and Rüter, A. (1975): Ober-
flächliche Knochenresorption um Implantate. *Med.
Orthop. Techn.*, 95:6–10.

182. Perren, S. M., Rahn B.A. (1980): Biomechanics of
fracture healing. *Can. J. Surg.*, 20:228–231.

183. Perrin, T., Dorr, L. D., Perry, J., Gronley, J., and Hull,
D. B. (1985): Functional evaluation of total hip arthro-
plasty with five- to ten-year follow-up evaluation. *Clin.
Orthop.*, 195:252–260.

184. Petty, W., Miller, G. J., and Piotrowski, G. (1980): *In
vitro* evaluation of the effect of acetabular prosthesis
implantation on human cadaver pelvis. *Bull. Pros.
Res.*, 17:80–89.

185. Pierson, J. L., and Harris, W. H. (1993): Extensive osteolysis behind an acetabular component that was well
fixed with cement—a case report. *J. Bone Joint Surg.*,
75-Am:305–315.

186. Pilliar, R. M., Lee, J. M., and Maniatopoulos, C.
(1986): Observation on the effect of movement on
bone ingrowth into porous-surfaced implants. *Clin.
Orthop. Rel. Res.*, 208:108–113.

187. Poss, R., Walker, P., Spector, M., Reilly, D. T., and
Robertson, D. D. (1988): Strategies for improving fix-
ation of femoral components in total hip arthroplasty.
Clin. Orthop., 235:181–194.

188. Prendergast, P. J., Huiskes, R., and Søballe, K. (1997):
Biophysical stimuli during tissue differentiation at implant interfaces. *J. Biomech.* (in press).

189. Pritchett, J. W. (1995): Femoral bone loss following hip
replacement. *Clin. Orthop. Rel. Res.*, 314:156–161.

190. Raab, S., Ahmed, A., and Provan, J. W. (1981): The quasistatic and fatigue performance of the implant/bone interface. *J. Biomed. Mater. Res.*, 15:159–182.

191. Radin, E. L., Rubin, C. T., Thrasher, E. L., Lanyon, L.
E., Crugnola, A. M., Schiller, A. S., Paul, I. L., and
Rose, R. M. (1982): Changes in the bone-cement interface after total hip replacement. *J. Bone Joint Surg.*,
64A:1188–1194.

192. Rapperport, D. J., Carter, D. R., and Schurman, D. J.
(1985): Contact finite element stress analysis of the hip
joint. *J. Orthop. Res.*, 3:435–446.

193. Reilly, D. T., and Burstein, A. H. (1975): The elastic
and ultimate properties of compact bone tissue. *J. Biomed.*, 8:393–405.

194. Renaudin, F., Lavst, F., Skalli, W., Pecheux, C., and
Schmitt, V. (1992): A 3D finite element model of
pelvis in side impact. *Proc. Eur. Soc. Biomech.*, 8:194.

195. Rice, J. C., Cowin, S. C., and Bowman, J. A. (1988):
On the dependence of the elasticity and strength of
cancellous bone on apparent density. *J. Biomech.*,
21:155–168.

196. Ries, M., Pugh, J., Au, J. C., Gurtowski, J., and Dee, R.
(1989): Cortical pelvic strains with varying size hemi-
arthroplasty in vitro. *J. Biomech.*, 22:775–780.

197. Ries, M. D., Gomez, M. A., Eckhoff, D. G., Lewis, D.
A., Brodie, M. R., and Wiedel, J. D. (1994): An *in vitro*
study of proximal femoral allograft strains in revision
hip arthroplasty. *Med. Eng. Phys.*, 16:292–296.

198. Roesler, H. (1987): The history of some fundamental

concepts in bone biomechanics. *J. Biomech.*, 20(11/12): 1025–1034.

199. Rohlmann, A., Cheal, J., Hayes, W. C., and Bergmann, G. (1988): A nonlinear finite element analysis of interface condition in porous coated hip endoprostheses. *J. Biomech.*, 21:605–611

200. Rosenthal, D., (1974): *Resistance and Deformation of Solid Media.* Pergamon Press, New York.

201. Ryd, L. (1986): Micromotion in knee arthroplasty. *Acta Orthop. Scand. [Suppl.]*, 220.

202. Saha, S., and Pal, S. (1984): Mechanical properties of bone cement: A review. *J. Biomed. Mater. Res.*, 18:435–462.

203. Saikko, V. O., Pavolainen, P. O., and Slätis, P. (1993): Wear of the polyethylene acetabular cup. Metallic and ceramic heads compared in a hip simulator. *Acta Orthop. Scand.*, 64:391–402.

204. Sanchez-Palencia, E. (1980): *Non-homogeneous Media and Vibration Theory.* Springer, Berlin.

205. Sandborn, P. M., Cook. S. D., Spires, W. P., and Kester, M. A. (1988): Tissue response to porous-coated implants lacking initial bone apposition. *J. Arthroplasty*, 3:337–346.

206. Schimmel, J. W., and Huiskes, R. (1988): Primary fit of the Lord cementless total hip. *Acta Orthop. Scand.*, 59:638–642.

207. Schmalzried, T. P., Kwong, L. M., Jasty, M., Sedlacek, R. C., Haire, T. C., O'Connor, D. O., Bragdon, C. R., Kabo, J. M., Malcolm, A. J., and Harris, W. H. (1992): The mechanism of loosening of cemented acetabular components in total hip arthroplasty. Analysis of specimens retrieved at autopsy. *Clin. Orthop.*, 274:60–78.

208. Schmitt, J., Lengsfeld, M., Alter, P., and Leppek, R. (1995): Use of voxel-oriented femur models for stress analysis. Generation, calculation and validation of CT-based FEM models. *Biomed. Tech. Berl.*, 40:175–181.

209. Schneider, E., Kinast, C., Eulenberger, J., Wyder, D., Eskilsson, G., and Perren, S. M. (1989): A comparative study of the initial stability of cementless hip prostheses. *Clin. Orthop.*, 248:200–209.

210. Schneider, E., Eulenberger, J., Steiner, W., Wyder, D., Friedman, R. J., and Perren, S. M. (1989): Experimental method for the *in vitro* testing of the initial stability of cementless hip prostheses. *J. Biomech.*, 22:735–744.

211. Schreurs, B. W., Buma, P., Huiskes, R., Slagter, J. L., and Slooff, T. J. (1994): Morsellized allografts for fixation of the hip prosthesis femoral component. A mechanical and histological study in the goat. *Acta Orthop. Scand.*, 65:267–275.

212. Selvik, G. (1989): *A roentgen stereophotogrammetric method for the study of the kinematics of the skeletal system.* Thesis, Lund, 1974. Reprinted as *Acta Orthop. Scand. [Suppl.]*, 232.

213. Shanbhag, A. S., Jacobs, J. J., Glant, T. T., Gilbert, J. L., Black, J., and Galante, J. O. (1994): Composition and morphology of wear debris in failed uncemented total hip replacement. *J. Bone Joint Surg.*, 76-Br:60–67.

213a.Skinner H.B., Kilgus D.J., Keyak J., Shimaoka E.E., Kim A.S., Tipton J.S. (1994) Correlation of computed finite element stresses to bone density after remodeling around cementless femoral implants. *Clin. Orthop.*, 305:178–189.

214. Snorrason, F., and Kärrholm, J. (1990): Primary stability of revision total hip arthroplasty: A roentgen stereophotogrammetric analysis. *J. Arthroplasty*, 5:217–229.

215. Snorrason, F., and Kärrholm, J. (1990): *Roentgen stereophotogrammetric analysis of acetabular prostheses.* Scientific Exhibit, 57th Annual Meeting AAOS, Feb. 8–12, New Orleans.

216. Søballe, K., Hansen, E. S. B., Rasmussen, H., Jørgensen, P. H., and Bunger, C. (1992): Tissue ingrowth into titanium and hydroxyapatite-coated implants during stable and unstable mechanical conditions. *J. Orthop. Res.*, 10:285–299.

217. Södeqvist, I., and Wedin, P. A. (1993): Determining the movements of the skeleton using well-configured markers. Technical Note. *J. Biomech.*, 26:1473–1477.

218. Spector, M., Shortkroff, S., Hsu, H. P., Lande, N., Sledge, C. B., and Thornhill, T. S. (1990): Tissue changes around loose prostheses. A canine model to investigate the effects of an antiinflammatory agent. *Clin. Orthop.*, 261:140–152.

219. Spilker, R. L., Donzelli, P. S., and Mow, V. C. (1992): A transversely isotropic biphasic finite element model of the meniscus. *J. Biomech.*, 25:1027–1046.

220. Stauffer, R. N. (1982): Ten-year follow-up study of total hip replacement. *J. Bone Joint Surg.*, 64A:983–990

221. Stone, J. L., Beaupré, G. S., and Hayes, W. C. (1983): Multiaxial strength characteristics of trabecular bone. *J. Biomech.*, 16:743–752.

222. Stone, M. H., Wilkinson, R., and Stother, I. G. (1989): Some factors affecting the strength of the cement–metal interface. *J. Bone Joint Surg.*, 71-Br:217–221.

223. Sugiyama, H., Whiteside, L. A., and Kaiser, A. D. (1989): Examination of rotational fixation of the femoral component in total hip arthroplasty. *Clin. Orthop.*, 249:122–128.

224. Tanner, K. E., Bonfield, W., Nunn, D., and Freeman, M. A. R. (1988): Rotational movement of femoral components of total hip replacements in response to an anteriorly applied load. *Eng. Med.*, 17:127–129.

225. Thanner, J., Freij-Larsson, C., Karrholm, J., and Malchau, H. (1995): Evaluation of Boneloc. Chemical and mechanical properties, and a randomized clinical study of 30 total hip arthroplasties. *Acta Orthop. Scand.*, 66:207–214.

226. Timoshenko, S. P. and Gere, J. M. (1977): *Mechanics of Materials.* Van Nostrand Reinhold, New York.

227. Turner, C. H., Cowin, S. C., Rho, J. Y., Ashman, R. B., and Rice, J. C. (1990): The fabric dependence of the orthotropic elastic constants of cancellous bone. *J. Biomech.*, 23:549–561.

228. Van Lenthe, H., de Waal Malefijt, M., and Huiskes, R. (1996): Distal femoral resorption after total knee arthroplasty. *Trans. ORS*, 21:152.

229. Van Rietbergen, B., Huiskes, R., Weinans, H., and Sumner, D. R. (1993): ESB Research Award 1992. The mechanism of bone remodeling and resorption around press-fitted THA stems. *J. Biomech.*, 26:369–382.

230. Van Rietbergen, B., Weinans, H., Huiskes, R., Odgaard A., and Kabel, J. (1995): A new method to determine trabecular bone elastic properties and loading using micromechanial finite element models. *J. Biomech.*, 28:69–81.

231. Van Rietbergen, B., Weinans, H., Polman, B. J. W., and Huiskes, R. (1996): Computational strategies for iterative solutions of large FEM applications employing voxel data. *Int. J. Num. Meth. Eng.* 39:2743–2767.

232. Van Rietbergen, B., Odgaard, A., Kabel, J., and Huiskes, R. (1996): The inherent mechanical quality of trabecular bone architecture can be accurately predicted from fabric and apparent density. *Trans. ORS,* 42:82.

233. Vasu, R., Carter, D. R., and Harris, W. H. (1982): Stress distributions in the acetabular region—I. before and after total joint replacement. *J. Biomech.,* 15:155–164.

234. Verdonschot, N. (1995): *Biomechanical faiure scenarios for cement total hip replacement.* Ph.D. thesis, Nijmegen University, The Netherlands.

235. Verdonschot, N. and Huiskes, R. (1990): FEM analyses of hip prostheses: validity of the 2-D side-plate model and the effects of torsion. In: *Proceedings 7th Meeting of the European Society of Biomechanics,* July 8–11, Arhus, Denmark, p. A20.

236. Verdonschot, N., and Huiskes, R. (1994): The creep behavior of hand-mixed Simplex P bone cement under cyclic tensile loading. *J. Appl. Biomater.,* 5:235–243.

237. Verdonschot, N., and Huiskes, R. (1995): Dynamic creep behavior of acrylic bone cement. *J. Biomed. Mater. Res.,* 29:575–581.

238. Verdonschot, N., and Huiskes, R. (1995): The application of continuum damage mechanics to pre-clinical testing of cemented hip prostheses; the effects of cement-stem debonding. In: *Second International Symposium on Computer Methods in Biomechanical & Biomedical Engineering,* edited by J. Middleton, pp. 25–33. Gordon and Breach, The Netherlands.

239. Verdonschot, N., and Huiskes, R. (1996): Subsidence of THA stems due to acrylic cement creep is exteremely sensitive to interface friction. *J. Biomech.* 29:1569–1575.

240. Verdonschot, N., and Huiskes, R. (1996): Mechanical effects of stem-cement interface characteristics in total hip replacement. *Clin. Orthop.* 329:326–336.

241. Verdonschot, N., and Huiskes, R. (1997): The cement debonding process of THA stems and its effects on cement stresses. *Clin. Orthop.* (in press).

242. Verdonschot, N., and Huiskes, R. (1997): The effects of bone cement creep on the mechanical endurance of femoral total hip reconstructions. *J. Bone Joint Surg.* (in press).

243. Verdonschot, N., and Huiskes, R. (1997): The effects of cement-stem debonding in THA on the long-term failure probability of cement. *J. Biomech.* (in press).

244. Verdonschot, N., Dalstra, M., and Huiskes, R. (1991): The relevance of implant telemetry for mechanical analyses of total hip arthroplasties. In: *Proceedings Book Workshop "Implantable Telemetry in Orthopaedics," Berlin.* Edited by Bergmann G, Graichen F, Rohlmann A. pp. 249–258. Freie Universitat Berlin, Berlin.

245. Verdonschot, N., Huiskes, R., and Freeman, M. A. R. (1993): Pre-clinical testing of hip prosthetic designs: a comparison of finite element calculations and laboratory tests. *J. Eng. Med.,* 207:149–154.

246. Walker, P. S., Schneeweis, D., Murphy, S., and Nelson, P. (1987): Strains and micromotions of press-fit femoral stem prostheses. *J. Biomech.,* 20:693–702.

247. Walker, P., Mai, S. F., Cobb, A. G., Bentley, G., and Hua, J. (1995): Prediction of clinical outcome of THR from migration measurements on standard radiographs. *J. Bone Joint Surg.,* 77-Br:705–714.

248. Weinans, H., Huiskes, R., and Grootenboer, H. J. (1990): Trends of mechanical consequences and modeling of a fibrous membrane around femoral hip prostheses. *J. Biomech.,* 23:991–1000.

249. Weinans, H., Huiskes, R., and Grootenboer, H. J. (1992): Effects of material properties of femoral hip components on bone remodeling. *J. Orthop. Res.,* 10:845–853.

250. Weinans, H., Huiskes, R., and Grootenboer, H. J. (1992): The behavior of adaptive bone-remodeling simulation models. *J. Biomech.,* 25:1425–1441.

251. Weinans, H., Huiskes, R., and Grootenboer, H. J. (1993): Quantitative analysis of bone reactions at implant–bone interfaces. *J. Biomech.,* 26:1271–1281.

252. Weinans, H., Huiskes, R., Van Rietbergen, B., Sumner, D. R., Turner, T. M., and Galante, J. O. (1993): Adaptive bone remodeling around bonded noncemented total hip arthroplasty: a comparison between animal experiments and computer simulation. *J. Orthop. Res.,* 11:500–513.

253. Weinans, H., Huiskes, R., and Grootenboer, H. J. (1994): Effects of fit and bonding characteristics of femoral stems on adaptive bone remodeling. *J. Biomech. Eng.,* 116:393–400.

254. Weinans, H., Igloria, R., Turner, T. M., Sumner, D. R., Natarajan, R. N., and Galante, J. O. (1995): Animal specific adaptive bone remodeling response to femoral hip components in dogs. *Trans. ORS,* 41:718.

255. Whiteside, L. A. (1989): The effect of stem fit on bone hypertrophy and pain relief in cementless total hip arthoplasty. *Clin. Orthop.,* 247:138–147.

256. Wiklund, I., Romanus, B., and Hunt, S. M. (1988): Self-assessed disability in patients with arthrosis of the hip joint. Reliability of the Swedish version of the Nottingham Health Profile. *Int. Disabil. Stud.,* 10:159–163.

257. Willert, H. G., Ludwig, J., and Semlitsch, M. (1974): Reaction of bone to methacrylate after hip arthroplasty. *J. Bone Joint Surg.,* 56-A:1368–1382.

258. Wolff, J. (1892): *Das Gesetz der Transformation der Knochen [The Law of Bone Remodeling].* Springer-Verlag, Berlin.

259. Wroblewski, B. M. (1988): Wear and loosening of the socket in the Charnley low-friction arthroplasty. *Orthop. Clin. North Am.,* 19:627–630.

260. Yelin, E. (1992): Arthritis. The cumulative impact of a common chronic condition. *Arthritis Rheum.,* 35: 489–497.

261. Yoon, Y. S., Jang, G. H., and Kim, Y. Y. (1989): Shape optimal design of the stem of a cement hip prosthesis to minimize stress concentration in the cement layer. *J. Biomechanics,* 22:1279–1284.

262. Young, R. J., and Lovell, P. A. (1991): *Introduction to Polymers.* The University Press, Cambridge.

263. Zhou, X. M., Walker, P. S., and Robertson, D. D. (1990): Effect of pres-fit femoral stems on strains in the femur. *J. Arthroplasty,* 5:71–82.

264. Zienkiewicz, O. C. (1977): *The Finite Element Method,* 3rd ed., McGraw-Hill, London.

Basic Orthopaedic Biomechanics, 2nd ed.,
edited by Van C. Mow and Wilson C. Hayes.
Lippincott–Raven Publishers, Philadelphia © 1997.

12

Biomechanical Principles of Total Knee Replacement Design

Peter S. Walker and Gordon W. Blunn

Centre for Biomedical Engineering, University College London, Royal National Orthopaedic Hospital Trust, Stanmore, Middlesex HA7 4LP, United Kingdom

THE EVOLUTION OF DESIGNS

Before the late 1960s, the treatments for arthritis of the knee were osteotomy, the interposition of metallic femoral condyles or tibial blocks, and uncemented metal hinges. In 1969, a cemented metal–plastic condylar replacement, the "polycentric," was developed by Gunston (41). This design, using the same cemented metal–plastic technology as devised for the hip by Charnley, was the forerunner of the modern-day condylar replacements. Since that time, the term "total knee replacement" (TKR) has taken on a broad meaning encompassing the replacement of the femoral, tibial, and patellofemoral bearing surfaces and including the complete mechanical replacement of the joint surfaces and ligaments with fixed and rotating hinges (Fig.

1). In parallel with the design of the TKRs has been the development of instrumentation and techniques that have probably had as much influence on the clinical outcome as the TKR components themselves.

Since 1969, TKR development has been an evolutionary process, relying on intuitive design, empirical data, and laboratory studies. As a result, the clinical outcomes of different designs have varied considerably. Paradoxically, some of the designs introduced in the 1970s have had successful long-term results, whereas some introduced more recently have exhibited serious problems. One might have expected the application of the engineering design process to have routinely led to increasingly successful designs. However, there are a number of reasons why this has not been the case. In the field of orthopaedic implants,

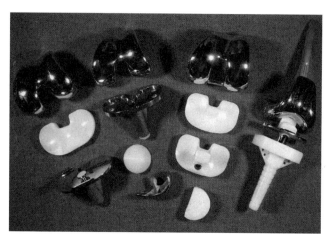

FIG. 1. Examples of total knee replacements. **Left,** mobile bearing; **left-center,** condylar replacement, patella button, and unicondylar; **right-center,** posterior stabilized and superstabilized; **right,** rotating hinge.

the art of design has often taken precedence, while science and analysis have been neglected. Although the design goals themselves might be well recognized, data on the mechanical conditions under which TKRs operate are far from complete. Testing equipment and appropriate analytic models have been lacking. In this chapter we establish a model for design that is applicable to orthopaedic implants such as TKRs and then apply the model to the design of different TKR systems.

CURRENT DESIGN FORMS

If varus–valgus stability is not required from the TKR, the most obvious design form is the standard "condylar replacement." However, within this form, there is a wide range of surface geometries and mechanisms for providing the laxity and stability characteristics. For analytic purposes, the geometry of the bearing surfaces can be parametrized (Fig. 2), enabling force–displacement characteristics and contact stresses to be calculated for a range of operating conditions (49,80). The status of the cruciate ligaments is an important factor. If both cruciates are retained, the bearing surfaces are required only to replicate the laxity and stability provided by the origi-

nal surfaces and the menisci. If one or both ligaments are absent, either as a result of the joint pathology or from a surgical preference to increase exposure or to simplify the procedure, this must be accounted for in the design of the surfaces.

In some design forms, a cam mechanism provides the stability and motion that would normally be provided by the ligaments. Typically, such cams have been configured to provide the progressive posterior displacement of the femur on the tibia with flexion, or to provide such displacement at the higher flexion range, in order to increase the maximum flexion angle obtained. A special design form of the condylar replacement is the mobile bearing or meniscal bearing type. This was originally introduced to minimize the wear of the plastic surfaces by maximizing contact area and allowing for anatomic displacements and rotations with preservation of the cruciate ligaments. However, more recent designs have allowed for the absence of one or both of the cruciate ligaments.

When varus–valgus stability is required, such mechanisms as a tibial post in a femoral housing or an axis connecting the femoral and tibial components have been used. Such means have been employed either as additions to the condylar replacement form or within a

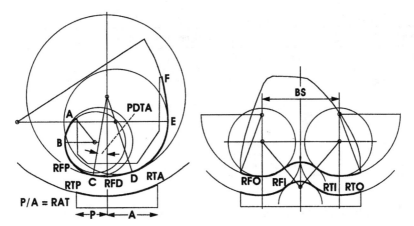

FIG. 2. Parametrized geometry of bearing surfaces. The sagittal profile consists of arcs AB, BC, CD, DE, and EF; PDTA is the posterior–distal transition angle.

more mechanistic design in which there is little physical resemblance to the articulations of a normal knee. Rather than merely allowing flexion–extension, many linked designs have sought to allow for internal–external rotation about the long axis of the tibia by various mechanisms; such structures are termed rotating hinges.

The above represent the design forms that are in widespread use or that are used for selected indications. However, new design forms could yet emerge. These might involve rolling rather than sliding, or entirely new materials. To date, the materials for TKR have been predominantly cobalt-chrome articulating on ultra-high molecular weight polyethylene (UHMWPE). Titanium alloy has been used but is not preferred because of its susceptibility to three-body abrasive wear. Ceramic, or metal with a ceramic coating, has been used for the femoral component, and some designs even use ceramic-on-ceramic, where the rationale is the reduction of friction and wear. For interfacing the components to the bone, acrylic cement continues to be the most popular method, but porous coatings of various types or macrotextures with hydroxyapatite (HA) coating are also being used. Regarding the mechanical means by which the components are attached to the bone, a wide range of pegs, posts, fins, and keels have been used. Screws have also been used to minimize interface micromotion

and facilitate bone ingrowth into porous surfaces. To expand the versatility, improve fit, restore the joint line, and enhance fixation where required, modular augments such as wedges, spacers, and stems have been developed. A range of implant sizes has also been available, although the optimum balance between achieving acceptable mechanics and an economical system remains an issue.

Instrumentation systems have generally become more complex, with numerous adjustments and means for attaching jigs to the bone. In general, the principle has been to attach the jigs based on bony landmarks and to utilize cutting guides on these jigs. The goals are to achieve anatomic limb alignment and to create a space for the components that will provide the correct geometric relations of the ligaments and muscles.

A MODEL FOR DESIGN

The goals of TKR design include relief of pain, restoration of function, durability for the life of the patient, and reliability. However, in order to utilize such criteria in a meaningful way for design purposes, their biomechanical implications must be specified (Table 1). The criteria are essentially targets against which a particular design can be measured. Any design form can then be optimized to more closely meet the ideal criteria.

TABLE 1. *Functional goals and the associated biomechanical criteria*

Functional goals	Biomechanical criteria
Relief of pain	Replacement of all articulating surfaces
	Interface micromotion less than 50 μm between components and bone
Restoration of function	Similar motion characteristics as in the normal knee
	Soft tissue lengths within normal range
	Similar laxity characteristics as in the normal knee
	The same or larger muscle lever arms as normal
Durability	Normal stresses at the interface and within the surrounding bone
	Minimal wear of the articulating surfaces (less than 0.05 mm depth per year)
Reliability	Insensitive to misalignment or size mismatch
	Function insensitive to different kinetics of patients

Designing for a biological environment introduces a number of complicating factors. However, even in standard engineering disciplines, the design process is not easily defined. The classical approach is to identify a need, specify the objectives, formulate different solutions, and select the solution most closely satisfying the objectives. This can be explained graphically (Fig. 3) and parallels the *total design* approach formulated by Pugh (73). The entire procedure comprises design and evaluation phases, with an iteration within the design phase and a further iteration between evaluation and design. In artificial joint design, however, although this design method can be used as a basis, there are other important considerations. The forces and kinematics are not known with any certainty and in any case vary from patient to patient. The properties of the structures into which the artificial joints are implanted, and their future remodeling, must be considered, but the remodeling rules for the biological materials are known only in general terms. The geometry of the biological structures such as the bones and soft tissues is highly variable. Finally, there is a variability introduced by the way in which the surgical procedure is carried out.

Before the design objectives can be stated, the problem or need must be defined. In the case of the arthritic or degenerate joint, the problem is to relieve pain and restore function. At this stage, it is important not to confuse a solution with the problem. For example, if the problem statement is to design an artificial joint to relieve pain and restore function, that would automatically exclude other solutions such as drugs or transplants. The objectives or design criteria are specified in order to satisfy the problem or need. An objective should be as general as possible while taking into account the practicalities of

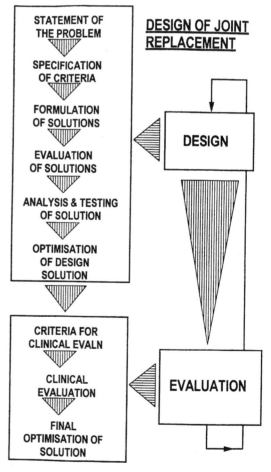

FIG. 3. The design process applicable to an implant such as a total knee replacement.

whatever design solutions are likely to be formulated. The objectives are divided into "musts" and "wants." Specifying the design criteria in this way is valuable because it provides an objective way of assessing any particular idea and can eliminate prejudice at a later stage.

In the process of design formulation, different solution possibilities are considered. For example, an artificial knee can range from an all-metal hinge to four pieces of plastic. The surgical technique can involve a major exposure with complete resection of the joint or only small components inserted arthroscopically. Each design form needs to be separate and distinct. At this stage, the design form as described may not be the optimum solution within that design form. In most instances, a final selection cannot usually be made with a single application of the design analysis matrix because further theoretical and experimental studies are likely to be required. However, experience and intuition are required to select those particular designs that merit further analysis because such analysis is likely to be costly and time consuming. The scoring system in the design analysis matrix is consistent with the Taguchi concept of robust engineering design (91). Designs with a high score for each objective will be "robust" and may require less subsequent evaluation.

Today, increasing efforts are being made to formulate meaningful preclinical evaluation methods. Such methods can be scientific experiments, theoretical analyses, or mechanical tests. Although scientific experiments are often justified and necessary for a particular design problem, at the stage of design formulation it is preferable that existing scientific data be utilized. The most widely used theoretical method is finite element analysis, but some models can include the rules for bone remodeling and use iteration to predict the final stable state. An example of an experimental method is the use of biological specimens to determine the surface strains on the bone, components, and cement, using strain gauges or photoelastic coating techniques. Cyclic load fatigue testing and long-term wear testing on joint simulators are essential parts of any implant development project. They can be considered as scientific experiments to test the hypothesis that the components will endure physiological loading conditions without failure, undue change of shape, or excessive wear. Such testing should be regarded as part of the design process as much as for final evaluation.

The degree to which human application constitutes "an experiment" depends on how many new or unknown features there are. Clinical follow-ups in humans must be regarded as a necessary part of the experimental plan to test the design hypothesis and modify the design if necessary. The reason is that it is impossible to predict complex clinical outcomes with any certainty. Herein lies an important difference between designing engineering components that can be tested under service conditions before being released generally and developing implant designs for which there is invariably an element of risk in the first implantations. Predictive methods of evaluation, where measurements taken in the short term predict the long-term outcome, are particularly valuable.

The evaluation of TKR designs requires a systematic application of the biomechanical criteria shown in Table 1.

RELIEF OF PAIN

Replacement of Articulating Surfaces

For localized lesions of the articular cartilage, restoration is feasible. If a varus or valgus deformity has not progressed too far, then redistribution of the forces by osteotomy can result in a medium- or even long-term solution. However, for severe surface destruction, there seems little alternative to a complete resurfacing with implanted components. Experience has shown that replacement of all of the bearing surfaces is needed to avoid pain and progressive degeneration. To provide data on the surface geometry of the knee, there have been a number of studies describing the sagittal femoral profiles in terms of spirals or circular arcs (37,74,111). Other studies have shown the close approximation of the posterior femoral condyles to spherical patches (53). Polynomial equations have been used to describe the entire surfaces (109), but it is only recently that accurate mapping methods capable of describing surfaces with complex geometries using surface patches (8) have been available. However, in the natural joint, the subtleties of motion that result from surface geometry are synergistic with soft tissue tensions, and it is unlikely that such a complex situation can be restored in an artificial joint. Partly for this reason, the surface geometry of TKRs has provided only a simplified representation of the complex three-dimensional shapes of the natural joint and motions of the menisci. Surface stresses are reduced in the natural knee by the menisci (1), and these are to a limited extent reproduced in meniscal bearing designs. Deformability of the menisci and the articular cartilage, which reduces stresses, is not reproduced in designs with metals, ceramics, or rigid plastics. The friction between the cartilage surfaces is insignificant but can have a major effect on the kinematics of the artificial joint.

Interface Motion

There is considerable clinical evidence that excess interface motion leads to bone resorption, component loosening, and pain (66). Interface motion can be defined as the displacements between adjacent reference points on the component and on the bone, at the femoral or tibial interfaces, in response to imposed forces across the joint. The important displacements are shear and distraction. In early studies, displacements between components and bone were measured directly or by using transducers fixed between pins or other markers fixed into the component and bone at different peripheral locations (101,103). The method was used to show the local deformations of plastic components and the peripheral distractions that occurred as a result of eccen-

tric loading. It was evident that displacements were caused by elastic deformations of both the component and the bone itself and that the nonuniformity and variability of the bone greatly influenced the results. The relative behavior of different tibial component designs, such as all-plastic versus a metal backing, a central post, two or four small side posts, and keels, was determined under a range of loading conditions (Fig. 4). For uncemented components relying on close bone apposition to achieve ingrowth, minimal interface micromotion is essential to prevent the formation of fibrous tissue. However, the unevenness of the prepared bone surfaces, amounting to 1.1 to 2.6 mm on different samples (93), and the variability of elastic properties of the cancellous bone result in greater motion than that seen with cemented components.

A similar method has been used to investigate uncemented components, showing the immediate advantages of screws in reducing implant–bone relative motion (95). One variation of the method has been to measure the displacements through holes in the component and bone to access the interface directly. A method for studying the motion at the interface at a macroscopic level was devised by Steege et al. (88), using a slab cut perpendicular to the component–bone interface. This technique recognized that the interface consisted of a complex three-dimensional geometry composed of trabeculae, intrusions of cement, and gaps. Cyclic forces were applied to the sections, and the motion was measured with a cine camera through a microscope. A complex pattern of motion at the irregular cement–bone interface was demonstrated along with crack propagation through both cement and bone itself.

Component–bone motion was actually measured during surgery by Yoshida et al. (110). For uncemented central stem components, a 200-N force applied at the posteromedial quadrant was able to produce axial compression from 30 to 270 μm and distraction from 0 to 250 μm for different component designs. Designs with screws showed the lowest displacement values. Such behavior

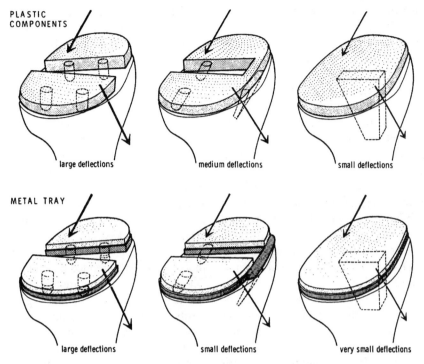

PLASTIC COMPONENTS

large deflections   medium deflections   small deflections

METAL TRAY

large deflections   small deflections   very small deflections

FIG. 4. A schematic representation of component–bone displacements, based on measurements at six locations around the periphery. One-piece metal-backed components produced the smallest displacements. (From Walker et al., ref. 101, with permission.)

can be attributed in large measure to the unevenness of the bone surface. When components that exhibited high values of relative motion were cemented, the motion was dramatically reduced.

Roentgen stereophotogrammetry (RSA) has been used successfully to study interface displacements *in vivo*. The method consists of the placement of 1-mm tantalum beads in the component and in the bone at surgery and then determining their three-dimensional coordinates from a special biplanar radiography system (84). Migration is defined as a change in component position over time, whereas implant–bone relative motion is the inducible displacement between loaded and unloaded conditions at a particular time. Displacements and rotations along and about particular axes can be calculated. The tilting of cemented and cementless tibial components was measured between standing and squatting (79). Typical inducible displacements and rotations were

0.5 mm and 1°, respectively. In squatting, a typical pattern was compression posteriorly and distraction anteriorly, displacements being higher with uncemented components. In another study, both the inducible displacements and the migrations of tibial components fixed with screws were less than for components without screws (78). Hence, the laboratory data cited above and the clinical data are consistent, adding to the accumulating evidence that well-designed laboratory studies can be predictive of clinical performance.

RESTORATION OF FUNCTION

Motion Characteristics

Motion refers to the three-dimensional behavior of the knee during specified loading conditions or during normal activities. The ideal situation is that the motion after prosthetic replacement is the same as that when the knee was in its normal intact state. To describe motion, it is necessary to establish suitable reference axes fixed in the femur, tibia, and patella. Among the different available methods, the system of Grood and Suntay (39) is particularly useful because of its ease of visualization, the inclusion of both rotations and displacements, and the analogy to the usual meaning of motions in clinical terms. The reference position is taken as 0° flexion when the long axes of the femur and tibia seen in the yz plane (sagittal) are parallel. If the femur is now flexed on the tibia, the three-dimensional motion can be described and used as a criterion for comparing the motion with a TKR implanted to normal motion. Such "passive motion" is defined as the motion that occurs when minimal forces and moments are applied to the joint. The motion can be described as a continuum of the six motion parameters (three rotations and three displacements) over time throughout the entire flexion range, although usually the parameters are plotted as a function of flexion angle.

One of the methods for determining motion under simple loading conditions is to apply a flexing moment to the knee and to equilibrate at a required angle of flexion using a force in the quadriceps (44). This method was applied in such a manner that the knee was continuously flexed and extended, and the motion parameters were recorded (77). As flexion increased from 0° to 120°, there was a posterior displacement of 8.6 mm of the femoral origin and an internal rotation of the tibia of 15°; the rate of change of these parameters was highest at zero flexion and reduced with flexion angle. The other displacements and rotations were much smaller in magnitude. The equations describing the motions as a function of flexion angle F (in degrees) were:

$$DISP = -0.128\,F + 4.796 \times 10^{-4}\,F$$

$$INTROT = 0.369\,F - 2.958 \times 10^{-3}\,F^2 + 7.660 \times 10^{-6}\,F^3$$

By calculating the lengths of the ligaments, it was found that the anterior–posterior (AP) displacement was primarily controlled by the tensions in the cruciate ligaments, whereas the axial rotation was controlled by all of the ligaments and the shape of the joint surfaces. Reproducing such motion with a TKR with close to normal sagittal profiles and preservation of both cruciate ligaments can be achieved (108). However, in the absence of the anterior collateral ligament (ACL), the AP displacement pattern is likely to be disrupted. Because the working lengths of ligaments are within a maximum of 15% strain (20), which represents only a few millimeters, it is likely to be difficult to achieve normal ligament lengths after TKR. Indeed, in gait studies, patients with an absent ACL adopt a compensatory motion pattern to reduce the flexing moment, which reduces the required quadriceps force; this is called "quad-avoidance" gait. The supposition is that reduced quadriceps force at the lower flexion angles will reduce the anterior shear force on the tibia (10).

Accurate measurement of the motion of the joint *in vivo* is difficult to do accurately. External measurement systems are subject to the well-known problem of the relative motion between the skin surface and the bones, although the motion itself may only be a few millimeters in many cases. In one study, direct measurement on normal subjects was achieved by attaching pins to the bones themselves (55). An average internal–external rotation range of 8° and an anterior–posterior translation of 10 mm during the stance phase of gait were recorded. In another study on normal subjects and on TKR patients, motion was measured using a three-space tracker system mounted on tightly fitting orthotic devices (32). For patients with a condylar replacement of moderate constraint, the AP displacement of the femoral origin relative to the tibia ranged from 9 to 14 mm during different activities, while the internal–external rotation range was 5° to 10°. The motion magnitudes were found to be similar to normal, but there was a much greater variation with the TKR patients, presumably reflecting the variable component sizes and placements and ligament tensions. Using the maximum flexion angle of the knee during stair ascending and descending as the variable, Andriacchi et al. (3,4) found that TKRs that preserved both cruciate ligaments were similar to the normal knee. At the other extreme, TKRs in which both cruciates were resected (total condylar, posterior stabilized) showed a much smaller flexion angle, and the angles of the limb segments and the body as a whole in the sagittal plane were abnormal so as to reduce the flexion moment on the knee. This was considered to be caused by a more anterior contact point on the tibial surface, which reduced the lever arm of the quadriceps.

Soft Tissue Lengths

Figure 5 shows some basic geometric factors that affect soft tissue lengths. A computer model of the knee with a TKR inserted was used to predict the motion as a function of several design variables (37). For tibial surfaces with relatively small sagittal radii, posterior displacement was reduced, and the maximum flexion was reduced in response to excessive tension in the posterior collateral ligament (PCL). When the tibial components had a larger sagittal radius or were sloped posteriorly, the motion became closer to normal. A further effect of the tension in the PCL relates to the level of the "joint line." It is common for this to be elevated at surgery because of the use of a thicker tibial component than the amount of bone resected. In cadaveric experiments (25), the maximum flexion angle was reduced with elevation in the joint line as a result of premature tightening of the PCL. When the PCL was resected, the flexion angle increased. Reduc-

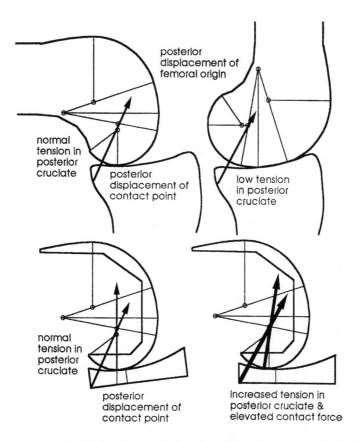

FIG. 5. Variables concerned with design, cruciate retention or absence, and surgical placement, which can affect the relative femoral–tibial position during functions.

tion of the height of the patella, corresponding to an elevation of the joint line, was also found to adversely affect stair climbing (69). The moments around the knee were significantly reduced, which is likely to be associated with a reduced quadriceps lever arm because of abnormal tracking on the patellar flange.

In flexion–extension of patients' knees under no load, knees with the PCL preserved showed the same internal–external rotation as in normal knees, whereas with the PCL absent, there was no rotation (48). In rising from a chair and sitting, implants with either preservation or sacrifice of the PCL showed rotation, but only half that of the normal knee. Hence, the rotational behavior is likely to be influenced by muscle directions as well as by the effect of the axial compressive forces on the asymmetric joint surfaces. Regarding AP translation, the tibial origin moved posteriorly in the first 30° of flexion regardless of the implant type and loading conditions. This was attributed to the femoral component remaining at the bottom of the tibial dish, the larger distal radius in early flexion promoting the posterior tibial displacement. Subsequently, there was no anterior tibial displacement, which would indicate femoral rollback in the absence of the PCL or with a loose PCL. Obviously, a tight PCL would induce rollback, indicating the dependence on surgical placement of the components. Experiments by Soudry et al. (86) illustrated the relative effects of the tibial surface geometry and the presence or absence of the PCL on the contact points. Preservation of the PCL maintained more central contact and reduced the "rocking moment" in the sagittal plane. Resection of the PCL resulted in anterior contact points and high anterior rocking moments in certain loading conditions. This has been counteracted with the posteriorly stabilized types of TKR.

It is thus evident that soft tissue lengths play a major role in the mechanics of the knee. Although most of the studies related to TKR have concentrated on the PCL, other soft tissue structures are likely to have an equally important effect. This was studied in relation to knee brace design, where the imposition of abnormal motion on a knee re-sulted in abnormal lengths and tensions in all of the major ligaments (104). In surgical practice, this has been well recognized, and the usual procedure is now to obtain the best possible component placements and soft tissue tensions using advanced instrumentation and to modify any obvious deficiencies by ligament releases.

Laxity Characteristics

Laxity is an important method of characterizing the knee joint. It essentially describes the force–displacement or torque–rotation relationships, the most relevant to TKR being the anterior–posterior (AP) and the internal–external rotational laxities. The magnitude of the laxity is defined between force limits, while the slope of the curve is defined as the stiffness (59). Around the neutral point, the stiffness is low, which can be related to the load-deflection characteristics of the restraining ligaments and other soft tissues, the initial lengths of the ligaments, which can be less than that necessary to generate forces, and the geometric orientation of the ligaments such that the applied displacements result in small length changes. For this reason the "neutral" position of the joint at any flexion angle is difficult to define because of its sensitivity to small forces. One way of addressing this is to measure the "envelope of motion" between defined torque or force limits (11). In this way, the need to identify this neutral position is avoided. The force–displacement curves have been found to vary with the flexion angle: the highest stiffnesses occur at zero flexion; stiffness reduces with flexion and remains reasonably constant after about 30° flexion.

The concept of "coupled motions" must be accounted for in the definition of the force–displacement curves (72). If the other degrees of freedom are held constant, the magnitudes of the displacements and the stiffnesses are greater than if the other degrees of freedom are unconstrained. Piziali et al. (72) proposed that the laxity characteristics could be described by a matrix of the form $F = Ku$, where F represents the input forces and moments, K the stiffness matrix, and u the displacement vector.

The inverse form of this equation is more relevant if displacements are required, but the form shown is more easily determined from an experimental point of view. A similar approach was adopted by Loch et al. (57), who recognized the problems of the nonlinear nature of the stiffness and hence chose to determine the constants in the stiffness matrix in a small region around an equilibrium position.

The presence of an axial force across the joint has been found to have an important effect on the laxity curves. In general, whether in AP or rotational tests, the magnitude of the laxity has reduced and the stiffness has increased as a result of the presence of axial force (46,58,106). This can be regarded as an important protective mechanism that reduces the forces in the ligaments and other soft tissues. This effect has been attributed primarily to the concavity of the upper tibia on the medial side and to a lesser extent to the increased constraint from the menisci, the friction at the bearing surfaces, and the deformation of the surfaces. As will be described, the effect of compressive force on laxity and stability has major implications for TKR design.

It can be seen that many studies such as those above are retrospective in that they compare the laxity characteristics of TKR with normal. In an early study (105), an attempt was made to specifically design the radii of the artificial surfaces in order to provide the normal laxity characteristics. In this case, it was assumed that the surfaces would transmit the shear forces and torques (as well as the axial forces), and the radii were calculated to produce the normal laxities. The surfaces were generally similar to those shown in Fig. 2. In a later study (96), this concept of surface design was expanded to include the normal translations and rotations as well as the laxities, resulting in more complex surface geometries (Fig. 6). Such a study was considered to provide a rational approach, given that a wide range of AP and rotary laxities were measured for contemporary TKRs (92).

However, such studies do not account for a number of other factors such as soft tissue restraint and friction at the joint surfaces. These factors were included in studies in which laxity was measured on patients with different designs of TKR. Carrying out a Lachman test at ± 100 N on patients with total knees ranging from low to high constraint gave anterior–posterior displacements of 5 to 11 mm (89). These investigators also measured internal–external rotation at ± 5 Nm and obtained ranges from 40° to 50° at 20° flexion. In another study under similar test conditions, anterior–posterior displacements of only 5 to 7 mm were recorded (107). Testing patients with total knees of moderate to high constraint under half body weight and ± 100 N shear force produced anterior–posterior displacements of 6 to 8 mm, which were 25% to 35% less than under a zero-load condition (97). Testing the prosthetic components themselves under one body weight compression reduced the displacements to only 1 to 3 mm. The data were extrapolated to functional conditions to provide estimates of 3 to 5 mm for level walking and 4 to 7 mm for stair activities. A theoretical analysis indicated that the friction between the bearing surfaces significantly reduced the anterior–posterior displacements. This effect was extreme when small acrylic particles were trapped between the surfaces, reducing the displacements to about 1 mm. These studies demonstrate that the anterior–posterior displacements are reduced not only by the compressive force but also by friction. In addition, the indication is that under functional loads, for moderate to high constraint designs of knee replacement, the displacements are sufficiently small because of the condylar geometry and the friction, that soft tissue restraints would play a minor role. At the same time, it is important to recognize that the soft tissue restraints would be important in the unloaded phases of gait and other activities.

DURABILITY

Interface and Bone Stresses

The ideal situation is one in which the stresses in the bone around the implant components are the same as those in the intact joint. However, this goal needs to be seen in

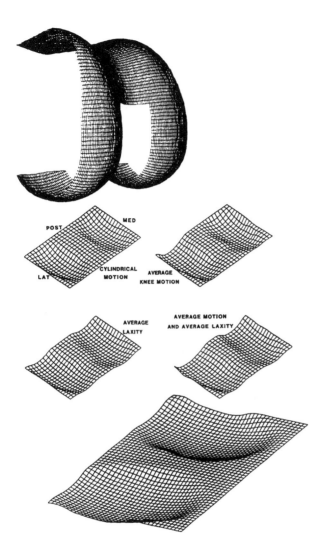

FIG. 6. Surface geometry of tibial surface generated by computer, based on the required motions and laxities, given an initial femoral surface geometry. (From Walker, ref. 96, with permission.)

relation to the pathologic status of the knee. Because of the arthritic process, the geometry and the properties of the femur, tibia, and patella are substantially modified. In a typical osteoarthritic knee with varus deformity, there is a depression on the medial side of the tibia, dense subchondral bone medially, and porotic bone laterally. Even after TKR and re-alignment of the limb, the bone density does not revert to normal in up to 2 years of follow-up, although there is some increase in density of the previously "unloaded" side (47). Hence, analyses of the effects of tibial components that use bone properties of a normal knee must be seen in this light.

One of the most widely used types of tibial component design uses a flat plate covering the tibial surface with a central peg for stabilization. A two-dimensional finite element analysis (FEA) model was used to compare the bone stesses among no peg, a standard peg, and a long peg, as well as the effect of metal backing (65). The results were particularly significant under conditions of loading on one condyle only (Fig. 7). For an all-plastic component, without a peg, the bone stresses resembled normal. With a central peg, the stresses were reduced under the plate because of some force transmission down the length of the peg, the effect being

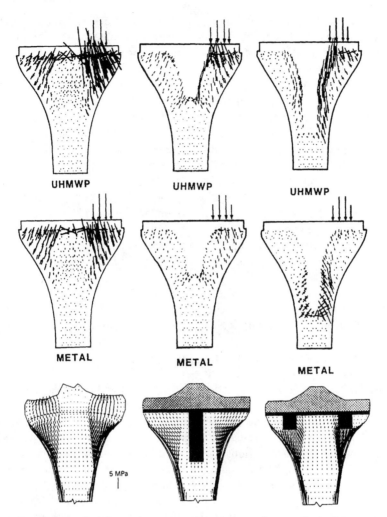

FIG. 7. Top row, maximum tensile and compressive stresses for an all-plastic component. **Middle row,** as above for a metal tray component. **Bottom row,** as above for intact tibia, and two metal tray component designs. (Adapted from Vasu et al., ref. 94, with permission.)

more pronounced with the longer peg. For a metal backing, the effect was to reduce the stresses on the loaded side by creating a more uniform distribution around the entire component, but with the long peg, there was considerable proximal stress protection because of the proximity of the lower end of the stem to cortical bone. Such results are dependent on other variables such as the assumed thickness of the cortical bone, especially in the extreme proximal region, and whether the component covers this rim. In the latter case, cancellous bone stresses are reduced for metal backing but not for an all-plastic component.

Experimental data can also be used to demonstrate how proximal cortical strains vary with component design. Bourne and Finlay (19) and Reilly et al. (75) found that a metal plate that completely covered the upper surface produced normal strains. However, when cortical contact was absent, there were reduced stresses in the cortical bone, suggesting overstressing of cancellous bone. Central metal stems reduce stresses in the proximal cortex in a pronounced way for a stem that reaches the cortex. Hence, to achieve the goal of normal cancellous and cortical bone stresses proximally, the ideal would appear to be a metal-backed design that covers the upper surface and with a central stem in the region of 30 mm in length. However, a metal component without rim contact and with a bulky or long stem would run the risk of seriously reduced peripheral stresses. All-plastic components carry the risk of overstressing the cancellous bone, and the consequences of this have been observed clinically. Another condition that can exacerbate proximal stress protection for an uncemented central stem is one in which the stem is rigidly fixed and the plateau surface is unfixed, such as would occur with a fibrous tissue interface (27). This situation can also apply to a cemented component where there is good cement penetration around the peg but poor penetration on the surface.

Another component design that has become widely used is the metal tray type with two or four short posts. Vasu et al. (94) carried out an FEA study of this type and found that there were higher than normal bone stresses in the region of the ends of the posts, with some stress protection in other regions, including peripherally (Fig. 7). These authors went on to show that an epiphyseal-based design had more favorable bone and interface stresses. However, some authors have pointed out that the optimum design would be one in which the stiffness of the upper plate would be intermediate between that made from all plastic or metal and could even have a variable stiffness over the surface (42).

Interface shear stresses and the stresses in the cement are a further consideration with any design, and these are generally higher for components of lower stiffness (34). Higher cement stresses especially occur with eccentric loading. Slight increases occur if the component does not completely cover the bone surface. Under physiological loading conditions, cracks are found in the cement mantle, primarily in association with voids or inclusions (38). Voids are more prone to crack propagation, which indicates that vacuum mixing and other techniques that remove bubbles are an advantage. Anecdotally, tibial components removed for loosening or infection do not show evidence of fragmentation of the cement mantle, although no systematic study has been reported. The conditions for an ideal cement mantle involve adequate penetration into cancellous bone to achieve a strong shear and tensile bond and adequate thickness at the surface to avoid cracking (52). In any analytic approach, the work of Angelides et al. (6) regarding the appropriate elements to use at boundaries should be noted.

Although reduced stresses are likely to lead to osteopenia, there is evidence that excessive stress at the interface can lead to bone resorption. It is notable that such a phenomenon needs to be viewed at a local level, where the implant, including cement, shares interfaces with individual trabeculae over a boundary of complex geometry. For example, resorption has been viewed as a process of bone replacement by fibrous tissue where relative motion is also present and includes progressive trabecular microfracture and local bone densification associated with local healing. In a gross sense, interface bone resorption has been detected for all components studied, as evidenced by a relative change of position between component and bone over time. Such a phenomenon is vitally important to the definition of fixation. Because bone resorption inevitably occurs around components, successful fixation must now be regarded as resorption and change in component position at a tolerable level that reaches an asymptotic limit at a reasonable time period.

The relative motion phenomenon has been studied in detail using roentgen stereophotogrammetry (RSA), developed by Selvik (84). In a key study, the migration patterns of the same design of TKR were compared over 2 years for cemented and uncemented (porous coated) applications used in RA and OA patients (67). The tibial component design was a Tricon M with a metal plate and two plastic posts. The relative motions were measured along and about a Cartesian axis system, and the maximum motion of any point and the maximum vertical lift-off of a peripheral point were determined (Fig. 8).

The typical behavior with all of these measurements was a migration rate that decreased with time, almost reaching zero at 1 to 2 years. The maximum migration distances were around 1 mm but were less than 0.5 mm along the individual axes. The rotations were just under 1°. The method has been used in a number of studies to compare different designs or design features and has been found to be exceedingly sensitive. A striking finding has been that components for which the migration reached a limit were clinically successful in subsequent follow-up, whereas when the migration rate was continuous up to 2 years, there was almost invariably symptomatic failure subsequently. This migration method, which has been used in hips as well as knees, is an invaluable method for identifying potentially unsatisfactory component designs at a short follow-up time.

Wear and Damage of the Articulating Surfaces

In metal–plastic condylar replacement designs, in order to allow for adequate AP and rotational laxity, and because of the reduced sagittal femoral radius in flexion, there is only partial conformity of the bearing surfaces, which results in higher than ideal stresses. In this situation, wear and mechanical damage of the plastic are an important concern. An indication of the severity of the plastic wear and the relative amounts of different types of wear can be obtained from retrieval studies (14,15, 22,56). The studies by Blunn et al. (15) comprised over 300 retrievals of a range of knee designs obtained from a number of European centers. Over a third of the cases had a follow-up in the range of 10 to 20 years.

Three main types of wear were observed on the plastic. The first was adhesive wear, occurring at local contact points between the metal and the plastic. Typically this generated small particles and shreds in the range 0.1 to 10 μm as well as thin sheets up to about 10 μm in width. Abrasive wear resulted from the cutting of the plastic surface by hard points on the femoral surface or by particles. In two-body abrasion, the roughness is integral with the hard surface, such as a carbide inclusion or a scratch. In three-body abrasion, interposed particles of metal, acrylic cement, bone, or other material cause the surface cutting. Fi-

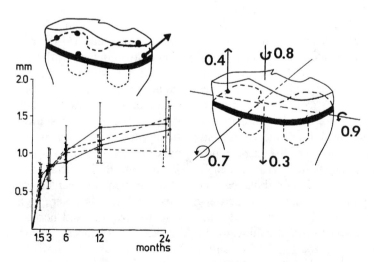

FIG. 8. The maximum total point motion (MTPM) plotted over time for OA and RA cases and the migrations (mm) and rotations (degrees) about the three axes are shown at 2 years. (Adapted from Nilsson et al., ref.67, with permission.)

nally, there was delamination wear, which is a fatigue phenomenon in which high subsurface stresses lead to cracks propagating within the plastic, the cracks eventually coalescing and reaching the surface. This typically resulted in surface destruction to depths of several millimeters, even down to the metal baseplate.

In many tibial components, especially of low to moderate conformity, a well-defined wear area was observed, often appearing shiny with fine scratches. This type of wear was both adhesive and abrasive. The depression at the surface was partly from deformation occurring early in use, when the high contact stresses exceeded the yield point of the plastic. The surface wear then proceeded steadily over time in proportion to the applied compressive force and the sliding distance. The rate of wear was usually much smaller than for hip replacement, probably because of the lower sliding distances involved during typical gait cycles. Based on scanning electron microscope (SEM) studies of retrieved specimens, the surface wear occurred at microscopic adhesive points. When there was sufficient boundary lubrication, the plastic surface displayed fine ripples with spacing from 2 to 10 µm, the contact points being at the peaks of these ripples. Thin sections viewed under polarized light, showed that there was a buildup of strain energy at these contact points to a depth of 40 µm (23). When this energy reached a critical level, particles were released from the surface. This type of wear resulted in very small particles and shreds, of around 1 µm and less in size, consistent with the study of Schmalzried et al. (82).

When the lubrication was less effective, as with "dilute" synovial fluid, the contact involved much larger areas of the surface, producing surface skins or sheets around 1 to 10 µm in thickness (16). These skins became progressively detached from the underlying surface and frequently fragmented into smaller regions, sometimes attaching to the femoral component in the form of a transfer film. A number of studies have shown that surface wear of this type can be reduced by using a femoral surface that is harder than

cobalt-chrome and that has a lower contact angle, making the surface more wettable (16,26). Examples of such materials are the ceramics aluminum oxide and zirconium oxide. The surface is more resistant to becoming scratched, which decreases abrasive wear (26), and the transfer films and adhesive wear are much less pronounced. This correlates with the finding in the laboratory that small increases in surface roughness of the hard counterface lead to a large increase in the wear of the polymer (30).

However, the most severe type of wear was delamination, causing destruction of the plastic to a depth of several millimeters. The important characteristic of delamination is that it is time dependent, and it is misleading to judge the wear resistance of a particular design in a relatively short-term follow-up. The earliest visible sign of delamination is an opaque region or blister, indicative of subsurface cracking but at this stage not involving the surface. Typical sections through a delaminating area of plastic show multiple cracks oriented horizontally and then curving upward toward the surface (Fig. 9). The subsurface cracks can be related to the stresses and strains within the material. Polarized light microscopy of thin sections of plastic showed that a region of high residual shear stress occurred below the surface, usually between 1 and 2 mm, the region where the cracks originated (14). For cylindrical or spherical contacts, the principal shear stresses are of magnitude 0.3 times the maximum surface contact stress and occur at a depth of 0.4 times the total contact width (50). In the example shown, with a 6-mm-thick plastic component, the depth of the maximum Von Mises stress is approximately 2 mm beneath the surface (Fig.10). The maximum principal direct stresses also occur on this midline. However, high shear stresses oriented parallel and perpendicularly to the surface occur beneath the edge of the contact, oriented at 90° to the horizontal, with magnitude and depth similar to those noted above. For tractive forces over the surface under sliding conditions, the magnitude of the shear

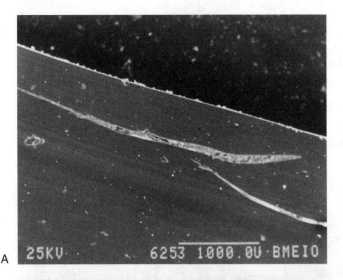

A

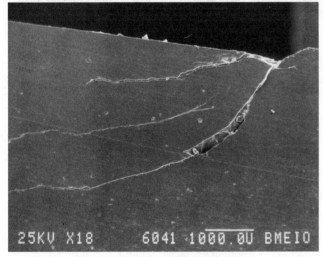

B

FIG. 9. Typical sections through the plastic in a region showing an impending blister at the surface. The subsurface cracks and intergranular defects are evident.

stress on the midaxis increases, and the region moves toward the surface (90).

In such a sliding situation, a particular location under the surface experiences first a shear stress at the leading end of the contact oriented parallel to the xz axes. When the location is under the center of the contact area, the shear stress is oriented at 45° to the horizontal. Finally, with further sliding, the orientation of the shear stress at the trailing end of the contact area is along the xz axes in an opposite direction to that at the leading edge. This cycle of subsurface shear stresses is analogous to reverse bending, which is the

most deleterious condition for initiation and propagation of a crack.

The radial tensile stresses on the surface of the plastic just outside the contact zone are also of significance. The magnitude of the stress is 0.13 times the maximum contact stress, but this increases at the trailing edge in sliding or tractive rolling conditions. It is likely that these stresses are responsible for the cracks that are frequently observed at the plastic surface because they contribute to the fragmentation of surface filaments and skins. However, of relevance to delamination wear is the fact that these surface cracks can coalesce with the sub-

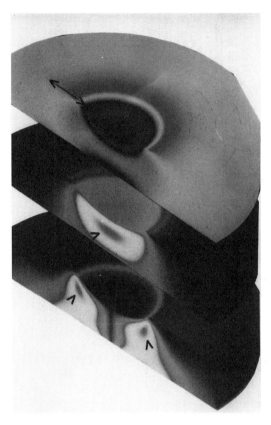

FIG. 10. The stresses in a 6-mm layer of plastic for a spherical contact where the relative radii of curvature are representative of a TKR in flexion. **Top,** maximum radial tensile stress at the surface; **center,** maximum Von Mises stress directly below the center of contact; **bottom,** maximum shear stress on the section, beneath the edge of the contact. (Analysis and graphics by S. Culligan, *Biomedical Engineering.*)

surface cracks to release large particles of plastic. Several authors have calculated the effect of the femoral and tibial component geometries on the maximum surface and subsurface stresses. The elevation of stresses in an elastic layer on a rigid substrate has been known for some time (61). For the particular configuration of an Insall–Burstein knee, Bartel et al. (9) used an elasticity solution to compute the changes in surface stress with plastic thickness. For unit stresses with a 10-mm-thick plastic layer, the stresses for 8-mm and 6-mm thick-

nesses were 1.09 and 1.26, respectively. However, the relative geometry of the femoral and tibial surfaces plays a major role in determining the contact stresses (Fig. 11). When the femoral and tibial radii differed by 5 mm in both planes (avoiding complete conformity), the stress was minimum. With this minimum value defined as unity, increasing the plastic radius towards infinite (flat) in either plane led to a 1.8 stress value. A completely flat plastic produced a 2.3 stress value. Hence, it is apparent that the relative radii of curvature can have a much greater effect on the surface (and subsurface) stresses than the thickness of the plastic layer. This was further illustrated by Jin et al. (49) in an elasticity analysis of TKRs modeled as elliptical bodies in contact (Fig. 12).

In retrieval specimens, polyethylene without visible defects was rarely seen to have cracks or delamination wear, even for flat plastic components, and hence, at least for the follow-up times considered, in order for the subsurface stresses to produce delamination wear, there needs to be a site for the initiation of cracks. There is good evidence that these sites are intergranular defects where inadequate bonding has taken place between polyethylene granules during the extrusion or molding processes (14,22,56). In retrieved specimens, localized regions of high shear strain can be seen around the corner points of these granules, from which cracks can be seen to emanate. Once a crack has initiated in this way, it can propagate using the energy provided at the crack tip by the cyclic stresses (31). Multiple cracks can occur if there are sufficient numbers of defects in the regions of high shear stress.

Another processing defect known to result in early delamination is hot-pressing, where the surface of the component is compressed under high temperature, causing the material to flow to form the surface shape. This produces a level below the surface where the material properties abruptly change, resulting in an increased propensity for subsurface cracking (13).

The potential adverse effects of γ-irradiation on UHMWPE were pointed out as early as 1979 (68). These authors identified oxida-

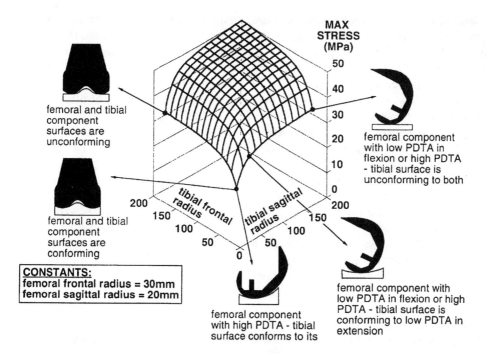

FIG. 11. Calculated values of maximum contact stress for a spectrum of relative radii of curvature. A thick plastic layer and constant modulus were assumed. (From Sathasivam and Walker, ref. 80, with permission.)

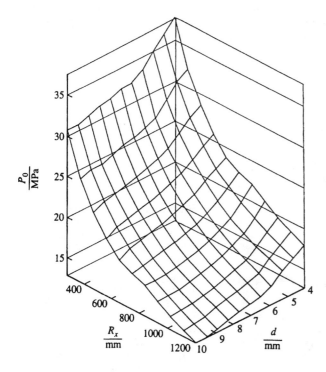

FIG. 12. A general elasticity contact theory applied to elliptical contacts relevant to TKR, showing the much greater effect of the relative radius of curvature R_x compared with plastic thickness d, on the maximum contact stress P_0. (From Jin et al., ref. 49, with permission.)

tive degradation, cross-linking, and exposure of carbonyl groups, leading to fluid absorption and reduced fatigue strength. This work was expanded on (76) to show the increased crystallinity and density that occurred with oxidation and the continuing process over time. These phenomena have been studied in much greater detail recently, and their significance to TKR has been highlighted. Very large increases in elastic modulus for only small increases in density were measured, which could significantly increase the contact stresses at and below the surface (54). The increase in oxidation with shelf time was also determined (18) and was associated with a severalfold elevation of wear rates (35).

Evidence for the validity of the above concerns has been shown in studies of sections of retrieved components (Fig. 13). On most components, there is a band of high oxidation peaking at about 1 mm below the surface, due to the gamma-irradiation process. Subsurface cracks oriented horizontally have been observed to occur beneath this oxidized layer, which approximately coincides in depth with the level of the maximum shear stresses. These two factors, particularly if combined with subsurface defects, lead to rapid propa-

gation of multiple subsurface cracks. At the edges of the contact region, the cracks curve upwards towards the surface, to meet cracks emanating from the surface. It is evident that this process can lead to complete fragmentation of the surface layer of plastic.

In addition to material properties, mechanical factors play a major role in wear behavior. In designs in which the frontal plane geometry is flat, under varus–valgus moments, edge loading with high stresses can occur. This can have serious consequences when the polyethylene is thin and where there is no metallic rail to restrain the plastic peripherally. It can lead to tensile cracks at the sides that can result in large fragments being broken off (40). Another disadvantage of flat plastic surfaces with low constraint is that the contact point locations during activities are both variable and unpredictable. Although the ideal contact region is in the middle third of the plastic surface, small variations of tibial slope or posterior cruciate tension can result in abnormal contact locations and excessive sliding motions (7). The sliding results from anterior–posterior or internal–external rotation. This produces extensive wear over the surface as well as severe wear damage at the anterior or posterior of the plas-

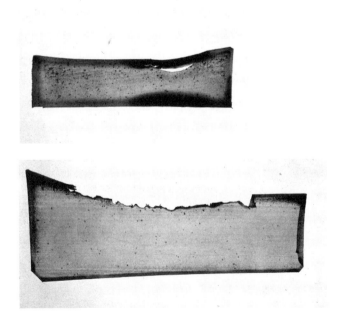

FIG. 13. Sections through retrieved plastic tibial components. The sections have been soaked in chlorosulfonic acid, which stains oxidized material. Note in top right, the region of maximum oxidation is below the surface consistent with γ-irradiation and exposure to air. **Top:** A subsurface crack has developed immediately beneath the oxidized (high-density, high-modulus) layer. **Bottom:** The surface has completely delaminated down to the lower level of the oxidized region.

tic. Wear studies on specimens have highlighted the increased wear caused by sliding, which is greatly reduced under rolling or when the contact point is in the same location (17).

At the other end of the spectrum, designs that have high constraint and hence large contact areas and low contact stresses have also exhibited delamination wear. The reason appears to be that high constraint prevents the natural movements of the joint from occurring. Thus, even though the condylar surfaces are providing more than adequate stability, this is at the expense of very high stresses on the plastic surface at the extremes of motion. Another exacerbating factor is that stresses are even higher if the components are not ideally aligned at surgery. Retrieval studies have shown that delamination can also occur in the intercondylar notch, a region that can resist internal or external rotation if it is improperly positioned (51). Because of the small width of the notch and the small and unconforming femoral and tibial radii, very high contact forces and stresses are developed. Sections viewed under polarized light show that high deformation stresses exist below the intercondylar radius, and these are clearly associated with subsurface cracks.

RELIABILITY

This is a most important functional criterion that has a major influence on the number of failures that occur, not because of the TKR design itself but because of variations in usage. These variations include the surgical placement and the patient's kinetics and activities. In general terms, TKR designs of both low and high constraint are less reliable than those in the middle range. Instrumentation systems with multiple parts and adjustments are more prone to technical errors by less experienced surgeons. Hinged designs are probably the most reliable from the point of view of achieving accurate alignment and stability, but their frequent use is avoided because a failure results in a major loss of bone. Reliability has received relatively little direct attention. However, it will assume a much greater importance in future because of health service

requirements of low cost and the use of products with a proven record.

DESIGN SYNTHESIS USING COMPUTER MODELS

An important potential method for TKR design is a computer knee model. Previous models have varied in their complexity and form and have included condylar and ligament geometries, soft tissue and bearing surface material properties, and muscle actions (5,12,24, 33,37,109). The equilibrium position of the femur on the tibia has been determined by equilibrium methods (12,109), by imposing defined motion parameters (37), by a minimum-energy method (33), or by a stochastic process (62). None of the above models takes friction into account, primarily because their main application was to the normal intact knee, where friction is small. However, in total knee replacements, the frictional forces are likely to attenuate the shear forces significantly.

In a recently developed knee model (81), the bearing surfaces of condylar replacement knees were defined using geometric parameters, notably the linear dimensions and the radii of curvature in the frontal and sagittal planes together with the locations of the centers of curvature (Fig. 2). Meshes of any required density were then generated to describe the surfaces. Coordinate systems were fixed in the femur and the tibia, coincident in extension, such that the transverse axis passed through the lowest points on the lateral and medial tibial surfaces and the anterior–posterior axis perpendicular to the long axis of the tibia. With the knee in extension, the lowest points on the lateral and medial femoral surfaces were located at the lowest points on the tibial surface. The tibial surface was considered fixed, and the femoral surface moved relatively. The applied forces and moments were defined relative to the tibial axis system and applied to the femoral component. For a given set of input forces and moments as a function of time, small time increments were chosen, and the equilibrium femoral–tibial position was determined using a modified Gauss–Seidel method.

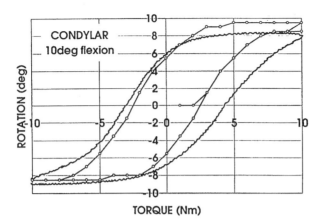

FIG. 14. Force–displacement curves for a TKR of moderate conformity for a simple AP drawer test at ±300 N. The curves show the agreement between the theory and the data from a knee-simulating machine.

The effects of friction and soft tissue restraint were found to be extremely important, such that to neglect these effects would result in major errors. For a simple AP laxity test, the predicted force–displacement and torque–rotation curves are shown in Fig. 14.

The close agreement between the data from the computer model and a knee simulator is evident. The finding that there was no displacement when the force direction changed, indicated by the flat lines at the top and bottom of the curves, resulted from friction, causing the surfaces to "stick" until there was sufficient force in the opposite direction to cause movement again. The friction itself considerably reduced the magnitudes of the laxity. The effect of the soft tissue restraints depended on the inherent constraint of the TKR. For designs of moderate constraint, there was only around 20% reduction in AP displacement by

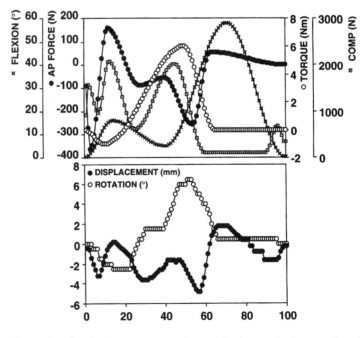

FIG. 15. Typical input data for the forces, moments, and flexion angle for a gait cycle. (Data from J. P. Paul.)

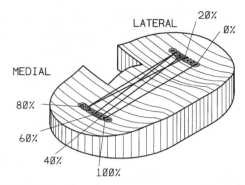

FIG. 16. Predicted contact pattern on the tibial surface for a moderately conforming condylar replacement with friction and soft tissue restraint accounted for. (Generated by S. Sathasivam, *Biomedical Engineering*.)

the restraints. However, for a design of low constraint, e.g., with a sagittal tibial radius of 120 mm, there was a 50% reduction.

The model could also be used to predict femoral–tibial motion and contact points for activity cycles (Fig. 15). In this example, the surfaces of a moderately constrained design were modeled using the mesh. Input of the gait cycle resulted in a complex response pattern of displacements and rotations that produced a changing contact pattern over the tibial surface (Fig. 16). Between successive increments, the motion was sliding, pure rolling, or tractive rolling. Each type of motion produced its own type of surface interaction, which would affect the wear. In addition, the changing pattern of stresses beneath the contact points would determine the likelihood of subsurface cracking and delamination. An addition to this approach is to compute the stresses in the plastic at each position, thereby producing a composite picture from which a wear probability index could be determined. This software has had a practical application for the design and manufacture of customized knees (Fig. 17) in which the anatomy is so abnormal that standard knee designs are not applicable. The surface-generating software was extended to include all surfaces of the components, while special CNC code enabled the parts to be manufactured from stainless steel.

TESTING METHODS

Mechanical Testing

Mechanical testing is an essential part of the design process. Such testing can also be regarded as one of many ways in which a TKR is characterized and evaluated. In princi-

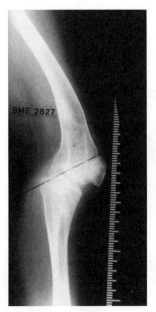
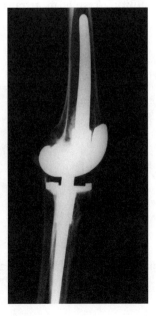

A,B

FIG. 17. The computer model applied to the design and manufacture of a customized stabilizer TKR for a patient with severely abnormal anatomy. (Produced by S. Sathasivam, *Biomedical Engineering*.)

ple, this requires the imposition of physiological forces and moments for an appropriate number of cycles. Fracture of tibial baseplates has been a problem with certain designs, and although it can be prevented today, consideration of this issue with each new design is necessary. Fracture of the femoral component has been rare, although a late failure mode has emerged whereby bone resorption behind the posterior femoral condyle has resulted in fracture-inducing increases in stresses in the metal. Fractures have been encountered in hinged designs, usually of the axle itself, of the axle mountings on the tibial component, or of the intramedullary stem. Most often these have occurred when the patient has been heavy or very active or where the gait pattern had led to high varus or hyperextension moments. Plastic tibial inserts of condylar replacements have fractured, usually in thin and relatively flat designs, and stabilizer posts have gradually eroded and eventually fractured. Polyethylene fractures or gross deformities have even occurred in mobile bearing designs as a result of excessive overhang of the plastic beyond its track or from inadequate femoral–tibial stability.

There is a need for a generalized approach to a complete and methodical evaluation of implant designs. Testing to failure by the application of a single force is of limited utility because most of the failure modes such as plastic deformation or fatigue fracture involve the effects of repetitive loading. Hence, the baseline test should be to apply a cyclic force to components mounted so that appropriate combinations of forces and moments are applied (Fig. 18). If the force is applied offset and inclined to an axis system defined in the tibia, this results in forces and moments about each of the three axes. The magnitude of the force and the dimensional parameters can be determined from the available data on forces and moments at the knee, although the values to be used need to be carefully specified. Each patient has a different weight, activity level, gait pattern, and bone quality, and the available *in vivo* data, especially for the forces and moments in a range of activities, are limited. Specifying the test requires a statistical statement of the "performance index" that is being tested, whether representative of the "average patient" or of a certain upper percentile. A standard test could also include the majority of the cycles representative of walking, but with time periods representing other activities.

If the applied force is offset and inclined, the major loading component should be vertical and typically have a magnitude of three times body weight. The AP shear component results in a translation of the femoral–tibial

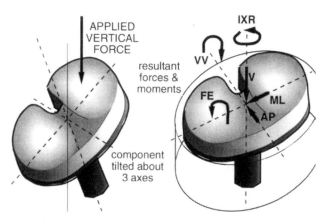

FIG. 18. The basis for a mechanical testing arrangement using a uniaxial cyclic force. The component is displaced and rotated relative to the force vector to achieve the required magnitudes of the forces and moments.

contact point posterior of center, possibly deforming plastic in that region. The medial-lateral shear component can cause gradual subluxation because of plastic deformation. A medial offset to the force giving a varus moment produces typically higher medial than lateral force, which can lead to tibial tray fracture or deformation of plastic. An increase in the varus moment, such as to cause lift-off, tests the strength of the axles or posts in superstabilized designs. The internal–external torque increases the posterior position of the femoral condyle on one side, leading to deformation of plastic and other problems as a result. For linked designs, a hyperextension moment tests the mechanical stops, which have shown problems in some designs.

The number of cycles of loading should reflect a realistic time of service, typically at least 10 years. Based on data from Seedhom and Wallbridge (83), the average subject makes 1.8 million steps per year, and hence a standard test should apply 20 million loading cycles. If heating or viscoelastic effects are not a major consideration, testing can be carried out at say 5 Hz, giving a continuous testing time of 46 days for 10 years' simulation. Regarding the practical test arrangement, this can be accomplished with a single-axis cyclic load machine, preferably multichannel. The tibial component or femoral–tibial component assembly is inclined about three axes and displaced in the horizontal plane so as to produce the required values of the forces and moments. In order to allow for elastic deformation and progressive deformation of materials, there needs to be suitable lack of constraint of the mounting of the components.

Simplified Wear Testing

If a TKR utilizes new or improved materials, wear testing is required, for which a screening test using a simplifed mechanical arrangement is applicable. Clarke (21) reviewed the early methods for wear screening. One of these methods used the curved side of a rotating metal disk loaded against a flat plastic disk, resulting in a contact area that increased, and hence a contact pressure that decreased, with time. Reduction of pressure with time also occurred in other methods such as where a reciprocating metal toroid was loaded against a dished plastic specimen (98). A standard method for total joints was developed by McKellop and others (60) in which a polymeric pin was loaded against a reciprocating metal plate with bovine serum as lubricant. The contact pressure in this standard test was only 3.5 MPa, however, and therefore more applicable to hips than to knees. In addition, even though the frictional shear stress changed direction in each cycle, the same area of plastic slid across the metal track, as opposed to periodic loading of the plastic, which would have been more representative of total knee designs. Both Clarke (21) and McKellop (60) pointed out that there could be no universal method suitable for joints as different as the hip and the knee, and hence, it would seem necessary to develop a simple wear model that would apply specifically to knees. The importance of this was shown by the different sizes and morphologies of wear particles between the hip and the knee (82), and a review of the types of surface damage and a means for quantifying them has recently been done (43). The criteria for such a test method are that the geometry and kinematic conditions resemble those of total knee replacements and that the wear and damage patterns on the bearing surfaces and the morphology and size of the wear particles be comparable with *in vivo* data.

Recently, a test method has been proposed as being representative of the wear conditions in TKR (100). The test consisted of an axially loaded metallic femoral indentor and a reciprocating ultrahigh-molecular-weight polyethylene (UHMWPE) flat disk that represented the tibial component (Fig. 19). The relative radii of curvature in combination with the applied force produce similar contact stresses to that calculated for *in vivo* conditions. To validate the method, a number of the test parameters were varied to determine their effects on the wear and surface damage: these parame-

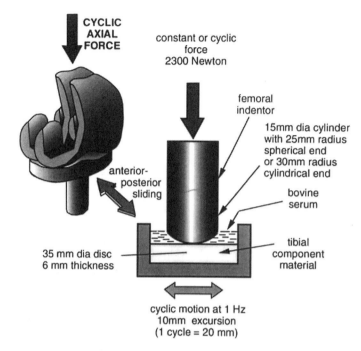

FIG. 19. A simplified wear test applicable to TKR for screening of new material pairs.

ters included the effect of conformity by vary-ing the radii of the femoral surface, use of dis-tilled water or serum as a lubricant, different femoral materials, and different types of UHMWPE. The different morphologies of the surface wear of the UHMWPE were similar to those seen on retrieved total knee replace-ments. Transfer films of UHMWPE were ob-served on the cobalt-chrome indentors for both serum and distilled water lubrication, al-though this film was more extensive for dis-tilled water. The lowest wear rate was ob-served when stabilized zirconium oxide on zirconium was used on the femoral side, which was attributed to greater wettability, surface hardness, and immunity to oxidative wear (26). Tests using cobalt-chrome femoral cylinders and different grades of UHMWPE showed different wear rates. Of these polyeth-ylenes, GUR 415 showed less wear than both RCH 1000 and UHMWPE containing numer-ous fusion defects. A test such as this is best utilized as a comparative evaluation method in which the reference materials are cobalt-chrome on GUR 415 UHMWPE. If neces-sary, the conformity and geometry of the

femoral indentor can be chosen to be applica-ble to a particular knee design.

Knee Simulators

The main purpose of a knee-simulating ma-chine is to perform long-term wear evaluation. An early form of simulator was the rig de-signed by Harding et al. (44) for static testing in which the tibia was clamped at a chosen flexion angle to the vertical, a weight was at-tached to the femur to apply a flexion moment, and the length of the quadriceps was adjusted to achieve the desired flexion angle, the force in the quadriceps providing equilibrium. Rovick et al. (77) constructed a dynamic form of this same system in which the quadriceps was wound in and out and three-dimensional motion was monitored. Shaw and Murray (85) were the first to use this configuration in a ma-chine capable of long-term testing. Hersh et al. (45) developed the concept further, using ser-vohydraulics and more sophisticated inputs and feedbacks. In a second type of simulator design, the required forces and motions are ap-plied directly to the femur or tibia without any simulation of muscle action. Simulators of this type have been designed by Walker and Hsieh (102), Stallforth and Ungethum (87), Paul et al. (71), Dowson et al. (29), Pappas et al. (70), and DiAngelo and Harrington (28). These designs have used various schemes of constraint and inputs.

The above types have their advantages and disadvantages. In the first type, the ground-to-foot reaction force is applied, for which there are accurate data, the geometry of the lower limb is reproduced, and the quadriceps action and patellofemoral mechanism are simulated. This means that a prosthetic patellofemoral joint is required, which adds complexity and the possibility of failure in long-term testing. The AP shear force is determined by the applied force vector, which in this case passes through the hip and ankle, implying zero moment about the hip and a knee moment that is a direct function of flexion angle. In contrast, in normal gait, in the first half of the stance phase, there is a flexing moment on the hip, which reverses to an extension moment in the second half of stance (10). Thus, the AP femoral–tibial shear forces are not strictly reproduced, and there is no restraint to simulate the cruciates and other ligaments.

The second simulator design is a more "mechanistic" approach in which the required joint forces, moments, and motions are input directly. However, the specific values for the forces and motions have involved a number of simplifying assumptions (63,64). The problem of dealing with the input of anterior–posterior forces and internal–external torques, together with the motions that would result, is more difficult than for the first type of simulator. The motions need to be either constrained or limited in some way or, alternatively, a simulation of soft tissue restraint provided. Merely inputting rotations and displacements is invalid because it does not account for differences in constraint between different TKR designs.

A simulator can be specified using first principles. For the femoral and tibial components, relative to global axes defined at some reference position such as zero flexion, there are six possible degrees of freedom, three rotations, and three translations. A suitable axis system is that described by Grood and Suntay (39) (Fig. 20). Flexion–extension is about a transverse axis through the femur. Varus–valgus rotation is defined about an axis perpendicular to the transverse axis. Anterior–posterior displacement is represented by motion of

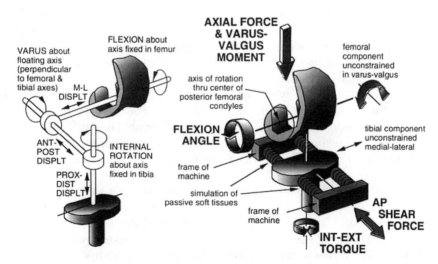

FIG. 20. The coordinate system of Grood and Suntay (39) used as the basis for a knee simulator. The schematic for a simulator showing the constraints and soft tissue simulation is shown.

the tibia along this perpendicular axis. Internal–external rotation is about the long axis of the tibia. To simulate the physiological conditions, apart from flexion–extension, which needs to be controlled in order to simulate any required activity, all of the other five degrees of freedom need to be unconstrained.

A number of forces and moments need to be imposed by the machine in a controlled waveform. The axial force FY applied in line with the tibial axis is the largest force with an immediate sharp peak in the stance phase followed by two shallower maxima, each of magnitude two to four times body weight. There is an unequal distribution of the force on the medial and lateral condyles, MY, in the ratio of around 2:1, a factor that can be approximated by a constant offset of the line of action of the compressive force. The anterior–posterior force FZ and the internal–external torque MY significantly affect the sliding and rotation patterns between the joint surfaces and need to be controlled as inputs. The medial–lateral force FX is sufficiently small that it can be neglected.

A machine based on the above scheme (Fig. 20) has been designed and used to evaluate TKR designs (99). The tibial component is mounted at the top of a long cylindrical beam, at the bottom of which is a low-friction spherical bearing. This allows the tibial component to move in a horizontal plane and to rotate about a vertical axis with minimal resistance. The internal–external torque and the anterior–posterior shear force are applied to the cylindrical beam. At the front and back of the container for the tibial component are four elastomeric springs or "bumpers," which simulate the average stiffness of the soft tissues, particularly the cruciate ligaments, for both anterior–posterior displacement and internal–external rotation. For designs in which one or both cruciates are intended to be resected, bumpers of reduced strength can be used (2,36).

The femoral component is fixed on a shaft such that the average center of curvature of the distal–posterior radii of the component is aligned with the axis of the shaft, so that dur-ing flexion–extension the lowest points on the femoral condyles are in approximately the same location in the AP direction. The ends of the shaft are in slider bearings, allowing unrestrained vertical movement and varus–valgus rotation of the femoral component. One end of the shaft is extended for attachment of a crank to apply flexion–extension. The vertical force on the femoral component is applied by two arms resting on the shaft at either side of the component. These arms are pivoted at their center in the machine framework. The arms are connected at the back by a transverse beam, with spherical bearings to allow each arm to pivot independently, allowing varus–valgus movement.

In the specification for the design, it was proposed that the various force and motion inputs were necessary to provide realistic kinematics. In turn, realistic wear patterns can be produced only if the kinematics are realistic. The regions of the bearing surfaces subject to sliding conditions, and the subsurface material subject to shear stresses (which can produce delamination wear), are clearly dependent on the kinematics during activity. Hence, to reproduce realistic kinematics and wear patterns, the input of AP forces and torques as well as the compressive forces is essential. The variability in kinematics between different total knee designs was clearly demonstrated in experiments in which ratios of displacements and rotations spanned more than a 2:1 range. The soft tissue restraints, simulated by the elastomeric bumpers, play an important role in the design of the simulating machine. If they were not present, the displacements and rotations of the less constrained designs would be unrealistically large. For example, for a design of low constraint (with flat or shallow tibial surfaces), it is obvious that the restraints would be needed to prevent dislocation. An important consideration in practical testing is the number of cycles of loading that are required. In a study of activities of typical individuals receiving TKR, it was found that each limb was subjected to 1.5 to 2.0 million steps per year (83). Hence, to predict performance in a 10- to 20-year follow-up would require around 30 million cycles,

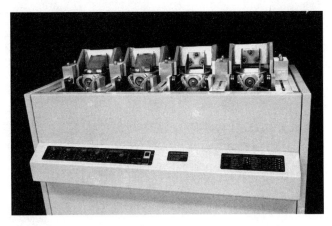

FIG. 21. A four-channel knee-simulating machine. The forces, moments, and flexion–extension are computer controlled and powered by pneumatics. All parameters are electronically monitored.

which would take almost 1 year of continuous running. Hence, multistation machines (Fig. 21) and accelerated testing are essential.

CONCLUSIONS

In this chapter, total knee replacement has been described in the context of a systematic engineering design problem. In reality, such an approach is not always applicable because of the many additional factors that are not necessarily under the control of a single designer. For example, the "designer" may be the coordinator of a design group, the members of which do not necessarily subscribe to a systematic or objective approach, and where the flow of information is sometimes erratic and unpredictable. Commercial or marketing interests may result in a choice of solutions for which experience is readily available to avoid working through new concepts that may require research, time, and expense. However, the most important step in the design process is the rigorous testing of the final product in both preclinical and clinical trials, with the expectation of design modifications from each stage.

At this time, the indicators are that knee design will proceed incrementally based on new knowledge and technology. Data on the forces and moments in the knee from telemetrized knee replacements, coupled with *in vivo* ligament force measurements, will facilitate the rational design of surfaces and cams to achieve optimum mechanics. In order to determine whether a new design is functionally superior, improved gait analysis and knee modeling will be used. One of these methods will be cine digital radiography, in which the three-dimensional orientations of the femoral and tibial components will be determined using pattern recognition techniques. In terms of durability, improved methods of processing and sterilizing of polyethylene will extend its useful life before the onset of delamination wear. Mobile bearing knees will be used more frequently, and new design forms will emerge that will result in a matching of the stiffness characteristics of the normal knee. It is also possible that rolling-element bearings will be designed. Technical aids for improving surgical technique will be more widespread. Pressure patterns of contact obtained during surgery will enable the surgeon to optimize component alignments. Milling cutters will enable the preparation of accurate surfaces to obtain osseointegration consistently. Robotically assisted cutting tools may even come into practical application. Finally, biological solutions are already making inroads into the replacement of ligaments, menisci, and cartilage surfaces and may even be applied to the entire joints themselves.

Acknowledgments

The authors wish to thank the Department of Health UK, the North-East Thames Health Authority, and the Bristol-Myers Squibb/Zimmer Foundation for support of much of the work reported in this chapter.

REFERENCES

1. Ahmed, A. M., and Burke, D. L. (1983): *In vitro* measurement of static pressure distribution in synovial joints—Part I: Tibial surface of the knee. *J. Biomech. Eng.,* 105(3):216–225.
2. Amis, A. A., and Dawkins, G. P. C. (1991): Functional anatomy of the anterior cruciate ligament. Fibre bundle actions related to ligament replacements and injuries. *J. Bone Joint Surg.,* 73-B(2):260–267.
3. Andriacchi, T. P. (1993): Functional analysis of pre- and post-knee surgery: total knee arthroplasty and ACL reconstruction. *J. Biomech. Eng.,* 115:575–581.
4. Andriacchi, T. P., Galante, J. O., and Fermier, R. W. (1982): The influence of total knee-replacement on walking and stair climbing. *J. Bone Joint Surg.,* 64-A:1328–1335.
5. Andriacchi, T. P., Mikosz, R. P., Hampton, S. J., and Galante, J. O. (1983): Model studies of stiffness characteristics of the human knee joint. *J. Biomech.,* 16(1):23–29.
6. Angelides, M., Shirazi-Adl, A., Shrivastava, S. C., and Ahmed, A. M. (1988): A stress compatible finite element for implant/cement interface analyses. *J. Biomech. Eng.,* 110:42–49.
7. Arima, J., Martin, J. W., White, S. E., McCarthy, D. S., and Whiteside, L. A. (1994): Partial posterior cruciate ligament release and knee kinematics after total knee arthroplasty. *Trans. Orthop. Res. Soc.,* 19:87.
8. Ateshian, G. A., Kwak, S. D., Soslowsky, L. J., and Mow, V. C. (1994): A stereophotogrammetric method for determining *in situ* contact areas in diarthrodial joints, and a comparison with other methods. *J. Biomech.,* 27(1):111–124.
9. Bartel, D. L., Burstein, A. H., Toda, M. D., and Edwards, D. L. (1985): The effect of conformity and plastic thickness on contact stresses in metal-backed plastic implants. *J. Biomech. Eng.,* 107:193–199.
10. Berchuck, M., Andriacchi, T. P., Bach, B. R., and Reider, B. (1990): Gait adaptations by patients who have a deficient anterior cruciate ligament. *J. Bone Joint Surg.,* 72-A(6):871–877.
11. Blankevoort, L., Huiskes, R., and de Lange, A. (1988): The envelope of passive knee joint motion. *J. Biomech.,* 21:705–720.
12. Blankevoort, L., Kuiper, J. H., Huiskes, R., and Grootenboer, H. J. (1991): Articular contact in a three-dimensional model of the knee. *J. Biomech.,* 24(11):1019–1031.
13. Bloebaum, R. D., Nelson, K., Dorr, L. D., Hoffmann, A. A., and Lyman, D. J. (1991): Investigation of early surface delamination observed in retrieved heat-pressed tibial inserts. *Clin. Orthop. Rel. Res.,* 269:120–127.
14. Blunn, G. W., Joshi, A. B., Lilley, P. A., et al. (1992): Polyethylene wear in unicondylar knee prostheses. *Acta Orthop. Scand.,* 63:247–255.
15. Blunn, G. W., Joshi, A. B., Minns, J., et al. (1997): Wear in retrieved condylar knee replacements. *J. Arthroplasty* (in press).
16. Blunn, G. W., Lilley, P. A., and Walker, P. S. (1994): Variability of the wear of ultra high molecular weight polyethylene in simulated total knee replacement. *Trans. Orthop. Res. Soc.,* 19:94.
17. Blunn, G. W., Walker, P. S., Joshi, A., and Hardinge, K. (1991): The dominance of cyclic sliding in producing wear in total knee replacement. *Clin. Orthop. Rel. Res.,* 273:253–260.
18. Bostrum, M. P. G., Bennett, A. P., Rimnac, C. M., and Wright, T. M. (1994): Degradation in polyethylene as a result of sterilization, shelf storage, and *in vivo* use. *Trans. Orthop. Res. Soc.,* 19:288.
19. Bourne, R. B., and Finlay, J. B. (1986): The influence of tibial component intramedullary stems and implant–cortex contact on the strain distribution of the proximal tibia following total knee arthroplasty. *Clin. Orthop. Rel. Res.,* 208:95–99.
20. Butler, D. L., Kay, M. D., and Stouffer, D. C. (1986): Comparison of material properties in fascicle–bone units from human patellar tendon and knee ligaments. *J. Biomech.,* 19(6):425–432.
21. Clarke, I. C. (1981): Wear of artificial joint materials. Friction and wear studies: validity of wear-screening protocols. *Eng. Med.,* 10:115–122.
22. Collier, J. P. M., Mayor, M. B., McNamara, J. L., Surprenant, V. A., and Jenson, R. E. (1991): Analysis of the failure of 122 polyethylene inserts from uncemented tibial knee components. *Clin. Orthop. Rel. Res.,* 273:232–242.
23. Cooper, J. R., Dowson, D., and Fisher, J. (1991): Birefringent studies of polyethylene wear specimens and acetabular cups. *Wear,* 151:391–402.
24. Crowninshield, R. D., Pope, M. H., and Johnson, R. J. (1976): An analytical model of the knee. *J. Biomech.,* 9:397–405.
25. Cummings, J. F., Carpenter, C. W., Grood, E. S., Leach, D. U., and Manley, M. T. (1990): Joint line elevation of a total knee replacement results in reduction of knee flexion. *Trans. Orthop. Res. Soc.,* 1990;15:280.
26. Davidson, J. A., Poggie, R. A., and Mishra, A. K. (1994): Abrasive wear of ceramic, metal and UHMWPE bearing surfaces from third-body bone, PMMA bone cement and titanium debris. *Biomed. Mater. Eng.,* 4:1–17.
27. Dawson, J. M., and Bartel, D. L. (1992): Consequences of an interference fit on the fixation of porous-coated tibial components in total knee replacement. *J. Bone Joint Surg.,* 74-A(2):233–238.
28. DiAngelo, D. J., and Harrington, I. J. (1992): Design of a dynamic multi-purpose joint simulator. *Adv. Bioeng. ASME,* BED-22:107–110.
29. Dowson, D., Gillis, B. J., and Atkinson, J. R. (1985): Penetration of metallic femoral components into polymeric tibial components observed in a knee joint simulator. *Am. Chem. Soc. Symp. Ser.,* 287:215–228.
30. Dowson, D., Taheri, S., and Wallbridge, N. C. (1987): The role of counterface imperfections in the wear of polyethylene. *Wear,* 119:277–293.

31. Elbert, K. E., Wright, T. M., Rimnac, C. M., et al. (1994): Fatigue crack propagation behavior of UHMWPE under mixed mode conditions. *J. Biomed. Mater. Res.*, 28:181–187.

32. El-Nahass, B., Madson, M. M., and Walker, P. S. (1991): Motion of the knee after condylar resurfacing—an *in-vivo* study. *J. Biomech.*, 24:1107–1117.

33. Essinger, J. R., Leyvraz, P. F., Heegard, J. H., and Robertson, D. D. (1989): A mathematical model for the evaluation of the behaviour during flexion of condylar-type knee prostheses. *J. Biomech.*, 22:1229–1241.

34. Finlay, J. B., Hardie, W. R., Bourne, R. B., and Chris, A. D. (1991): Deformation of the cement mantle of tibial components following total knee arthroplasty: a laboratory study. *Proc. Inst. Mech. Eng.*, 205(H4):211–217.

35. Fisher, J., Hailey, J. L., Chan, K. L., Shaw, D., and Stone, M. (1995): The effect of ageing following irradiation on the wear of UHMWPE. *Trans. Orthop. Res. Soc.*, 20:120.

36. Fukubayashi, T., Torzilli, P. A., Sherman, M. F., and Warren, R. F. (1982): An *in-vitro* biomechical evaluation of anterior–posterior motion of the knee. Tibial displacement, rotation and torque. *J. Bone Joint Surg.*, 64-A:258–264.

37. Garg, A., and Walker, P. S. (1990): Prediction of total knee motion using a three-dimensional computer-graphics model. *J. Biomech.*, 23(1):45–48.

38. Gharpuray, V. M., Keer, L. M., and Lewis, J. L. (1990): Cracks emanating from circular voids or elastic inclusions in PMMA near a bone–implant interface. *J. Biomech. Eng.*, 112:22–28.

39. Grood, E. S., and Suntay, W. J. (1983): A joint coordinate system for the clinical description of three-dimensional motions: application to the knee. *J. Biomech. Eng.*, 105:136–144.

40. Gunsallus, K. L., and Bartel, D. L. (1992): Stresses and surface damage in PCA and total condylar polyethylene components. *Trans. Orthop. Res. Soc.*, 17:329.

41. Gunston, F. H. (1971): Polycentric knee arthroplasty. Prosthetic simulation of normal knee movement. *J. Bone Joint Surg.*, 53-B(2):272–277.

42. Hahn, D. L., Cooke, F. W., and McQueen, D. A. (1990): Dichotomy in improved total knee arthroplasty tibial plateau component longevity: prosthesis stiffness. *Trans. Orthop. Res. Soc.*, 15:472.

43. Hansson, C. M., Reedan, J., Kennedy, L. A., and Cooke, T. D. V. (1995): A quantitative technique for reporting surface degradation patterns of UHMWPE components of retrieved total knee replacements. *J. Appl. Biomater.*, 6:9–18.

44. Harding, M. L., Harding, L., and Goodfellow, J. W. (1977): A preliminary report of a simple rig to aid study of the functional anatomy of the cadaver human knee joint. *J. Biomech.*, 10:517–523.

45. Hersh, J. F., Hillberry, B. M., and Kettelkamp, D. B. (1981): Laboratory knee simulation testing: preliminary results on three prostheses. *Trans. Orthop. Res. Soc.*, 6:211.

46. Hsieh, H.-H., and Walker, P. S. (1976): Stabilizing mechanisms of the loaded and unloaded knee joint. *J. Bone Joint Surg.*, 1976;58-A:87–93.

47. Hvid, I., Bentzen, S. M., and Jørgensen, J. (1988): Remodeling of the tibial plateau after knee replacement. CT bone densitometry. *Acta Orthop. Scand.*, 59(5):567–573.

48. Ishii, Y., Terajima, K., Bechtold, J. E., and Gustilo, R. B. (1993): Comparison of knee joint laxity after total knee replacement with posterior cruciate retaining and substituting prostheses. *Trans. Orthop. Res. Soc.*, 18:429.

49. Jin, Z. M., Stewart, T., Auger, D. D., and Dowson, D. (1995): Contact pressure prediction in total knee joint replacements. Part 2: application to the design of total knee joint replacements. *Proc. Inst. Mech. Engrs.*, 209(H1):9–15.

50. Johnson, K. L. (1985): *Contact Mechanics*. Cambridge University Press, Cambridge.

51. Justin, D. F., Mann, J. W., and Winters, T. F. (1992): Evaluation of tibial component with external rotation of the intercondylar eminence. *Trans. Orthop. Res. Soc.*, 17:20.

52. Krause, W. R., Krug, W., and Miller, J. (1982): Strength of the cement–bone interface. *Clin. Orthop.*, 163:290–299.

53. Kurosawa, H., Walker, P. S., Abe, S., Garg, A., and Hunter, T. (1985): Geometry and motion of the knee for implant and orthotic design. *J. Biomech.*, 18(7):487–499.

54. Kurtz, S. M., Rimnac, C. M., and Bartel, D. I. (1994): A bilinear material model for UHMWPE in total joint replacements. *Trans. Orthop. Res. Soc.*, 19:289.

55. Lafortune, M. A., Cavanagh, P. R., Sommer, H. J., and Kalenak, A. (1992): Three-dimensional kinematics of the human knee during walking. *J. Biomech.*, 25(4):347–357.

56. Landy, M. M., and Walker, P. S. (1988): Wear of ultrahigh-molecular-weight polyethylene components in 90 retrieved knee prostheses. *J. Arthroplasty [Suppl.]*, 3:S73–S85.

57. Loch, D. A., Luo, Z., Lewis, J. L., and Stewart, N. J. (1992): A theoretical model of the knee and ACL: theory and experimental verification. *J. Biomech.*, 25(1):81–90.

58. Markolf, K. L., Bargar, W. L., Shoemaker, S. C., and Amstutz, H. C. (1981): The role of joint load in knee stability. *J. Bone Joint Surg.*, 63-A(4):570–585.

59. Markolf, K. L., Graff-Radford, A., and Amstutz, H. C. (1978): *In vivo* knee stability. *J. Bone Joint Surg.*, 60-A(5):664–678.

60. McKellop, H., Clarke, I., Markolf, K., and Amstutz, H. (1981): Friction and wear properties of polymer, metal and ceramic prosthetic joint materials evaluated on a multi-channel screening device. *J. Biomed. Mater. Res.*, 15:619–653.

61. Meijers, P. (1968): The contact problem of a rigid cylinder on an elastic layer. *Appl. Sci. Res.*, 18:353–383.

62. Mikosz, R. P., Andriacchi, T. P., and Andersson, G. B. J. (1988): Model analysis of factors influencing the prediction of muscle forces at the knee. *J. Orthop. Res.*, 6(2):205–214.

63. Morrison, J. B. (1969): Function of the knee joint in various activities. *Biomed. Eng.*, 4(12):573–580.

64. Morrison, J. B. (1970): The mechanics of the knee joint in relation to normal walking. *J. Biomech.*, 3:51–61.

65. Murase, K., Crowninshield, R. D., Pedersen, D. R., and Chang, T.-S. (1983): An analysis of tibial component design in total knee arthroplasty. *J. Biomech.*, 16(1):13–22.

66. Nafei, A., Nielsen, S., Kristensen, O., and Hvid, I. (1992): The press-fit Kinemax knee arthroplasty. *J. Bone Joint Surg.*, 74-B(2):243–246.

67. Nilsson, K. G., Kärrholm, J., Ekelund, L., and Magnusson, P. (1991): Evaluation of micromotion in cemented vs uncemented knee arthroplasty in osteoarthrosis and rheumatoid arthritis. Randomized study using Roentgen stereophotogrammetric analysis. *J. Arthroplasty,* 6(3):265–278.

68. Nusbaum, H. J., and Rose, R. M. (1979): The effects of radiation sterilization on the properties of ultrahigh molecular weight polyethylene. *J. Biomed. Mater. Res,* 13:557–576.

69. Olsen, C. L., Martell, J. M., Rosenberg, A. G., and Andriacchi, T. P. (1992): The relationship between changes in patellar height and function following total knee replacement (TKR). *Orthop. Res. Soc.,* 17:272.

70. Pappas, M. J., Makris, G., and Buechel, F. F. (1992): Wear in prosthetic knee joints. Scientific exhibit. *Proc. Am. Acad. Orthop. Surg., 59th Annual Meeting,* Washington, DC.

71. Paul, I., Chernack, R., Manzi, S. F., Rose, R. M., Radin, E. L., and Simon, S. R. (1980): *Total knee prosthesis deterioration.* Massachusetts Institute of Technology (Mechanical Engineering Department), Industrial Liaison Program, Cambridge, MA.

72. Piziali, R. L., Rastegar, J. C., and Nagel, D. A. (1977): Measurement of nonlinear, coupled stiffness characteristics of the human knee. *J. Biomech.,* 10:45–51.

73. Pugh, S. (1991): *Total Design. Integrated Methods for Successful Product Engineering.* Addison-Wesley, Wokingham.

74. Rehder, U. (1983): Technical note. Morphological studies on the symmetry of the human knee joint: femoral condyles. *J. Biomech.,* 16(5):351–361.

75. Reilly, D., Walker, P. S., Ben-Dov, M., and Ewald, F. C. (1982): Effects of tibial components on load transfer in the upper tibia. *Clin. Orthop.,* 165:273–282.

76. Roe, R.-J., Grood, E. S., Shastri, R., Gosselin, C. A., Noyes, F. R. (1981): Effect of radiation sterilization and aging on ultrahigh molecular weight polyethylene. *J. Biomed. Mater. Res.,* 15:209–230.

77. Rovick, J. S., Reuben, J. D., Schrager, R. J., and Walker, P. S. (1991): Relation between knee motion and ligament length patterns. *Clin. Biomech.,* 6(4):213–220.

78. Ryd, L., Carlsson, L., and Herberts, P. (1993): Micromotion of a noncemented tibial component with screw fixation. *Clin. Orthop. Rel. Res.,* 295:218–225.

79. Ryd, L., and Toksvig-Larsen, S. (1993): Early postoperative fixation of tibial components: An *in vivo* Roentgen stereophotogrammetric analysis. *J. Orthop. Res.,* 11:142–148.

80. Sathasivam, S., and Walker, P. S. (1994): Optimization of the bearing surface geometry of total knees. *J. Biomech.,* 27(3):255–264.

81. Sathasivam, S., and Walker, P. S. (1997): A computer model with surface friction for the prediction of total knee kinematics. *J. Biomech.,* 30:177–184.

82. Schmalzried, T. P., Jasty, M., Rosenberg, A., and Harris, W. H. (1994): Polyethylene wear debris and tissue reactions in knee as compared to hip replacement. *J. Appl. Biomater.,* 5:185–190.

83. Seedhom, B. B., and Wallbridge, N. C. (1985): Walking activities and wear of prostheses. *Wear,* 44:838–843.

84. Selvik, G. (1989): Roentgen stereophotogrammetry: a method for the study of the kinematics of the skeletal system. *Acta Orthop. Scand. [Suppl.],* 232:1.

85. Shaw, J. A., and Murray, D. G. (1973): Knee joint simulator. *Clin. Orthop.,* 94:15–23.

86. Soudry, M., Walker, P. S., Reilly, D. T., Kurosawa, H., and Sledge, C. B. (1986): Effects of total knee replacement design on femoral–tibial contact conditions. *J. Arthroplasty,* 1:35–45.

87. Stallforth, H., and Ungethum, M. (1978): Tribological investigation of total knee joint prostheses. *Biomed. Technol.,* 23:295–304.

88. Steege, J. W., Lewis, J. L., Keer, L. M., and Wixson, R. L. (1987): Crack propagation at the bone–cement interface. *Trans. Orthop. Res. Soc.,* 12:54.

89. Stein, A., Flemming, B., Pope, M. H., and Howe, J. G. (1988): Total knee arthroplasty kinematics: An *in vivo* evaluation of four different designs. *J. Arthroplasty [Suppl.]:*S31–S36.

90. Suh, N. P. (1986): *Tribophysics.* Prentice-Hall, Englewood Cliffs, NJ.

91. Taguchi, G. (1993): *Taguchi on Robust Technology Development. Bringing Quality Engineering Upstream.* ASME Press, New York.

92. Thatcher, J. C., Zhou, X.-M., and Walker, P. S. (1987): Inherent laxity in total knee prostheses. *J. Arthroplasty,* 2(3):199–207.

93. Toksvig-Larsen, S., and Ryd, L. (1994): Surface characteristics following tibial preparation during total knee arthroplasty. *J. Arthroplasty,* 9(1):63–66.

94. Vasu, R., Carter, D. R., Schurman, D. J., and Beaupré, G. S. (1986): Epiphyseal-based designs for tibial plateau components—I. Stress analysis in the frontal plane. *J. Biomech.,* 19(8):647–662.

95. Volz, R. G., Nisbet, J. K., Lee, R. W., and McMurtry, M. G. (1988): The mechanical stability of various noncemented tibial components. *Clin. Orthop. Rel. Res.,* 226:38–42.

96. Walker, P. S. (1988): Bearing surface design in total knee replacement. *Eng. Med.,* 17(4):149–156.

97. Walker, P. S., Ambarek, M. S., Morris, J, R., Olanlokun, K., and Cobb, A. (1995): Anterior–posterior stability in partially conforming condylar knee replacement. *Clin. Orthop. Rel. Res.,* 310:87–97.

98. Walker, P. S., Ben Dov, M., Askew, M. J., and Pugh, T. (1981): The deformation and wear of plastic components in artificial knee joints: an experimental study. *Eng. Med.,* 10:33–38.

99. Walker, P. S., Blunn, G. W., Broome, D. R., Perry, J., Watkins, A., Sathasivam, S., Dewar, M. E., and Paul, J. P. (1997): A knee simulating machine for performance evaluation of total knee replacements. *J. Biomechanics,* 30:83–89.

100. Walker, P. S., Blunn, G. W., and Lilley, P. A. (1996): Wear testing of materials and surfaces for total knee replacement. *J. Appl. Biomater.* 33:159–175.

101. Walker, P. S., Greene, D., Reilly, D., Thatcher, J., Ben-Dov, M., and Ewald, F. C. (1981): Fixation of tibial components of knee prostheses. *J. Bone Joint Surg.,* 63-A(2):258–267.

102. Walker, P. S., and Hsieh, H.-H. (1977): Conformity in condylar replacement knee prostheses. *J. Bone Joint Surg,* 59-B:222–228.

103. Walker, P. S., Ranawat, C., and Insall, J. (1976): Fixation of the tibial components of condylar replacement knee prostheses. *J. Biomech.,* 9:269–275.

104. Walker, P. S., Rovick, J. S., and Robertson, D. D. (1988):

The effects of knee brace hinge design and placement on joint mechanics. *J. Biomech.,* 21(11):965–974.

105. Walker, P. S., Wang, C.-J., and Masse, Y. (1974): Joint laxity as a criterion for the design of condylar knee prostheses. *Inst. Mech. Engrs.,* CP16:22–29.

106. Wang, C., and Walker, P. S. (1974): Rotary laxity of the human knee joint. *J. Bone Joint Surg.,* 56-A(1):161–170.

107. Warren, P. J., Olanlokun, T. K., Cobb, A. G., Walker, P. S., and Iverson, B. F. (1994): Laxity and function in knee replacements. *Clin. Orthop. Rel. Res.,* 305:200–208.

108. Weinstein, J. N., Andriacchi, T. P., and Galante, J. (1986): Factors influencing walking and stairclimbing following unicompartmental knee arthroplasty. *J. Arthroplasty,* 1(2):109–115.

109. Wismans, J., Veldpaus, F., Janssen, J., Huson, A., and Struben, P. (1980): A three-dimensional mathematical model of the knee joint. *J. Biomech.,* 13(8):677–685.

110. Yoshida, K., Asada, K., and Sakane, H. (1993): Intra-operative measurement of tibial component micro-movement in total knee arthroplasty. In: *Micromovement in Orthopaedics,* edited by A. R. Turner-Smith, pp. 124–139. Clarendon Press, Oxford.

111. Zoghi, M., Hefzy, M. S., Fu, K. C., and Jackson, W. T. (1992): A three-dimensional morphometrical study of the distal human femur. *J. Eng. Med.,* 206(3):147–157.

Subject Index

Note: Figures and tables are represented by *f* and *t* respectively.